Sonography Scanning

PRINCIPLES AND PROTOCOLS

Sonography Scanning

PRINCIPLES AND PROTOCOLS

FIFTH EDITION

M. Robert De Jong, RDMS, RDCS, RVT, FAIUM, FSDMS
Owner
Bob De Jong, LLC
Ultrasound Educational Services
Baltimore, Maryland

ELSEVIER

3251 Riverport Lane
St. Louis, Missouri 63043

SONOGRAPHY SCANNING: PRINCIPLES AND PROTOCOLS,
FIFTH EDITION

ISBN: 978-0-3235-9738-8

Notices

Knowledge and best practice in this field are constantly changing. As new research and experience broaden our understanding, changes in research methods, professional practices, or medical treatment may become necessary.

Practitioners and researchers must always rely on their own experience and knowledge in evaluating and using any information, methods, compounds, or experiments described herein. In using such information or methods they should be mindful of their own safety and the safety of others, including parties for whom they have a professional responsibility.

With respect to any drug or pharmaceutical products identified, readers are advised to check the most current information provided (i) on procedures featured or (ii) by the manufacturer of each product to be administered, to verify the recommended dose or formula, the method and duration of administration, and contraindications. It is the responsibility of practitioners, relying on their own experience and knowledge of their patients, to make diagnoses, to determine dosages and the best treatment for each individual patient, and to take all appropriate safety precautions.

To the fullest extent of the law, neither the Publisher nor the authors, contributors, or editors, assume any liability for any injury and/or damage to persons or property as a matter of products liability, negligence or otherwise, or from any use or operation of any methods, products, instructions, or ideas contained in the material herein.

Library of Congress Control Number: 2020937024

Executive Content Strategist: Sonya Seigafuse
Senior Content Development Manager: Luke Held
Content Development Specialist: John Tomedi
Marketing Manager: Ed Major
Publishing Services Manager: Shereen Jameel
Senior Project Manager: Kamatchi Madhavan
Designer: Renee Duenow

Working together
to grow libraries in
developing countries

ELSEVIER | Book Aid International

www.elsevier.com • www.bookaid.org

Printed in India

Last digit is the print number: 9 8 7 6 5 4

To Linda,
for her love and support of my career these past 45 years.
Love changes everything.

Contributors

M. Robert De Jong, RDMS, RDCS, RVT, FAIUM, FSDMS
Owner
Bob De Jong, LLC
Ultrasound Educational Services
Where an image is more than a picture
Baltimore, Maryland
Chapter 1: Understanding Protocols and How They Are Determined; Chapter 2: Scanning Planes and Scanning Methods; Chapter 3: Scanning Protocol for Abnormal Findings and Pathology; Chapter 4: Abdominal Aorta Scanning Protocol; Chapter 5: Inferior Vena Cava Scanning Protocol; Chapter 6: Liver Scanning Protocol; Chapter 7: Gallbladder and Biliary Tract Scanning Protocol; Chapter 8: Pancreas Scanning Protocol; Chapter 9: Renal Scanning Protocol; Chapter 10: Spleen Scanning Protocol; Chapter 11: Image Protocols for Full and Limited Studies of the Abdomen; Chapter 15: Male Pelvis Scanning Protocol for the Prostate Gland, Scrotum, and Penis; Chapter 16: Thyroid Scanning Protocol; Chapter 20: Abdominal Doppler and Doppler Techniques

Aubrey Justin Rybyinski, BS, RDMS, RVT
Senior Clinical Manager
Vascular Laboratory
Navix Diagnostix
Taunton, Massachusetts
Chapter 21: Cerebrovascular Duplex Scanning Protocol; Chapter 22: Peripheral Arterial and Venous Duplex Scanning Protocols

Shannon Trebes, RDMS, RVT
Senior Sonographer II
Obstetrics and Gynecology
Johns Hopkins Hospital
Baltimore, Maryland
Chapter 14: Obstetric Scanning Protocol for First, Second, and Third Trimesters

Tricia Turner, BS, RDMS, RVT
Program Director
Diagnostic Medical Sonography
South Hills School of Business & Technology
State College, Pennsylvania
Chapter 12: Female Pelvis Scanning Protocol; Chapter 13: Transvaginal Sonography; Chapter 17: Breast Scanning Protocol

Ashley Upton, BSDI, RDMS, RVT, RVS
Pediatric Sonographer
Ultrasound
Texas Children's Hospital
Houston, Texas
Chapter 18: Neonatal Brain, Spine, and Hip Scanning Protocol

Ted Whitten, BA, RDMS, RVT, FSDMS
Ultrasound Practitioner
Sonography Department
Elliot Hospital
Manchester, New Hampshire
Chapter 18: Neonatal Brain, Spine, and Hip Scanning Protocol; Chapter 19: Musculoskeletal Scanning Protocol for Rotator Cuff, Carpal Tunnel, and Achilles Tendon

It is an honor that I was once again asked to revise a textbook loved and used by many students, teachers, and sonographers. I have been a sonographer since 1976, and it is my hope that some of the tips and tricks I have learned over the years will help students and anyone reading this book be better sonographers. I wanted to add some new sections, including liver elastography, neonatal hips and spine, and neck mapping. Unfortunately, that meant some material had to be cut to make room for the new material. It was not an easy decision, but I decided to eliminate the echocardiography section. The main reason I decided to not include these chapters is that the field of echocardiography has exploded with new technologies, and I felt it would not be fair to the reader to have a basic chapter, nor would it give the echocardiography profession the justice it deserves. I also agreed with Shannon to combine the obstetrics chapter with the obstetric transvaginal scanning chapter, because very rarely would just a transvaginal examination be ordered for a pregnancy, but it would be performed at the time of the transabdominal study to clarify findings.

One of the most frustrating things for a student is understanding why it appears that every sonographer scans a patient differently, giving the impression that they are following different protocols. In addition, there is the conflict between the protocol they learn in school and the one the sonographer follows in the clinical rotations. It is my hope that by reading this book the student understands that all studies have a basic protocol as defined by the ultrasound societies and accrediting organizations, which allows the department to add additional images that it may require for the practice. Some sonographers may prefer to start with transverse images, whereas others prefer to begin with longitudinal images, which can add to the confusion. The bottom line is that sonographers document the required images by the end of the study. Sonography is unique in that it allows some freedom in image order and expansion of the protocol as needed when pathologic findings are present. As sonographers, we develop our own style of scanning over the years.

Sonography is the most operator-dependent modality, and the skills and knowledge of the sonographer will determine the quality and findings of the sonographic images. As sonographers, we constantly use our critical thinking skills to optimize images and determine which images to document to provide a complete study to radiologists or sonologists, so they can determine if the study is normal or if a pathologic condition is present. Sonographers must know what a normal organ or Doppler signal looks like so they can determine if what they are seeing is abnormal. A sonographer needs a good understanding of sonographic principles and instrumentation to obtain high-quality images. The ultrasound unit can only do so much for the image, and the sonographer must take the image to the next level by adjusting the proper controls and choosing the correct transducer type and frequency.

All of the chapters follow a similar structure and are divided into three sections. The chapter begins by starting with a review of anatomy and physiology, followed by the sonographic appearance of the organ and any normal variants. The next section deals with scanning the organ: discussing patient prep, appropriate transducers, and the right patient position or positions to use while scanning. Rounding out this section are discussion of breathing techniques needed and technical tips for a successful study. The final section is the protocol for the study. All protocols were current at the time of writing the book and are based on the American Institute of Ultrasound in Medicine (AIUM) practice parameters and the Intersocietal Accreditation Commission Vascular Testing (IAC-VT) standards. The AIUM protocols were not created solely by the AIUM but have been created and approved jointly by the major ultrasound, radiology and other medical organizations that use ultrasound in their daily practice. This makes following a protocol much easier than deciding whether to follow the AIUM or ACR protocol, for example. The IAC-VT standards are only for vascular examinations and are very similar if not identical to the AIUM guidelines.

What's New

This edition has been updated to reflect current required minimum images for sonographic examinations based on the AIUM guidelines and IAC-VT standards at the time of publication. There are all new images to illustrate the images required for protocols and some examples of common pathologic conditions that might be found incidentally. With the increase of information and images, the review questions have been moved online. In addition, you will notice that the survey information has been removed. With current constraints on the amount of time to complete a sonogram, sonographers do not have the time to perform a whole protocol before they start documenting images. Many sonographers start the examination and see what unfolds as they are scanning. Some sonographers may do a quick survey before starting the documentation process by maybe scanning the organ in one plane, usually transverse. It does not make you a poorer sonographer if you do not do a survey scan before you start the examination. To be honest, I never did a pre-scan survey. If the purpose of the sonogram is to verify or clarify findings from another imaging study, I would pay special attention to the area in question when I examined that area. Usually at the end of the study I would document a few images using a split screen technique and obtain longitudinal and transverse images of any mass or pathologic finding with measurements. I would also add any images at the end as needed to document areas of pain or concern, again in longitudinal and transverse planes, that were not evaluated with the normal protocol images.

It is my hope as you journey along your road to becoming a great sonographer that this book will help you in your travels.

M. Robert De Jong, RDMS, RDCS, RVT, FAIUM, FSDMS

Acknowledgments

They say it takes a village to raise a child, but I will add that it also takes a village to publish a book. First, I want to thank Sonya Seigafuse, Executive Content Strategist, Education Content for Elsevier, for believing in me and giving me this opportunity. I would also like to thank Luke Held, Senior Content Development Manager, Elsevier Education, Reference, and Continuity, for getting me started, and John Tomedi of Spring Hollow Press for helping and guiding me along this journey and giving me his insightful advice, as well as a little prodding. Thanks to Kamatchi Madhavan, Senior Project Manager, Health Content Management, Elsevier, and her team for creating these incredible looking chapters from words and images. I could have not asked for better contributors: Shannon Trebes, Ted Whitten, Trish Turner, Ashley Upton, and Aubrey Rybyinski, all of whom did an incredible job revising the material. I also want to thank Jeanine Rybyinski, Liz Ladrido, Marianna Holman, Tara Cielma and Blake Randles for their incredible image contributions.

I would not be who I am today, not only as a sonographer but who I am in the sonography community, if it were not for the mentoring and most importantly the friendship of the following sonographers: Marveen Craig, Anne Jones, Marsha Neumyer, and Frank West. I have been truly blessed to have these legends of sonography molding and guiding me along my path to becoming a sonographer. Thanks also go out to all my former staff at Hopkins for allowing me to be away from them as I became involved in our profession. They were the best staff and team that any manager could ever hope to be a part of or to lead.

I also want to thank Dr. Ulrike Hamper, sonologist extraordinaire, for challenging me to be a better sonographer and for getting me involved with the AIUM, SRU and RSNA, introducing me to the best radiologists in the country, many who supported me in my career as a speaker or hands-on instructor at national meetings. I want to thank Dr. Bob Gayler for his support over the years and who indirectly inspired me to take on this project. Finally to my first and best ever manager who molded me into the manager/leader that I became, Mr Michael Reese.

Two physicians encouraged me in this project while treating me as a patient. They were Dr. Bashir Zikria and Dr. Sheera Lerman Zohar, both of whom guided me through some rough times, always asking me how the book was coming along.

Last but most important is my family. My parents, Bob and Doris, for instilling in me my faith In God as well as good work ethics. My two sons, Alex and Daniel, for their understanding why dad seemed to be always working and their incredible support and love. I am so proud of the men they have become. A little unusual, but to my cat Maggie, for sitting with me as I typed away until the wee hours of the morning, sometimes helping me type with her paws on the keyboard! To my wife Linda; God has given me a partner for life and a best friend. We have survived many ups and downs these past 45-plus years, but our love for each other is stronger than ever. Your understanding of why I was chained to the computer for countless hours, days, weeks, and months and ignoring you pretty much all day truly helped me not to feel as guilty. You have always been the wind beneath my wings.

M. Robert De Jong, RDMS, RDCS, RVT, FAIUM, FSDMS

Contents

Understanding Protocols and How They Are Determined

M. Robert DeJong

Key Words

Accreditation
As Low As Reasonably Achievable (ALARA)
Case presentation
Congenital anomaly
Current Procedural Terminology (CPT) code
Decubitus
Electronic Medical Record (EMR)
Ergonomics
Health Insurance Portability And Accountability Act (HIPAA)
Identification (ID) bracelet
Pathologic condition
Personal Protection Equipment (PPE)
Protocol
Scope of practice
Sonographer
Sonologist

Objectives

At the end of this chapter, the reader will be able to:

- List the organizations that determine which images are needed for a protocol
- Discuss the difference between a complete and limited Current Procedural Terminology (CPT) code
- Discuss how congenital anomalies and pathologic conditions can influence the final protocol
- Define ultrasound terms used to describe the ultrasound appearance of structures

Who and What Determines a Protocol

Protocols can be very frustrating to a student or a new employee. What exactly is a protocol? In ultrasound a **protocol** determines the images needed to ensure that a diagnosis can be made or verify that an organ is normal. The **sonographer**, using sound waves to create images of the body, is responsible for obtaining the images of a protocol. Although protocols may differ among laboratories, all have a core of similarity. For example, hospital A may require the right kidney to be fully imaged in a right upper quadrant (RUQ) examination, whereas hospital B may require only a long-axis image of the right kidney with a measurement. What is the reason for these differences? Shouldn't protocols be uniform across the country?

Ultrasound Organizations

The good news is that our national ultrasound organizations and those medical organizations that use ultrasound, such as The American College of Obstetricians and Gynecologists (ACOG), are working with the ultrasound **accreditation** organizations that evaluate the ultrasound practice for the quality of their studies, reports, and policies to help standardize ultrasound protocols. These organizations include the American Institute of Ultrasound in Medicine (AIUM), Society of Radiologists in Ultrasound (SRU), American College of Radiology (ACR), Society of Pediatric Radiologists (SPR), the Society for Maternal-Fetal Medicine (SMFM), Society of Interventional Radiology (SIR), and ACOG. For protocols in which the sonographic examination may be performed by different specialties, the organization associated with that protocol was invited for collaboration. For example, for any urology-related protocols, the American Urologic Association (AUA) had input because some urologists perform ultrasound examinations in their office.

Accrediting Organizations

The common denominator of protocols is the requirements of the accreditation organizations, because their standards will require a minimum set of images to be accredited by that organization. Accreditation is required for reimbursement by some insurance companies. A department may add additional images or views to the protocol, but they may not delete required images. Accrediting organizations include the AIUM, ACR, and Intersocietal Accreditation Commission–Vascular Testing (IAC-VT). The ACR and IAC-VT provide accreditation for laboratories or departments that perform vascular examinations, and the AIUM for departments that perform ultrasound examinations that are not vascular. The AIUM has vascular protocols on their web site but they do not offer vascular accreditation through AIUM accreditaion. Working with IAC, they provide accreditation for all aspects of ultrasound accreditation. The ACR accredits both vascular and nonvascular examinations, and most radiology ultrasound departments prefer ACR accreditation, as they offer accreditation for all the imaging modalities in a radiology department. Most vascular laboratories receive their accreditation through IAC-VT, and nonimaging departments that perform their own ultrasound examinations, such as urology and endocrine departments, achieve accreditation through the AIUM. Protocols and accreditaion standards should be checked annually and can be found on each of the organization's web site.

Coding

Another aspect that influences protocols is the billing codes that are sent to the insurance companies, called the Current Procedural Terminology codes, or, more commonly, **CPT codes**. The main purpose of the CPT code is to define what constitutes a complete versus a limited ultrasound examination. The internal code used by the ultrasound department, such as US123, which is used to order a renal ultrasound, is mapped to CPT code 76775. The 76775 code, not the US123 code, is sent to the insurance company for billing. The CPT code 76775 is used to bill an "ultrasound, retroperitoneal (e.g., renal, aorta, nodes), real time, with image documentation, limited." The CPT book defines which images are needed to legally bill for a complete study. A complete retroperitoneal study, 76770, is defined as follows: a complete ultrasound examination of the retroperitoneum consists of real-time scans of the kidneys, abdominal aorta, common iliac artery origins, and inferior vena cava, including any demonstrated retroperitoneal abnormality. Alternatively, if clinical history suggests a urinary tract pathologic condition, complete evaluation of the kidneys and urinary bladder also comprises a complete retroperitoneal ultrasound. This means that if your department bills 76770 for a renal ultrasound and the bladder is not imaged or mentioned in the final report, the insurance company will reject the bill, since the CPT code submitted was by definition a complete study and a limited study was performed. Once rejected, the department may not be able to bill again for the study. If a practice is caught billing for complete studies when only performing limited studies, they are heavily fined. The structures that need to be imaged to constitute a complete study are found in the CPT book and should be checked with each new edition to update protocols as needed.

FUTURE OF IMAGE STORAGE: As technology evolves, our protocols evolve also. Some laboratories now include video clips of the anatomy along with still images, whereas other laboratories take only video clips. With volume imaging, some laboratories acquire volumes of data and "slice and dice" the data like computed tomography (CT) and magnetic resonance imaging (MRI). There will be new ways to document and store the images as the industry evolves.

How Congenital Anomalies and Pathology Influence the Protocol

The sonographer must be knowledgeable and aware of congenital anomalies, because these will require adjusting the protocol. A

congenital anomaly is defined as something that is unusual or different at birth, such as a choledochal cyst or ectopic kidney. If a sonographer discovers a kidney is not in its correct location, this cannot be ignored, but rather the protocol should be expanded into the pelvic region to locate the missing kidney. If the kidney in the normal position is normal in size, there is a second kidney somewhere in the body, as a solitary kidney would be increased in size.

The protocol will be expanded when a **pathologic condition** is found. An example would be in the finding of unsuspected liver metastases; in this case the protocol should be expanded to try to determine the primary tumor and look for abdominal lymph nodes. Another example is when ascites is discovered on a RUQ ultrasound examination. Once ascites is discovered, the full extent of the fluid should be documented, which will entail scanning the flanks, the pelvic area, and the left upper quadrant (LUQ). Sometimes an obvious cause for the patient's symptoms is not diagnosed, and the sonographer needs to keep looking. For example, if a patient presents with bilateral leg swelling, yet no deep vein thrombosis (DVT) is found in the leg veins, the sonographer should expand the protocol to image the inferior vena cava to look for a central clot.

Nonimage Aspects of Protocols

Protocols do not just tell the sonographer what images are needed but also inform the sonographer about patient positions, transducer types and frequencies, required patient preps, and other information. In addition, protocols may tell the sonographer how to alter the protocol when congenital anomalies or pathologic conditions are present and what images are needed for short-term follow-up examinations.

Protocol: Patient Positions and Scanning Planes

Protocols will describe the best patient position to obtain the needed images and any specific patient positions required. For example, a protocol for the gallbladder will have the patient start in a supine position and require, depending on the patient's condition, turning the patient into a left lateral **decubitus** position, also called a right side up (RSU) position. A decubitus position is when the patient lies on their side, with the side that is on the table, or down, stated before the word "decubitus." Other patient positions include prone, oblique, and erect views. Various patient positions are illustrated in Fig. 1.1.

All protocols will require images obtained in at least two planes, usually the longitudinal and transverse planes. Other imaging planes may include oblique, coronal, sagittal, and the long axis of the organ.

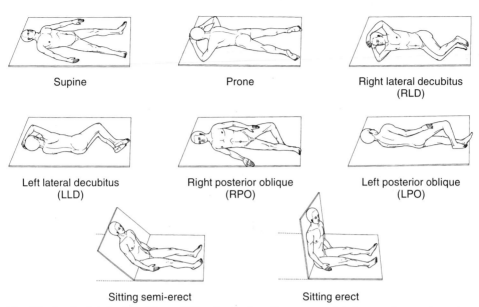

Fig. 1.1 Standard Patient Positions. Different patient positions are used during an ultrasound examination depending on the area of interest being evaluated. The best patient position is determined by what will produce the optimal view. It is standard practice to use different patient positions during a study to evaluate various structures. Note that any change in patient position must be noted on the images as part of standard labeling.

Protocols: Documentation

As technology grows and the cost of storing images on a server is decreasing, documentation of ultrasound studies is changing. One limiting factor is the size of video clips that the picture archiving and communication system (PACS) can play, although this is no longer an issue with modern PACS. The number of images required for documentation may change between ultrasound departments. This is especially true with the increasing number of departments integrating video clips into their protocols. The sonographer may obtain these video clips while assessing the anatomy to determine whether the organs seen are normal or affected by a pathologic condition. Using a scanning protocol is essential for methodical and organized documentation and for future comparable studies. Follow a scanning protocol as you would follow steps in a recipe.

The Sonographer and the Patient

- Dress according to the department's guidelines. Many institutions are adopting department color-coded uniforms or scrubs so the area the employee works in can be easily identified. For example, diagnostic imaging personnel, no matter what department they work for, may wear blue uniforms, and nurses may wear green uniforms. Make sure you know the guidelines for, wearing jewelry, visible body piercings, and tattoos. If you are allowed to wear street clothes, make sure you know what is acceptable and what is not acceptable to wear. Gel and body fluids can stain your clothes (I cannot begin to count my gel-stained ties), so make sure these are clothes that can be washed; stain-removal laundry products can help with gel stains. Consider investing in a few laboratory coats if you are allowed to wear them. Remember that your identification badge is part of your uniform and should be worn at all times while on the job and displayed so your name can be easily seen. You are a representative of the place where you work, so dress accordingly.

- Introduce yourself to your patient as soon as possible, which may be when you go to the waiting area to escort them back to the scanning room.
- Make sure you have the correct patient by checking the inpatient **identification (ID) bracelet**; some hospitals and outpatient centers are also placing them on outpatients. The typical ID bracelet displays the patient's full name, date of birth, and hospital identification or medical record number. If the patient does not have an ID bracelet, identify the patient as required by your place of employment. Some departments will not let you scan an inpatient who is missing their ID bracelet until one is placed on the patient. Although usually on the patient's wrist, they may be found in other places on the patient's body, such as their ankle.
- Briefly explain the examination to the patient in layman's terms. For example, tell the patient that he or she will need to roll on the left side when instructed, as opposed to needing to roll into a decubitus position. Be sure to ask if the patient has any questions or concerns before beginning the examination. Make sure that you speak clearly and at a slow pace.
- When indicated, obtain a brief medical history from either the patient or the patient's **EMR** and obtain any needed lab values and operative or other imaging reports. The EMR replaces the patient's physical chart and contains information on the patient such as physical findings, vital signs, operative notes, laboratory values, imaging reports, and physician notes, among other information. Avoid using medical terms a patient may not understand when asking questions about history pertinent to the examination.
- Always be professional, courteous, and respectful to your patients, co-workers, and other staff.
- When in public areas, do not discuss patient information or tell patient stories. Be careful with what you put on social media about work and using social media as a place to complain, especially about a patient that you scanned. People have lost their jobs over improper social media content. As remote as it seems, your comments can be seen as a HIPAA violation. **HIPAA** is a U.S. law designed to provide privacy standards to protect patient medical records and other health-related and personal information that the patient or guardian provided to health plans, doctors, hospitals, and other health

care providers. As difficult as it may be, never tell patients or their family member about the sonographic findings or give your opinion on the study results, no matter how much they beg or threaten you. One solution is to have the **sonologist**, the doctor who interprets the ultrasound examination, talk to the patient or family member. Talk to an experienced staff member on how to handle these situations. Remember that only physicians can legally render a diagnosis, and it is against the sonographer's scope of practice, which can be found on the Society of Diagnostic Medical Sonography (SDMS) website. In health care, a **scope of practice** informs a person of the procedures, actions, and processes that a health care practitioner is permitted to do in keeping within the confines of their profession.

Clinical Safety for the Patient and the Sonographer

- Be familiar with your institution's standard precautions protocol and whom to call if there are any questions, especially the proper procedure to follow and whom to call if you are stuck by a dirty needle.
- Be familiar with isolation policies and where to locate **PPE**, which includes gowns, gloves, masks, and eye protection. The sonographer will also need to know how to disinfect the equipment and transducers, which parts of the ultrasound unit can be wiped down, what disinfecting agents to use, and where to find them. Not all disinfection products can be used on ultrasound units or transducers. The sonographer needs to learn where on the manufacturer's website to find the information on disinfecting products. Note that different products may be needed to disinfect the ultrasound unit and the transducers. Failure to use the proper products can damage the equipment and void any warranties. Finally, the sonographer needs to know how to safely use the disinfecting products, what PPE is needed, and how to dispose of the used product. The infection prevention department and the safety officers are great resources.
- Be familiar with the sonographer's role in sterile procedures. This may include prepping the transducer, including how to attach the proper biopsy attachment, opening sterile kits, and determining a safe approach to the area being biopsied.
- Be familiar with assisting the patient into a hospital gown in a professional manner that helps preserve patient modesty.
- When helping a patient into or out of a wheelchair, be certain that both brakes are locked and the leg supports and footrests are pushed out of the way. Know the correct and safe way to assist the patient.
- Assist the patient with any medical equipment attachments such as an intravenous (IV) pole and/or Foley catheter bag.
- Ensure the scanning table and stretcher brakes are locked and the other side of the stretcher's rail is elevated when assisting a patient on to or off a stretcher.

- Have a handled step stool available for patients who require assistance to get up onto the scanning table.
- If the patient is already on a stretcher, avoid bumping into walls when wheeling the stretcher into the examination room. If the stretcher is difficult to move, get someone to help you, not only for the patient's safety but also for your own. It can be very easy to hurt your back or shoulders when struggling with a stretcher. After the stretcher is situated, set the brakes.
- Drape the patient properly for the examination and make sure he or she is as comfortable as possible.
- Invasive procedures require informing the patient about the details of the procedure, risks, and alternative methods to obtain the same information. The consent process is performed by the physician performing or assisting with the procedure. The patient must sign an informed consent form before the procedure can take place. The informed consent must have a witness, which can be the sonographer. A family member or guardian can sign the consent form for a minor or a family member that is unable to understand the explanation and sign for themselves.
- It is highly recommended that all endovaginal procedures be chaperoned by another health care professional, even if the sonographer is a woman. The chaperone must be employed by the hospital or facility and can never be a family member. Some institutions make having a chaperone present mandatory. The chaperone needs to be documented per the department's policy. With current EMR systems, there is usually a place to document this information. Chaperones are present to protect not only the patient but also the sonographer performing the examination. Female sonographers have been successfully sued by patients for "inappropriate" use of the transvaginal transducer.
- The sonographer needs to know what to do if a patient needs to be left alone in the examination room. Minimally the sonographer needs to raise both side rails, make sure the scanning table or stretcher is locked, and give the patient a call bell.

The Importance of Ergonomics

- **Ergonomics** in ultrasound is concerned with designing equipment, determining proper workflow, the sonographer's position while scanning, and proper use of scanning accessories so that the sonographer can perform their job functions safely. Sonographers are at risk for injury, especially of their muscles, nerves, ligaments, and tendons, when they do not scan in an ergonomic manner. With scanning all day there is a fair amount of repetitiveness that can lead to stress or musculoskeletal (MSK) injuries.

- To reduce work-related musculoskeletal disorders (WRMSDs) and scanning in pain, the sonographer needs to understand how to properly adjust the height of the ultrasound unit, correctly adjust the monitor and keyboard, and how to position the patient, their body, and the scanning chair, if used. The monitor and control panel should be ergonomically designed so the height and tilt can be adjusted to accommodate standing or seated users and the height of the sonographer.
- To protect himself or herself, the sonographer needs to learn proper body mechanics when moving the patient, ultrasound equipment, stretchers, and wheelchairs.
- The sonographer needs to learn how to use wedges and cushion blocks to assist in positioning the patient.
- Cable support devices should be used to reduce wrist and forearm torque while holding the transducer. Scanning support sponges should be used to offer support for the sonographer while scanning.
- Scanning chairs should be ergonomically designed to help the sonographer maintain proper posture and to allow for easy movement. Chairs should be height adjustable and include an adjustable lumbar support to encourage an upright posture. They should swivel, allowing easy rotation from patient to machine without affecting body alignment.
- Scanning tables should be specifically designed for the comfort of both the patient and the sonographer. The height of the table should be adjustable with the ability to place the patient in Trendelenburg or reverse Trendelenburg position. For ergonomic vaginal scanning, there should be stirrups available and the end of the table should either lower or have a cutout.

Scanning Tips

- Select the proper transducer or transducers needed to perform the ultrasound study and have them on the unit for quick access.
- Use a coupling agent such as gel, preferably warmed, to remove the air between the transducer and the surface of the patient's skin.
- The amount of transducer pressure exerted on the patient is an important aspect of scanning. When increasing the amount of transducer pressure, such as to push gas out of the way, warn the patient before pressing.
- Have an understanding of the controls used to create the image. These include but are not limited to overall gain, time-gain compensation (TGC), image contrast, field of view or depth, and focusing. These controls are used mainly to optimize the gray-scale image. The sonographer also needs to know how to adjust the controls used to optimize the spectral and color Doppler aspects of the examination.

- Remember to use the proper amount of output power, following the **ALARA** principle (*as low as reasonably achievable*). It is important to have enough power to create good images. If too low an output power is used, it may be difficult to see deep structures without increasing the far gain, which will increase noise in the image and decrease resolution. Using the proper preset for the exam will ensure that you cannot increase the power into unsafe levels.

Image Documentation

- The following information must be included on all images:
  - Patient name and identification number or medical record number
  - Date and time of study
  - Scanning site (name of hospital, outpatient facility, or private office)
  - Name or initials of the person performing the ultrasound examination
  - Area of body being scanned or the organ being scanned: for example, right kidney, left lower quadrant (LLQ)
  - Patient position: for example, supine, RSU
  - Scanning plane such as longitudinal, transverse, or coronal
  - If using abbreviations such as *long* for longitudinal, *rt* for right, or *kid* for kidney, make sure they are the accepted abbreviations used in the department. It can be confusing if one sonographer abbreviates the right kidney as *rt kid* and another sonographer uses *r ren* for right renal.
- Labeling of the image should be confined to the margins surrounding the image. Try not to label over the image unless you take the very same image without any labels. Labels could cover important diagnostic information for the interpreting physician; however, they can help the sonologist understand the image. A good example is annotating the word *bowel* over an area of bowel that could be mistaken for possible pathology because the sonographer can see the peristalsis.

Scanning Tips

- Normal anatomy and pathology must be scanned in at least two planes, usually longitudinal or sagittal and transverse. Single-plane representation of a structure will not properly demonstrate the entire organ or area. Any pathology must be scanned in at least two imaging planes to ensure that the pathologic area seen is real and that an artifact did not create the suspect area.

- It is impractical to take an ultrasound image every 1 or 2 cm through a structure. Therefore, the representative images that are given to the sonologist for a diagnostic interpretation must accurately represent the normalcy or any pathology or abnormality present. The use of video clips may help the sonologist with their interpretation of the static images. A good use of a video clip is to demonstrate peristalsis when bowel is creating false pathology.

Presenting an Examination to the Sonologist

- In a **case presentation**, the sonographer will present the images, patient history, details of the study, any technical issues, any patient issues such as patient's inability to hold their breath, and their impression of the study to the interpreting sonologist.
- The sonographer should start out by stating the reason for the examination and the patient history.
- Tell the sonologist about any relevant laboratory test results and any known correlative information such as reports from other imaging modality studies.
- Be able to discuss the techniques used.
- Be able to describe the ultrasound findings using appropriate sonographic terminology (Box 1.1).
- Inform the sonologist of any technical or patient issues.

Describing Sonographic Findings

- After a study is completed, some departments may require the sonographer to complete any worksheets or provide technical observations with a written summary of the ultrasound findings. Written documentation of any type almost always becomes part of a patient's medical record. The sonographer's technical impression should be documented in such a way as not to be legally compromising. Usually the sonographer's worksheet is looked at as a preliminary impression rather than a final one. Using ultrasound terminology, the report should include the echogenicity, size, location, and relationship to other structures of any abnormal findings. The sonographer should be very careful in providing a diagnosis either written or verbally, as this is outside the scope of practice for a sonographer. For example, the sonographer can state that there are multiple hypoechoic areas seen in the liver as opposed to stating that liver metastases are seen.
- It is important to note that if a sonographer fails to mention an abnormality in his or her technical observation but demonstrates the abnormality on the images, he or she has performed within the legal guidelines of the scope of practice for diagnostic medical sonographers.

Box 1.1   Ultrasound Descriptors

Ultrasound Imaging Terminology

- *Anechoic:* Neither possessing nor producing echoes; without internal echoes, such as a cyst.
- *Artifacts:* Echoes that do not correspond to real structures.
- *Complex:* The ultrasound appearance of a heterogeneous structure with both cystic and solid components, such as a necrotic mass.
- *Cystic:* A fluid-filled structure that does not produce any echoes, such as a normal gall bladder.
- *Echogenicity:* The characteristic of tissue to reflect sound waves and produce echoes. For example, the thyroid has a medium gray echogenicity.
- *Heterogeneous:* A structure that produces echoes of various amplitudes. The normal kidney is a heterogeneous organ because it is composed of echoes of various brightnesses.
- *Homogeneous:* A structure that is composed of similar echo brightness. The thyroid is a homogenous organ.
- *Hyperechoic:* More echogenic than the surrounding tissue. A hemangioma is a hyperechoic mass in the liver.
- *Hypoechoic:* Less echogenic than the surrounding tissue. Liver metastases are usually hypoechoic.
- *Isoechoic:* Areas having similar echogenicity are said to be isoechoic to each other. It can be difficult to see prostate cancer because the cancer tissue is isoechoic to the normal prostate tissue.

Labeling and Scan Orientation Terminology

- *Anterior:* Situated in front of or in the forward part of an organ.
- *Caudal:* Denoting a position more toward the feet of the body.
- *Cephalic:* Denoting a position more toward the head of the body.
- *Distal:* A position farther from any point of reference; opposite of proximal.
- *Lateral:* A position farther from the median plane or midline of the body or a structure.
- *Medial:* Pertaining to the middle; closer to the median plane or midline of a body or structure.
- *Posterior:* Situated behind or in the back part of, at, or toward the rear.
- *Proximal:* A position nearer to any point of reference.
- *Superior:* Situated upward or above; toward the head end of the body.

Positioning Terminology

- *Decubitus:* Lying on a horizontal surface, designated according to the portion of the body resting on the surface; therefore, in left lateral decubitus, the patient is lying on the left side.
- *Prone:* Lying face downward. The patient will be on their stomach.
- *Sagittal:* A vertical plane that separates the body into left and right sections; midsagittal describes a plane that separates the body into equal left and right halves.
- *Supine:* Lying on the back.
- *Trendelenburg position:* A position in which the patient is lying on their back inclined at an angle of 30 to 45 degrees so that the feet are higher than the head.

CHAPTER 2

Scanning Planes and Scanning Methods

M. Robert DeJong

Key Words

Angle of incidence	Orientation
Axial views	Positional orientation
Coronal planes	Pressure
Focal zone	Sagittal planes
Long axis	Short axis
Longitudinal views	Transverse planes
Measurement	
Oblique orientation	

Objectives

At the end of this chapter, you will be able to:

- Define the key words.
- Explain the way ultrasound uses body and scanning planes to image the body.
- Differentiate between scanning planes and views.
- Interpret scanning planes.
- Apply scanning methods and manipulate the transducer.
- Produce accurate measurements.
- Identify surface landmarks.

Labeling the Image

How does a sonographer evaluate the sonographic image? First, they need to know the plane used to obtain the image. Was it from a supine or a coronal approach? Second, they need to know the scanning plane used to obtain the image. Was it from a longitudinal or transverse plane? Remember that the transducer is like a flashlight and only sees what is in the path of the sound beam and some structures need to be seen to understand the orientation of the image. Finally, knowing the normal sonographic appearance of the structures and organs on the image is key to understanding if the image is normal or if pathology is present.

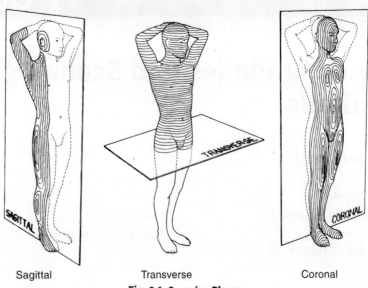

| Sagittal | Transverse | Coronal |

Fig. 2.1 Scanning Planes.

Anatomic Planes

The scanning planes used in sonography are the same as the anatomic body planes (Fig. 2.1). The plane from which the image is taken depends on the location of the transducer and the orientation of the sound beam as it enters the body.

- *Sagittal planes:* The mid or median sagittal plane divides the body into equal right and left sections. This is usually called midline (ML) on the image. Parasagittal planes are parallel planes to the right or left of midline. With the transducer in a longitudinal or sagittal position, these planes would be obtained by moving the transducer to the right or left side of the patient's body. For this book's purpose, unless noted, the term *sagittal* implies a parasagittal plane.
- *Transverse planes:* Divides the body into superior and inferior sections and is perpendicular to the sagittal plane. The transducer is turned 90 degrees and is moved up toward the head or down toward the feet on the patient's body.
- *Coronal planes:* Divides the body into anterior and posterior sections. This plane is obtained from scanning along the side of the patient, with the transducer pointing to the opposite side of the body when scanning abdominally. The coronal plane is also obtained with transvaginal and three-dimensional (3D) imaging.

Scanning Planes Overview

Scanning planes are used to establish the direction from which the ultrasound beam enters the body and the anatomic portion of anatomy being visualized from that direction.

Scanning planes are often from an **oblique orientation**, that is, slanted or angled, by slightly twisting or rotating the transducer. The degree of the oblique is determined by how the structure of interest lies in the body. Most body structures lie at a slight angle; they usually do not lie in a straight line up and down or straight across the body. An oblique scanning plane often affords visualization of the longest length of a structure.

Body structures must be viewed in planes, usually longitudinally and axially. **Longitudinal views** show a structure's length and depth. **Axial views** show width and depth. Most people use the term *transverse* for axial views. For example, the sonographer may mark an image of the liver as RT Trans liver.

Sonographers will also use the terms *sagittal* (sag) and *longitudinal* (long) interchangeably. For example, the sonographer will obtain images of the aorta from a sagittal plane but will annotate the image Long Aorta.

Ultrasound Scanning Planes

Sagittal

Scanning in a **sagittal plane** (Fig. 2.2) means that the ultrasound beam is entering the body from either an anterior approach, with the patient in the supine position, or a posterior approach, with the patient in the prone position. Usually the transducer is perpendicular to the floor. The body structures being imaged in this direction are evaluated in the following directions:

- Anterior
- Posterior
- Superior
- Inferior

NOTE: Medial and lateral are not seen on a sagittal scan, and the transducer must be moved either to the right or left of a sagittal plane to visualize adjacent anatomy in the parasagittal planes.

Transverse

The **transverse plane** (Fig. 2.3) is 90 degrees to the sagittal plane and indicates that the ultrasound beam is entering the body from either an anterior or posterior direction. Usually the sound beam is perpendicular to the floor or slightly angled toward the head or the feet. The body structures in this direction are evaluated in the following

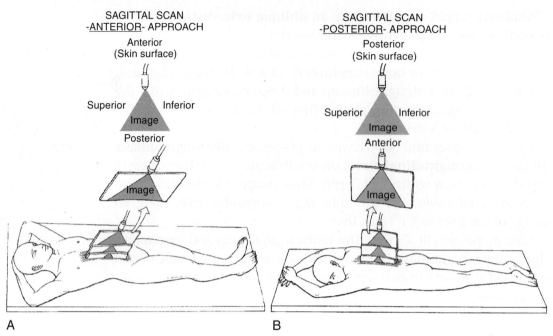

Fig. 2.2 A, Sagittal scan, anterior approach. **B,** Sagittal scan, posterior approach.

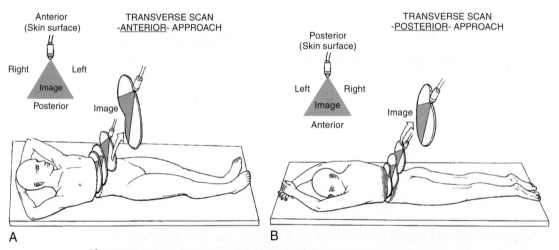

Fig. 2.3 A, Transverse scan, anterior approach. **B,** Transverse scan, posterior approach.

directions, when the beam is entering from an anterior or posterior direction:

- Anterior
- Posterior
- Medial
- Lateral

NOTE: Superior and inferior are not seen on a transverse scan, and the transducer must be moved either superiorly or inferiorly from a transverse plane to visualize adjacent anatomy.

Coronal Scanning Plane

Scanning in a **coronal plane** means that the ultrasound beam is entering the body from either a right or left lateral direction. This is accomplished by placing the transducer along the side of the patient's body (Fig. 2.4). Both longitudinal and transverse images can be obtained in a coronal plane. One of the main reasons to scan in this plane is to scan under bowel or between ribs. Most liver images are obtained from a variation of a coronal plane because this allows the sonographer to see the largest amount of the liver parenchyma.

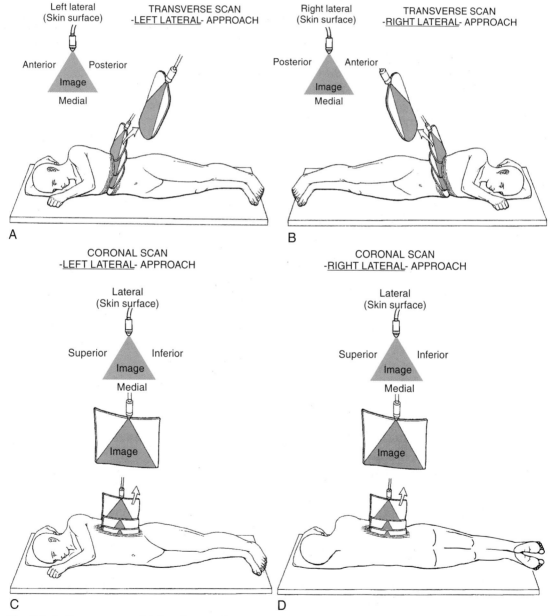

Fig. 2.4 A, Transverse scan, left lateral approach. **B,** Transverse scan, right lateral approach. **C,** Coronal scan, left lateral approach. **D,** Coronal scan, right lateral approach.

Scanning Planes and Anatomy Seen

The body structures being visualized from a longitudinal or long axis approach evaluate the following aspect of structures and organs:

- Anterior
- Posterior
- Superior
- Inferior

The body structures being visualized from a transverse approach evaluate the following aspect of structures and organs:

- Medial
- Lateral
- Superior
- Inferior

Scanning

The primary role of a sonographer is to provide interpretable images for diagnosis to a physician. This goal depends totally on the skills of the operator. Becoming an accomplished sonographer happens with practice, development of good scanning methods, knowing how to optimize the image, good critical thinking skills, and knowledge of anatomy and pathologic conditions.

Transducers

- Much has been accomplished with regard to the various types and designs of transducers used in diagnostic ultrasound. The new types and styles offer better penetration, better resolution, and better Doppler sensitivity. Also, ergonomically designed transducers assist the sonographer in producing optimal images and providing enhanced patient care while helping to protect the sonographer's joints.
- Transducers come in a variety of shapes and sizes. The shape of the transducer determines the field of view, and the frequency (MHz) of the sound waves emitted determines how deep the sound waves penetrate and the resolution of the image.
- The depth of the structure being imaged ultimately determines which transducer should be used. Low-frequency transducers have the most penetration, but their resolution is not as good as that of high-frequency transducers, which have less penetration, are used for more superficial structures, and have better resolution.
- The letter refers to the type of transducer and the numbers to the emitted frequencies. Some common diagnostic ultrasound transducers include:
  - *Curved linear array:* These are the most common type of transducer used in abdominal, obstetric, and gynecologic imaging.

Frequencies can range from a high of 10 MHz to a low of 2 MHz. An example of this transducer is a C5-2, which tells the sonographer that the transducer is a curved linear array (C) and will emit a range of frequencies from 2 to 5 MHz.

- *Vector/sector array:* These transducers are used when a low frequency is required, to scan between the ribs and in pediatrics. Vector transducers are either in the low-frequency range, V4-1, or a higher frequency range, S12-4, for scanning the newborn or infant, since the transducer can scan easily between the ribs. The V tells the sonographer it is a vector array, and the S is a sector array transducer.

- *Linear array:* These transducers display the largest amount of tissue beneath the transducer and are used for imaging superficial structures such as the thyroid, breast, and scrotum. They are also used for Doppler examinations, such as the carotid artery, lower extremity vessels, and musculoskeletal examinations. Two commonly used transducers are the L12-5 for carotid examinations and L18-5 for the thyroid. The L denotes that this is a linear array transducer.

- *Transvaginal and Transrectal:* These transducers have a small scanning head at the end of a long shaft for insertion into the vagina or rectum. Some companies have two separate transducers, and some use the same transducer. If there is a separate transrectal transducer, it is usually thinner. A C9-3 endovaginal transducer is used to obtain better resolution of the pelvic organs. A C12-5 is used to image the prostate. Since these are curved linear array transducers, they will be identified with a C, although some dedicated endovaginal transduces will be marked as EV9-3, with EV for endovaginal.

- *Hockey stick:* These transducers resemble a small "hockey stick" and are used primarily for intraoperative imaging and musculoskeletal (MSK) studies because of their small size. An L12-5 would be used to scan during a carotid endarterectomy. The L is used because it is a type of linear array.

- *Three-dimensional imaging (3D):* 3D ultrasound is now used in a variety of applications besides obstetrics and gynecology, including evaluating liver masses and vasculature, thyroid pathology, arterial disease, and other applications. These transducers are usually designated as a 3D transducer such as 3D9-3. New 3D transducers are now all electronic with no moving parts.

- Older transducers use a **focal zone**, which is where the sound beam is narrow to improve resolution. A transducer's focal zone is usually indicated by a small triangle, line, or other mark just to the right of the image. When scanning, every effort should be made to position the area of interest in the focused area to obtain the best images. Newer transducer technologies do not use focal zones.

Scanning Techniques

Sonographers will hold the transducer in various ways. I prefer to hold the transducer like a pencil, with my little finger touching the skin. I use my finger as a guide. I think this also allows better control of the transducer, especially for small movements. Think of the transducer as a fulcrum; holding the transducer higher on the handle will cause bigger movements of the transducer as opposed to holding it closer to the transducer head with the same amount of motion. Other sonographers hold the transducer on the handle portion. The correct way is whichever way allows you to scan and obtain the best images without causing you to scan in pain.

Scanning should be a series of fluid motions involving a combination of angling, rotating, and moving the transducer. Transducers can be easily maneuvered into different positions, providing multiple options for thoroughly evaluating an area of interest and obtaining the best images (Fig. 2.5).

The **angle of incidence** is the angle at which the sound beam strikes the surface (interface) of a structure. When the sound beam angle is perpendicular to the interface, the transducer will receive all of the echoes, which will also ensure that the true amplitude of the reflecting structure is determined. Remember that the intensity of the echo determines its shade of gray. When the sound beam hits the interface at an angle that is not 90 degrees, some of the echoes will reflect away from the transducer and not be processed. This may result in some structures not being displayed or the wrong amplitude processed, resulting in an incorrect shade of gray.

Applying the correct amount of **pressure** with the transducer can help improve image quality. Typically, pressure should be applied evenly and lightly, but in some cases more pressure is needed to get close to the structure or push gas out of the way. Always tell your patient when and why you need to apply pressure. For example, you might say, "Mr. Smith, I need to push some gas out of the way to see your pancreas better. Let me know if I push too hard or if it causes you pain."

Positional orientation of the transducer is needed to determine that the transducer is in the correct orientation to the image on the screen. For example, if you hold the transducer 180 degrees in the wrong orientation, the transverse images will look like the patient has situs inversus, which is a congenital condition when the organs are on the opposite side of the body from their normal side. The manufacturer will have something on the transducer, such as a groove, indentation, or light, that, when the transducer is held properly, will correspond to their trademark on the screen. A quick way is to hold the transducer in a transverse plane and touch the end of the

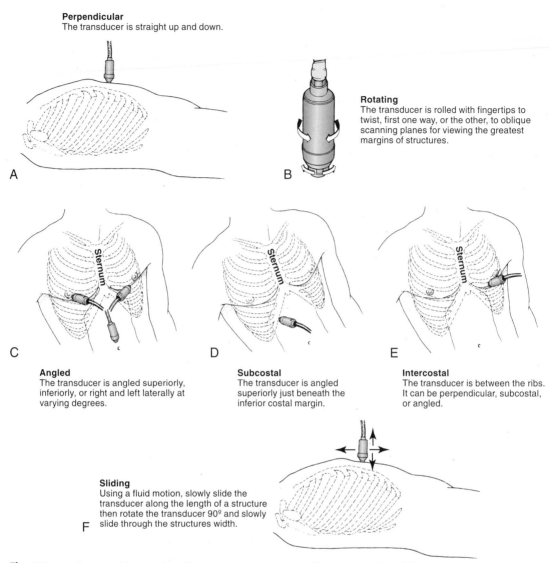

Perpendicular
The transducer is straight up and down.

A

Rotating
The transducer is rolled with fingertips to twist, first one way, or the other, to oblique scanning planes for viewing the greatest margins of structures.

B

C

Angled
The transducer is angled superiorly, inferiorly, or right and left laterally at varying degrees.

D

Subcostal
The transducer is angled superiorly just beneath the inferior costal margin.

E

Intercostal
The transducer is between the ribs. It can be perpendicular, subcostal, or angled.

Sliding
Using a fluid motion, slowly slide the transducer along the length of a structure then rotate the transducer 90° and slowly slide through the structures width.

F

Fig. 2.5 Transducer Positions and Motions. Transducers can be easily manipulated into different positions and motions for optimal imaging. They include the following: **A,** Perpendicular. **B,** Rotating. **C,** Angled. **D,** Subcostal. **E,** Intercostal, **F,** Sliding.

transducer. If the echoes created by your finger are displayed at what appears to be the other end of the transducer, you are holding the transducer the wrong way and need to turn it 180° so that it is in the correct orientation.

How to Take Accurate Measurements

Accurate and reproducible measurements are critical for good patient care. This is especially true when a patient returns for a follow-up and another sonographer performs the ultrasound exam and gets a different measurement that does not correlate with the previous measurement. For example, the first sonographer measures the right kidney as

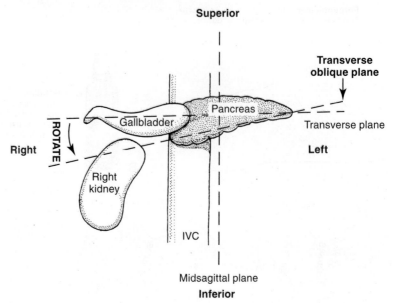

Superior

Transverse
oblique plane

Pancreas

Gallbladder

Transverse plane

Right

ROTATE

Left

Right
kidney

IVC

Midsagittal plane

Inferior

Fig. 2.6 Pancreas long axis would be seen in a transverse oblique scanning plane. The sonographer can resolve the long axis by slightly rotating the transducer and scanning through the pancreas until the long axis is resolved, as demonstrated in this figure. *IVC,* Inferior vena cava.

8.6 cm, which is small for a kidney. The patient returns in 3 months for a follow-up renal measurement, and this time another sonographer measures the right kidney as 10.2 cm, which is normal. After carefully measuring the kidney again and maybe even having someone else obtain a measurement, it is determined that the 10.2 cm measurement is correct. Small, diseased kidneys will not grow, so that means the first time it was incorrectly measured. How do you explain this to the referring physician? This makes the sonographer and the department appear incompetent.

Most organs do not lie perfectly in a parasagittal plane but rather in an oblique plane. To do an accurate measurement, the sonographer needs to scan according to how a structure is oriented within the body. The **orientation**, which is the position of the organ in the body, is determined by its **long axis**, which is the maximum length of a structure. The long axis of a structure can be seen in any scanning plane depending on how that structure lies in the body. For example, the pancreas lies obliquely in the abdomen with the head inferior in the C-loop of the duodenum and the tail more superior in the hilum of the spleen; therefore, its long axis is seen in a transverse oblique scanning plane (Fig. 2.6). This is accomplished by holding the transducer in a transverse plane and then very slowly rotating it counterclockwise until the entire length of the pancreas is seen.

In a true sagittal plane, the length of the kidney cannot be determined because the kidney lies in an oblique plane with the lower

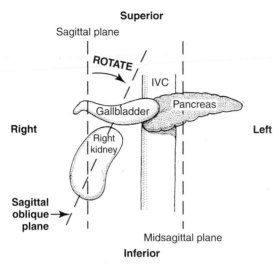

Fig. 2.7 Right kidney long axis would be seen in a sagittal oblique scanning plane. Note how the long axis is resolved by slightly rotating the transducer. *IVC,* Inferior vena cava.

poles more anterior and lateral than upper poles. Therefore, the sagittal plane must be at an oblique plane to match the angle of the kidney (Fig. 2.7). Starting with the transducer in a sagittal plane, slowly rotate the transducer clockwise until the entire length of the kidney is seen.

The long axis of the gallbladder is variable and can be seen in any of the three scanning planes, including transverse (Fig. 2.8). Once the orientation of the gallbladder has been determined, rotate the transducer until the long axis of the gallbladder is seen.

From the long axis of the organ, slowly rotate the transducer 90 degrees into the **short axis** plane for width measurements, which are taken at a structure's widest margins.

For an accurate width **measurement** of structures, begin by scanning perpendicular to the structure, slightly rotating the transducer until the widest part of the organ or structure is seen and a true representation of its size can be determined. Some organs, such as the kidneys, do not lie parallel in the body but rather at an angle; therefore, the transducer must be tilted, that is, toward the head or the feet, until it is perpendicular to the organ. For example, in obtaining a true transverse view of the kidney, the transducer needs to be tilted toward the feet. If the transducer is not tilted, it will be cutting the kidney obliquely and cause the kidney to be overmeasured. Accurate measurements are very important for patients undergoing some types of therapy to determine whether the mass or other pathologic condition has grown or shrunk in size. Sloppy or incorrectly measuring will have a direct effect on the care of the patient as well as reflect on your skills as a sonographer.

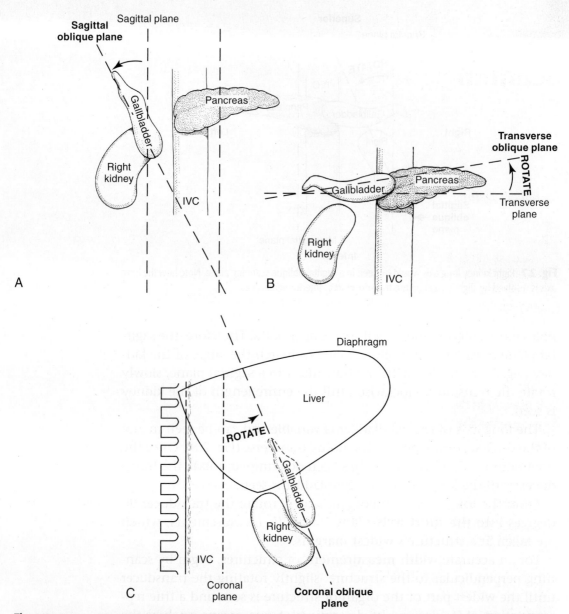

Fig. 2.8 The orientation (longitudinal lie/long axis) of the gallbladder (GB) is variable because it can lie in different positions throughout the abdomen. As illustrated in the figures, once the orientation is determined, the sonographer can slightly rotate the transducer, scanning through and evaluating the GB, until the long axis is established. **A,** GB long axis will be seen in a sagittal oblique plane. **B,** GB long axis will be visualized in a transverse oblique plane. **C,** GB long axis will be seen in a coronal longitudinal plane. *IVC,* Inferior vena cava.

CHAPTER 3

Scanning Protocol for Abnormal Findings and Pathologic Conditions

M. Robert DeJong

Keywords

Acoustic shadow	Homogeneous
Calculi	Mass
Complex	Necrosis
Cystic	Septations
Diffuse disease	Simple cyst
Enhancement	Solid
Heterogeneous	

Objectives

At the end of this chapter, you will be able to:

- Define the key words.
- Discuss the sonographic image in ultrasound terminology.
- Discuss how artifacts can help with the diagnosis.
- List the sonographic criteria of a simple cyst.
- Discuss how to present sonographic findings to the interpreting physicians.
- Explain the need to demonstrate pathologic conditions in two planes.

Evaluating Abnormal Findings or Pathologic Conditions

Proper Communication of the Results of the Examination

Our role as a sonographer is to differentiate normal tissue from abnormal tissue and to be able to properly discuss these findings with the sonologist. The term *sonologist* is used to describe the person that is interpreting the sonographic study, because a variety of physicians can interpret them—for example, radiologists, obstetricians, vascular surgeons, urologists, and cardiologists. As sonographers, we cannot make a diagnosis; therefore, we must learn to communicate these sonographic findings appropriately and within our scope of practice, as detailed on the website of the Society of Diagnostic Medical Sonography (https://www.sdms.org/about/who-we-are/scope-of-practice).

For example, the sonographer should not tell the clinician that the patient has a high-grade carotid stenosis. The sonographer should instead inform the clinician that there is echogenic material seen within the bulb and proximal internal carotid, with a peak systolic velocity of 230 cm/s and an end-diastolic velocity of 101 cm/s. By describing the findings like this the sonographer is not telling the physician that there is a greater than 70% stenosis, but that something is abnormal and they can either wait for the report or seek out the sonologist. The sonologist may not agree with the sonographer's diagnosis based on information obtained from the patient's medical history and report a different degree of stenosis. This will cause confusion for the referring physician with a change in diagnosis. This is a good teaching moment for the sonographer to learn why the sonologist did not agree with their interpretation.

Sonographic Terminology

Like other industries, sonography uses special terminology to discuss the sonographic image. Looking at the image, the sonographer will describe the organ and any pathologic area seen within and outside the organ. The parenchyma of an organ can be described as **homogeneous** when it is a uniform texture with the same shades of gray throughout, or as **heterogeneous** when there are a variety of shades from black to gray to white. For example, a normal liver would be described as homogenous (Fig. 3.1). If the liver has metastatic disease and contains multiple hypoechoic areas, this liver would be described as heterogenous (Fig. 3.2) because it has lost that uniform appearance.

When a change in echo texture is seen, it must be evaluated to determine whether it is localized (Fig. 3.3) or diffuse (Fig. 3.4).

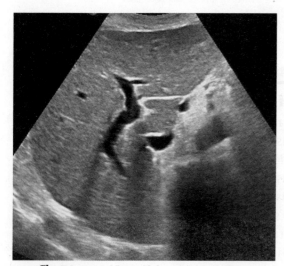

Fig. 3.1 Normal liver with homogenous texture.

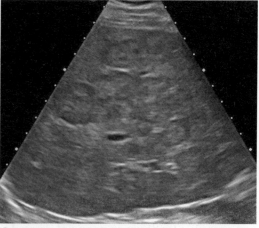

Fig. 3.2 Liver with heterogenous texture resulting from metastatic disease.

Localized disease is when the **mass** or masses are easily seen and have borders that can be defined and measured. **Diffuse disease** is when the entire organ is affected either by an infiltrative disease, such as metastatic disease of the liver or Hashimoto's disease of the thyroid, or by a process that affects all the cells of the organ, such as a fatty or cirrhotic liver (Fig. 3.5).

A mass is characterized according to its composition as **solid**, which is all tissue; **cystic**, which is fluid filled; or **complex**, which has both tissue and fluid components. Solid masses can be homogenous or heterogenous in appearance, while complex masses have a variety of appearances and contain both solid and cystic parts.

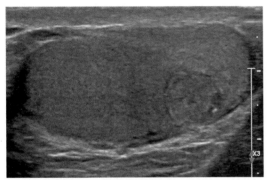

Fig. 3.3 Localized mass in the testicle.

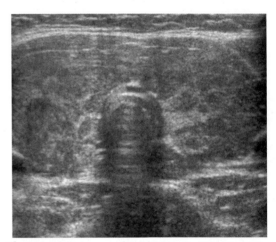

Fig. 3.4 A heterogenous thyroid due to Hashimoto's disease.

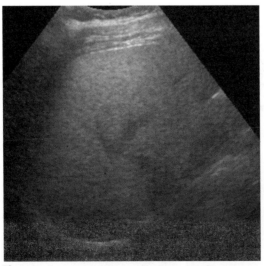

Fig. 3.5 The liver is heterogenous due to fatty liver disease.

Solid masses are further described by their echogenic relationship to the normal surrounding tissue as hypoechoic (Fig. 3.6), hyperechoic (Fig. 3.7), or isoechoic (Fig. 3.8). *Hypoechoic* is when the echo brightness of the mass is not as bright as the normal tissue (see Fig. 3.6); for example, there is a hypoechoic mass seen in the liver. A similar term is *less echogenic,* but this term is normally used when the entire organ does not have its characteristic brightness; for example, the pancreas is less echogenic than the liver, compatible with pancreatitis (Fig. 3.9). *Hyperechoic* is when the mass is brighter than the normal tissue; for example, a 2-cm hyperechoic mass is seen in the liver, compatible with a hemangioma (Fig. 3.10). *More echogenic* describes when a structure is brighter than normal; for example, the kidneys

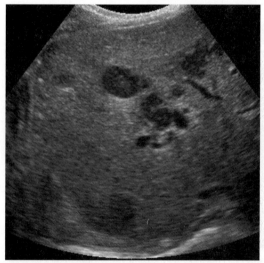

Fig. 3.6 Hypoechoic lesions in the liver from metastatic disease.

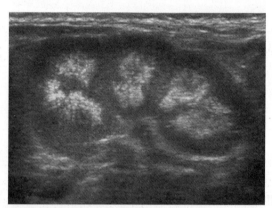

Fig. 3.7 Hyperechoic pyramids in the kidney compatible with nephrocalcinosis.

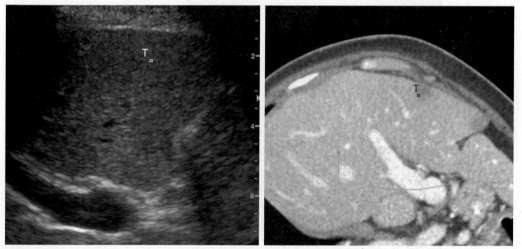

Fig. 3.8 Isoechoic mass in the liver that can be seen with fusion imaging using the patient's magnetic resonance image. The T with the small *box* on both images corresponds to the mass.

are more echogenic than the liver and spleen, compatible with medical renal disease (Fig. 3.11). *Isoechoic* masses are the hardest type of masses to appreciate because their echogenicity is the same as or very close to the normal echogenicity of the organ. With isoechoic masses the sonographer needs to look for secondary signs such as a bulge in the capsule, displaced vessels, or an abnormal area of vascularity (Fig. 3.12). Contrast ultrasound can be helpful in identifying isoechoic lesions.

Documenting Abnormal Findings and Pathologic Conditions

When a pathologic area or condition is discovered, the sonographer will integrate images of the pathologic area into the protocol. Additional images of the pathologic area can be obtained after

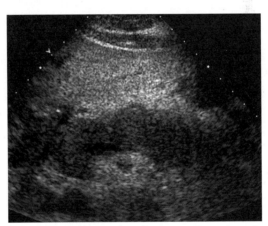

Fig. 3.9 Patient with acute pancreatitis. Note how the pancreas is now less echogenic than the liver.

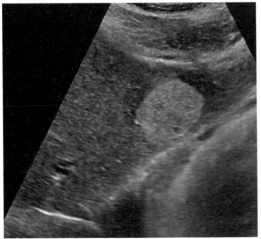

Fig. 3.10 Hyperechoic mass in the liver compatible with a hemangioma.

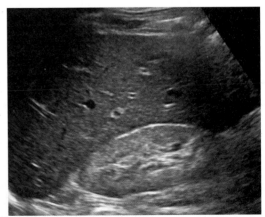

Fig. 3.11 The kidney and liver have reversed their normal relationship, with the kidney now being more echogenic than the liver, compatible with medical renal disease.

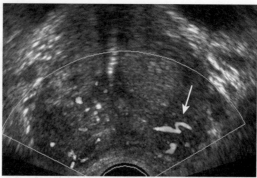

Fig. 3.12 An area of abnormal vascularity *(arrow)* in the prostate that helped to identify where to perform the biopsy, which turned out to be cancer.

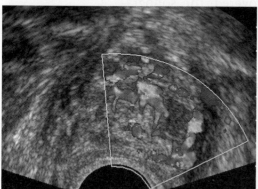

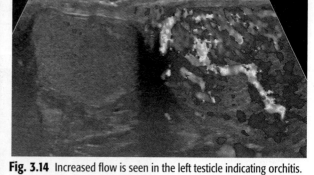

Fig. 3.14 Increased flow is seen in the left testicle indicating orchitis.

Fig. 3.13 Increased flow is seen in the area of a prostate abscess.

completion of the protocol, as needed. It is important that a full protocol is performed and the study is not limited to only the pathologic area that is found. The documented images need to show the extent of the pathologic area, organ or organs affected, sonographic characteristics, accurate measurements, any additional abnormal findings that may or may not be related to the initial findings, and, when appropriate, color and spectral Doppler images to determine the vascularity of the mass or abnormal area. A good example is the increased flow seen with an abscess (Fig. 3.13) or inflammation (Fig. 3.14). Taking a video clip can be very helpful for the sonologist to understand the relationship between normal and abnormal anatomy. Proper annotation is important for the sonologist to understand where the image was taken. Annotation should include the scanning plane (longitudinal, transverse, oblique, etc.), the side of the body (right or left), and the organ (Fig. 3.15). Sometimes the sonographer may need to be a little descriptive about where the image is from and how it was obtained. If no pathologic area is seen, the sonographer may annotate this region as the area of concern or area of pain (Fig. 3.16). For vascular and obstetric examinations,

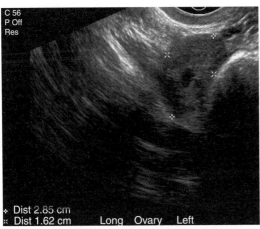

Fig. 3.15 Longitudinal endovaginal image of the left ovary.

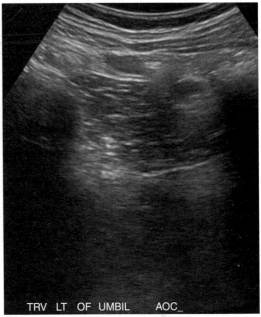

Fig. 3.16 *UMBIL* stands for umbilicus and *AOC* for area of concern. Peristalsis was seen in real time, and no pathologic area is seen.

annotation will be more descriptive: right femoral vein proximal, transverse left bulb, fetal kidneys, biparietal diameter, placenta, lower uterine segment (Fig. 3.17).

All pathologic findings must be documented in at least two scanning planes. This is to demonstrate that the abnormal area is pathologic, because the abnormal area seen in a single plane may be created by an artifact. Therefore, when an organ looks normal in one plane and shows a mass in another plane, the sonographer needs to go back to the first plane and demonstrate the mass. This usually occurs because the mass interacts with the sound beam at poor angles of reflection, resulting in the mass appearing isoechoic, whereas in the second plane the mass is interacting with the sound beam at more perpendicular angles, resulting in better reflections.

You can document an abnormality without knowing exactly what it is, because it is difficult to be familiar with every pathologic condition that can be demonstrated with sonography. The goal of the sonographer is to provide the physician with images demonstrating normal tissue and organs and images showing the extent of any pathologic area seen. The required images are a small representation of what a sonographer sees during a study, and the images should provide the interpreting physician with technically accurate information concerning the areas being scanned. Combining the pathophysiology knowledge of the sonologist with the sonographic knowledge

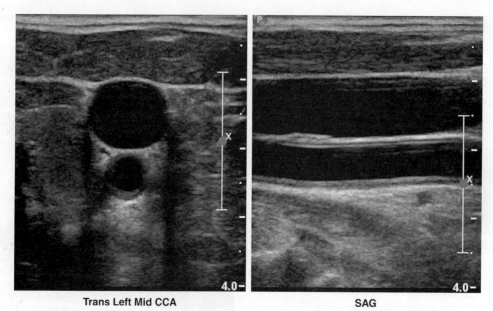

Trans Left Mid CCA   SAG

Fig. 3.17 Left mid–common carotid artery *(CCA)* in both transverse and sagittal *(SAG)* planes.

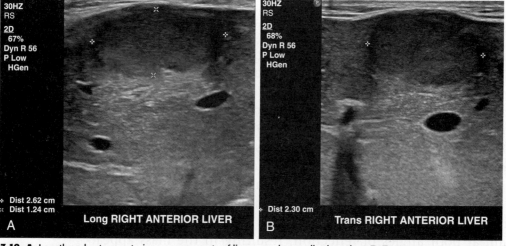

Fig. 3.18 A, Length and anteroposterior measurements of liver mass in a pediatric patient. **B,** Transverse measurements of the same liver mass, which was a hepatoblastoma.

of the sonographer can result in a more accurate diagnosis for the patient and teaching opportunities for both the sonographer and the sonologist. This will help increase the knowledge of pathologic conditions and abnormal findings for the sonographer.

Once a mass or lesion is found, the sonographer should carefully measure the length, width, and anteroposterior (AP) dimensions (Fig 3.18A, B). Images should be taken with and without measurements, because a caliper or the dotted lines may obscure part of the image. This is easily accomplished by documenting an image without the measurements, performing the measurements on the same image,

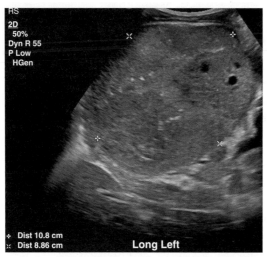

Fig. 3.19 Long-axis view with measurements of a neuroblastoma in a 3-year-old patient.

and then documenting it again. Most masses will not be parallel to the floor, and thus the sonographer needs to determine the true length of the mass. The AP measurement should be perpendicular to the length measurement (Fig. 3.19), and the width measurement should be 90 degrees from the length measurement. Calipers are placed from outer edge to outer edge. Sloppy or incorrect measuring techniques will result in confusion, especially when follow-up examinations are needed to help determine whether a mass is enlarging or shrinking. This is especially crucial for patients receiving treatment to try to shrink a mass.

One challenging situation with pathologic findings is when you see the *effect* of the pathologic condition but you do not see the pathologic condition itself. For example, isolated dilated ducts are seen in the liver but no obvious stone or mass is seen. One possibility is a cholangiocarcinoma, which is a tumor arising from bile duct cells and rarely seen by ultrasound. The dilated ducts that are obstructed from the tumor are seen, but not the tumor itself (Fig. 3.20). A more common example is when a stone causes hydronephrosis, but the stone is not visualized because it is in a part of the ureter that is obscured by bowel. To verify this, the bladder is evaluated with color Doppler looking for a ureteral jet. If none is seen, complete obstruction is suspected. If a weak jet is seen, a nonobstructive stone is suspected. It is seeing these indirect signs that make sonography interesting and challenging.

Helpful Artifacts

Most artifacts can cause problems determining whether there is truly a pathologic area present. Not all artifacts are troublesome; some actually can be helpful for diagnosing. As a sonographer, it is important

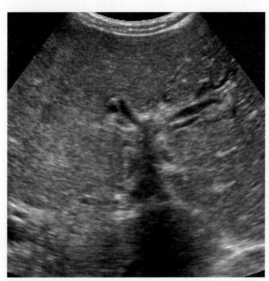

Fig. 3.20 Patient with dilated right and left common hepatic ducts. No stones or masses were seen. Computed tomography demonstrated a Klatskin's tumor.

to not only recognize artifacts but also understand how they are created so they may be explained.

Some disease processes can cause the formation of **calculi**, often called stones, which are caused by a concretion of material, usually mineral salts, that forms in an organ or duct. With ultrasound, stones are recognized by the **acoustic shadow** produced by the sound beam passing through a highly attenuative structure that absorbs the sound beam, leaving no sound beam to interact with the deeper tissue, thus creating a black space—a shadow—under the stone. The acoustic shadow is usually referred to as a good artifact because it helps identify and locate stones (Fig. 3.21).

Another helpful artifact is acoustic **enhancement**, which is kind of like the opposite of an acoustic shadow, because it is caused by the sound beam going through a low-attenuating substance, such as fluid, causing the echoes under the fluid to be brighter than echoes on either side of the fluid-filled structure. Some solid-appearing masses may exhibit enhancement, thereby identifying the mass as fluid filled rather than solid tissue. A good example is an abscess, which can look like a solid mass; however, the enhancement artifact tells us that it contains fluid and not solid tissue (Fig. 3.22).

Describing the Sonographic Appearance of Abnormal Findings and Pathologic Conditions

One of the biggest challenges a sonographer faces is a patient or patient's family member asking what the sonographer sees. So how does a sonographer answer these questions while staying within the scope of practice for a sonographer? As discussed earlier in this

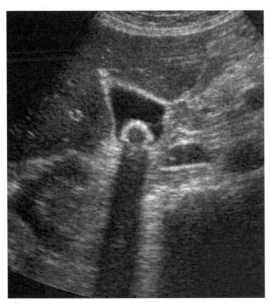

Fig. 3.21 An example of an acoustic shadow caused by a gallstone.

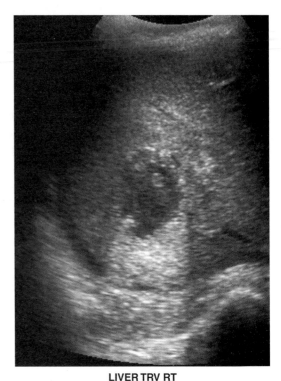

LIVER TRV RT

Fig. 3.22 A solid-appearing mass is seen in the liver. The enhancement under the mass indicates that this is not a solid mass but contains fluid and is compatible with an abscess.

chapter, a sonographer cannot make a diagnosis; they can only describe their findings using sonographic terminology. This will be beyond the understanding of the patient and will cause confusion and potentially unnecessary concern that something is wrong. A good way to get out of this situation is to say something like, "The radiologist will evaluate the images and correlate them with your lab values, other imaging studies and your medical history to come up with an accurate report for your doctor." The sonographer must also be careful what they say to the referring physician. It is important to remember that the sonologist will determine the final diagnosis. The danger with the sonographer giving the diagnosis is that the sonologist may disagree and have a different final diagnosis. This will cause confusion to the patient's physician. There is also the possibility that the physician will act on the sonographer's diagnosis and potentially treat the patient incorrectly. This could put the sonographer in legal liability for going outside their scope of practice. One of the most challenging situations occurs when the fetus has no heartbeat or has a congenital anomaly. The patient may suspect something is wrong, especially if she had a prior normal ultrasound with this or another pregnancy or is there to determine whether the fetus is viable. It can be difficult trying to dodge answering the mother's questions.

However, it is important to let the sonologist discuss the results with the patient, because the sonologist will be more knowledgeable with answering the patient's questions. At this point the sonographer is there for moral support.

As sonographers, we should describe our findings in sonographic terms. For example, instead of saying that a mass is seen in the liver, the sonographer should say that a 2-cm hypoechoic area is seen within the right lobe of the liver. Instead of saying that the patient has an abdominal aortic aneurysm, the sonographer should say that the distal aorta measures 5 cm in diameter. Telling a patient that he or she has gallstones may not seem like a big deal; however, there is no way of knowing how the patient will react to this news or how the referring physician will react when the patient tells them that the sonographer already told them that they have gallstones. The physician may get upset and possibly complain to the radiologist or the sonographer's manager about them giving the patient information that should have come from the physician. The sonographer should understand what the department allows the sonographer to say to the referring physician, especially when the interpreting physician is not available. This can be stressful to the sonographer, especially when the referring physician is standing over the sonographer's shoulder asking what the examination shows. Even in these situations the sonographer needs to describe the findings in sonographic terms. For example, the sonographer is scanning a renal transplant in a patient who has sudden onset of anuria. The sonographer does not see any flow in the renal artery. Instead of saying to the physician that there is renal artery thrombosis, the sonographer should tell the physician that no color Doppler is seen in the kidney or in the main renal artery. This may seem like saying the same thing, but the difference is that the sonographer is not making a diagnosis of renal artery thrombosis, but rather is describing the sonographic findings of not seeing any color Doppler in the kidney or artery. Most physicians will understand the significance of these findings and then will have the information needed to try to save the transplant.

Cysts should be described as fluid-containing structures with posterior acoustic enhancement and stones as echogenic structures causing an acoustic shadow. Cirrhosis of the liver would be described as the liver is heterogeneous in texture with nodularity seen along the capsule. Any ascites should be described as free fluid and its location identified. To describe a deep venous thrombosis, the sonographer should state that the vein walls do not touch with compression and that the vein is distended with low-level echoes or simply say that the vein is noncompressible. When discussing your case with the radiologist or sonologist, it is usually permissible to talk directly about the disease to them: the patient has fibroids, there are enlarged lymph nodes in the neck, there is a deep venous thrombosis in the popliteal vein, or the fetus appears to have spina bifida.

Describing Pathologic Areas

Sonography cannot definitively distinguish between malignant and benign masses, even though some masses may have benign or malignant characteristics.

Solid Masses

Solid masses are described in terms of their echogenicity and can be variable in appearance. They can appear hyperechoic, hypoechoic, or isoechoic to the organ parenchyma. They also can be characterized as anechoic, homogeneous, or heterogeneous. Anechoic does not always indicate that the mass is a cyst, which is why the absence of enhancement points to the mass being solid. In some masses the walls may be poorly defined and the contour can appear irregular. The sonographer could describe a thyroid mass as follows: A 0.4-cm hypoechoic, homogenous, well-defined mass is seen in the mid left lobe of the thyroid gland, or as a 2.3-cm heterogenous or complex mass seen in the upper pole of the right lobe of the thyroid gland.

Cystic Masses

Cystic masses are described as being either a simple cyst or a complicated cyst. To be considered a **simple cyst**, the following sonographic criteria must be met:
1. It should be round or oval in shape.
2. There should be no internal echoes.
3. The walls must be well defined, thin, and smooth.
4. The mass must exhibit posterior acoustic enhancement (Fig. 3.23).

   If one of these criteria is not met, the cyst is called a complex cyst. A complex cyst will display one or more of the following: **septations**, which are thin septums, in the cyst; echoes in the cyst, especially at the bottom; tissue or nodules inside; or irregular walls. Note that echoes at the top of the cyst usually are caused by reverberation artifact, because particles will not float to the top of the cyst. Echoes at the bottom of the cyst can be true echoes from infection or hemorrhage or artifactual echoes from a slice thickness artifact (Fig. 3.24). It is important that the sonographer determine whether the echoes are real or an artifact. The sonographer should describe a simple cyst as follows: A 3-cm cystic structure is seen in the lower pole of the right kidney with good acoustic enhancement. A complex cyst would be described as follows: A 2.2-cm cystic structure containing septations is seen in the upper pole of the right kidney (Fig. 3.25). Or low-level echoes are seen in a 2.8-cm cystic structure in the mid-pole of the left kidney.

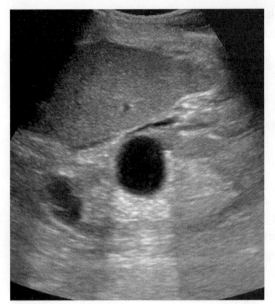

Fig. 3.23 A renal cyst demonstrating the classic signs of a cyst.

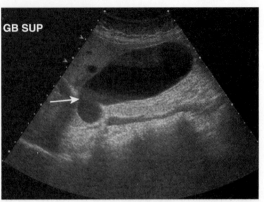

Fig. 3.24 A reverberation artifact is seen at the top of the gallbladder and a slice thickness artifact *(arrow)* at the bottom of the gallbladder.

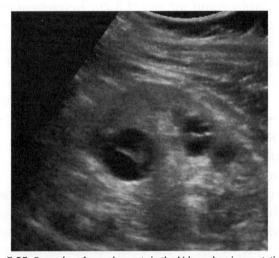

Fig. 3.25 Examples of complex cysts in the kidney showing septations.

Complex Masses

Complex masses contain both fluid and solid components. Complex masses may be primarily cystic or primarily solid. The internal composition of a complex mass may change with time. For example, a solid mass on follow-up now has cystic components compatible with areas of **necrosis**, or dead tissue. A sonographer should describe a complex mass as follows: A 7.9-cm complex mass is seen in the right lobe of the liver.

Scanning Tips

There will be times when a sonographer misses a pathologic area. Sometimes the sonographer is concentrating on documenting a pathologic finding and does not see another pathologic condition is present. I call this situation "wearing blinders" and intend that in a positive way. I have done this myself multiple times in my career. For example, a sonographer working up a pancreatic head mass, liver metastases, and distended gallbladder might miss the parapancreatic nodes. The radiologist notices them and asks the sonographer about them. Be truthful and admit to overlooking them and offer to go take some images of that area. Never lie to the sonologist with statements such as: "That was bowel," "It's nothing," or "It's an artifact." If the sonologist goes into the room to scan the patient or watch you scan and finds that the area is pathologic, you have lost some respect with the sonologist and your future scans may be doubted. Admit that you missed it and go back and work up that area. It is very easy to have an unusual finding and focus on it or identify an extensive pathologic area and miss other pathology. Don't be upset at yourself but learn from the experience. We've all been there.

Make sure that all pathologic areas are documented in at least two planes. Use color Doppler as needed to document any vascularity; however, also obtain a spectral Doppler signal image because the sonologist will not be able to determine whether the vessel is an artery or a vein. Nor can the sonologist evaluate flow characteristics, such as whether this is a high- or low-resistance arterial signal or if venous flow is continuous or pulsatile. Color Doppler imaging tells part of the story, but to get the whole story, a spectral Doppler signal image is needed.

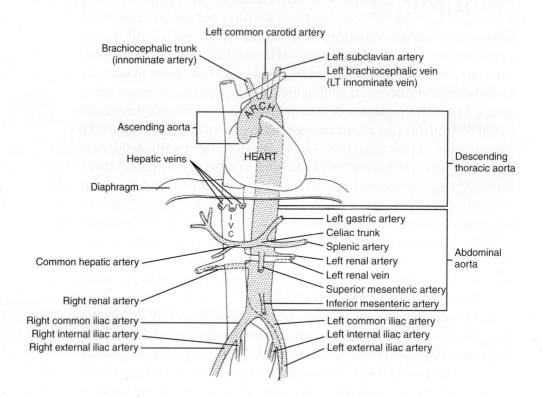

Left common carotid artery

Brachiocephalic trunk
(innominate artery)

Left subclavian artery

Left brachiocephalic vein
(LT innominate vein)

ARCH

Ascending aorta

Descending
thoracic aorta

HEART

Hepatic veins

Diaphragm

IVC

Left gastric artery

Celiac trunk

Splenic artery

Common hepatic artery

Left renal artery

Left renal vein

Abdominal
aorta

Superior mesenteric artery

Right renal artery

Inferior mesenteric artery

Right common iliac artery

Left common iliac artery

Right internal iliac artery

Left internal iliac artery

Right external iliac artery

Left external iliac artery

CHAPTER 4

Abdominal Aorta Scanning Protocol

M. Robert DeJong

Keywords

Abdominal aorta	Mid
Anteroposterior (AP) diameter	Proximal
Aorta	Renal arteries
Celiac artery (CA)	Superior mesenteric artery
Common iliac arteries	(SMA)
Distal	Tortuous
Left renal artery (LRA)	Width

Objectives

At the end of this chapter, you will be able to:

- Define the key words.
- Identify the sonographic appearance of the aorta.
- List the transducer options for scanning the aorta.
- Describe patient prep for an abdominal aorta study.
- Identify the order and exact locations to take representative images of the aorta.
- Discuss how to locate the common iliac arteries.
- Discuss the importance of identifying the renal arteries.
- Describe how to accurately measure a normal aorta and an aorta with an aneurysm.

Overview

Aorta Anatomy

Sonographic exams of the aorta can be performed in both radiology and vascular lab departments. Some cardiology departments may do them also. They may also be performed by physicians in the Emergency Department (ED). The **aorta** is the largest artery and is responsible for providing oxygenated blood to the body. It originates from the left ventricle of the heart at the aortic valves; becomes the ascending aorta; makes a U-turn, called the aortic arch; continues down the chest cavity, called the descending aorta; pierces the diaphragm, where it is then called the abdominal aorta; and ends at the aortic bifurcation, where it branches into the two common iliac arteries. The descending aorta is divided into two sections; above the diaphragm it is called the thoracic aorta and below the diaphragm the abdominal aorta. The abdominal aorta can be further divided into suprarenal and infrarenal sections (Fig. 4.1).

Thoracic Aorta

The ascending aorta rises from the heart and is about 2 inches long. The coronary arteries branch off of the ascending aorta to supply blood to the heart. The aortic arch curves over the heart and connects the ascending aorta with the descending aorta. The arteries that arise from the arch are the brachiocephalic artery, the left carotid artery, and the left subclavian artery. These arteries supply blood to the head, neck, and upper extremities. The descending thoracic aorta travels down through the chest. Its small branches supply blood to the lungs, thoracic esophagus, ribs, diaphragm, and the pericardium.

Abdominal Aorta

The **abdominal aorta** begins at the diaphragm and ends around the level of the umbilicus, where it divides to become the paired common iliac arteries. The first branch that can be seen by ultrasound is the **celiac artery** (CA), also known as the celiac trunk or celiac axis. It arises from the anterior wall of the aorta around the level of T12 and behind the median arcuate ligament. The CA provides oxygenated blood to the stomach, esophagus, liver, spleen, pancreas, and superior portions of the duodenum. The celiac trunk trifurcates into the following three arteries: the left gastric artery, common hepatic artery, and splenic artery. (*Note*: The first true branches of the aorta are the inferior phrenic arteries that supply blood to the diaphragm

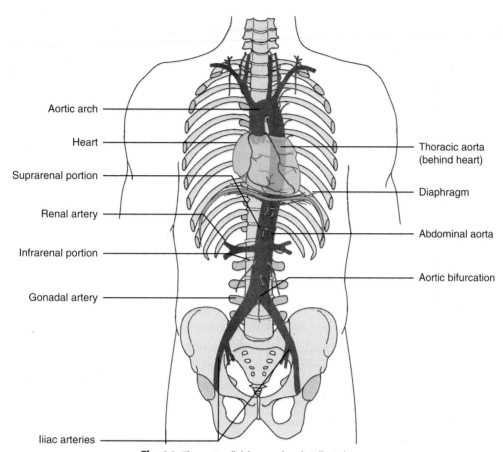

Fig. 4.1 The aorta: divisions and main tributaries.

and a branch to the adrenal gland.) The next anterior branch is the **superior mesenteric artery** (SMA), which can be found approximately 1 cm below the CA and supplies blood to the head of the pancreas, parts of the duodenum and jejunum, ileum, cecum, appendix, and segments of the ascending and transverse colon. The **renal arteries** are the first lateral branches off of the aorta that can be seen with ultrasound and supply blood to the kidneys and ureter; it is one of the three arteries that supplies blood to the adrenal gland. The renal arteries are seen just past the origin of the SMA. Superior to the renal artery is the middle suprarenal artery. Inferior to the renal arteries are the gonadal arteries that supply blood to the testicles or ovaries. The next branches are the posterolateral branches, which are the lumbar arteries that supply blood to the spinal cord, abdominal wall, vertebral canal, and the muscles of the back. The final anterior branch is the inferior mesenteric artery (IMA), which supplies blood to the descending colon, sigmoid colon, rectum, and anastomosing branches to Riolan's arcade, which provides an anastomosis between the superior and inferior mesenteric circulation. The end of the abdominal aorta branches into the paired **common iliac arteries**, which supply blood to the lower extremities and pelvic organs.

The abdominal aorta runs retroperitoneally just anterior and to the left of the spine and bifurcates into the common iliac arteries anterior to the body of the fourth lumbar vertebra. The normal diameter of the abdominal aorta is less than 3 cm and gradually tapers in size toward the bifurcation. An aortic diameter greater than 3 cm is suspicious for an abdominal aortic aneurysm (AAA). The aorta can become very **tortuous**, or twisted, with age and disease.

Arterial Wall Anatomy

Like all arteries, the aorta's wall has three layers. The tunica intima is the innermost layer composed of endothelial cells and provides a smooth surface for blood flow. The tunica media is the middle layer and is composed of smooth muscle cells and elastic tissue and collagen, which allows the aorta to expand and contract with each heartbeat. The tunica adventitia is the outer layer and is composed of collagen and external elastic lamina to provide additional support and structure to the aorta.

Sonographic Appearance

The aorta is a tubular structure with echogenic walls and an anechoic lumen. It is immediately anterior to the spine and a little to the left of midline.

The long axis of the aorta is seen in a sagittal plane and transverse images in the transverse plane. In longitudinal views the aorta is seen as a long tube-like structure, whereas in transverse views it has a round or circular appearance.

It can be easy to mistake the inferior vena cava (IVC) for the aorta in a longitudinal image, especially if the IVC is prominent. Look for walls that are pulsating, bright, and thicker and anterior branching vessels to ensure that you are imaging the aorta. The IVC also can be distinguished from the aorta as it runs through the liver and empties into the right atrium. Using your sonographer's imagination, the aorta looks like a frown as it dives under the liver or as a straight tube, whereas the IVC looks like a smile as it turns up to empty into the heart (Fig. 4.2).

Aortic Sections

- The **proximal**, closest to the origin, portion of the abdominal aorta is the portion of the aorta from the diaphragm to the celiac trunk.

- The **mid** portion of the abdominal aorta is from the CA to the renal arteries.
- The **distal**, farthest from origin, portion of the abdominal aorta is past the renal arteries to the bifurcation.

Ultrasound of the Aorta

Our goal for an aorta ultrasound is to visualize the entire length of the abdominal aorta looking for any disease or abnormalities, the most common being a AAA (pronounced "triple A"). Many AAAs are found incidentally with ultrasound and computed tomography (CT), some as large as 8 to 10 cm. If an unexpected aneurysm is discovered, the sonologist may need to call the referring physician while the patient waits, especially if it is 5 cm or greater in diameter. A less common reason is to evaluate for a dissection. This is when blood penetrates the intima layer and enters the media layer. This creates two lumens called the true lumen and the false lumen. The dissection can involve the entire aorta and extend into its branches. It is important to see if the flap is interfering with flow to either kidney.

Patient Prep
The patient should fast (nothing by mouth [NPO]) for at least 6 to 8 hours before the ultrasound study to reduce bowel gas and be scheduled in the morning. The patients may take medications with water or other clear liquids. If the patient has eaten, still attempt the examination, because the patient is NPO to reduce bowel gas and not for physiologic reasons. Studies to rule out a AAA are true medical emergencies, and prep is irrelevant.

Transducer
The most common transducer used is a curved linear array that includes a 3–3.5 MHz frequency in its bandwidth. Newer technologies are expanding the bandwidth, allowing for lower frequencies in curved array transducers. For larger patients a sector/vector array transducer may be needed that includes a 2–2.5 MHz frequency in its bandwidth. A curved array transducer is best for pushing gas out of the way because of its larger footprint and is more comfortable for the patient than a sector/vector array when pressing gas out of the way.

Breathing Technique
The aorta may be scanned with the patient breathing normally, also called quiet breathing. Deep, held inspiration or having the patient stop breathing at the end of expiration may also be helpful. Sometimes a combination of different breathing techniques is needed to visualize the entire aorta to obtain an adequate study.

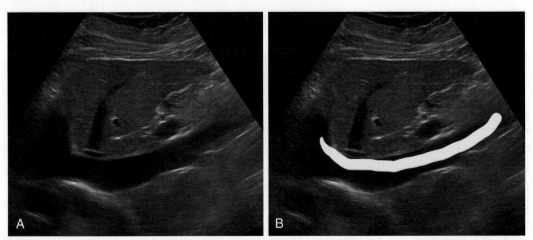

Fig. 4.2 A, A normal inferior vena cava (IVC) going through the liver. Note how it turns up to enter the right atrium. **B,** Same image showing the IVC smile.

Patient Position

Most patients can be scanned with them in the supine position. If unable to see the aorta or parts of the aorta, other possible patient positions are as follows: (1) a coronal plane approach from the right side; (2) a right lateral decubitus, also known as left side up; (3) a left or right posterior oblique; (4) a left lateral decubitus, or right side up; (5) a coronal approach from the left side; or (6) the patient in a semierect position. Different patient positions should be used to try to see the entire aorta (Fig. 4.3).

Technical Tips

The lumen of the aorta should be echo free. If echoes are present inside the lumen, true echoes need to be distinguished from echoes caused by artifacts, because true echoes should not be removed. There are different ways to "clean up" the aorta. It is important to ensure that the echoes inside the aorta are artifacts and do not represent thrombus or other pathologic condition. The easiest way is to turn on harmonics, if it is not already activated, and compound imaging. Decreasing the dynamic range will make the image more black and white, eliminating low-level gray echoes, and may also clean up the image. Other technical tips include tapping back the time-gain compensation (TGC) pods at the depth of the aorta, checking the position of the focal zone and turning down the overall gain. Sometimes gently pressing with the transducer will help clean up the aorta because the aorta will be closer to the transducer. If it is hard to see the mid to distal aorta, using a curved linear array transducer rock the transducer side to side while gently pressing on the abdomen. Be sure to warn the patient first. A linear artifact can be seen in the lumen of the aorta

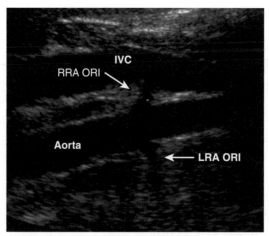

Fig. 4.3 A view of the abdominal aorta at the level of the renal arteries. This view is obtained by placing the transducer on the right side of the patient and lining up the liver, inferior vena cava *(IVC)*, and aorta in a coronal plane. It can be referred to as the "banana peel" view. *LRA ORI,* Left renal artery origin; *RRA ORI,* right renal artery origin.

on some patients. This is most likely a type of mirror artifact. This echo will move with the pulsations of the aortic wall. This should not be mistaken for a dissection. A true dissection is a thin echogenic line that moves independently of the pulsations of the aorta.

Required Images

Abdominal Aorta Protocol

The required images are a small representation of what a sonographer visualizes during a study. The images should provide interpreting physicians with technically accurate images for them to be able to make a diagnosis. While scanning, experiment using different amounts of transducer pressure, keeping the patient's comfort in mind, to help improve the image.

An adequate examination should include the following:

1. Longitudinal views of the aorta at proximal, mid, and distal levels and the proximal portions of the common iliac arteries.
2. Transverse views of the proximal, mid, and distal aorta and the origin of the common iliac arteries.

Aorta • Longitudinal Images

1. Begin scanning with the transducer at the midline of the body, just inferior to the xiphoid process of the sternum. Slightly move or angle the transducer to the patient's left and identify the proximal aorta just posterior to the liver. Document the image with and without an antereoposterior (AP), height, measurement. Note how the cursors are perpendicular to the aortic walls. Some departments

may allow documenting just one image as long as the calipers do not interfere with the image.

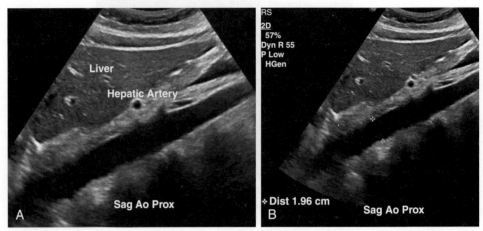

Suggested Annotation: **SAG AO PROX**

NOTE: Annotation will be determined by the department and may be different from what is suggested here. Some departments will use the automatic annotations that are built into the machine or use their customized annotations. This helps with standardization among sonographers in the same department.

2. Slide the transducer inferiorly until the aorta's anterior branches, the CA and the SMA, are about mid-image. Document the image. If it was difficult to measure the proximal portion of the aorta, a measurement could be obtained on this image at the level above the CA.

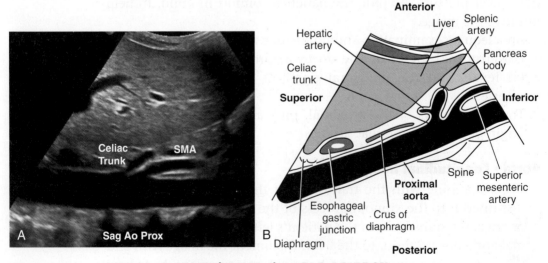

Suggested Annotation: **SAG AO PROX**

3. Slide the transducer inferiorly following the length of the aorta. Keep your eyes on the screen, using the image as a guide. With the SMA at the left edge of the image, stop and document the aorta at this level. This image will include the area of the renal arteries. Most AAAs are infrarenal; thus, this is an important area at which an AP measurement needs to be obtained. Document the image with and without calipers. The right image demonstrates how to correctly measure the aorta from outer wall to outer wall.

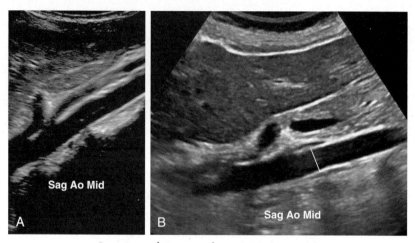

Suggested Annotation: **SAG AO MID**

4. Continue to slide the transducer to the distal portion of the aorta to the level of the bifurcation, usually seen just superior to the umbilicus. Measure the AP diameter at this level and document with and without calipers.

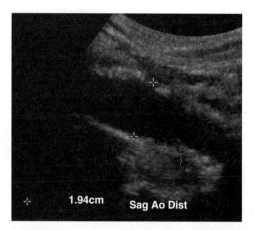

Suggested Annotation: **SAG AO DST**

SCANNING TIP: If the aorta is better seen in a transverse view, turn the transducer into a longitudinal view while maintaining pressure until the aorta is visualized in long axis.

5. With the transducer at the distal aorta, slightly rotate the transducer clockwise until the proximal part of the right common iliac artery (ILA) is seen. Measure the AP diameter at this level and document with and without calipers.

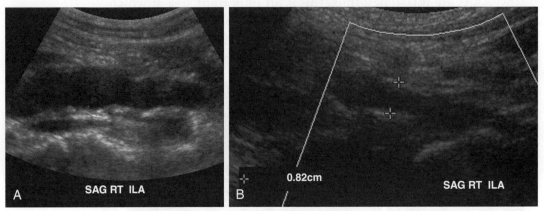

Suggested Annotation: **SAG RT ILA, IL A, or IA**

NOTE: *ILA* usually refers to the interlobar arteries in the kidney. As you can see, there are various ways to annotate the iliac artery: ILA, IL A, or IA. Use the annotation that your department prefers.

6. Slightly rotate the transducer counterclockwise until the proximal part of the left common iliac artery is seen. Measure the AP diameter at this level and document with and without calipers.

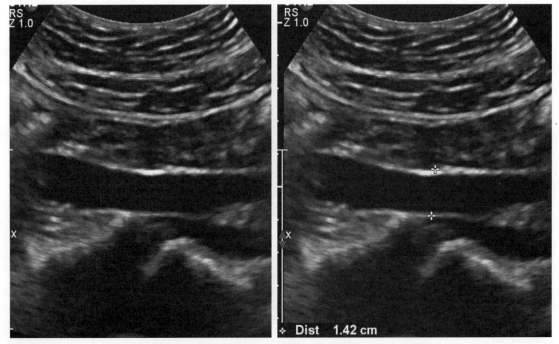

Suggested Annotation: **SAG LT ILA, IL A, or IA**

SCANNING TIP: If the iliac arteries are difficult to see, turn the transducer in a transverse position. Start scanning right above the umbilicus and slowly move the transducer toward the feet until you see two smaller circles. Keeping your eye on the iliac artery rotate the transducer until you have the long axis of the artery. Repeat for the other side.

Aorta • Transverse Images

1. Begin scanning with the transducer in a transverse scanning plane just inferior to the xiphoid process. Identify the aorta just to the left of midline and anterior to the spine as a round, anechoic structure. If having difficulty obtaining the transverse image, turn the transducer back into a longitudinal position and identify the proximal aorta. From that position, slowly rotate the transducer 90 degrees into the transverse plane. Measure the **width** of the aorta at this level and document with and without calipers. On some patients it may be difficult to see the very proximal portion of the aorta because of overlying bowel gas, especially if the patient has a liver that is higher in the abdomen and does not extend past the xiphoid or has a small left lobe.

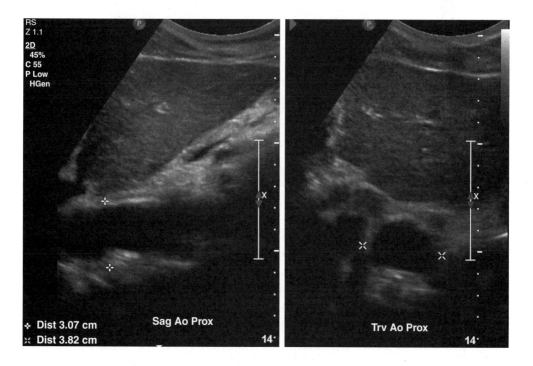

The sonographer used a dual screen to show the proximal aorta in both sagittal and transverse planes with measurements.
Suggested annotation: TRV or TRANS AO PROX

SCANNING TIP: Some sonographers may also measure the AP diameter again. This can be confusing because usually these two measurements are slightly different. In a transverse plane it is difficult for the sonologist to verify that the transducer has been tilted so that the aorta is perpendicular to the sound beam. TRV or TRANS are both common ways to annotate transverse. Use the one that is used in your department.

2. Slowly slide the transducer toward the feet while keeping your eyes on the screen and using the image as a guide. Slowly scan down to the level of the CA and SMA. Freeze and document the image with the SMA visible in the image. Unless unable to obtain a proximal measurement, there is no need to measure again; however, some departments may require this area also to be measured.

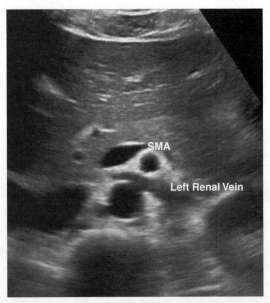

Suggested Annotation: **TRV or TRANS AO PROX**

3. Continue to slide the transducer toward the feet until you are at the level of the renal arteries. Use the left renal vein where it courses between the aorta and SMA as a landmark if the renal arteries are not clearly seen. Use color Doppler to assist with finding the renal arteries if needed. Measure the width of the aorta at this level and document with and without calipers. The left image is a color Doppler scan to locate the renal arteries. The right is the same image with color Doppler removed and the aorta measured. Because most aortic aneurysms are infrarenal, this is an important view.

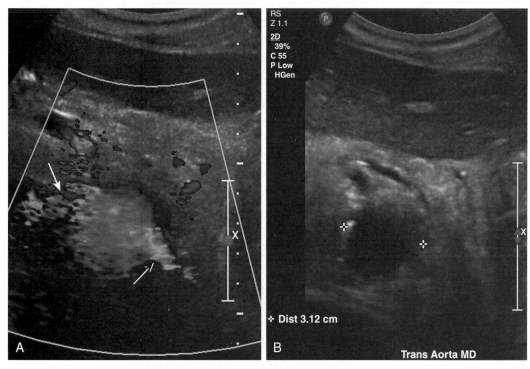

Suggested Annotation: **TRV or TRANS AO MID**

4. Continue to slide the transducer toward the feet until you are at the level of the bifurcation, just above the umbilicus. Here the view will change from one large round structure, the aorta, to two small round structures, the iliac arteries, one seen on each side of midline. Slowly scan toward the head until the aorta is seen again. Measure the width of the aorta at this level and document with and without calipers.

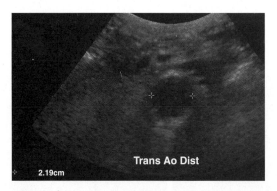

Suggested Annotation: **TRV or TRANS AO DIST**

SCANNING TIP: If the aorta is covered with bowel gas, slowly apply pressure while rocking the transducer from side to side until the aorta is seen or it causes the patient too much discomfort. If there is a AAA present, the aneurysm will be displacing the bowel from the inside and thus not require a lot of transducer pressure. If a AAA is present while applying a lot of pressure, slowly decrease pressure until the aorta disappears. Now lightly apply pressure until it is seen again and obtain the needed images.

5. Slide the transducer back down until the two small circles representing the iliac arteries are seen. They usually both can be seen in one image. Measure the width of the iliac arteries and document with and without calipers.

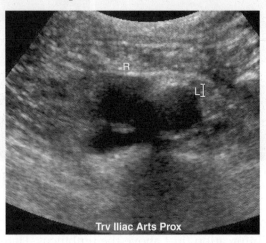

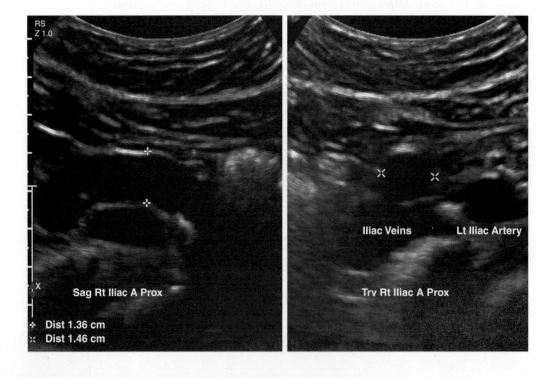

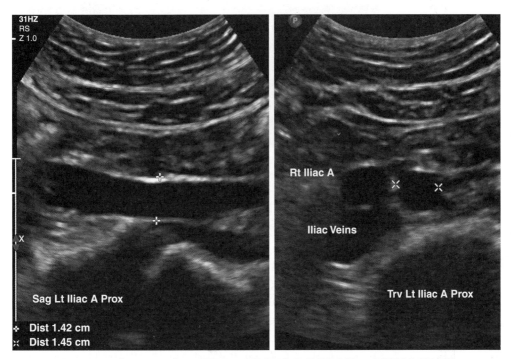

Suggested Annotation: **TRV or TRANS ILA PROX or TRV IA PROX**

Color Doppler

Color Doppler may be used to outline the lumen of the aorta when thrombus is present or to help with the diagnosis of a dissection to determine the true and false lumens. If a AAA or dissection is present, some departments may require a color Doppler image of the kidneys to evaluate flow and perfusion.

How to Measure the Aorta

Typically, measurements of the diameter of the aorta are documented at different levels to assess for any areas of dilatation. These images are from the proximal, mid, and distal aspects of the aorta. The entire length of the aorta should be seen on the longitudinal images.

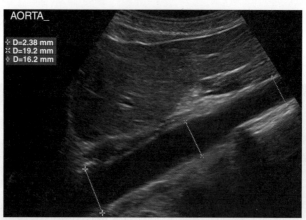

Fig. 4.4 Long axis of a normal aorta showing measurements at proximal, mid, and distal levels. Notice how the aorta tapers in size. Sag Ao Dist - Sagittal Aorta Distal.

A diameter of the abdominal aorta greater than 3 cm or the diameter of an iliac artery greater than 1.5 cm is diagnostic for the presence of an aneurysm.

In longitudinal images the aorta is measured in the AP dimension. If a AAA is present, the length of the aneurysm is also measured and the diameter just before the aneurysm. The largest AP diameter of the aneurysm is documented. When measuring the anteroposterior diameter of the aorta, it is important for the transducer to be perpendicular to the walls of the aorta and not the floor. The aorta can become tortuous with age or if there is a AAA present, so the sonographer must be careful in measuring to provide accurate measurements. Measuring perpendicular to the floor when the aorta is tortuous and not running parallel to the floor will cause the diameter to be falsely increased in size. Measure from the outer wall to the outer wall. Do not measure from the edge of the thrombus to the opposite wall or outer wall to inner wall (Fig. 4.5).

In transverse images the width of the aorta is measured. Some sonographers may measure the AP diameter again, but this can be confusing, especially for the interpreting physician, because the measurements may not match. Because the aorta is not parallel to the floor at all times, measuring the AP in a transverse view will cause overestimation of the size, even in a normal aorta. To accurately measure the AP dimension in a transverse view, start in a longitudinal plane and note how the aorta is angled. Now rotate and tilt the transducer to be truly perpendicular to the walls of the aorta. If an aneurysm is present, the widest diameter should also be measured and documented.

The size of the abdominal aorta is routinely measured and documented because most ultrasound studies of the aorta are performed to rule out an aneurysm. The biggest risk factor for rupture of an

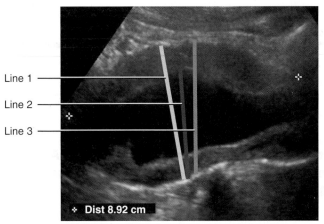

Fig. 4.5 Abdominal aortic aneurysm (AAA) with the length measured. Line 3 demonstrates incorrectly measuring the aneurysm because it is being measured perpendicular to the floor. Line 2 demonstrates incorrect measuring from the inner edge of the thrombus to the outer edge of the far wall. Line 1 demonstrates proper measuring perpendicular to the walls of the aorta. Line 3 will falsely increase the size of the aneurysm, and line 2 would falsely decrease the size of the aneurysm. If incorrect measuring technique is not corrected, it will be more difficult in follow-up to determine whether the AAA is increasing in size and by how much.

aneurysm is its size. Aneurysms over 5 cm have the greatest risk of rupturing. The risks are increased as the aneurysm increases in size. Note that the most common location for a AAA is infrarenal. If an aneurysm is present, it is required to have an image of one of the renal arteries. Using color Doppler will aid in finding the renal arteries. Treatment may be changed if an aneurysm is at the level of the renal arteries or higher.

The size and growth of a AAA plays an important part in planning treatment. Aneurysms do not shrink in size; therefore, if a follow-up measurement is smaller than the previous study, the measuring techniques of both studies need to be evaluated. If the prior study is unavailable, remeasure the AAA to verify your results or have another sonographer perform the measurements blinded to your measurements. Improper measurement will directly affect patient care. The physician is looking for an increase in the size of the aneurysm, because that will determine whether the patient needs surgery, an interventional procedure, or continued monitoring of growth with shorter intervals between ultrasound studies. Do not fudge your measurements to protect the previous sonographer. You will look incompetent if a third study is ordered and that sonographer measures correctly, or if the patient is sent for CT, where it is determined that you measured the aneurysm incorrectly. More importantly, this is very poor patient care and could jeopardize the patient's life.

Screening Protocol to Rule Out an Abdominal Aortic Aneurysm

Some patients are allowed to have a one-time screening of their aorta to rule out a AAA as part of The Welcome to Medicare package. A screening examination is just that; it is not a complete study and has a special CPT (billing) code.

American Institute of Ultrasound in Medicine, American College of Radiology, and Society of Radiologists in Ultrasound (AIUM/ACR/SRU) Protocol

The required images for the AIUM/ACR/SRU protocol are as follows:
1. Longitudinal images:
   a. Proximal near the celiac artery
   b. Mid below the SMA near the level of the renal arteries
   c. Distal above the iliac bifurcation
2. Transverse images:
   a. Proximal near the celiac artery
   b. Mid near the level of the renal arteries
   c. Distal above the iliac bifurcation
3. Measurements
   a. Anteroposterior measurement of the aorta is sufficient to determine whether an aortic aneurysm exists according to current criteria.
   b. If an aneurysm is present, its greatest dimension should be reported.
   c. If no aneurysm is identified, the largest diameter of the abdominal aorta should be reported.

This examination is gray-scale images only and requires just one AP measurement of the largest diameter. Color or spectral Doppler is not required. If an aneurysm is discovered, the maximal size and location of the aneurysm and its relationship to the renal arteries should be documented. If needed, the patient's physician might order a complete aortic ultrasound while the patient is still there.

Intersocietal Accreditation Commission (IAC) Vascular Testing's Protocol

The IAC Vascular Testing's protocol is as follows:
1. One transverse image (defined as perpendicular to the long axis of the aorta) with the single widest outer wall to outer wall diameter measurement.
2. Abnormal examination:
   a. One transverse image (defined as perpendicular to the long axis of the aorta) with the single widest outer wall to outer wall diameter measurement. This is usually an AP measurement, but sometimes the aneurysm may be in the width.

b. One transverse image (defined as perpendicular to the long axis of the aorta) with the single widest outer wall to outer wall diameter measurement of a nondilated segment for comparison.

This is a much simpler protocol than the AIUM version and is basically one image on a normal examination with a measurement.

Protocols from the major ultrasound and accreditation organizations can change, so it is important to review them annually and implement them by the given date.

Finding an Unexpected Abdominal Aortic Aneurysm

Many a sonographer has discovered a AAA on a patient incidentally while scanning the patient for reasons not related to the aorta, for example a renal or gallbladder ultrasound study. When this happens, measure the widest AP diameter. If the aneurysm is greater than 5 cm the findings need to be reported to the referring physician while the patient is still present. If you have not finished the examination, excuse yourself and notify the sonologist. Have the referring doctor's name and phone number to give to the sonologist. While the sonologist is notifying the referring physician, return to the patient and finish the ordered examination. Return to the sonologist and see if he or she has made contact with the patient's doctor. Aneurysms greater than 6 cm are at risk for rupture, so in these patients it is very important to make contact with the patient's doctor because of the very high risk for aortic rupture. Make sure that the patient waits until someone has talked to the doctor so instructions on what to tell the patient are given. The usual options are to send the patient home, to the physician's office, or to the emergency department. The physician might place an order for a stat, dedicated aorta ultrasound and/or CT of the aorta.

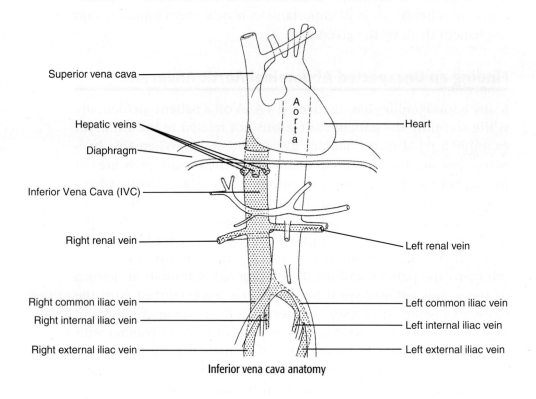

Inferior vena cava anatomy

CHAPTER 5

Inferior Vena Cava Scanning Protocol

M. Robert DeJong

Keywords

Common iliac veins	Proximal IVC
Distal IVC	Renal veins
Hepatic veins	Retroperitoneum
Iliac veins	Left adrenal vein
Inferior vena cava (IVC)	Gonadal veins
Mid IVC	

Objectives

At the end of this chapter, you will be able to:

- Define the key words.
- List the branches of the inferior vena cava (IVC).
- Distinguish the sonographic appearance between the IVC and the aorta.
- Describe the different transducer types and frequencies used for scanning the IVC.
- Discuss the images needed for a sonographic examination of the IVC.

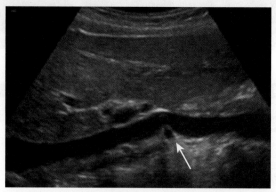

Fig. 5.1 Normal proximal to mid–inferior vena cava (IVC). The *small circle* (arrow) posterior to the IVC is the right renal artery.

Overview

Anatomy and Function

Ultrasound of the IVC is usually performed in both the radiology and vascular lab departments. The **inferior vena cava** (IVC) is the largest vein in the body and is formed by the union of the right and left **common iliac veins** around the level of L5. It returns unoxygenated blood from the lower extremities, the reproductive organs, the kidneys, and the adrenal glands to the heart. The gut and abdominal organs do not drain into the IVC but drain into the portal venous system. The portal system eventually drains into the IVC via the **hepatic veins**.

The IVC runs vertically in the body just to the right of the spine and the aorta in the **retroperitoneum**. It will run posteriorly to the right lobe of the liver to pass through the diaphragm at the level of T8 on its way to the right atrium of the heart (Fig. 5.1).

Because the IVC is on the right side of the body, the right **renal veins**, gonadal veins, and adrenal veins can easily drain directly into the IVC. Because the aorta is in the way, the left renal vein has to get past it to get to the IVC, usually coursing anterior to the aorta. The **left adrenal vein** and left gonadal vein will also need to get past the aorta, so they empty into the left renal vein.

The IVC does not contain valves, and forward flow to the heart is caused by the different pressures created by the diaphragm during the respiratory cycle.

Describing the order of the branches of the IVC from the **proximal IVC** to the **mid IVC** to the **distal IVC** can be confusing because their order starts where the two **iliac veins** join to form the IVC around the level of the umbilicus. Anatomically this is the proximal, close to origin, IVC. Therefore, the order of the branches begins above the umbilicus and goes superiorly toward the heart. The major veins that drain directly into the IVC in order are the following:

1. Common iliac veins
2. Lumbar veins
3. Right ovarian or testicular vein (generically called the gonadal vein)

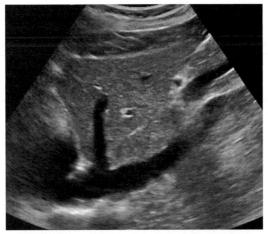

Fig. 5.2 The intrahepatic portion of the inferior vena cava as it empties into the right atrium.

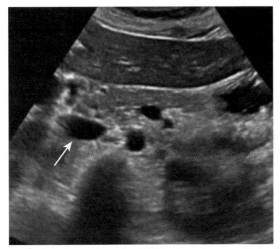

Fig. 5.3 Transverse image of an oval or elliptical inferior vena cava at the level of the kidneys.

4. Renal veins (the left adrenal and gonadal vein drain into the left renal vein)
5. Right adrenal vein
6. Hepatic veins
7. Inferior phrenic veins

The IVC consists of three layers, as follows: the intima layer, which is the most innermost, followed by the media and finally the outer layer called the adventitia.

Sonographic Appearance

The IVC in long axis appears as an anechoic tube with thin echogenic walls, is anterior and to the right of the spine, courses posterior to the right lobe of the liver, and has slight pulsations with respirations (Fig. 5.2). In transverse it can appear as a circle, oval, or elliptical structure (Fig. 5.3). During real-time evaluation, the IVC demonstrates variation in diameter with respiration. The IVC is seen to decrease in size with inspiration and return to normal or baseline diameter during expiration. The right renal artery will appear as a small circle posterior to the IVC (see Fig. 5.1). In short axis or transverse sections, the IVC is seen as an ovoid structure lateral to the aorta and anterior to the spine.

Ultrasound of the Inferior Vena Cava

Patient Prep

The patient should fast for at least 6 to 8 hours before the ultrasound examination to help reduce abdominal gas. If the patient has eaten, still attempt the examination.

Transducer

A curved linear array that has a 3–3.5 MHz frequency is used. Sector/vector array with a 3–3.5 MHz frequency may be necessary to get between the ribs if needed.

Breathing Technique

Normal respiration is preferred or have the patient stop breathing when you see the IVC. Remember that if the patient takes a deep breath and holds it, the IVC will decrease in size or collapse.

Patient Position

Start the patient in the supine position. If needed, turn the patient into a left posterior oblique and/or a left lateral decubitus position.

Required Images

Ultrasound of the IVC is not a common request. It is usually requested to look for a thrombus or an extension of a thrombus from an iliac or renal vein (Fig. 5.4) or to evaluate an IVC filter (Fig. 5.5). Currently

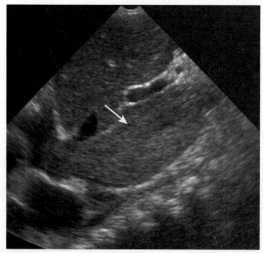

Fig. 5.4 Longitudinal image of an IVC filled with thrombus that extends into the right atrium *(arrow)*. The clot originated in the right renal vein and propagated into the IVC.

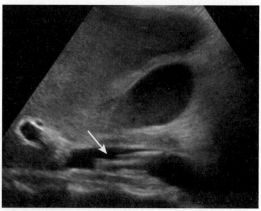

Fig. 5.5 Longitudinal of mid IVC demonstrating a normal IVC filter *(arrow)*.

there are no guidelines available. The main purpose of the examination will be to answer the clinical question.

Inferior Vena Cava • Longitudinal Images

The entire IVC should be documented from the sternum to the bifurcation. Typically, no measurements are required. Some laboratories will not use anatomic labeling but will label the part of the IVC closest to the heart as proximal and closest to the umbilicus as distal.

> **NOTE:** Be certain that you are imaging the IVC and not the aorta. The aorta will pulsate, whereas the IVC undulates with respiration. The IVC will go through the liver, whereas the aorta runs posteriorly. If still uncertain, have the patient sniff, which will momentarily cause the IVC to collapse. If still uncertain after the sniff, obtain a Doppler signal to verify the vessel.

1. Longitudinal image of the proximal or intrahepatic portion of the liver.

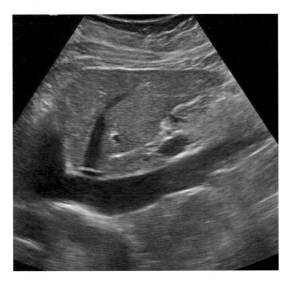

Suggested annotation: IVC SAG PROX or IVC LONG PROX

2. Longitudinal image of the mid IVC at the level of the renal veins.

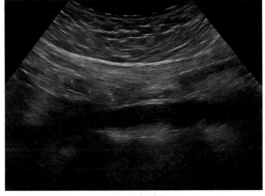

Courtesy Ted Whitten.

Suggested annotation: IVC SAG MID or IVC LONG MID

3. Longitudinal image of the distal IVC.

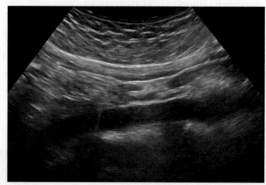

Courtesy Ted Whitten.

Suggested annotation: IVC SAG DIST or IVC LONG DIST

4. Longitudinal image of each common iliac vein. This can be accomplished by rotating the transducer and identifying the iliac vein where it empties into the IVC.

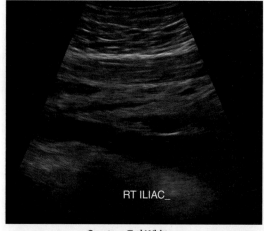

RT ILIAC_

Courtesy Ted Whitten.

Suggested annotation: SAG RT ILIAC VEIN or SAG LT ILIAC VEIN

Inferior Vena Cava • Transverse Images

1. Transverse image of the proximal IVC to include the hepatic veins.

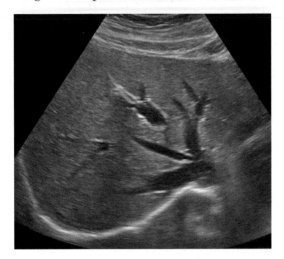

Suggested annotation: IVC TRV PROX

2. Transverse image of the mid IVC at the level of the renal veins.

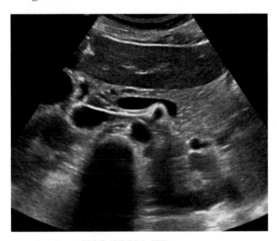

Suggested annotation: IVC TRV MID

3. Transverse image of the distal IVC right above the level where the iliac veins form the IVC.

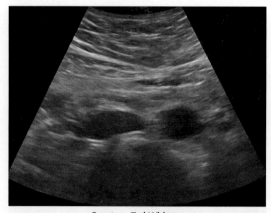

Courtesy Ted Whitten.

Suggested annotation: IVC SAG DIST

4. Transverse image of the common iliac veins either separately or together. It is usually very easy to obtain an image of both common iliac veins right before they join to form the IVC. The *arrow* indicates the transverse iliac vein.

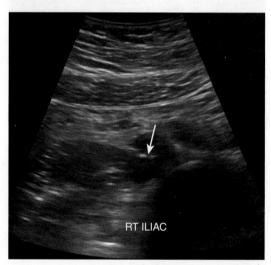

Courtesy Ted Whitten.

Suggested annotation: IVC TRV RT AND LT ILIAC VEINS or TRV RT ILIAC VEIN or TRV LT ILIAC VEIN.

Required Images When the Inferior Vena Cava Is Part of Another Study

If the IVC is included in any of the abdominal protocols, the required images may be different. In a right upper quadrant or liver sonogram, just the intrahepatic portion is imaged. In a complete abdominal sonogram, just the proximal and distal portions are documented unless there is pathology in the IVC. (Note: If a thrombus is found in the IVC, the sonographer should include images of the hepatic veins, renal veins, and both common iliac veins to show any extension of the thrombus.)

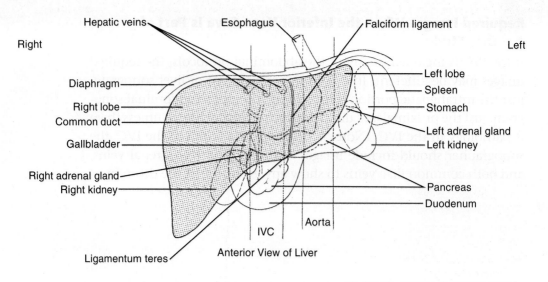

Anterior View of Liver

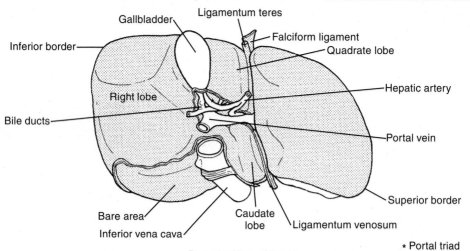

Posterior View of the Liver

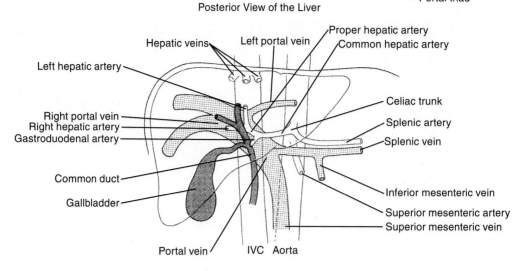

Liver Vasculature

CHAPTER 6

Liver Scanning Protocol

M. Robert DeJong

Keywords

Caudate lobe
Common hepatic artery
Elastography
Falciform ligament
Glisson's capsule
Hepatic ducts
Hepatic veins
Intraperitoneal
Left lobe
Left intersegmental fissure
Ligamentum teres

Ligamentum venosum
Main lobar fissure
Middle hepatic vein
Porta hepatis
Portal triad
Portal vein
Right hepatic artery
Right lobe

Objectives

At the end of this chapter, you will be able to:

- Define the keywords.
- Identify the three lobes of the liver
- Describe the transducer options for scanning the liver.
- List the various suggested breathing techniques for patients when scanning the liver.
- List the suggested patient positions when scanning the liver.
- Describe the patient prep for a liver study.
- Distinguish normal variants of the liver.
- Explain the order and locations to take representative images of the liver.

Overview

Ultrasound of the liver is usually performed in the radiology department. Dedicated ultrasound scans of the liver are usually performed to evaluate the liver for any pathologic conditions not associated with the biliary system. Reasons can include to look for a liver mass, metastatic disease, abscess, or hematoma or to clarify and help characterize an abnormal area seen on computed tomography (CT) or magnetic resonance imaging (MRI). When the biliary system does not need to be evaluated, the patient does not have to be on nothing per mouth (NPO) status, although it is preferred so that the biliary system can be evaluated. An examination to look for a hematoma after a biopsy, a procedure, or trauma is an urgent examination, especially if there is concern for active bleeding, and these patients do not need to follow a prep.

Anatomy

The liver is an intraperitoneal organ and is the largest organ in the abdomen, the second largest organ in the body, and the largest gland in the body with both exocrine and endocrine functions. (The skin is the largest organ of the body.) It measures approximately 13 to 15 cm in length and weighs between 1400 and 1600 grams. It is triangular in shape and occupies the right hypochondrium, most of the epigastric, and part of the left hypochondrium regions. The liver is covered by the peritoneum except for an area at the dome of the liver called the bare area where the liver is attached to the diaphragm. A layer of connective tissue called Glisson's capsule surrounds the liver and the portal triad, which consists of a branch of the hepatic artery, portal vein, and bile duct. Glisson's capsule is highly reflective on ultrasound (Fig. 6.1). The liver is composed primarily of hepatocytes along with bile duct and vascular cells. The liver is organized into functional units known as lobules. These lobules are hexagonal in shape and are composed of hepatocytes that are arranged into columns called cords and separated by the vascular sinusoids. The parenchyma of the liver is composed of these hepatocyte cords. The portal triads are located at the vertices of each hexagonal-shaped lobule with the lobule receiving blood from both the hepatic artery and the portal vein. This mixture of blood goes into the sinusoids and then drains into a central vein located in the middle of each lobule. These central veins unite to eventually drain into the larger hepatic veins, which drain into the inferior vena cava (IVC). The lobules are lined with the phagocytic Kupffer cells, which cleanse the blood of foreign materials and toxic substances (Fig. 6.2).

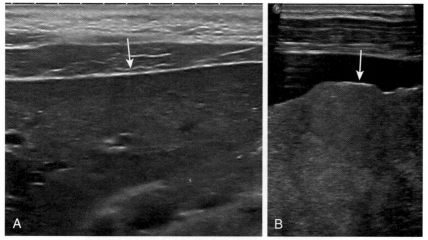

Fig. 6.1 Glisson's capsule. **A,** The *arrow* is pointing to Glisson's capsule in a normal patient using a high-frequency linear array transducer. **B,** The *arrow* is pointing to Glisson's capsule in a patient with ascites and cirrhosis of the liver using a high-frequency linear array transducer. Note how irregular the capsule is due to nodularity.

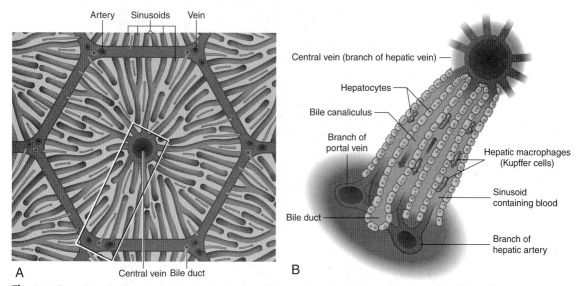

Fig. 6.2 Illustration of a hepatocyte showing the hexagonal shape, the portal triads, and the central draining vein. (From Grant A, Waugh A. Ross & Wilson *Anatomy and Physiology in Health and Illness,* 13th ed. Edinburgh, 2018, Elsevier.)

Liver Lobes and Segments

The right lobe is the largest lobe of the liver, occupying the right hypochondrium. It is bordered on the upper surface by the falciform ligament, which merges with the parietal peritoneum. Sonographically, the falciform ligament is not seen unless ascites is present, in which case it is seen as a thin hyperechoic structure between the liver and the abdominal wall (Fig. 6.3). The **falciform ligament** conducts the umbilical vein to the liver in the fetus. After birth, the umbilical vein

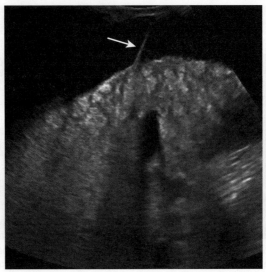

Fig. 6.3 The falciform ligament *(arrow)* is seen in this patient with a cirrhotic liver and ascites.

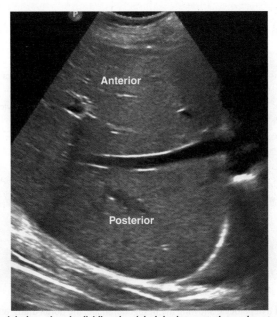

Fig. 6.4 The right hepatic vein dividing the right lobe into anterior and posterior segments.

atrophies and becomes the ligamentum teres. Inferior and posterior surfaces of the right lobe are marked by three fossae: the **porta hepatis**, gallbladder, and IVC. The right lobe is further divided into right anterior and posterior segments by the right hepatic vein (Fig. 6.4).

The **left lobe** lies in the epigastric and left hypochondriac regions. It is separated from the right lobe by the middle hepatic vein and the main lobar fissure. The left lobe is also further divided into two segments. The left hepatic vein and the ligamentum teres divide the left lobe into left lateral and medial segments. The ligamentum teres

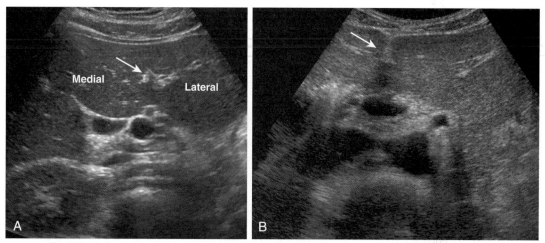

Fig. 6.5 The ligamentum teres *(arrows)* dividing the left lobe of the liver into medial and lateral segments.

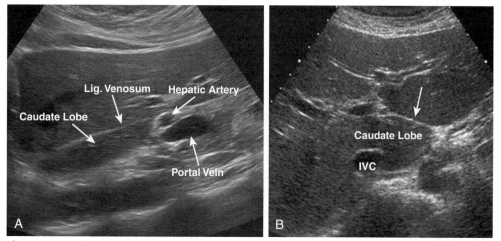

Fig. 6.6 A, Longitudinal image of the caudate lobe. **B,** Transverse image of the caudate lobe. The *arrow* is pointing to the ligamentum *(Lig.)* venosum. *IVC,* Inferior vena cava.

may be seen as an echogenic structure in the left lobe of the liver on a transverse image (Fig. 6.5). The ligamentum teres can have a variety of shapes, such as round or triangular, and may or may not cast an acoustic shadow.

The **caudate lobe** is the smallest lobe of the liver and is located on the posterior-superior surface of the right lobe. It is bounded by the main **portal vein** inferiorly, the IVC posteriorly, and the **ligamentum venosum**, which is the atrophied ductus venosus, anteriorly (Fig. 6.6).

Liver Segments

Using the Couinaud classification system of liver anatomy, the liver is divided into eight functional segments. These eight segments are formed horizontally by the portal vein where it bifurcates and

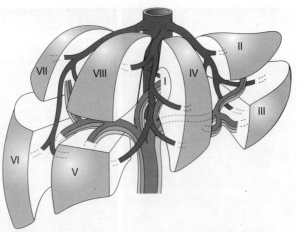

Fig. 6.7 A diagram of Couinaud's segmental liver anatomy. Segment 1 is seen behind segment 4. (From Ryan S, McNicholas M, Eustace S. *Anatomy for Diagnostic Imaging,* 3rd ed. Edinburgh, 2011, Saunders.)

becomes horizontal and vertically by the hepatic veins. Each segment has its own vascular inflow of both the portal vein and hepatic artery and the outflow of bile. The caudate lobe is segment one. The other segments are numbered counterclockwise starting with the left, with segments two through four and continuing onto the right lobe, which contains segments five through eight. The hepatic veins course intersegmentally, between the segments, whereas the portal veins course intrasegmentally through the segment, with the exception of the ascending portion of the left portal vein, which runs in the left intersegmental fissure. It is important to be familiar with Couinaud's classification because the CT or MRI report will discuss the mass in the appropriate segment. Therefore, when you read a CT or MRI report, you will understand where to look in the liver. For example, if the CT report reads that a mass is seen in segment 5, you will know that it is the right lobe, posterior segment. Just remembering which segments belong in each lobe is helpful.

The **main lobar fissure** divides the liver into right and left lobes. It is located in a line that joins the gallbladder and IVC and is seen as a bright echogenic line that runs from the right portal vein to the gallbladder fossa (Fig. 6.8). The middle hepatic vein courses within it superiorly. Sonographically, the middle hepatic vein separates the anterior segment of the right lobe from the medial segment of the left lobe (Fig. 6.9).

The right intersegmental fissure contains the right hepatic vein and is used to divide the right lobe into anterior and posterior segments (Fig. 6.10). The anterior segment contains segments 5 and 8, and the posterior segment contains segments 6 and 7.

The **left intersegmental fissure** contains the left hepatic vein, the **ligamentum teres,** and the ascending portion of the left portal vein. It divides the left lobe into medial and lateral segments. Sonographically,

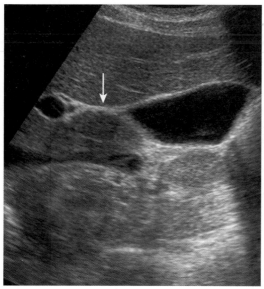

Fig. 6.8 The *arrow* is pointing to the main lobar fissure.

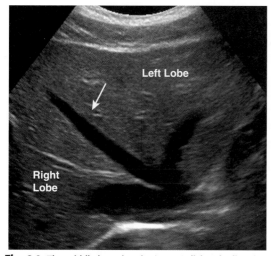

Fig. 6.9 The middle hepatic vein *(arrow)* diving the liver into right and left lobes.

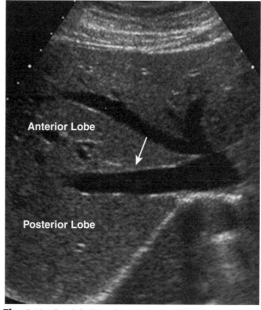

Fig. 6.10 The right hepatic vein *(arrow)* in a transverse image dividing the right lobe into anterior and posterior lobes.

the ligamentum teres (Fig. 6.11A) and left hepatic vein (see Fig. 6.11B) are used to divide the left lobe into medial and lateral segments. The medial segment contains segment 4, which also can be called the quadrate lobe, and the lateral segment contains segments 2 and 3.

Liver Ligaments and Fissures

Liver ligaments attach the liver to the diaphragm, stomach, anterior abdominal wall, and retroperitoneum. Liver ligaments are seen

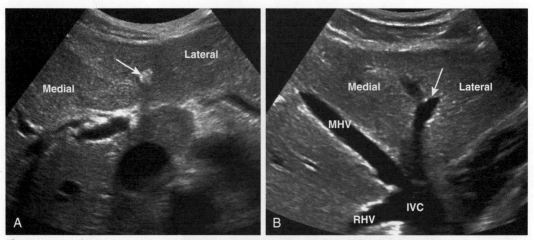

Fig. 6.11 A, The ligamentum teres *(arrow)* dividing the left lobe into medial and lateral lobes. Note how different this one looks than the examples in Fig. 6.5. The ligamentum teres can have different appearances. This one is casting an acoustic shadow. **B,** The left hepatic vein *(arrow)* dividing the left lobe into medial and lateral lobes. *IVC,* Inferior vena cava; *MHV,* middle hepatic vein; *RHV,* right hepatic vein.

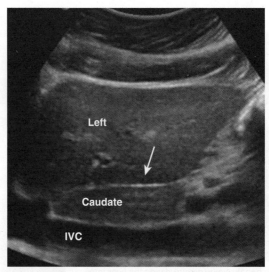

Fig. 6.12 The ligamentum venosum *(arrow)* separating the caudate lobe from the left lobe. *IVC,* Inferior vena cava.

with ultrasound because of their fat and collagen, which makes them hyperechoic relative to the hepatic parenchyma.

The falciform ligament is a sickle-shaped fold of peritoneum that extends from the umbilicus to the diaphragm, running along the liver's anterior surface and is continuous with the ligamentum teres, which is contained within its layers.

The ligamentum teres is the rounded termination of the falciform ligament and is the obliterated fetal umbilical vein. It can be used to divide the medial and lateral lobes of the left lobe of the liver.

The ligamentum venosum is the obliterated fetal ductus venosus and separates the caudate lobe from the left lobe (Fig. 6.12).

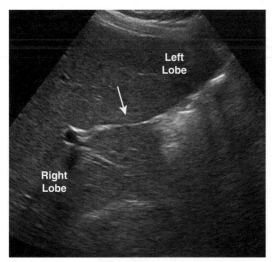

Fig. 6.13 The *arrow* is pointing to the main lobar fissure as it locates the gallbladder fossa in this patient with a cholecystectomy.

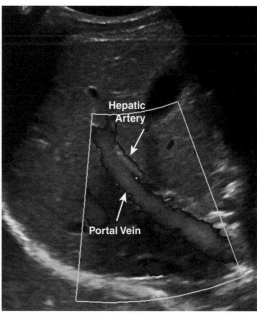

Fig. 6.14 A grayscale version of a color Doppler image of the portal vein and hepatic artery as they bring blood into the liver. The hepatic artery is a brighter shade of gray because of its faster velocity.

The main lobar fissure is used to seperate the right lobe from the left lobe and is also used to find the gallbladder fossa (Fig. 6.13).

Liver Circulation

The liver has a dual blood supply consisting of the hepatic artery and portal vein (Fig. 6.14). Both vessels enter the hilum of the liver at the porta hepatis. The hepatic artery supplies oxygenated blood, which contributes 20% to 30% of the total hepatic blood supply. The portal vein contributes 70% to 80% of the hepatic blood supply and carries nutrients, various contaminants, and partially oxygenated blood. The two vessels mix their blood in the sinusoids. The hepatocytes take oxygen and nutrients from this blood mixture and eliminate any waste products, stores vitamins and minerals, and produces bile. The blood then drains into the central hepatic vein of the lobule.

The portal vein is formed posterior to the neck of the pancreas by the confluence of the splenic and superior mesenteric veins. The portal circulation is separate from the systemic circulation, which is blood from the lower extremities and abdominal organs that drain directly into the IVC. The main portal vein divides into the right and left portal veins at the porta hepatis. The right portal vein divides into an anterior branch that lies centrally in the anterior segment and a posterior branch that lies centrally in the posterior segment of the right lobe. The left portal vein travels anteriorly, proximal to the falciform ligament and caudate lobe,

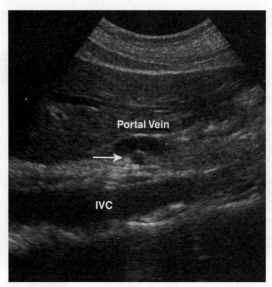

Fig. 6.15 The arrow is pointing to a replaced hepatic artery as it courses between the inferior vena cava and the portal vein. *IVC,* inferior vena cava.

giving off branches that travel in the medial and lateral segments of the left lobe. The caudate lobe receives portal branches from both the right and left portal veins.

The **common hepatic artery** is a branch of the celiac axis. The other branches of the celiac axis are the splenic artery and the left gastric artery. The common hepatic artery is seen coursing anteriorly to the portal vein and medially to the common bile duct. After it gives off the gastroduodenal artery (GDA) branch inferiorly, it becomes the proper hepatic artery. At the porta hepatis, the proper hepatic artery divides into the right and left hepatic arteries. The branches of the hepatic artery accompany the branches of the portal vein. Common anatomic variants include a replaced left hepatic artery, which originates from the left gastric artery; a replaced **right hepatic artery**, which originates from the superior mesenteric artery (SMA); and a replaced common hepatic artery, which originates from the SMA. In this variant the hepatic artery will be seen coursing between the portal vein and the IVC (Fig. 6.15). The caudate lobe receives branches from both the right and left hepatic arteries.

Blood perfuses through the sinusoids to enter the central hepatic vein and keeps joining larger veins until they become the main hepatic veins. There are generally three main hepatic veins that drain into the IVC: the right hepatic vein, the middle hepatic vein, and the left hepatic vein. The right hepatic vein drains the anterior and posterior segments of the right lobe. The middle hepatic vein drains the right anterior and the left medial lobes. The left hepatic vein drains the medial and lateral segments of the left lobe. The middle and left hepatic veins frequently join to form a common trunk. An inferior right hepatic vein, which drains the inferoposterior portion of the right lobe, is another variant and may be seen emptying directly into the IVC. The caudate lobe drains its blood directly into the IVC through the caudate veins.

Portal Triad Anatomy

The portal triad consists of a branch of the portal vein, a branch of the hepatic artery, and a bile duct contained within a layer of connective tissue, Glisson's capsule.

The **hepatic ducts** transport bile, a fluid made in the liver, to the bile ducts that convey the bile to the gallbladder for storage.

The porta hepatis is located medially in the hilum of the liver. It is here that the hepatic artery and portal vein enter the liver and the common bile duct exits the liver. The hepatic artery and common bile duct course anterior to the portal vein, with the common bile duct coursing laterally to the hepatic artery. Lymph nodes are also located in the region of the porta hepatis and may be the cause of biliary obstruction if they become enlarged.

Physiology

The liver has several major functions, which are classified as excretory, metabolic, storage, and synthetic. Specific functions include producing bile; metabolizing fats, carbohydrates, and proteins; storing carbohydrates, vitamins, and lipids; synthesizing major proteins; detoxifying ammonia and other harmful chemicals; assisting in the formation of lymph fluid; and regulating blood volume and body heat.

Sonographic Appearance

The time-gain compensation (TGC) and overall gain are adjusted so that the normal liver texture is a homogeneous gray scale, with echo brightness slightly greater than normal renal cortex and slightly less than normal pancreatic tissue (Fig. 6.16).

> **Echogenicity** of soft tissue in the abdomen is as follows: renal sinus > pancreas > spleen > liver > renal cortex.

Hepatic and portal vessels can be distinguished from each other by the following sonographic characteristics: (1) **hepatic veins** are larger in diameter at the diaphragm, whereas portal veins are larger near the porta hepatis; (2) hepatic vein branches point to the diaphragm, and portal vein branches point to the porta hepatis; (3) hepatic veins usually appear borderless, whereas portal vein walls are echogenic; and (4) Doppler signals from the hepatic veins display a multicomponent waveform, and portal veins exhibit continuous flow (Fig. 6.17). The large hepatic veins that are near the IVC will have what appears to be

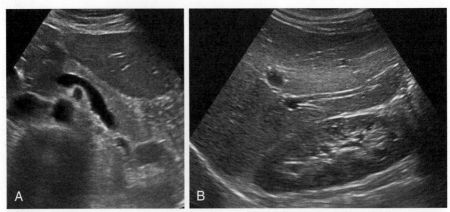

Fig. 6.16 Echogenicity comparisons to the liver. **A,** An image demonstrating that the pancreas is hyperechoic to the liver. **B,** An image demonstrating that the liver is hyperechoic to the kidney cortex. Note the band of bright echoes near the *top* of the image. This is caused by the focal zone being at that level. To correct, bring the focal zone down to the diaphragm or tap back the time-gain compensation in that area.

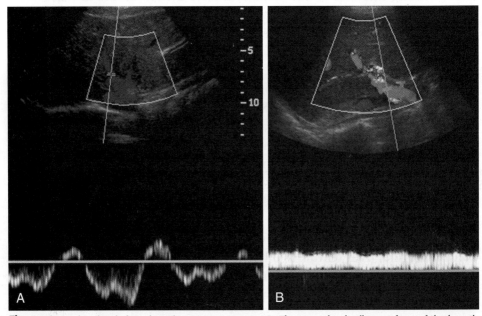

Fig. 6.17 Doppler signals from hepatic venous structures. **A,** The normal pulsatile waveform of the hepatic vein. **B,** The normal continuous waveform of the portal vein.

echogenic walls except that these are caused by specular reflections. If you insonate the hepatic vein at an angle, the echogenic wall will disappear (Fig. 6.18).

The most common anatomic variation of the liver is called a Reidel's lobe, which is an inferior extension of normal liver tissue of the right lobe. It is described as a downward finger-like or tongue-like projection of the anterior edge of the **right lobe** of the liver, which can extend in some patients to the level of the iliac crest. It is frequently seen in women and may present clinically as hepatomegaly or a liver or right kidney mass. Sonographically, a Reidel's lobe is seen in a sagittal plane and will display a normal echo and vascular

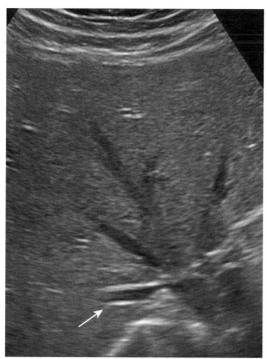

Fig. 6.18 An image demonstrating the echogenic walls of the portal veins and the nonechogenic walls of the hepatic veins. The right hepatic vein *(arrow)* appears to have echogenic walls as a result of a specular reflection.

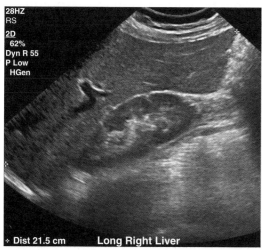

Fig. 6.19 A Reidel's lobe of the liver causing the liver to measure 21 cm.

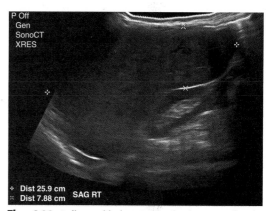

Fig. 6.20 A liver with hepatomegaly demonstrating increased length and anteroposterior measurements.

pattern as in the rest of the liver (Fig. 6.19). A Reidel's lobe should not be confused with hepatomegaly, because a Reidel's lobe will only increase the length of the liver, whereas in hepatomegaly both the length and anteroposterior (AP) measurements will be increased (Fig. 6.20).

Metastatic disease of the liver is more common than primary cancer. The liver is a very common site for metastatic disease (Fig. 6.21). There will be times when the sonographer will discover that there is

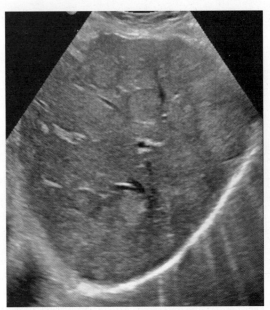

Fig. 6.21 A liver with metastatic disease demonstrating multiple hyperechoic masses. This patient had a colon primary.

metastatic disease in the liver that is unsuspected. After documenting the metastatic disease, the sonographer should try to locate the primary cancer. Images should be obtained of the pancreas to look for pancreatic cancer. The most common primary is in the gastrointestinal tract. Other sources that can be detected with ultrasound include the kidneys and ovaries. The sonographer should do a sweep following the large intestine to look for any large masses as well as evaluate the kidneys and the female pelvis. These should just be sweeps with no documentation unless something is found or if required by the department's protocol.

Some departments may obtain a portal vein signal to show that there is no portal hypertension (Fig. 6.22A). This may be required for patients with cirrhosis because they are at high risk to develop portal hypertension (see Fig. 6.22B).

Ultrasound of the Liver

Patient Prep

Patients should be fasting (NPO) for at least 6 to 8 hours before the examination to reduce bowel gas and allow maximum dilatation of the gallbladder. If the biliary system does not need to be evaluated, the patient is not required to be NPO, but it is preferred.

Transducer

A 3–3.5 MHZ curved linear array transducer is preferred. A lower-frequency transducer may be needed in obese patients or patients with a dense liver, whereas a higher-frequency transducer may be used in thin

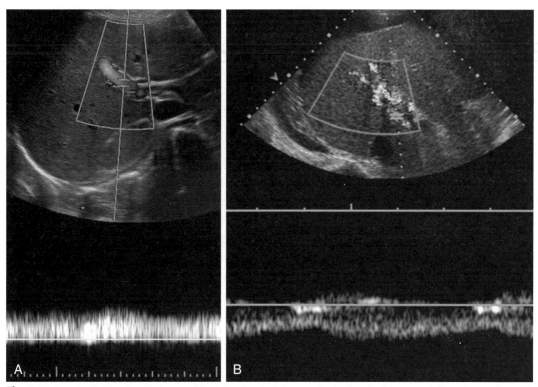

Fig. 6.22 Portal vein Doppler. **A,** A normal Doppler signal of the portal vein showing hepatopetal flow. **B,** A patient with reversed flow in the portal vein, hepatofugal flow; that is, it is leaving the liver. This patient has a cirrhotic liver, ascites, and portal hypertension.

patients, pediatric patients, or to evaluate structures in the near field. The TGC and overall gain are adjusted so that the normal liver texture is a homogeneous gray scale, with echo brightness slightly greater than normal renal cortex and slightly less than normal pancreatic tissue

The most common transducer used to scan the liver is a curved linear array transducer that has a 3.5 MHz frequency in its bandwidth. A sector/vector array transducer with lower frequencies in the 1–3 MHz range may be needed for a patient with a fatty liver, cirrhotic liver, or other reasons that prevent complete penetration of the liver. A linear array in the 5–7 MHz range can be used to evaluate the capsule of the liver. This is helpful in patients with cirrhosis to look at the nodularity of the liver.

Breathing Technique
Scanning is performed using a subcostal approach with the patient holding his or her breath in a deep inspiration or with intercostal views with the patient in suspended or quiet respiration.

Patient Position
Patients are scanned in a supine position to start and placed in other positions as needed, depending on the patient's body habitus. Scanning

is a combination of subcostal and intercostal views. Systematic, careful scans are performed in longitudinal and transverse planes, with oblique and decubitus views as needed to thoroughly evaluate liver size and shape, echogenicity, presence or absence of focal lesions, and presence of dilated biliary ducts. It is important to evaluate the liver completely when evaluating it for liver masses.

Technical Tips

To see the dome of the liver, place the transducer parallel to the ribs on the right side of the body just lateral to the xiphoid and angle it upward until the liver is no longer seen or appears small. The dome of the liver refers to the liver parenchyma close to the diaphragm. For some patients, to see the dome, the transducer may almost be flat on their abdomen, and you may have to gently push under and up below the ribs; just warn your patient. This can be performed with the patient in a deep inspiration or with quiet breathing. Then slowly raise the handle of the transducer off the skin, documenting the anatomy. A good view to see a lot of parenchyma is to place the transducer parallel to the ribs slightly medial to the right kidney and angle up under the ribs.

Liver Required Images

The following protocol is for evaluating only the liver. Reasons to scan just the liver include looking for a mass; clarifying an area seen on CT or MRI; evaluating polycystic disease, abscess, or hematoma; or following a mass after treatment. Some laboratories may routinely perform a right upper quadrant examination (see Chapter 11 for that protocol).

Liver • Longitudinal and Sagittal Images

1. Longitudinal image of the left lobe to include its inferior margin and the abdominal aorta.

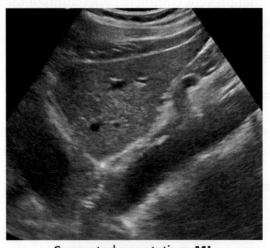

Suggested annotation: **ML**

2. Longitudinal images of the left lobe at 2 to 3 cm intervals until you are completely through the left lobe. The number of images taken will depend on the size of the left lobe.

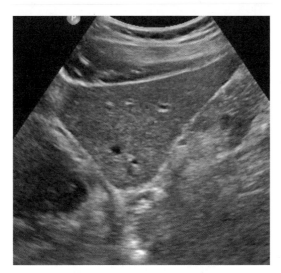

Suggested annotation: **SAG LT**

3. Longitudinal image of the **caudate lobe**.

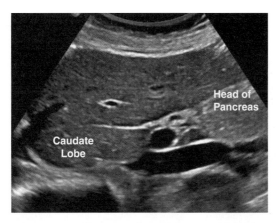

Suggested annotation: **SAG CAUDATE**

4. Longitudinal image of the right lobe just lateral to the IVC.

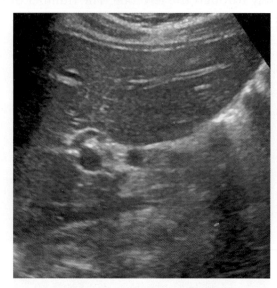

Suggested annotation: **SAG RT**

5. Longitudinal images of the right lobe at 2–3 cm intervals from the right hepatic vein to past the right kidney.

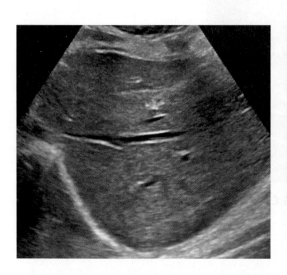 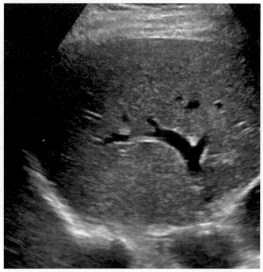

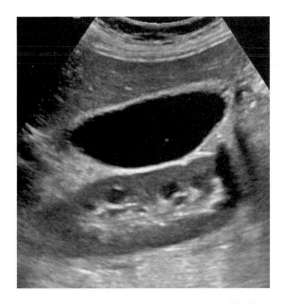

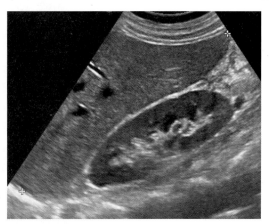

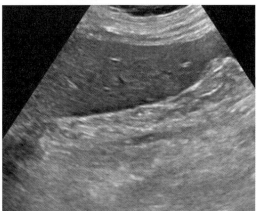

Suggested annotation: **SAG RT**

6. Longitudinal image of the right lobe to include the right kidney for parenchyma comparison.

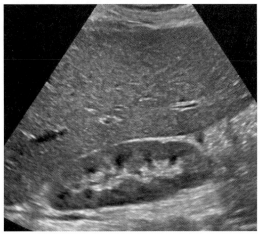

Suggested annotation: **LIVER / RT KIDNEY or RT KID**

7. Longitudinal image of the dome and the adjacent pleural space.

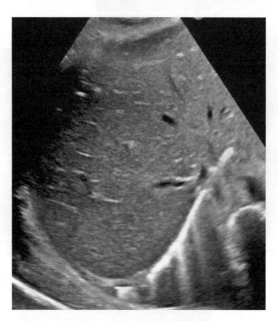

Suggested annotation: **SAG RT DOME**

8. Longitudinal image of the right lobe measuring the longest length. The liver is best measured at mid–right clavicle *(left image)*. If this is not possible, move the transducer to the edge of the body near the curve of the rib and angle medially until you determine the longest length *(right image)*. Note that the two measurements are very close.

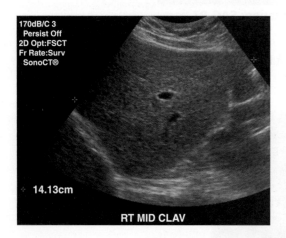

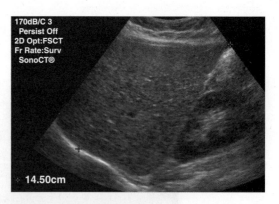

Suggested annotation: **LIVER or LIVER LENGTH**

Liver • Transverse Images

1. Transverse image of the left lobe to include its lateral margin.

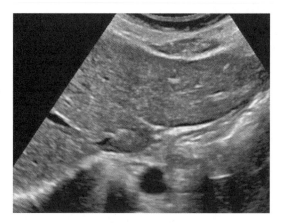

Suggested annotation: **TRV LT**

2. Transverse images of the left lobe to include the ligamentum teres (left image) or ascending branch of the left portal vein (right image).

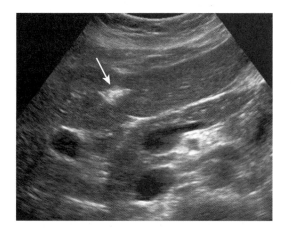 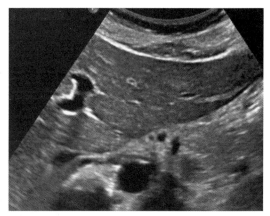

Suggested annotation: **TRV LT**

3. Transverse image to include the hepatic veins.

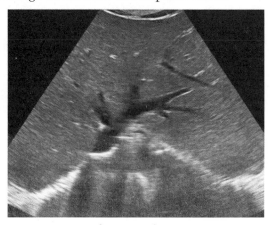

Suggested annotation: **TRV HVS**

4. Transverse images of the right lobe just past the hepatic veins. Right image demonstrates a mirror image artifact across the diaphragm.

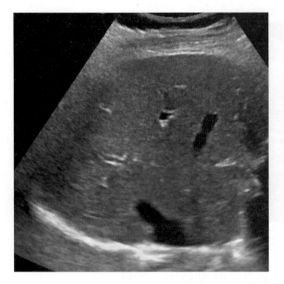
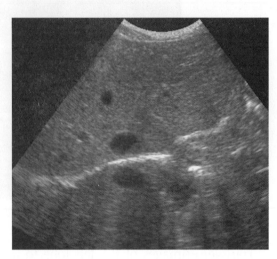

Suggested annotation: **TRV RT**

5. Transverse image of the right lobe to include (A) the main portal vein, (B) at the level of the right portal vein, and (C) color Doppler image of the main portal vein showing flow direction. Notice the 2 small liver cysts in A.

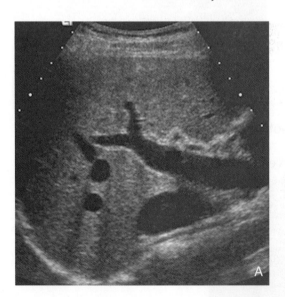
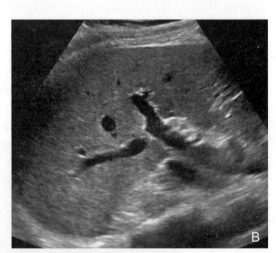

Suggested annotation: **TRV RT**

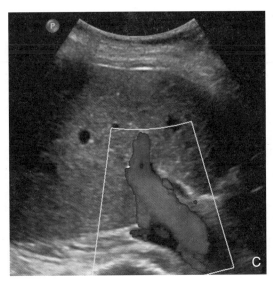

Suggested annotation: **TRV RT MPV**

6. Transverse images of the right lobe at 2–3 cm intervals until the upper pole of the right kidney is seen.

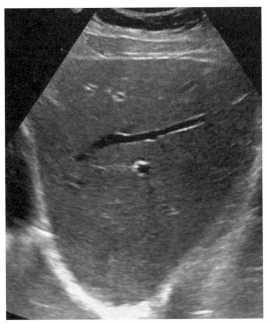
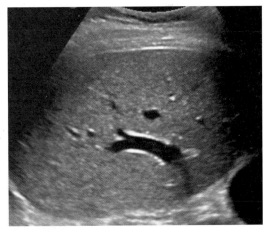

Suggested annotation: **TRV RT**

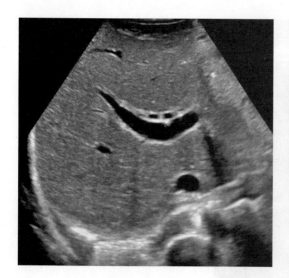

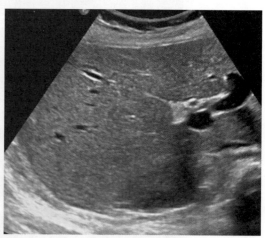

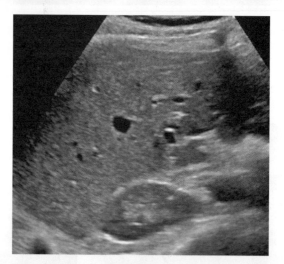

Suggested annotation: **TRV RT**

7. Transverse image of the right lobe to include mid–right kidney.

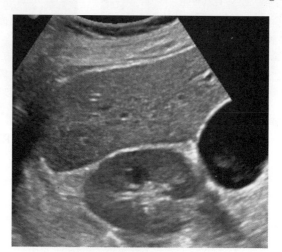

Suggested annotation: **TRV RT**

8. Transverse image of the right lateral lobe at 2-3 cm interval until out of liver.

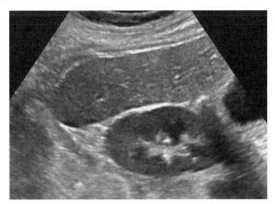

Suggested annotation: **TRV RT**

9. Transverse image of the right lateral lobe to include the gallbladder if visualized.

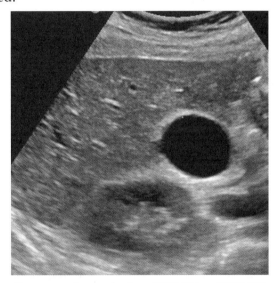

Suggested annotation: **TRV RT or TRV GB**

10. Transverse image of the right lateral lobe to include the dome and the adjacent pleural space.

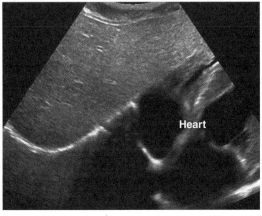

Suggested annotation: **TRV DOME**

Elastography of the Liver

Chronic liver disease can lead to liver fibrosis and liver failure. Chronic liver disease can be the result of viral hepatitis B, alcoholic liver disease, chronic hepatitis C, and, recently, nonalcoholic fatty liver disease (NAFLD) and Non-Alcoholic SteatoHepatits (NASH). The liver is the only organ that can repair damaged cells by making new cells. In chronic conditions, as the liver tries to continually repair itself, the attempts at repair result in fibrotic scar tissue. As the fibrosis progresses, there is increasing loss of liver function and the liver can become cirrhotic, resulting in portal hypertension and an increased risk for hepatocellular carcinoma (HCC). The staging of liver fibrosis is important to the clinician to evaluate for the progression or regression of the fibrosis if being treated. Until the development of **elastography**, a liver biopsy was required to stage the degree of fibrosis, which is an invasive procedure and has potential complications that can be severe. Although a liver biopsy is the gold standard, the biopsy sample is prone to sampling errors and there is also interobserver variability with interpretation.

Liver elastography is performed to stage the degree of fibrosis in patients with chronic liver disease. Another indication for liver elastography is to follow patients with fibrosis to observe their response to therapy treatments that can actually decrease fibrosis

Elastography uses a standard ultrasound transducer and unit that has elastography software installed. Shear wave elastography (SWE) is a type of elastography that uses a technique called acoustic radiation force impulse (ARFI; pronounced *arf e*). In physics, radiation is the transmission of energy in the form of waves through a medium and is not necessarily ionizing radiation. With SWE, a push pulse is sent into the tissue that compresses the tissue and produces sound waves that are perpendicular to the push pulse called shear waves. Next, detection pulses are sent out to measure the speed of the shear waves. The velocity of the shear wave is determined by the stiffness of the liver tissue. The stiffer the tissue, the faster the velocity of the shear wave. The result is displayed in meters per second (m/s) or megapascals (MPa). Meters per second is used more commonly in the United States because the U.S. Food and Drug Administration initially only allowed meters per second to be measured and reported. Most of the rest of the world uses megapascals. Elastography charts will display both values. Currently there is not a single chart that can be used across manufacturers, so each manufacturer has its own chart to determine the amount of fibrosis based on the speed of the shear waves. This means that it is important to use the exact make and model ultrasound machine for follow-up examinations. The ARFI pulse is quickly attenuated and is good only up to 6 to 8 cm.

Performing a Liver Elastography Examination

At the time of publication, the following information is based on the protocol to perform a liver elastography examination that is based on the Society of Radiologists in Ultrasound (SRU) Liver Elastography Consensus Panel from 2014. This article can be found for free online at https://pubs.rsna.org/doi/full/10.1148/radiol.2015150619.

Patient Prep

The patient should be NPO for 4 to 6 hours. A fibrotic liver in a non-fasting state will have falsely increased elastography values because eating food increases the blood flow to the liver, thus increasing its stiffness and overestimating the disease.

Patient Position

The patient should be in a supine position or in a slight 30-degree left posterior oblique position with the right arm raised over the head to open the rib space because an intercostal approach is used.

Transducer Position

The transducer is placed in an intercostal position, and a location is determined that is free of reverberations. Region of interest (ROI) placement: The box is placed at the liver 2 cm below Glisson's capsule, and not 2 cm from the skin surface, perpendicular to the capsule. The ROI should not include blood vessels, rib shadow, the diaphragm, the liver/kidney interface, the liver capsule, or any ligaments because this will cause inaccurate measurements. The ROI box is placed at segment 7 or 8 of the right lobe (Figs. 6.23 and 6.24).

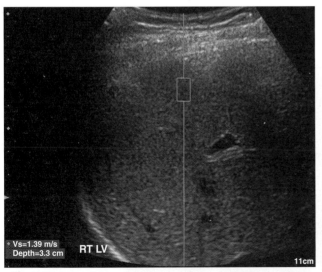

Fig. 6.23 Image demonstrating proper region of interest placement.

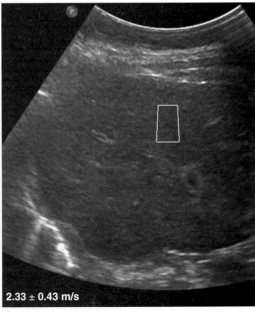

Fig. 6.24 Image demonstrating proper region of interest placement with a different unit. This patient has moderate to severe fibrosis.

Breathing Technique

The measurement is obtained on a neutral breath hold because deep inspiration or expiration will affect the measurement. Before each measurement, the patient should be asked to pause breathing in a neutral, relaxed state. They should not take a deep breath in or completely exhale but rather just stop breathing. The breath hold is only 1 to 2 seconds.

Measurements

Currently it is recommended to take 10 measurements from the same location, that is, not to move the ROI to different places in the liver. This may seem unusual, but research has shown that this method samples more liver tissue than a biopsy and yields a more accurate measurement. Because of the energy needed to create the push pulse, the transducer will need to cool down between samples. In Fig. 6.25, the *arrow* is pointing to the message that the unit is cooling. The unit will not allow any further measurements to be taken until it displays a message that the unit is ready. This takes only a few seconds. Errors in measurement should be deleted before finalizing the 10 measurements. For example, the patient took a deep breath or the machine gave an error value. The median value is used, not the mean or average value. The interquartile ratio (IQR) is also determined and also should be reported. The IQR looks at the variability in a dataset, based on dividing a dataset into quartiles. An IQR value of less than 0.30 suggests that the measurements are acceptable. If the IQR is greater than 0.30, the numbers should be evaluated and outliers deleted. New measurements should be obtained using the same area until there is a total of 10 good measurements. It may be that the numbers appear "all over

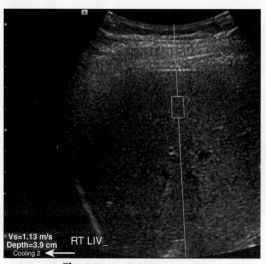

Fig. 6.25 Cool-down message.

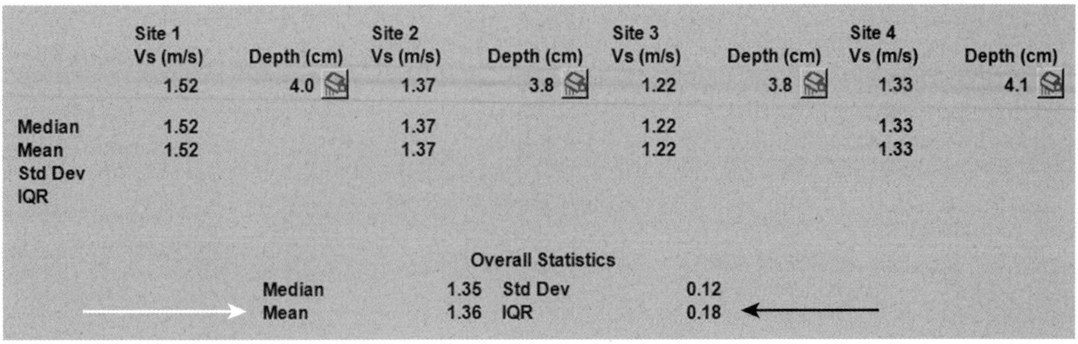

	Site 1 Vs (m/s)	Depth (cm)	Site 2 Vs (m/s)	Depth (cm)	Site 3 Vs (m/s)	Depth (cm)	Site 4 Vs (m/s)	Depth (cm)
	1.52	4.0	1.37	3.8	1.22	3.8	1.33	4.1
Median	1.52		1.37		1.22		1.33	
Mean	1.52		1.37		1.22		1.33	
Std Dev								
IQR								

Overall Statistics

Median	1.35	Std Dev	0.12
Mean	1.36	IQR	0.18

Fig. 6.26 An example of the results page from an elastography study. The *white arrow* is pointing to the mean value and the *black arrow* to the IQR.

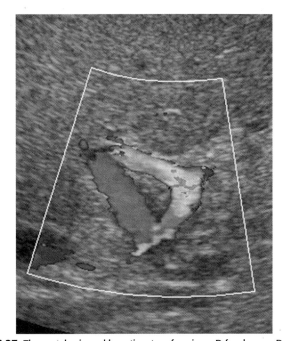

Fig. 6.27 The portal vein and hepatic artery forming a D for done or Doppler!

the place," which is why the IQR is important. The ultrasound unit should automatically determine the IQR (Fig. 6.26).

An elastography examination of the liver is usually a dedicated examination for just the elastography and usually takes 10 to 15 minutes to complete (Fig. 6.27). There is a special CPT code just for liver elastography.

NOTE: Just before publication a new elastography chart is being suggested, as well as new techniques, that will be for all makes of ultrasound equipment. The sonographer is advised to keep current as this exciting new technique continues to evolve. The RSNA web site is a good place to see updates at www.rsna.org
For the latest information go to https://pubs.rsna.org/doi/10.1148/radiol.2020192437.

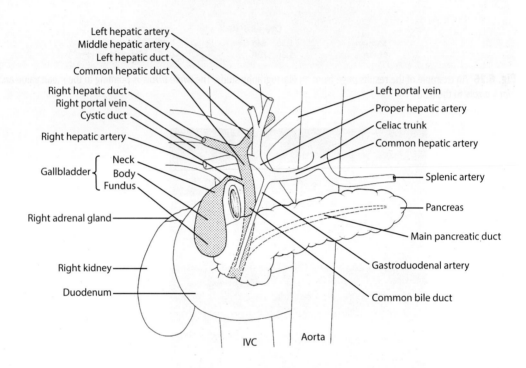

Left hepatic artery
Middle hepatic artery
Left hepatic duct
Common hepatic duct

Right hepatic duct
Right portal vein
Cystic duct

Right hepatic artery

Gallbladder { Neck
Body
Fundus

Right adrenal gland

Right kidney

Duodenum

Left portal vein
Proper hepatic artery
Celiac trunk
Common hepatic artery

Splenic artery

Pancreas

Main pancreatic duct

Gastroduodenal artery

Common bile duct

IVC   Aorta

CHAPTER 7

Gallbladder and Biliary Tract Scanning Protocol

M. Robert DeJong

Keywords

Ampulla of Vater	Left hepatic duct
Common bile duct (CBD)	Main lobar fissure (MLF)
Common duct	Main pancreatic duct
Common hepatic duct (CHD)	Porta hepatis
Cystic duct	Portal triad
Hepatic artery	Right hepatic duct

Objectives

At the end of this chapter, you will be able to:

- Define the keywords.
- List the patient positions needed when scanning the gallbladder.
- Describe the patient preparation for a gallbladder and biliary tract study.
- Discuss some of the major gallbladder and biliary tract normal variants.
- Explain the order and locations to take representative images of the gallbladder and biliary tract.

Overview

A sonogram of the gallbladder and biliary system is usually performed in the radiology department and is usually part of a right upper quadrant (RUQ) sonogram that includes the liver, gallbladder, pancreas, and right kidney. A dedicated ultrasound of the gallbladder and biliary system would be ordered to evaluate for pathologic conditions of the biliary system when there is no concern for a liver or pancreas pathologic condition. However, because the biliary system lies within the liver, images of the liver will be included as well as images of the pancreas when evaluating the distal **common bile duct** (CBD).

Anatomy

The biliary system consists of the gallbladder and biliary tree or ducts. The biliary system works closely with the liver and pancreas. The gallbladder stores and concentrates bile, and the biliary ducts drain the bile from the liver.

The gallbladder is located on the posterior and inferior portion of the liver and is closely related to the **main lobar fissure** (MLF) (Fig. 7.1). It is a pear-shaped sac variable in shape and volume and is normally located at the junction of segments 4 and 5 of the liver. The gallbladder wall consists of an inner epithelial mucosa, a muscular layer, and an outer serosal layer. The gallbladder is divided into three parts; the fundus, the body, and the neck (Fig. 7.2). The fundus of the gallbladder is the wide end that projects from the inferior edge of the liver. The body is the main part of the gallbladder lying in contact with the visceral surface of the liver. The narrow area of the gallbladder is called the neck; it tapers to become the **cystic duct** (Fig. 7.3). The cystic duct connects the gallbladder to the **common hepatic duct** (CHD). It is 2 to 4 cm in length and contains a series of mucosal folds that are continuous from the folds in the neck of the gallbladder, called the valves of Heister, which are not true valves because they do not control flow or have leaflets. Their purpose is to prevent the cystic duct from collapsing,

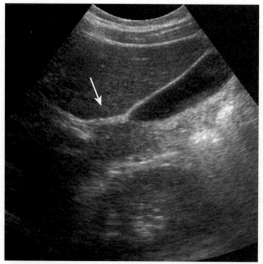

Fig. 7.1 The *arrow* is pointing to the main lobar fissure.

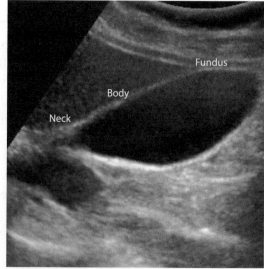

Fig. 7.2 An image demonstrating the neck, body, and fundus of a normal gallbladder.

allowing bile to pass easily into and out of the gallbladder. A fully distended gallbladder is usually 7 to 10 cm long and 3 to 4 cm in a transverse dimension (Fig. 7.4), with a wall thickness of less than 3 mm (Fig. 7.5).

Gallbladder Variations in Appearance

There are normal variants of the gallbladder that the sonographer needs to recognize. They include an intrahepatic gallbladder, a junctional fold (Fig. 7.6), and a Phrygian cap, which is a type of junctional fold. The Phrygian cap (Fig. 7.7) is a common variant and occurs when the fundus of the gallbladder folds on itself. Junctional folds may mimic septations, which are rare in the gallbladder. In some patients, a small outpouching of the wall of the gallbladder, called Hartmann's pouch, is seen at the junction of the neck of the gallbladder and the cystic duct. This is a place where stones may become stuck (Fig. 7.8).

Physiology

The gallbladder and biliary tract are considered accessories to the digestive system because they store and transport bile to the second portion of the duodenum to aid in the digestion process.

Bile is secreted by the hepatocytes into the smallest ductal branches, called bile canaliculi. These drain into the interlobar bile ducts, which join to former larger bile ducts until they become the right and left hepatic ducts. The right and left hepatic ducts join in the **porta hepatis**

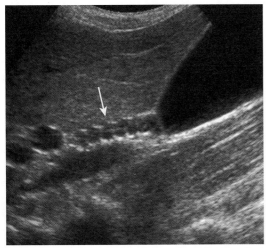

Fig. 7.3 The *arrow* is pointing to the valves of Heister in the cystic duct.

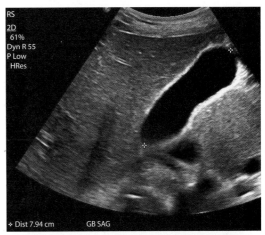

Fig. 7.4 Measurement of a normal gallbladder length.

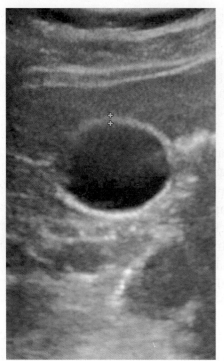

Fig. 7.5 Transverse image of the gallbladder showing proper technique for measuring the wall of the gallbladder.

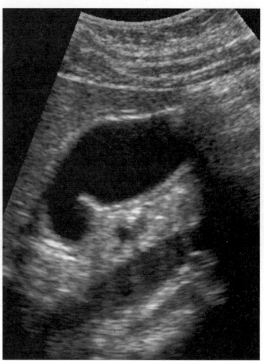

Fig. 7.6 An image of a junctional fold.

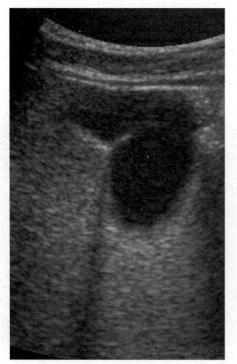

Fig. 7.7 An image of a Phrygian cap.

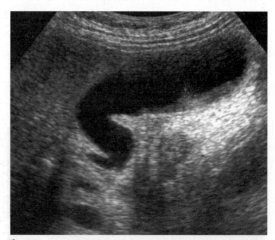

Fig. 7.8 An image of a gallbladder with a Hartmann's pouch.

to become the CHD. The CHD (Fig. 7.9) becomes the CBD where the cystic duct empties into the CHD. The CBD (Fig. 7.10) is approximately 8 to 10 cm in length and travels to join the **main pancreatic duct**, the duct of Wirsung, at the **ampulla of Vater**, which is surrounded by the sphincter of Oddi (Fig. 7.11). The sphincter of Oddi is a smooth muscle sphincter that controls the flow of bile and pancreatic juices into the duodenum and prevents reflux of duodenal content into the ducts. When the sphincter of Oddi is closed, bile is forced back into the gall-bladder, where it is stored and concentrated until needed. When food enters the duodenum, cholecystokinin is released, which causes the sphincter to relax, the gallbladder to contract, and bile and pancreatic enzymes to enter the duodenum. This is why the patient needs to fast, because the diameter of the CBD will be affected with the sphincter of Oddi relaxing, allowing bile to flow out of the duct and into the duo-denum. This will cause the duct to decrease in size, sometimes making it difficult to visualize. Normal **common duct** size is variable according to the amount of bile it contains and the patient's age. The common duct is known to enlarge with age as the duct loses tone. CHD is con-sidered normal up to 4 mm and the CBD up to 6 mm in diameter (Fig. 7.12). After a cholecystectomy, the common duct assumes bile storage function and is considered normal in size up to 10 mm. The cystic duct, CHD, and CBD are considered extrahepatic ducts because they are not enclosed by liver. Intrahepatic ducts are those ducts covered by liver tissue and include the right and left hepatic ducts and the smaller bile ducts in the liver.

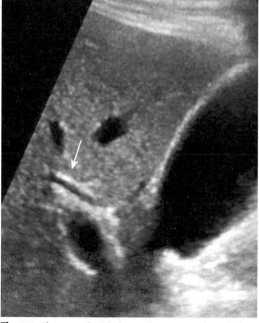

Fig. 7.9 The *arrow* is pointing to the common hepatic duct.

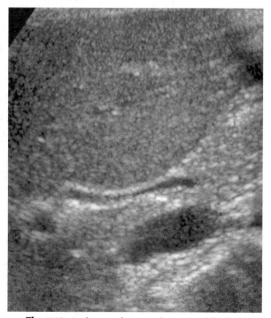

Fig. 7.10 An image of a normal common bile duct.

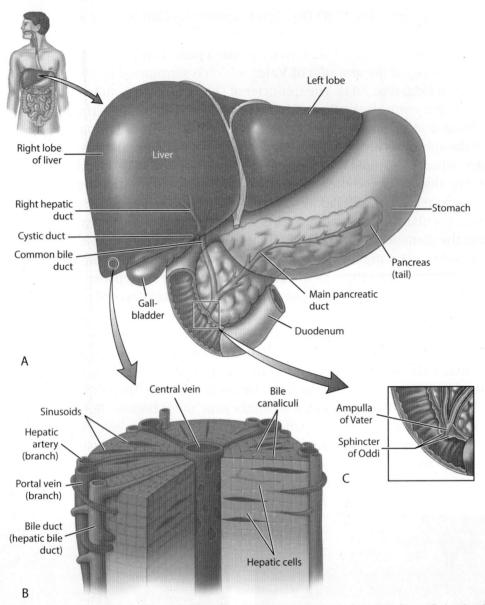

Fig. 7.11 A, Illustration of the liver, pancreas, duodenum, and biliary and pancreatic ducts. **B,** A liver cell showing the bile canaliculi and the portal triad. **C,** The second part of the duodenum illustrating the ampulla of Vater and the sphincter of Oddi. (From Lewis SL, Dirksen SR, Heitkemper MM, Bucher L, Harding MM. *Medical-Surgical Nursing: Assessment and Management of Clinical Problems,* 10th ed. St. Louis, 2017, Elsevier.)

Sonographic Appearance

An abdominal general preset should be used. The time-gain compensation and gain should be adjusted so the liver texture is a homogeneous gray scale and the normal gallbladder appears echo free.

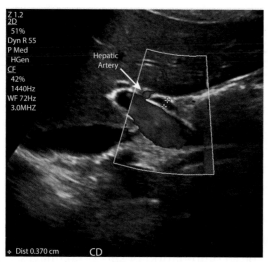

Fig. 7.12 A normal common duct being measured at the porta hepatis anterior to the portal vein.

Ultrasound of the Gallbladder and Biliary Tree

Patient Prep

To evaluate the biliary system, the patient needs to be on nothing by mouth (NPO) status for a minimum of 4 hours but preferably for 6 to 8 hours. This will allow the gallbladder to distend so it can be evaluated. Measurements of the wall of the gallbladder and CBD size are based on preprandial measurements. Stimulating the biliary system will cause the gallbladder to contract and the walls to thicken. As the sphincter of Oddi relaxes to allow the bile to flow into the duodenum, the CBD will decrease in size because the bile is not "dammed." This is why patients with a cholecystectomy should be NPO for at least 4 hours for proper measurements. Postprandial measurements are not accurate and may result in false-negative results. Having the patient properly prepped can be a challenge with some physicians, and explaining why the patient needs to be NPO may be required.

To evaluate for biliary atresia in newborn patients, it is very important that the child has been NPO for a minimum of 4 hours. Remember that if the child has been given something that would stimulate the gallbladder and biliary system, it may be difficult to locate the gallbladder or CBD. This will lead to a false-positive diagnosis, and the child might have to undergo another test unnecessarily and might require sedation. These infants will be upset and crying because of hunger, so it is important to quickly scan the liver for signs of dilated ducts, a gallbladder, and a CBD. That is the most important aspect of the examination. After obtaining those images, allow the child to drink and calm down before finishing the rest of the protocol. With the mother's consent I have even completed the examination while the child is breastfeeding.

Transducer

The most common transducer to use is a 2–5 MHZ curved linear array (Fig. 7.13). A sector/vector transducer may be needed to allow inter-costal access as needed. For pediatric patients, especially a newborn, a high-frequency sector array may be needed to get between the ribs. Once the initial scan is completed, the sonographer can switch to a higher-frequency transducer to improve resolution of the gallbladder and gallbladder wall and to bring out acoustic shadowing if stones are present (Fig. 7.14). For this part of the examination we are not worried about penetration because those images have already been documented.

Breathing Technique

Images obtained may be a combination of subcostal images, with the patient in deep inspiration or quiet breathing when using an inter-costal approach. Because the liver and gallbladder will fall forward in decubitus views, these are usually subcostal with the patient in quiet breathing or deep inspiration.

Patient Position

Longitudinal and transverse scans are required in both supine and decubitus positions. The examination begins with the patient supine and then turned into a left lateral decubitus (LLD) position, also called right side up (RSU). Decubitus views ensure that struc-tures inside the gallbladder are mobile, for example, a stone vs a polyp (Fig. 7.15), or that stones in the neck of the gallbladder are mobile (Fig. 7.16). With the decubitus position, sometimes stones can appear that were not seen with the patient supine or the stone

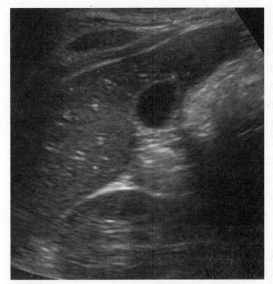

Fig. 7.13 The gallbladder and liver being scanned with a 3.5 MHz frequency.

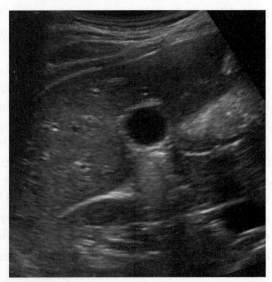

Fig. 7.14 The same image as Fig. 7.13 scanned with a 5 MHz frequency. Note the improvement of the resolution of the gall-bladder wall.

is brought into a better interaction with the sound beam, improving the acoustic shadow. To resolve any questions, the patient can sit up or the head of the stretcher can be raised to evaluate the gallbladder in the upright position. At times it can be challenging to distinguish between gallstones and shadowing from gas. Another position to try

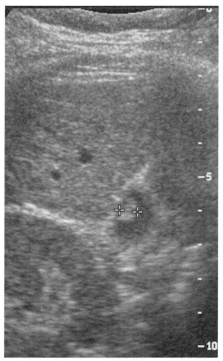

Fig. 7.15 A decubitus view demonstrating that the polyp is attached to the wall.

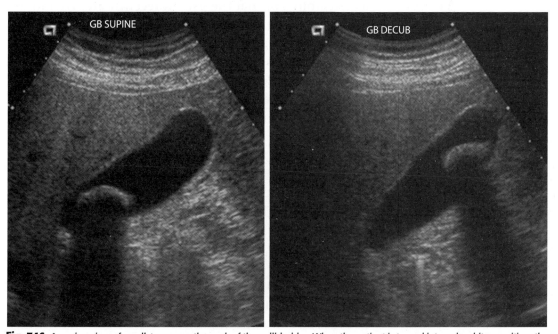

Fig. 7.16 A supine view of a gallstone near the neck of the gallbladder. When the patient is turned into a decubitus position, the stone moves down to the fundus, which is now the dependent part of the gallbladder.

is to have the patient turn into a right posterior oblique position so the stones will fall next to the liver parenchyma and separate them from the gas.

Technical Tips
Focal Zones

When taking images of the gallbladder, the focal zone should be moved up to the level of the gallbladder wall or just below it, especially when measuring it. The focal zone may also need to be optimized to bring out an acoustic shadow or other pathologic area.

Transducer Positions

Scanning is performed using either a subcostal approach with the patient holding their breath in a deep inspiration or with intercostal views with the patient in suspended or quiet respiration. Systematic, careful scans in both longitudinal and transverse planes in both supine and decubitus positions are required.

Importance of Verifying When and What the Patient Last Ate

It is essential to determine when patients last ate and what they had to eat and drink. Improper patient prep can lead to incorrect measurements of the gallbladder wall. For example, if a patient had a cup of coffee with cream in it 3 hours before the examination, it would be difficult to determine whether a thickened gallbladder wall is a postprandial response or the presence of a pathologic condition (Fig. 7.17). A nonvisualized gallbladder is indicative of gallbladder disease, cholecystectomy, or that the patient recently ate. To find the gallbladder fossa, locate the MLF because the distal portion will end in the gallbladder fossa (Fig. 7.18). This is also helpful in patients whose gallbladder has shrunk down to stones, displaying the wall echo shadow (WES) sign (Fig. 7.19). It is acceptable to scan a patient who has had something to eat or drink that would not stimulate the gallbladder or biliary system. Patients can also take any medications with sips of water or a clear liquid.

Mickey Mouse Sign

On transverse images through the porta hepatitis, the "Mickey Mouse" sign can be seen. The portal vein represents Mickey's head, and the bile duct represents Mickey's right ear and the **hepatic artery** Mickey's left ear (Fig. 7.20).

How to Properly Measure the Gallbladder Wall

Wall thickness measurements should be made where the wall is perpendicular to the sound beam, using the anterior wall or at the area

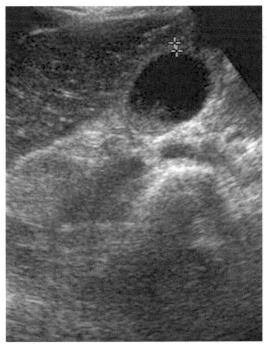

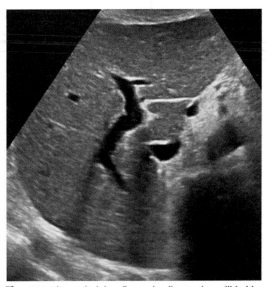

Fig. 7.18 The main lobar fissure leading to the gallbladder fossa on this patient with a cholecystectomy.

Fig. 7.17 Postprandial image of a patient with a thickened gallbladder wall. There is also sludge seen, making it difficult to determine whether the wall is thickened because disease.

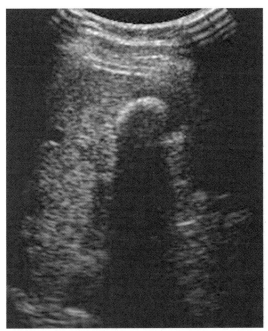

Fig. 7.19 A transverse image of the gallbladder showing a gallbladder contracted down to stones and demonstrating the web echo shadow sign.

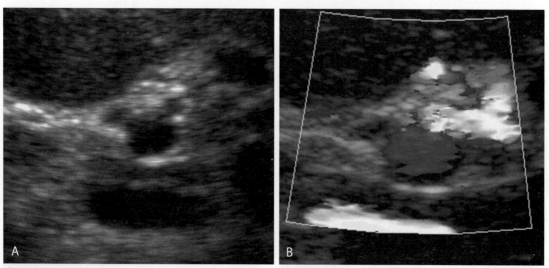

Fig. 7.20 A hidden Mickey! The "Mickey Mouse" sign. **A,** Gray-scale image of the portal triad. Mickey's head is the portal vein, his left ear (as you look at him) the common duct, and his right ear the hepatic artery. **B,** A color Doppler image showing flow in the hepatic artery. A way to remember that the artery is medial is with HAM—hepatic artery medial.

in question if irregular wall thickening is present (Fig. 7.21). Axial resolution is better than lateral resolution, so measuring a side wall may overestimate the measurement (Fig. 7.22).

Intrahepatic Duct Dilatation

When the smaller intrahepatic duct is dilated, the appearance is called the parallel channel or double channel sign. The anterior structure is the dilated bile duct, and the posterior structure is the portal vein. Acoustic enhancement may be demonstrated. A color Doppler image should be obtained to show that the dilated structures are not vascular (Fig. 7.23).

Murphy's Sign

A positive Murphy's sign (MS) is caused by blockage of the cystic duct usually by a stone. This causes a buildup of pressure inside the gallbladder, leading to inflammation and potentially ischemia of the gallbladder wall. A positive (+) MS is very suggestive of cholecystitis. Testing for a + MS can be tricky. The patient is in pain, and a positive response does not mean it is from the gallbladder. Often the patient will say yes just to try to get some pain medications. I would press at multiple locations to make sure that it was a true + MS and that the patient was not in the same amount of pain no matter where I pressed, as follows:

1. Locate the gallbladder in a transverse plane.
2. Starting in the left upper quadrant (LUQ), press as you watch the patient's response. I would usually observe the patient from the corner of my eye for signs of any reaction.

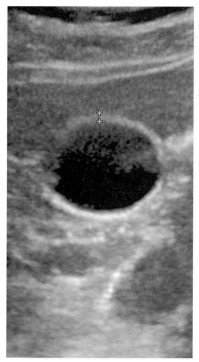

Fig. 7.21 The proper method of measuring the gallbladder wall.

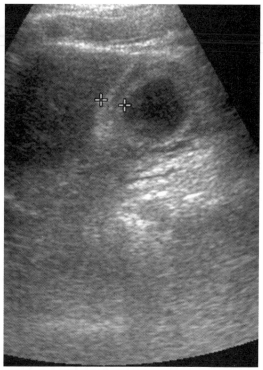

Fig. 7.22 The gallbladder wall being measured improperly as the lateral wall is being measured and not the anterior wall. The wall thickening appears to be circumferential.

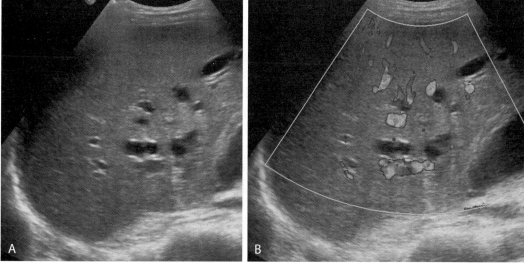

FIG. 7.23 Dilated biliary ducts in the liver on a patient with a pancreatic head mass. **A,** A gray-scale image of the dilated ducts. **B,** A color Doppler image differentiating the dilated ducts from the vascular structures.

3. Continue moving over to the midline at 4–5 cm intervals until you go past the gallbladder, making sure that one compression is over the gallbladder.
4. If there was a noticeable difference when pressing over the gallbladder, I would ask the patient where it hurt worse, here, over the gallbladder, or here, somewhere near midline. If the

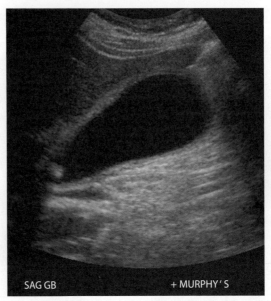

SAG GB   + MURPHY'S

Fig. 7.24 A patient with acute cholecystitis. Note the stone in the neck of the gallbladder. On decubitus views, the stone did not move. The patient had a positive Murphy's sign.

patient said over the gallbladder, I would mark it as a + MS (Fig. 7.24).

5. If there was not a noticeable difference when pressing over the gallbladder, I would ask the patient where it hurt the worse and press at that spot, over the gallbladder, and at two or three different spots. If the patient could not pinpoint the gallbladder as the most painful area, I would mark it as a negative (–) MS. This was helpful in patients who had pain no matter where I pressed to pinpoint that over the gallbladder was not the most sensitive area.

Fig. 7.25A to C illustrates that the gallbladder can have thickened walls and not be painful to the patient.

Artifacts That Can Lead to a Misdiagnosis

The sonographer should be aware of two artifacts that could possibly lead to a misdiagnosis. The first is slice thickness artifact, which causes echoes to be produced at the bottom of the gallbladder. These echoes can be mistaken for sludge (Fig. 7.26). The best way to prove whether the echoes are real is to scan in a transverse plan and turn the patient in an LLD position while scanning. If unable to scan while the patient is turning, once the patient is in an LLD position, quickly find the gallbladder again scanning transversely. If the echoes are caused by sludge, you will see them as they are layering to the dependent portion of the gallbladder (Fig. 7.27). If they are caused by an artifact, they will either disappear or be there immediately. (Historical note: Gallbladder sludge was first described by ultrasound in the 1970s.)

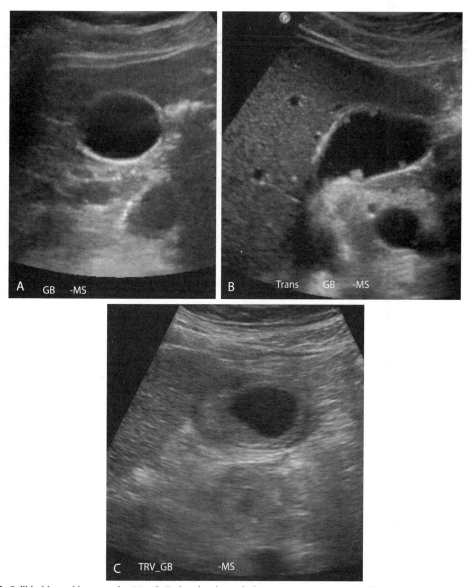

Fig. 7.25 Gallbladders with a negative Murphy's sign despite pathology present. **A,** Normal gallbladder. **B,** Patient with cholesterolosis, or strawberry gallbladder. **C,** Very thickened walls as a result of acquired immunodeficiency syndrome cholangiopathy.

The second artifact is a type of refraction artifact, called an edge refraction shadow, that is caused by the edge of a curved wall, which casts an acoustic shadow. It is important not to mistake this artifact for a stone. The quickest way to differentiate is to follow the shadow up to its origin and see the cause. If a stone is not seen, you know the shadow is being caused by an artifact (Fig. 7.28). Although reverberations may be seen at the top of the gallbladder, these echoes will not be mistaken for pathology because there is not a pathologic condition that would float to the top of the gallbladder.

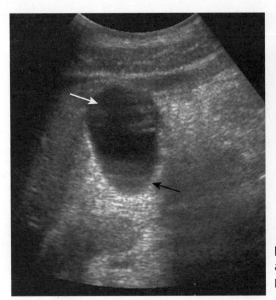

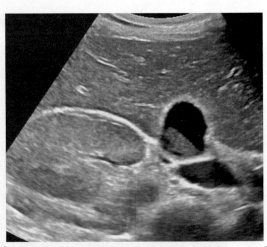

Fig. 7.27 A patient with biliary sludge. Note that it is at an angle as it settles to the dependent portion of the gallbladder when the patient was turned into left lateral decubitus position.

Fig. 7.26 An image demonstrating both reverberations *(white arrow)* and slice thickness *(black arrow)* artifacts.

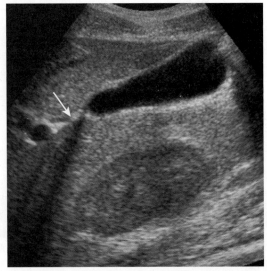

Fig. 7.28 The *arrow* is pointing to an acoustic shadow caused by edge refraction. When you follow the shadow to its origin (arrow), it is coming from the wall and not a stone.

Common Bile Duct Tips

When it is difficult to see the lumen of the CBD, do not assume it is because of an artifact but rather suspect cholangitis. Cholangitis is an inflammation of the bile duct system and in most cases is caused by a bacterial infection. Sonographically, thickening of the extrahepatic biliary duct walls is seen (Fig. 7.29). Dilated bile ducts also may be seen in the liver.

To help distinguish if a dilated CBD is due to a distal stone or pancreatic head mass, look at the shape of the duct distally. If it is pointed (Fig. 7.30), it is because the mass is compressing the duct. If the duct remains the same diameter, it may be due to a distal CBD or ampulla

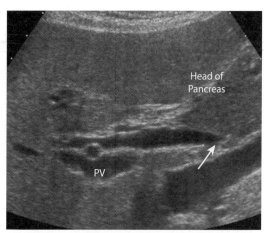

Fig. 7.30 The *arrow* is pointing to the tapering of the common bile duct being caused by a pancreatic head mass. *PV,* Portal vein.

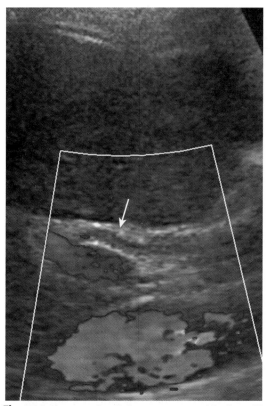

Fig. 7.29 The *arrow* is pointing to a common bile duct with no lumen resulting from thickened walls in this patient with ascending cholangitis.

of Vater tumor (Fig. 7.31). Carefully scan down from the head of the pancreas transversely looking for the stone. Gently push gas out of the way (Fig. 7.32).

Gallbladder and Biliary Tract Required Images

Systematic scans should be performed in both planes to evaluate for the presence of dilated biliary ducts and the size, shape, and contents of the gallbladder; the thickness of the gallbladder wall; and the diameter of the CBD at the level of the main portal vein at the porta hepatis and at the head of the pancreas. Any pathologic areas needs to be documented in at least two planes. *Note:* Sonographically it is difficult to tell where the CHD becomes the CBD because the cystic duct is usually difficult to visualize, especially where it joins the common duct. Usually CD or CBD is used to annotate the bile duct in the region of the porta hepatitis. The following is just required images to evaluate the gallbladder and biliary tract. Typically these images will be incorporated with the images for the liver protocol. Otherwise, a few images of the liver to show that there is or is not dilated ducts.

In some ultrasound departments, a video clip sweeping through the gallbladder in both longitudinal and transverse planes also may be required.

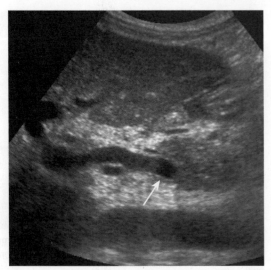

Fig. 7.31 The *arrow* is pointing to the common bile duct (CBD) as it passes through the head of the pancreas. Note how the duct is a constant diameter on this patient with a distal CBD stone.

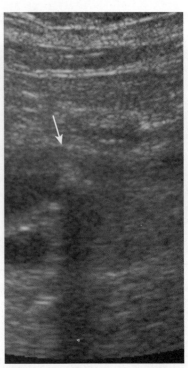

Fig. 7.32 Same patient as in Fig. 7.31. The *arrow* is pointing to the distal stone that was past the pancreatic head. Although not a "pretty" image it is diagnostic and that is what is important.

Gallbladder and Biliary Tract • Longitudinal Images

The gallbladder must be documented in two different patient positions.

1. Long-axis image of the gallbladder with measurement.

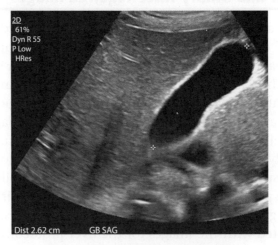

Suggested annotation: **GB SAG**

2. Multiple longitudinal images through the gallbladder.

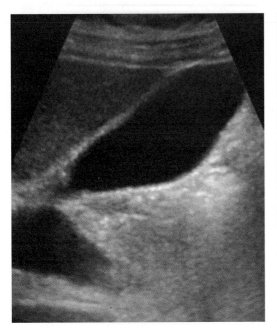 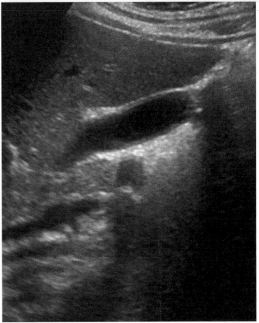

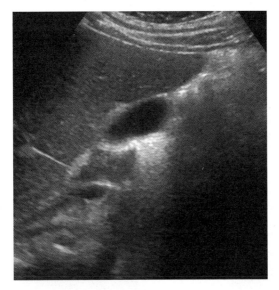

Suggested annotation: **GB SAG**

3. Long axis of CD/CBD with and without measurement. (Some laboratories label the duct seen as CBD even though it may be the CHD, whereas other laboratories just label it CD.)

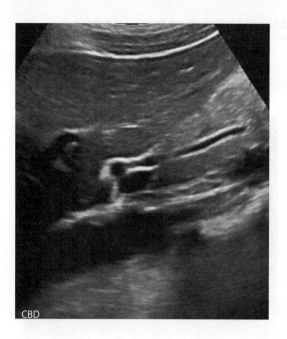

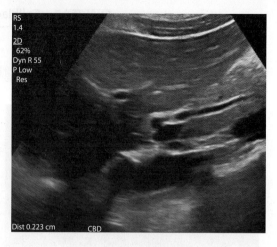

Suggested annotation: **CBD or CD**

> **SCANNING TIP:** To help visualize the duct better for measurements, magnify the area with a write zoom as opposed to a read zoom to maintain resolution.

Gallbladder and Biliary Tract • Transverse Images

1. Multiple transverse images of the gallbladder from the neck to the fundus.

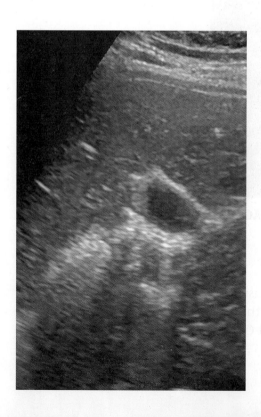

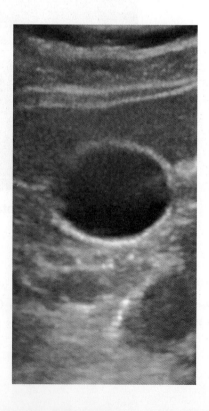

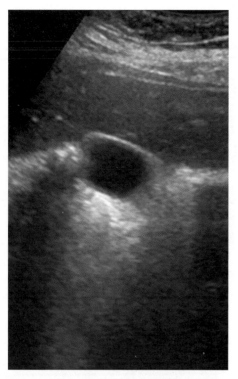

Suggested annotation: **GB TRV or TRANS**

2. Measurement of the gallbladder wall thickness.

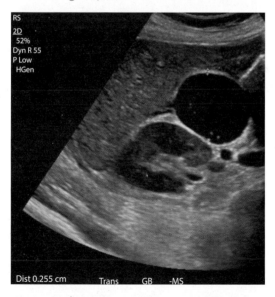

Suggested annotation: **GB WALL**

3. Image demonstrating the results of Murphy's sign (MS). This patient had multiple gallstones but did not have a + MS, which was expected because there were no clinical signs of cholecystitis.

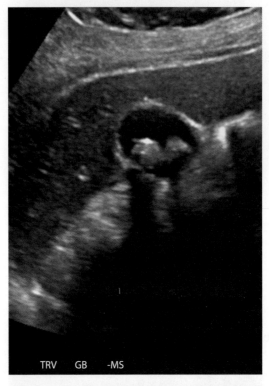

Suggested annotation: **either + MS or − MS**

4. Transverse of CBD, if possible, demonstrating the "Mickey Mouse" sign. The box around the **portal triad** is defining the area for a write zoom (see Fig. 7.20).

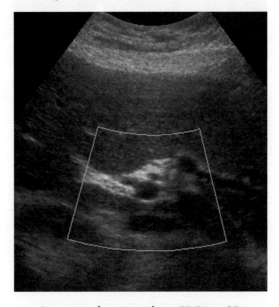

Suggested annotation: **CBD or CD**

5. Transverse of CBD *(arrow)* at the head of the pancreas with and without a measurement.

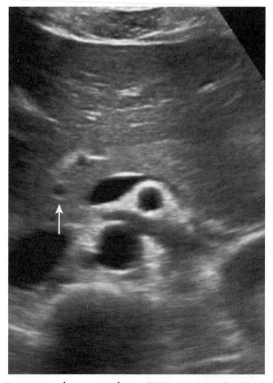

Suggested annotation: **CBD AT PANC HEAD**

Gallbladder and Biliary Tract • Longitudinal Images With Patient in LLD or RSU*

1. Multiple longitudinal images through the gallbladder.

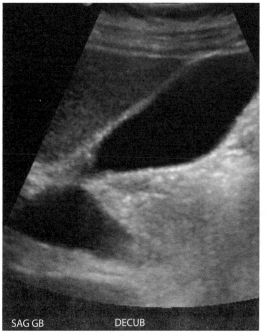

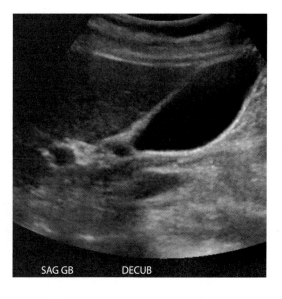

Suggested annotation: **GB SAG LLD, DECUB or RSU**

*Some laboratories annotate LLD, whereas others use RSU.

2. Long axis of CD/CBD with and without measurement.

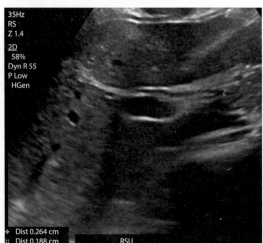

Suggested annotation: **CBD or CD LLD or RSU**

Gallbladder and Biliary Tract • Transverse Images With Patient in LLD or RSU

1. Multiple transverse images of the gallbladder from the neck to the fundus.

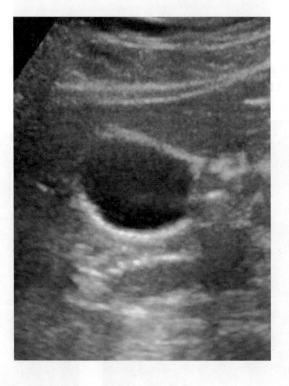

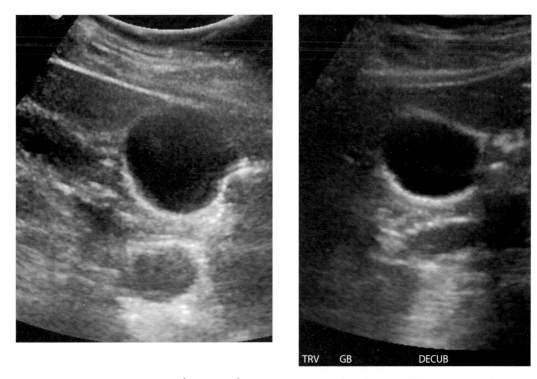

Suggested annotation: **GB TRV LLD, DECUB or RSU**

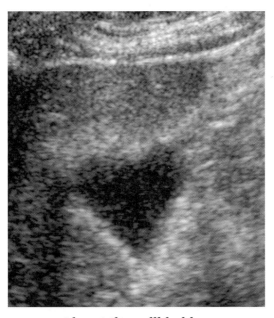

I heart the gallbladder.

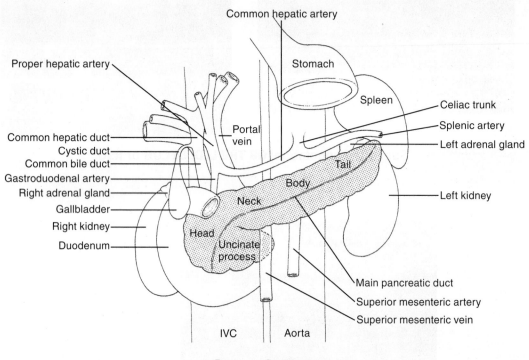

Pancreas Anatomy

CHAPTER 8

Pancreas Scanning Protocol

M. Robert DeJong

Keywords

Common bile duct (CBD)	Portal splenic confluence
Endocrine	Portal vein
Exocrine	Retroperitoneal
Gastroduodenal artery	Santorini's duct
Pancreatic body	Splenic vein
Pancreatic head	Superior mesenteric artery
Pancreatic neck	Superior mesenteric vein
Pancreatic tail	Wirsung's duct
Pancreatic uncinate process	

Objectives

At the end of this chapter, you will be able to:

- Define the keywords.
- Discuss the sonographic appearance of the pancreas.
- List the vessels that help define the pancreatic borders.
- Discuss the different sections of the pancreas.
- Discuss the endocrine and exocrine functions of the pancreas.
- List the names of the pancreatic ducts.
- Describe the patient prep for a pancreas study.
- Explain the order and locations to take representative images of the pancreas.

Overview

Anatomy

The pancreas is typically scanned in the radiology department. It is a *retroperitoneal* organ located in the epigastrium and left hypochondrium. It occupies the anterior pararenal space and lies obliquely between the C-loop of the duodenum and the splenic hilum (Fig. 8.1). It has both *endocrine* and *exocrine* functions. The size and shape of the pancreas may vary, with the length being approximately 12 to 15 cm.

The pancreatic head is the most inferior portion lying within the curve of the duodenum, called the C-loop. It lies anterior to the inferior vena cava (IVC) and inferior to the caudate lobe and *portal vein*. The *common bile duct* (CBD) marks the posterolateral border and passes through a groove posterior to the *pancreatic head*. The

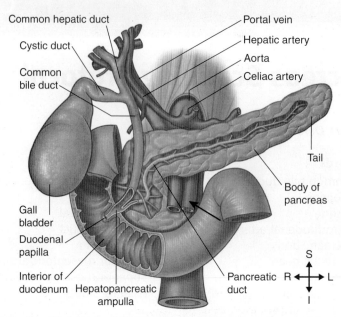

Fig. 8.1 Illustration of the pancreas, biliary system, and vascular structures around the pancreas. The *black arrow* is pointing to the superior mesenteric artery and vein. (Modified from Grant A, Waugh A. *Ross & Wilson Anatomy and Physiology in Health and Illness,* 13th ed. Edinburgh, 2018, Elsevier.)

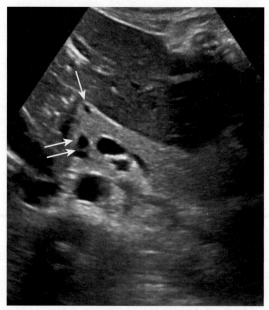

Fig. 8.2 Long axis of the pancreas. The *single arrow* is pointing to the gastroduodenal artery and the *double arrows* to the common bile duct. To remember which one is which, they are alphabetical: *A* on top for artery and *B* on the bottom for bile duct.

gastroduodenal artery (GDA) (Fig. 8.2), a branch of the common hepatic artery, marks the anterolateral border. The *pancreatic unci-nate process* is a posteromedial extension of the head of the pancreas and is the only part of the pancreas to pass posteriorly to the *superior*

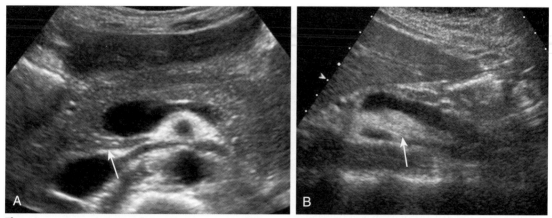

Fig. 8.3 A, The *arrow* is pointing to the uncinate process scanning in a transverse plane. **B,** The *arrow* is pointing to the uncinate process scanning in a sagittal plane.

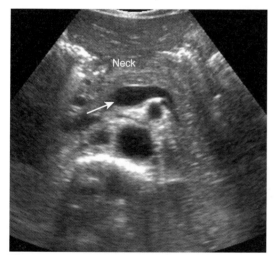

Fig. 8.4 Image of the area of the neck of the pancreas. The *arrow* is pointing to the portal confluence.

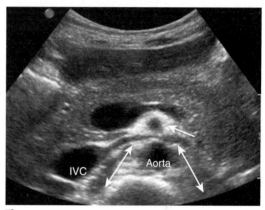

Fig. 8.5 An image of the body of the pancreas as it drapes over the splenic vein, superior mesenteric artery *(single arrow)*, left renal vein *(double-headed arrows)*, and aorta.

mesenteric vein (SMV) (Fig. 8.3). The anteroposterior (AP) diameter of the head is approximately 20 to 30 mm.

The pancreatic neck lies between the head and body and is anterior to the superior mesenteric vessels. The *splenic vein* and SMV join together posterior to the neck to form the portal vein (Fig. 8.4). It is 10 to 20 mm in AP diameter.

The pancreatic body is the largest section of the gland and curves slightly anteriorly as it extends over the aorta, *superior mesenteric artery*, and lumbar spine (Fig. 8.5). The splenic vein marks the posterior border and the splenic artery the superior border. We can see the pancreas and the splenic vein in the same image; however, the splenic artery is not seen with pancreatic tissue except in a sagittal plane (Fig. 8.6). The AP diameter of the body is approximately 20 to 30 mm.

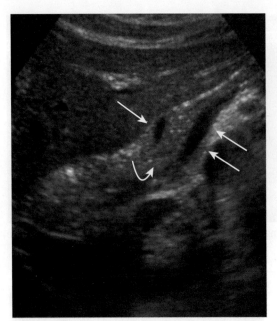

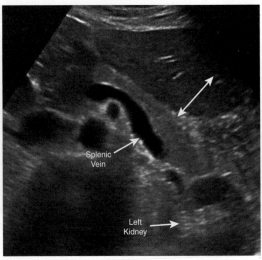

Fig. 8.7 Evaluating the tail of the pancreas *(double-headed arrow)*.

Fig. 8.6 Scanning in a sagittal plane to evaluate the pancreas in its transverse plane. The *single arrow* is pointing to the splenic artery, the *curved arrow* to the *pancreatic body*, and the *double arrows* to the splenic vein.

The ***pancreatic tail*** is the most superior aspect, is in close contact with the hilum of the spleen, and lies anterior to the splenic vein and left kidney (Fig. 8.7). It measures approximately 10 to 20 mm in the AP dimension.

The main pancreatic duct, ***Wirsung's duct***, begins in the tail of the pancreas and receives branches in a herringbone fashion. At the head of the pancreas it turns inferiorly to pierce the posteromedial wall of the second part of the duodenum joining the CBD (Fig. 8.8). An accessory pancreatic duct, ***Santorini's duct***, drains the anterior portion of the head of the pancreas. It may join the main pancreatic duct but usually empties directly into the duodenum at the minor duodenal papilla.

Physiology

The main functions of the pancreas are to secrete the digestive enzymes in the pancreatic juice, which is its exocrine function, and the secretion of glucagon and insulin into the blood, which is its endocrine function. Remember that exocrine glands need a duct to deliver their product, whereas endocrine glands secret their product through the walls directly into the bloodstream by the osmosis process; thus, there are no ducts associated with the islets of Langerhans.

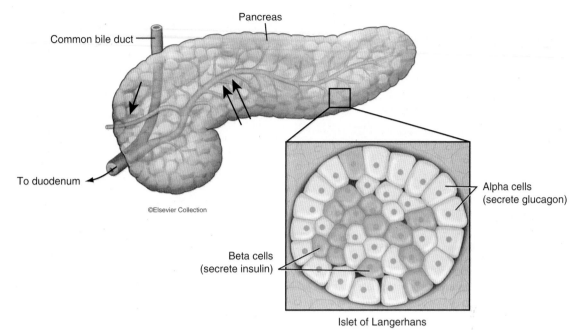

Fig. 8.8 Illustration of the pancreatic ductal system showing both Wirsung's duct *(double arrows)* and Santorini's duct *(single arrow)*. Note how curvy the duct is, which is why it is usually seen in short segments. This drawing also shows how the smaller ducts resemble fish bones. An islet of Langerhans cell is enlarged. (© Elsevier Collection.)

The majority of the pancreas is exocrine tissue and is composed of acini cells, ductules, and ducts. The pancreas is a main source of digestive enzymes that are synthesized in the acinar cells. They include the following:

- Amylase for the digestion of starch
- Lipase for the digestion of lipids
- Peptidases for the digestion of proteins

Pancreatic juice also contains sodium bicarbonate to neutralize gastric acid. When chyme (partially digested food) enters the duodenum, it stimulates the release of cholecystokinin, which stimulates the gallbladder to contract, and secretin, which is responsible for the release of sodium bicarbonate. If the acinar cells are damaged and not producing pancreatic juice, the patient will have digestive issues.

The endocrine cells of the pancreas are the islets of Langerhans and are scattered throughout the pancreas like little islands. Their main purpose is to produce the hormone insulin. Failure to produce sufficient amounts of insulin leads to diabetes mellitus.

Sonographic Appearance

Hints on Finding the Pancreas

To locate pancreatic tissue, it is necessary to identify the superior mesenteric artery, splenic vein, and ***portal splenic confluence***. Observing peristalsis in the duodenum is helpful in delineating the lateral border of the

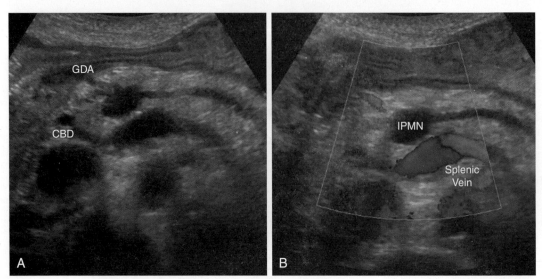

Fig. 8.9 A, A patient with intraductal papillary mucinous neoplasm *(IPMN)* in the head of the pancreas. Note the dilated pancreatic duct going into the cyst. The gastroduodenal artery *(GDA)* and common bile duct *(CBD)* are very nicely seen. **B,** Color Doppler, seen in gray scale here, confirms the GDA. Note that inside the splenic vein are two different shades of gray. This is because the center of the transducer senses flow direction. The light gray is coming from the spleen toward the middle of the transducer. The darker gray is going to the portal confluence and the liver and is flowing away from the middle of the transducer.

head of the pancreas and to avoid mistaking the duodenum for a mass or part of the pancreas. The splenic vein runs along the posterior margin of the pancreas body and tail and helps in identifying the pancreas. The splenic vein joins with the SMV directly posterior to the *pancreatic neck* to form the portal vein. The head of the pancreas is identified as it sits anterior to the IVC. The GDA marks the anterolateral border, and the CBD marks the posterolateral border of the head of the pancreas (Fig. 8.9).

The pancreatic duct is usually seen in short segments, because of its tortuosity, within the body of the pancreas as two parallel echogenic lines measuring less than 2 to 3 mm (Fig. 8.10). Care should be taken not to mistake vascular structures or the posterior wall of the stomach for the pancreatic duct (Fig. 8.11). If unsure, turn on color Doppler to verify that it is not a vessel. Identifying pancreatic tissue on both sides of the duct will verify that it is truly the duct.

If there is too much gas obscuring the pancreas, the patient may be given water to distend the stomach (Fig. 8.12). The fluid-filled stomach then can be used as an acoustic window. If still unable to see the pancreas, turn the patient into both right and left oblique positions and/or in a semi-upright position to change the position of the water and gas to try to improve visualization. With some patients it is not possible to visualize the pancreas, and some sonographers will take an image showing the gas and label it "area of pancreas" to document that they tried to see the pancreas (Fig. 8.13).

A fatty pancreas is fat accumulation in the pancreas and is usually an incidental finding during abdominal ultrasound examinations.

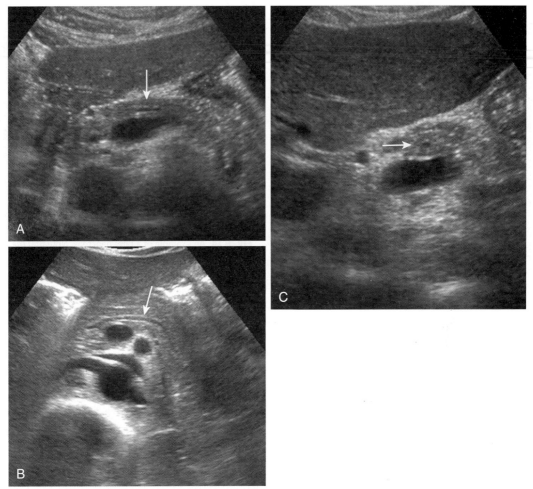

Fig. 8.10 A, The *arrow* is pointing to a segment of the pancreatic duct. **B,** Another patient in whom the duct *(arrow)* is seen almost in its entirety. **C,** The pancreas is seen in its transverse plane. The *arrow* is pointing to the pancreatic duct. Note how it is surrounded by pancreatic tissue.

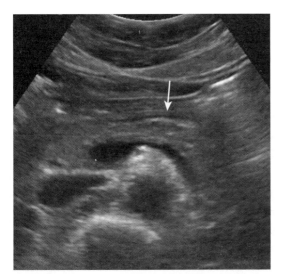

Fig. 8.11 The *arrow* is pointing to the posterior wall of the stomach. Because there is no pancreatic tissue above this tubular appearing structure, it cannot be the pancreatic duct. The anterior wall of the stomach can be seen superiorly, confirming that this is the posterior wall.

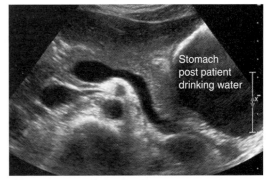

Fig. 8.12 The patient was given water to drink, which helped visualize the tail of the pancreas.

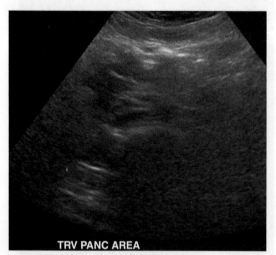

TRV PANC AREA

Fig. 8.13 The area of the pancreas has gas overlying it, making it difficult to see the pancreas.

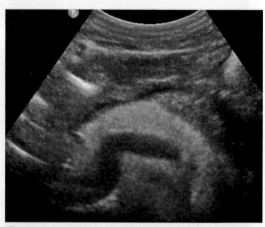

Fig. 8.14 An example of a fatty pancreas. Note that the pancreas is normal in size and shape.

Fatty pancreas can be seen in elderly patients, obese patients, and other metabolic diseases. On ultrasound, the pancreas is normal in size and shape, with a very bright white echo texture (Fig. 8.14).

Pancreas Relationships to Other Organs and Blood Vessels
- *Head:* Anterior to IVC, lateral to portal vein in a transverse plane and posterior in a sagittal plane, anteromedial to GDA, posteromedial to CBD, and medial to the duodenum (Fig. 8.15)
- *Uncinate process:* Anterior to IVC, posterior to SMV
- *Body:* Anterior to SMA, aorta, splenic vein, SMV, left renal vein, and spine; posterior to the left lobe of liver, stomach, and splenic artery
- *Tail:* Medial to hilum of spleen, anterior to left kidney, superior to splenic vein and left renal vein

Ultrasound of the Pancreas

Because of the difficulties that can be encountered imaging a pancreas, dedicated sonograms of the pancreas are rarely ordered and the pancreas is included as part of a right upper quadrant (RUQ) examination (Fig. 8.16). When scanning the pancreas, it is important to remember that the long axis of the pancreas is in a transverse oblique plane and transverse images of the pancreas are in a sagittal plane. Patients are scanned in the supine position with transverse oblique scans to image the long axis of the pancreas. Longitudinal scans are especially useful in evaluating the head of the pancreas.

The time-gain compensation and gain should be adjusted so that the pancreatic texture is homogeneous and has an echo brightness that is slightly greater than that of the liver. The echo texture of the pancreas is coarser than that of the liver. The echogenicity of the pancreas may increase with age because of fatty replacement and may also decrease in size.

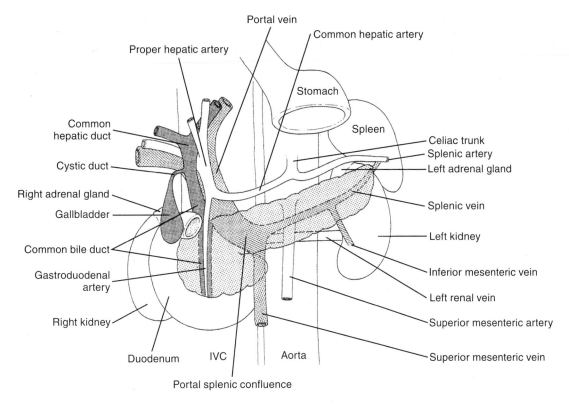

Fig. 8.15 Illustration of the vascular structures around the pancreas and other organs. Note the splenic artery on the superior border of the pancreas and the splenic vein on the posterior (indicated by *dotted line*) border.

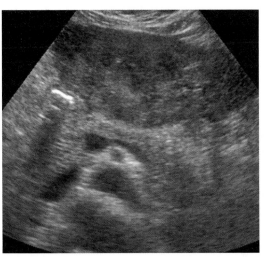

Fig. 8.16 A patient with metastatic disease of the liver (multiple hypoechoic lesions). The pancreas is well seen, eliminating the pancreas as the site of the primary cancer.

Patient Prep

Because of the surrounding bowel and stomach, visualization of the pancreas can be difficult. Having the patient fast 6 to 8 hours may help in reducing bowel gas.

Transducer

A curved linear array transducer that emits a 3–3.5 MHz frequency should be used. A curved linear array transducer that emits a 5 MHz frequency may be used in pediatric patients, thin patients, or when better resolution is needed. Like the gallbladder, the pancreas is closer to the surface, and a higher-frequency transducer can be used to increase resolution if needed. A curved linear array transducer is preferred because it allows the sonographer to gently rock the transducer side to side while gently pressing the gas out of the way. Pressing with a vector/sector array is uncomfortable for the patient because of the small footprint.

Breathing Technique

The pancreas is best visualized with the patient in a deep inspiration, scanning from a subxiphoid approach, using the left lobe of the liver as an acoustic window and angling the transducer caudally. Sometimes having the patient take a deep breath and push out the stomach is helpful.

Patient Position

For an ultrasound examination of the pancreas, the patient should be started in the supine position. If having difficulty seeing the pancreas, sometimes raising the head of the bed at least 60 degrees and scanning with the patient in a semi-upright position can be helpful because this might cause the liver to drop a littler lower in the abdomen.

Pancreas Required Images

The required images are a small representation of what a sonographer visualizes during a study. Therefore, the images should provide the interpreting physician with technically accurate information to be able to make a diagnosis. While scanning, try using different amounts of transducer pressure over the area of the pancreas, keeping patient comfort in mind, to help improve visualization of the pancreas. Scanning should include evaluating the pancreas for size, shape, contour, duct diameter, and echo texture. Attention should be given to observe for any focal areas of enlargement, masses, or calcifications. The walls of the duct should be smooth and parallel in a normal patient.

Pancreas • Long Axis Views From a Transverse Oblique Plane

1. Multiple views of the pancreas demonstrating as much of the pancreas as possible. Images should include views of the head, neck, uncinate process, body, and tail. The head, neck, and uncinate process can be seen in the same image. Usually measurements of the pancreas are not routinely obtained, although some departments will measure the AP measurement of the head routinely.

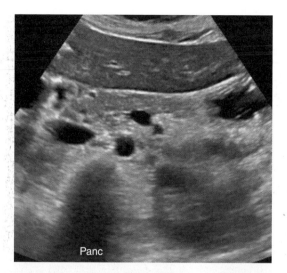

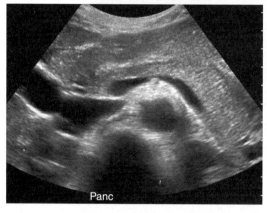

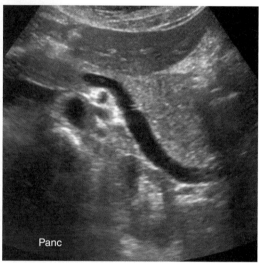

Suggested annotation: **PANC or PANCREAS**

2. Image of the head demonstrating the GDA and CBD.

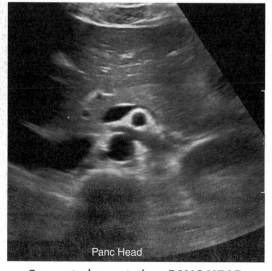

Suggested annotation: **PANC HEAD**

3. Image of the pancreatic duct with and without a measurement *(optional)*.

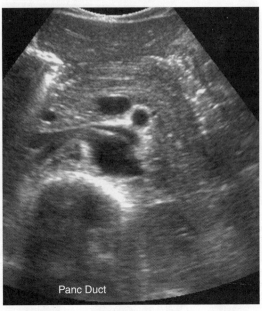

Suggested annotation: **PANC DUCT**

Pancreas • Transverse Views From a Sagittal Plane

1. Image of the head of the pancreas.

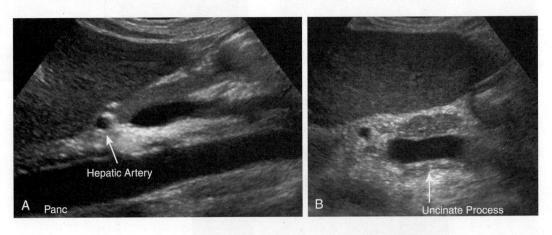

Suggested annotation: **PANC HEAD**

2. Multiple images of the pancreas through the body and tail when it can be seen. The pancreatic tissue should be seen between the splenic artery and the splenic vein.

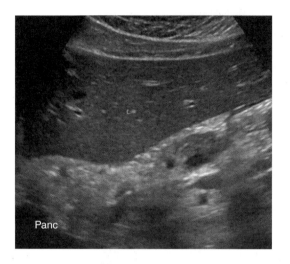

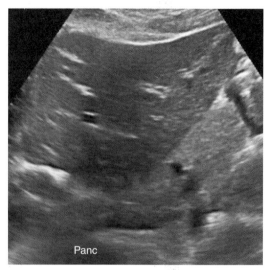

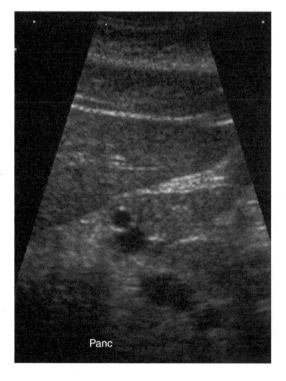

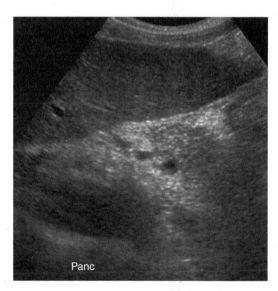

Suggested annotation: **PANC**

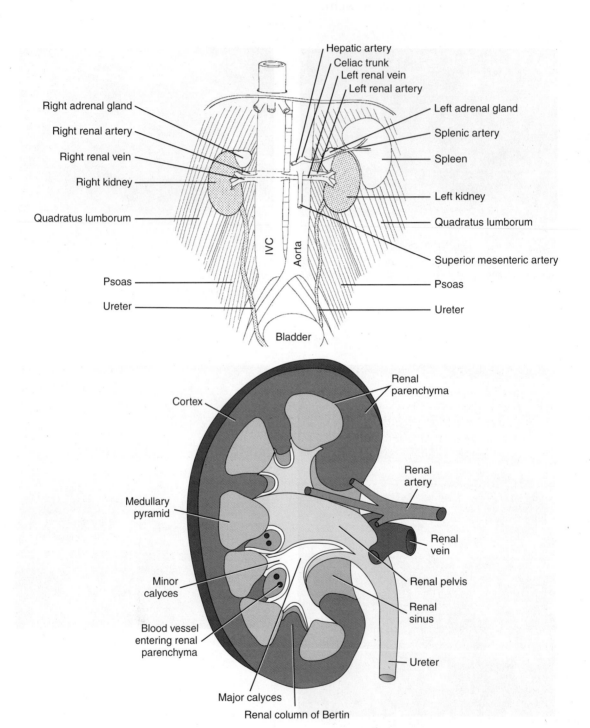

CHAPTER 9

Renal Scanning Protocol

M. Robert De Jong

Key Words

Collecting system	Renal capsule
Columns of Bertin	Renal cortex
Gerota's fascia	Renal hilum
Major calyces	Renal parenchyma
Medullary pyramid	Renal pelvis
Minor calyces	Renal sinus
Morison's pouch	Ureter
Nephron	

Objectives

At the end of this chapter, you will be able to:
- Define the keywords.
- Describe the anatomy of the kidneys.
- Distinguish the sonographic appearance of the kidneys and its normal variants.
- Describe the transducer options for scanning the kidneys.
- Discuss the normal difference in size between the kidneys and major causes if there is a discrepancy.
- List the suggested patient positions when scanning the kidneys.
- Describe the patient prep for a renal study.
- Explain the order and exact locations to take representative images of the kidneys.

Overview

Ultrasound of the kidneys is performed in the radiology department and can also be performed by urology practices. Ultrasound is typically the test of choice when suspecting a renal pathologic condition, because there is no radiation or nephrotoxic contrast needed. It is also portable and therefore can go to the units when a patient cannot come down to the department. It can easily determine whether the patient has hydronephrosis and is useful for searching for renal stones, although smaller stones and stones in the mid-**ureter** may be difficult to visualize. Ultrasound can be used to guide renal biopsies needed to diagnosis the cause of medical renal disease and can be used to evaluate for post biopsy complications such as hematomas and arteriovenous fistulas.

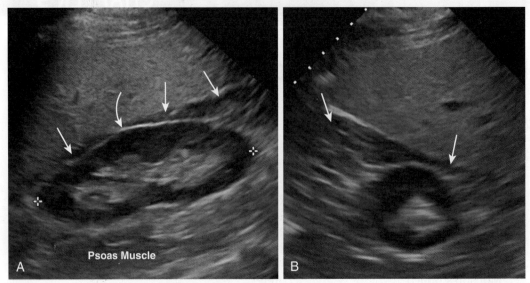

Fig. 9.1 A, Longitudinal view of a normal right kidney. The *straight arrows* are pointing to the pararenal fat. The *curved arrow* is pointing to the renal capsule. **B,** Transverse of a normal right kidney. The *arrows* are pointing to the pararenal fat.

The sonographer needs to be aware of the different renal variants and anomalies so as not to mistake them for a pathologic condition.

Anatomy

The kidneys are retroperitoneal organs located in the perirenal space. They are surrounded by an inner fibrous capsule called the renal or true capsule, a middle layer of perinephric fat, an outer layer of fibroareolar tissue that also surrounds the adrenal gland, called **Gerota's fascia**, and finally an outer layer of pararenal fat (Fig. 9.1). The kidneys lie in an oblique plane on each side of the vertebral column, about the level of T12 and L3-4. The upper renal pole is more medial and posterior than the lower pole, which causes the kidneys to lie in an oblique plane as well as to be tilted, with the lower pole closer to the skin. The psoas muscle is posterior and medial to the kidneys, the quadratus lumborum muscle is posterior and lateral to the kidneys, and the transversus abdominis muscle is deeper and lateral to the kidneys. The right kidney is posterior to the liver and lateral to the gallbladder. The left kidney is inferior and medial to the spleen. Because of the right lobe of the liver, the right kidney is lower than the left kidney.

Normal kidneys have an average length of 9 to 12 cm (Fig. 9.2), with the left kidney usually slightly larger than the right. The accepted difference between the two kidneys is 2 cm. The most common cause for one kidney to be longer than the other is a duplicated **collecting system** (Fig. 9.3), and renal artery thrombosis is the most common cause for one kidney to be smaller (Fig. 9.4). With renal parenchymal disease, such as patients with chronic renal failure, both kidneys will decrease in size (Fig. 9.5). If there is a size discrepancy, the sonographer should

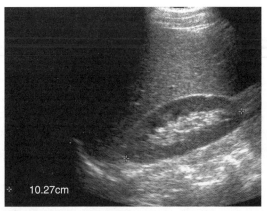

Fig. 9.2 A normal kidney measuring in the normal range.

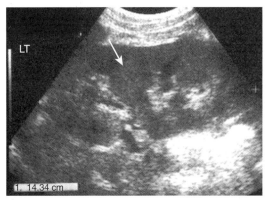

Fig. 9.3 An image of a kidney with a duplicated collecting system. The kidney measures over 14 cm. The *arrow* is pointing to the break between the two collecting systems.

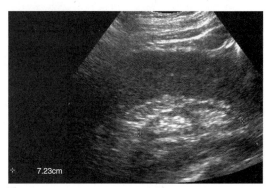

Fig. 9.4 A small kidney measuring 7.2 cm caused by renal artery thrombosis. Color or power Doppler failed to show any internal flow.

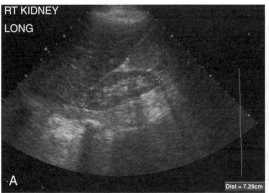

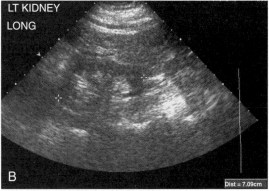

Fig. 9.5 Bilateral small kidneys resulting from chronic renal failure.

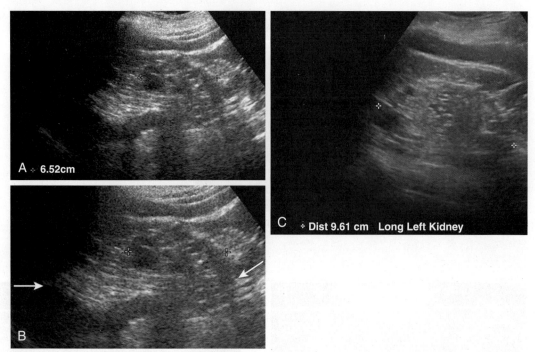

Fig. 9.6 A, The left kidney is measured incorrectly, which made it appear as if it was 4 cm shorter than the right, which measured 10.8 cm. **B,** The *arrows* show the correct locations to place the cursors. **C,** The kidney is now measured correctly and is now just 1.2 cm shorter than the right.

reevaluate the measurements and the quality of the images, ensuring that both poles are well seen and measured correctly (Fig. 9.6).

The size of pediatric kidneys will depend on the age of the child. At birth the kidneys will measure 4.5 to 5 cm (Fig. 9.7), obtaining a normal adult size at about 15 years of age. Remembering that the length of a newborn kidney's size is about half the size of an adult's kidney will help differentiate a normal infant from a newborn with infantile polycystic kidney disease (IPCKD), because the echogenicity of the two can be similar; however, the lengths are very different, with the infant with IPCKD having larger kidneys of more than 9 cm in length (Fig. 9.8).

The medial border of the kidney is concave, and it is here that the renal hilum is located. The **renal hilum** is where the renal artery and nerves enter the kidney and the renal vein and ureter exit the kidney.

The **renal parenchyma** is composed of two layers, the cortex and the medulla. The cortex is the outer portion of the renal parenchyma, lies under the **renal capsule**, and contains millions of **nephrons**, which are the microscopic functional units of the kidney that form urine. The cortex contains the renal corpuscles, glomerulus, and proximal and distal convoluted tubules of the nephron. Filtration occurs in the **renal cortex**. The medulla is the inner portion of the renal parenchyma and contains the loop of Henle, which is where reabsorption takes place. The medulla also contains 10 to 14 renal pyramids,

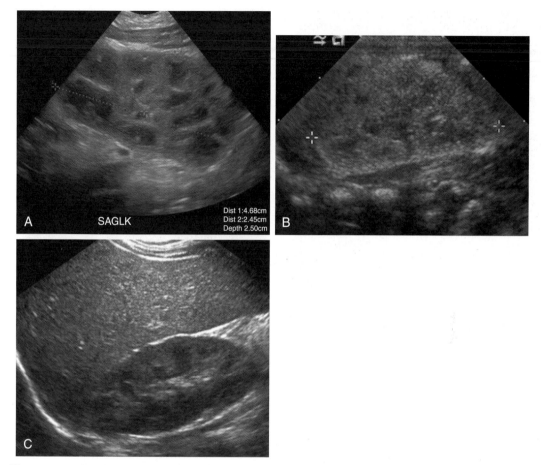

Fig. 9.7 Examples of normal kidneys in newborn patients. **A,** Note the echogenicity of the kidneys. **B,** The parenchymal echoes are as echogenic as the sinus echoes. **C,** An image of a normal kidney in a 9-month-old patient. The kidney now has the sonographic appearance of a normal adult kidney.

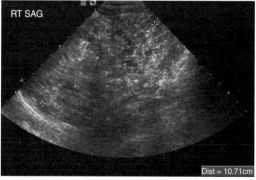

Fig. 9.8 A patient with infantile polycystic kidney disease (IPCKD). Note how the kidney is echogenic, similar to the normal kidneys in Fig. 9.7. However, this kidney measures over 10 cm, which is the length of an adult kidney.

which are separated by extensions of cortical tissue, called **columns of Bertin**, or renal columns, which extend inward to the renal sinus. The base of the **medulla pyramid** is along the corticomedullary junction, and the apex, referred to as the renal papilla, points toward the renal sinus. The papilla fits into the cuplike cavity of a minor calyx. There

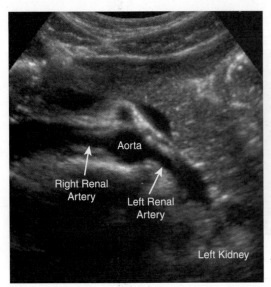

Fig. 9.9 An image of the origin of the main renal arteries with the patient in the supine position. Note how close the left kidney is to the aorta.

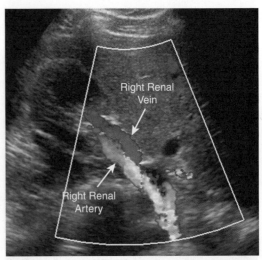

Fig. 9.10 An image showing the relationship between the renal artery and vein. The vein is a dark gray and the artery a light gray.

are 7 to 14 minor calyces. Four or five **minor calyces** unite to form two to three **major calyces**, which unite to form the **renal pelvis**.

The **renal sinus** is the central portion of the kidney and contains the major and minor calyces, the renal pelvis, renal vessels, fat, nerves, and lymphatics. The fat in the sinus is an extension of the perirenal fat. The renal pelvis is a urine reservoir formed by the expanded superior end of the ureter and receives urine from the major calyces. The urine then travels down the ureter to be stored in the urinary bladder.

The kidneys receive their blood supply from the renal arteries, which arise from the lateral borders of the aorta, just inferior to the superior mesenteric artery (SMA) (Fig. 9.9). The renal arteries travel posteriorly to the renal veins (Fig. 9.10). The right renal artery goes posteriorly to the inferior vena cava (IVC) on its way to the kidney and can be seen as a small circle posterior to the IVC in a sagittal plane (Fig. 9.11). The left renal artery is shorter in length. The renal arteries divide into segmental arteries shortly before or after entering the renal hilum. The segmental arteries give off the interlobar branches, which run between the pyramids. These divide into the arcuate arteries at the corticomedullary junction. The arcuate arteries then give off the interlobular branches, which course through the cortex toward the surface of the kidney and divide into the numerous branches that supply the nephrons (Fig. 9.12). Approximately 20% to 30% of the cardiac output enters the renal arteries.

The kidneys are drained by the renal veins. The left renal vein goes between the SMA and aorta to reach the IVC (Fig. 9.13). A common variant is a retroaortic left renal vein, where the vein courses posterior to the aorta (Fig. 9.14). The right renal vein is shorter than the left one.

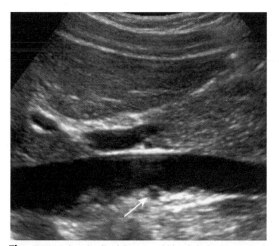

Fig. 9.11 A longitudinal image of the inferior vena cava (IVC). The *arrow* is pointing to a *small circle* posterior to the IVC that is the right renal artery. Because the long axis of the artery is in a transverse plain, the artery is seen transversely in a sagittal plane.

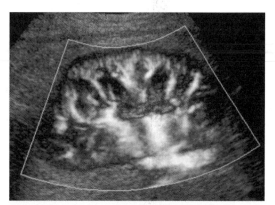

Fig. 9.12 A power Doppler image demonstrating the vascularity of the kidney. Flow is seen out to the capsule.

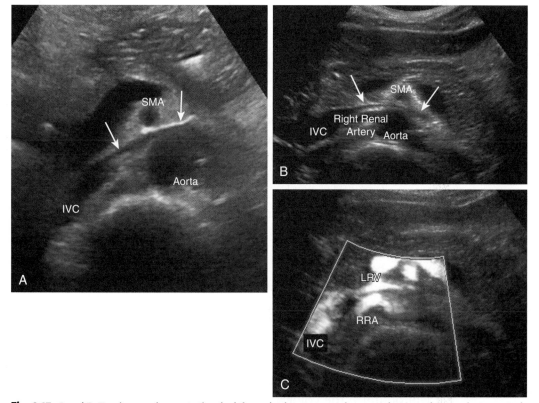

Fig. 9.13 A and **B,** Two images demonstrating the left renal vein, arrows, as it courses between the superior mesenteric artery *(SMA)* and the aorta on its way to the inferior vena cava *(IVC)*. **C,** A power Doppler image of the left renal vein *(LRV)* at this level. Note the exceptional spatial resolution that allows the LRV to be seen separate from the right renal artery *(RRA)*.

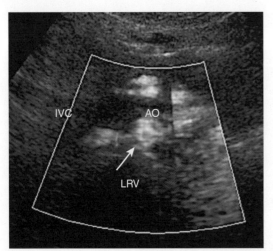

Fig. 9.14 A power Doppler image with the arrow pointing to a retroaortic left renal vein *(LRV)*. Power Doppler allows flow to be visualized even at 90-degree angles. *AO,* Aorta; *IVC,* inferior vena cava.

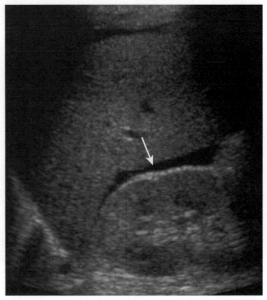

Fig. 9.15 The *arrow* is pointing to a small amount of ascites that is seen in Morison's pouch, which is the most dependent portion of the upper abdomen.

This space between the right kidney and the liver is **Morison's pouch**. This space is important because it is a potential site for abnormal collections of fluid, such as ascites (Fig. 9.15).

Physiology

The nephron is the basic functional unit of the kidney and is composed of the glomerulus, tubules, renal corpuscle, and collecting ducts. Urine is formed by the filtration of blood in the nephron, where substances needed by the body are returned to the blood and waste products and excessive water pass into the collecting ducts as urine. Urine drains from the collecting tubule into a minor calyx, which in turn empties into a major calyx. Urine then flows into the renal pelvis and ureter to empty into the urinary bladder. The bladder stores the urine before it is excreted from the body through the urethra. The calyces, renal pelvis, ureters, bladder, and most of the urethra are lined by waterproof transitional epithelium and have an outer layer of connective tissue and smooth muscle.

Sonographic Appearance

When performing a renal sonogram, the renal preset should be used. The machine will optimize the gray scale needed, but more importantly it will optimize the color and power Doppler sensitivity for a kidney. Using a general setting, the color is more optimized for the liver and the finer renal vasculature may be difficult to appreciate (Fig. 9.16). The time-gain compensation (TGC) and overall gain should be adjusted so the renal cortex is hypoechoic to the normal liver and spleen echogenicity.

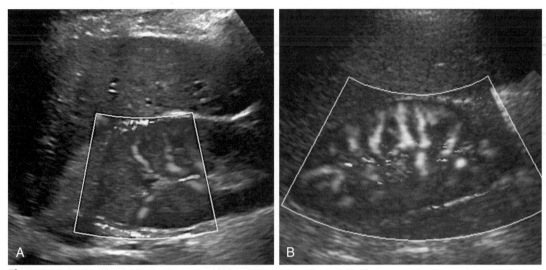

Fig. 9.16 A, A color Doppler image of a normal kidney using a general preset. **B,** The same patient now using a renal preset. Note the improved flow. Although not seen on these images, the other controls such as color velocity scale and color gain were the same.

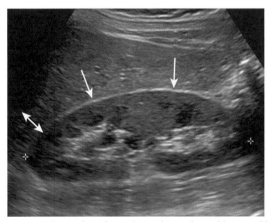

Fig. 9.17 The *arrows* are pointing to the echogenic renal capsule on this normal kidney. Note that the capsule is not appreciated at the level of the *double arrow* because of a critical angle on this specular reflection.

The kidney is oval with a smooth contour and surrounded by an echogenic capsule (Fig. 9.17). The cortex should be symmetric in thickness, about 6 mm, with a medium-to low-level homogeneous echogenicity. The normal renal cortex is less echogenic than the normal liver. The medullary portions may be indistinct from the cortex. The pyramids are seen as hypoechoic, inverted, triangular structures that are less echogenic than the renal cortex (Fig. 9.18). The arcuate arteries may be seen as small, bright, pulsating echoes at the corticomedullary junction. The renal sinus will appear as an oval, highly echogenic structure in the center of the kidney (Fig. 9.19). This bright echogenicity is caused by the fat and the multiple interfaces from the calyces, renal pelvis, vessels, and lymphatics. The normal renal sinus

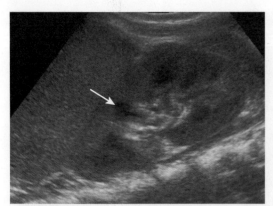

Fig. 9.18 The *arrow* is pointing to one of the multiple renal pyramids.

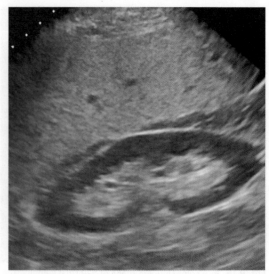

Fig. 9.19 A normal kidney demonstrating the normal echogenicity relationships of the kidney and liver.

should be more echogenic than both the normal renal cortex and the normal liver. The renal cortex is the least echogenic structure in the upper abdomen, and the renal sinus is the most echogenic structure. If the patient is well hydrated, the renal pelvis may be visualized as a lighter gray echo pattern inside the echogenic renal sinus.

With the orientation of the kidney in a vertically oblique plane in the body, the long axis of the kidney is seen in an oblique sagittal scanning plane and oblique coronal scanning plane, with the kidney appearing elliptical. In a transverse image the kidney appears round, with the renal hilum seen medially. A transverse kidney at the midpole may show the renal vein exiting the renal hilum. So as not to confuse with mild hydronephrosis, color Doppler should be used to prove that these tubular structures are vascular (Fig. 9.20). The ureters are not normally visualized with ultrasound unless dilated.

Normal Variants

There are times when the kidney or renal sinus complex will not have its signature oval, smooth shape; however, the kidneys will be in their normal place in the body.

Columns of Bertin

Prominent or hypertrophied columns of Bertin are double layers of renal cortex between the renal pyramids, widening the space between them (Fig. 9.21). They are characterized by being isoechoic to and continuous with the normal renal cortex. Columns of Bertin may indent the renal sinus and mimic a duplicated collecting system. Care should be taken not to mistake a very prominent column of Bertin for a duplicated kidney. If it is truly a duplicated kidney, it will be longer than usual and in the transverse view only cortical tissue will be seen between the two poles.

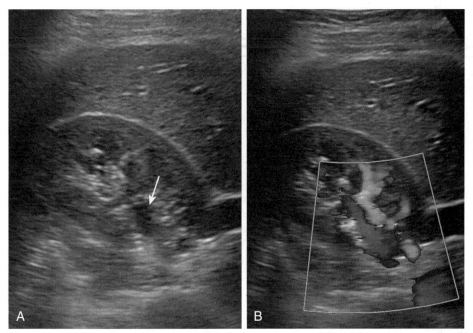

Fig. 9.20 A, The *arrow* is pointing to a small dilated tubular structure at the renal hilum. **B,** The same image using color Doppler. The structure fills in with color and was the renal vein, represented by the darker gray.

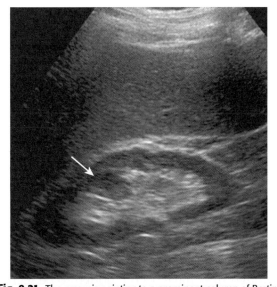

Fig. 9.21 The *arrow* is pointing to a prominent column of Bertin.

Dromedary Hump

A dromedary hump is a benign anatomic variant that gets its name because it resembles the hump of a dromedary camel. It is a prominent focal bulge on the lateral border of the left kidney, giving it a triangular shape (Fig. 9.22). It is caused by the splenic impression onto the superolateral left kidney and is seen in the mid-pole of the kidney. This area will have the same echo texture as surrounding kidney tissue and demonstrate normal parenchymal flow patterns with color or power

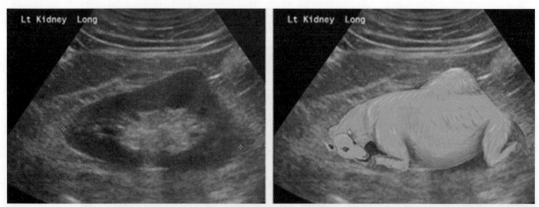

Fig. 9.22 An image of a left kidney with a dromedary hump. At https://onlinelibrary.wiley.com/doi/full/10.1111/1754-9485.20_12784 is an image of a kidney next to a camel superimposed over the kidney that is sitting on the ground. It illustrates the appearance of the kidney with a dromedary hump. (From Xiang H, Han J, Ridley WE, Ridley LJ. *Dromedary hump: anatomic variant. Journal of medical imaging and radiation oncology.* 2018;62(S1):72.)

Doppler. A dromedary hump may mimic the appearance of a renal mass and is considered a renal pseudotumor. This is why interrogating the area with color or power Doppler is needed, because a renal mass will show only peripheral flow and possibly scattered internal flow.

Fetal Lobulations

Persistent fetal lobulations give the kidney a bumpy contour, as opposed to a smooth contour, and causes the surface of the kidney to appear as several lobules instead of smooth, flat, and continuous (Fig. 9.23). Embryologically, the kidneys originate as distinct lobules that fuse together as they develop. With fetal lobulations there is incomplete fusion of the developing renal lobules. Like the dromedary hump, fetal lobulations can be worrisome for a renal mass, and color or power Doppler should be used to document normal parenchymal flow.

Junctional Parenchymal Defect

A junctional parenchymal defect produces a hyperechoic, wedge-shaped defect that extends from the capsule to the renal sinus, near the junction of the upper and middle poles usually in the right kidney (Fig. 9.24), although they have been reported to be seen posteriorly in the lower pole of the right and left kidneys. The defect is the extension of sinus fat into the cortex as a result of partial fusion of two embryonic parenchymatous masses called renunculi. The defects occur at the junction of the renunculi, which is where the term junctional parenchymal defect comes from. They should not be mistaken for renal scars.

Extrarenal Pelvis

An extrarenal pelvis is an anatomic variant when part of the renal pelvis is located outside the renal hilum. It appears dilated as opposed to the normal intrarenal pelvis, which is surrounded by sinus fat that

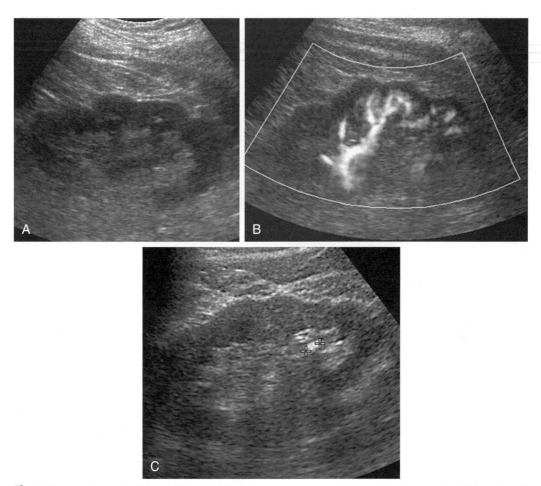

Fig. 9.23 A, An image of a kidney with fetal lobulations. **B,** A power Doppler image showing normal renal flow through the "bumpy" areas of the kidney. **C,** Another example of a kidney with fetal lobulations. This patient also has a small kidney stone seen between the cursors. The fetal lobulation was discovered while scanning the patient to evaluate for kidney stones based on the patient's history.

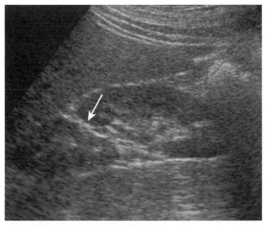

Fig. 9.24 The *arrow* is pointing to an echogenic line that represents a junctional parenchymal defect.

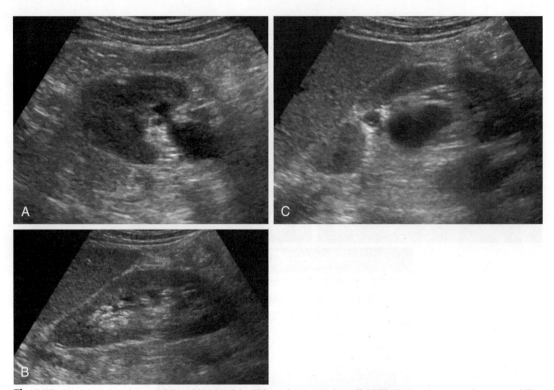

Fig. 9.25 A, A transverse image of the mid-pole of the kidney demonstrating a fluid filled structure. **B,** An image at midline of the same kidney. **C,** An image angled medially showing the fluid-filled structure compatible with an extrarenal pelvis. Good documentation is needed so as not to mistake the fluid as mild hydronephrosis.

helps keep it compressed. An extrarenal pelvis is asymptomatic and usually an incidental finding. An extrarenal pelvis is best appreciated in a transverse image of the kidney (Fig. 9.25). A midline longitudinal image will show a normal-looking kidney. When the transducer is aimed at the lateral portion of the kidney, it will also appear normal. However, when the transducer is aimed at the medial portion of the kidney some fluid will be seen in the area of the renal pelvis. Sonography will demonstrate a central cystic area lying partially or entirely outside of the renal pelvis on a transverse mid-pole image. In transverse images the upper and lower poles will appear normal. Care should be taken not to mistake an extrarenal pelvis for hydronephrosis by noting lack of dilated calyces, parenchymal thinning, or hydroureter. With a normal midline image that does not show any fluid or dilatation, mistaking an extra renal pelvis for hydronephrosis should not be too difficult.

Duplication of the Collecting System
Duplication of the collecting system, also known as a duplex collecting system, is one of the most common congenital renal abnormalities. It is an anatomic variation of the ureter and pyelocaliceal

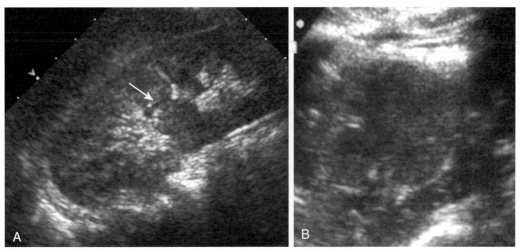

Fig. 9.26 A, The *arrow* is pointing to the break between the two poles in a kidney with a duplicated collecting system. **B,** A transverse image through the area of the *arrow* that demonstrates only normal parenchymal tissue and no central sinus echoes.

system, can be unilateral or bilateral, and is found more frequently in women. A duplicated collecting system can be associated with a variety of other congenital abnormalities of the urinary and genital systems, such as a didelphic uterus in women. On sonography a duplicated collecting system appears as two separate and distinct collecting systems, separated by normal parenchymal tissue. The kidney is larger than normal, usually greater than 13 to 14 cm in length. Transverse scans will confirm this anomaly by observing the disappearance and reappearance of the renal sinus echoes while scanning from the upper to the lower poles (Fig. 9.26). A prominent column of Bertin may mimic a duplicated collecting system but will display continual renal sinus echoes, although they may be thin, as well as a normal renal length.

A duplicated collecting system is characterized by an incomplete fusion of the upper and lower poles, which are separated by renal parenchyma. This results in a variety of complete or incomplete duplications of the collecting system. The variations can include duplication of the renal pelvis with a bifid ureter where the two ureters unite before emptying into the bladder or two separate ureters that drain independently into the bladder. Most duplicated systems are asymptomatic with no issues with renal function and are incidental findings. Symptomatic patients can present with infection, reflux, or obstruction. Any complications are usually related to abnormal implantation of one or both ureters and can include the upper pole ureter, forming a ureterocele in the bladder (Fig. 9.27) that leads to obstructive hydronephrosis and renal dysplasia, with the lower pole ureter having a short intravesical segment that results in vesicoureteral reflux.

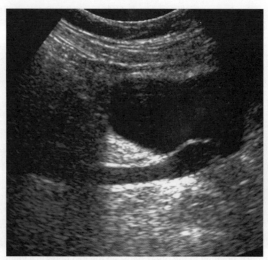

Fig. 9.27 A patient with a duplicated collecting system with a ureterocele from the upper pole ureter.

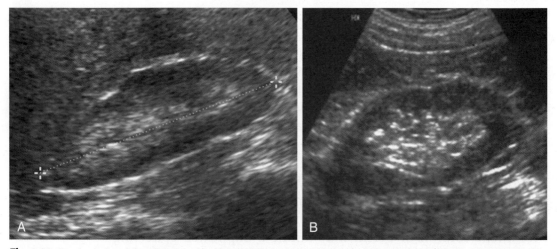

Fig. 9.28 Two examples of sinus lipomatosis. Although there appears to be cortical thinning, the kidney function is normal.

Sinus Lipomatosis

Renal sinus lipomatosis refers to a condition in which there is excessive fat in the renal sinus, often seen as an enlarged echogenic central sinus with what appears to be cortical thinning (Fig. 9.28). There is a benign proliferation of central fat in the renal sinus that is considered characteristic. It usually is seen in the sixth and seventh decade and occurs with advanced age, obesity, and exposure to corticosteroids. Renal sinus lipomatosis has no clinical significance and is usually found incidentally.

Vascular Variants

Multiple (accessory, supernumerary) renal arteries can occur in 10% to 30% of the population, either unilaterally (Fig. 9.29) or bilaterally.

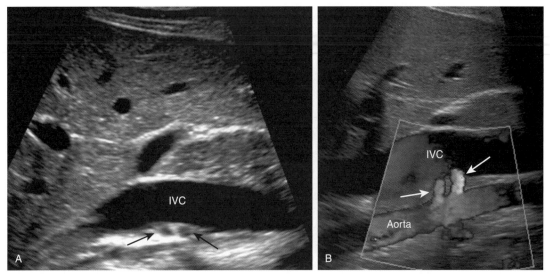

Fig. 9.29 A, A longitudinal image through the inferior vena cava (IVC) with the *arrows* pointing to two right renal arteries. This is a great view to help document the number of renal arteries if they are close together. **B,** This image was obtained from a coronal plane in which the transducer was placed along the side of the patient and manipulated until the aorta and IVC are in the same plane. The *arrows* are pointing to two right renal arteries.

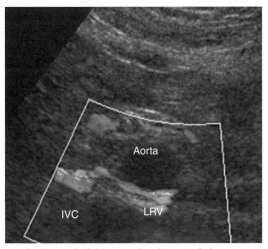

Fig. 9.30 A power Doppler image of a left retroaortic vein. *IVC,* Inferior vena cava; *LRV,* left renal vein.

These accessory renal arteries may be difficult to locate because they can originate from the aorta above or below the main artery, iliac artery, and SMA, among other locations. They are more common on the left.

Renal vein variants can occur in from 2% to 40% of the population. Variants include multiple renal veins, a retroaortic left renal vein, in which the vein goes under the aorta as opposed to over (Fig. 9.30), and a circumaortic left renal vein, in which an accessory

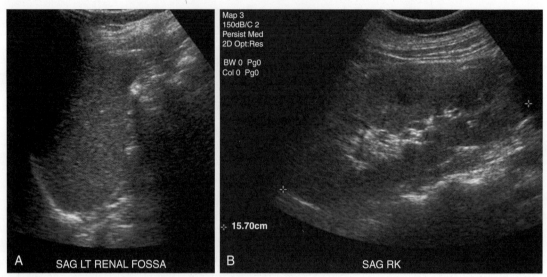

Fig. 9.31 **A,** An image of the spleen in the area of the left kidney, which is not seen. **B,** This is the same patient showing a right kidney that has hypertrophied to compensate for doing the work of two kidneys.

left renal vein passes posterior to the aorta as the normal left renal vein passes anterior to the aorta.

Renal Anomalies

Renal anomalies are different from normal variants, with the kidney shape usually normal but the kidney is in the wrong location or missing.

Renal Agenesis

Renal agenesis is the failure of a kidney and ureter to develop and is seen more commonly in males. Unilateral renal agenesis causes hypertrophy, or enlargement, of the contralateral kidney (Fig. 9.31). Bilateral renal agenesis is usually detected *in utero* and is usually incompatible with life. Ultrasound was not widely available 40 to 50 years ago, and it is thought that people with only one kidney were born with a multicystic dysplastic kidney (MCDK) that regressed because MCDK is more common than renal agenesis. Patients with renal agenesis can have other genitourinary anomalies. For example, a man might have ipsilateral seminal vesicle agenesis (Fig. 9.32) and women may have uterine malformations. It will be helpful for patients to know that they have only one kidney. When performing a pelvic or prostate ultrasound and an anomaly is seen, the sonographer might take one longitudinal image of each kidney to document the presence of both kidneys or the absence of one kidney.

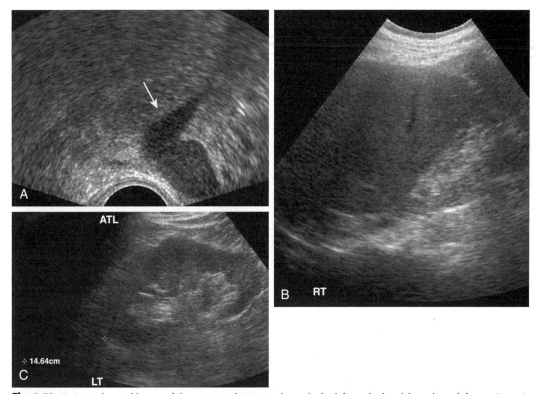

Fig. 9.32 A, An endorectal image of the prostate demonstrating only the left seminal vesicle and vas deferens *(arrow).* **B,** The same patient showing the absence of a right kidney compatible with the ipsilateral missing seminal vesicles. **C,** The same patient showing a hypertrophied left kidney that also has a dromedary hump.

Ectopic Kidney

An ectopic kidney, or renal ectopia, is when a kidney does not completely ascend to its usual position in the upper abdomen. During fetal development, the kidneys first appear as buds in the pelvic area near the bladder. As the fetal kidneys continue to develop, they ascend gradually toward their normal position in the retroperitoneum. Sometimes, one of the kidneys fails to completely ascend and may stop anywhere along the path or it may remain in the pelvis. Failure to visualize a kidney in the renal fossa should prompt a search in the pelvic area. Pelvic kidneys can be felt as a pelvic mass, and the patient may be referred for a pelvic sonogram (Fig. 9.33). Pelvic kidneys also have a higher incidence of infection. In most cases, people with an ectopic kidney have no complaints and it is an incidental finding. In other cases, the ectopic kidney may create urinary problems, such as urine blockage, infection, or urinary stones.

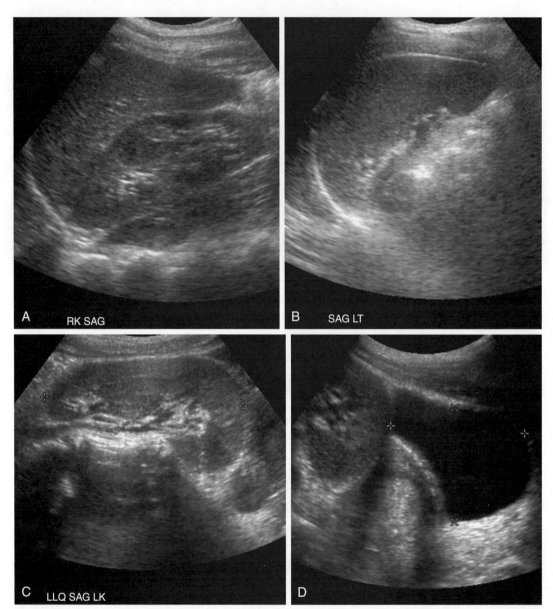

Fig. 9.33 **A,** A right kidney that is normal in length. **B,** The same patient with an image of the left upper quadrant that only shows the spleen. **C,** Because the right kidney was normal in length, a search for the left kidney was initiated. The kidney was found in the left lower quadrant. **D,** The same patient showing the left kidney superior to the bladder.

SCANNING TIP When only one kidney is found, there is a clue to know if there is just one kidney or if there is an ectopic kidney. Remember that if there is only one functioning kidney, that kidney will become bigger to compensate for doing the work of both kidneys. If the found kidney is normal in size, that means that there is another kidney somewhere and an effort should be made to find its location.

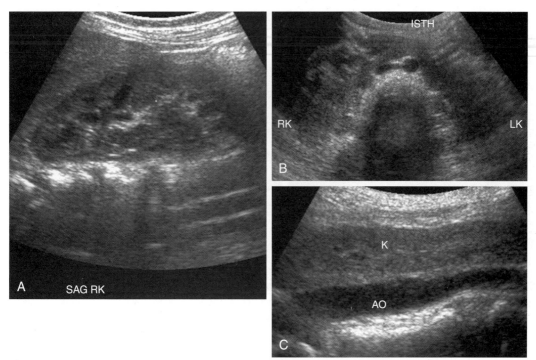

Fig. 9.34 A, A longitudinal image of the right kidney in a patient with a horseshoe kidney. Because there is no lower pole, the lower pole is not appreciated. **B,** A transverse image of the isthmus *(ISTH)* and kidneys *(K)*. **C,** A longitudinal image of the aorta *(AO)* showing the isthmus. The pulsations of the aorta are passed through the isthmus to the skin surface, creating the suspicion that the patient has an abdominal aortic aneurysm.

Fusion Abnormalities

The two main types of fusion abnormalities of the kidney are horseshoe kidney and crossed fused ectopia, which is when both kidneys are on the same side of the body.

Horseshoe Kidneys

A horseshoe kidney is the most common type of renal fusion anomaly. It consists of two distinct functioning kidneys on either side of the midline, connected at their lower poles, or rarely at their upper poles, by an isthmus of functioning renal parenchyma that crosses the midline of the body anterior to the great vessels (Fig. 9.34). The inferior mesenteric artery stops the ascent of the kidneys, causing them to stop just superior to the umbilicus. Usually the kidneys are closer to midline, and patients may be referred for ultrasound evaluation of a pulsatile abdominal mass with a request to look for an abdominal aortic aneurysm (AAA). It is more common in men, often asymptomatic, and usually diagnosed incidentally. Because these kidneys are "out in the open" and not protected by the ribs or fat layers, they are more prone to injury. It is recommended that patients with horseshoe kidneys refrain from playing rough contact sports.

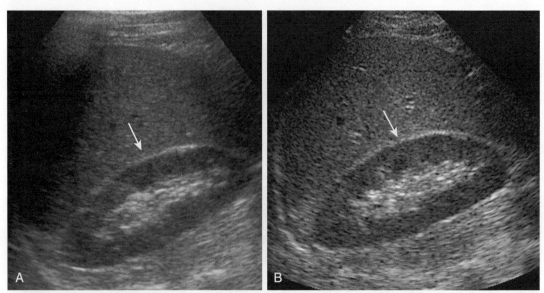

Fig. 9.35 A, The right kidney using a curved linear array transducer. **B,** The same kidney using a vector array transducer. Note the lack of rib shadowing; however, because the transducer is a lower frequency, the resolution is not as good as the higher-frequency curved linear array transducer. The *arrows* are both pointing to the kidney capsule.

Crossed Ectopia

An ectopic kidney may cross over the midline and become fused with the contralateral kidney on the same side of the body. When a crossover does occur, the two kidneys grow together and may become fused. This is called crossed renal ectopia. Patients are most often asymptomatic. A left-to-right crossing is more common, and there is a male predilection with a 2:1 male-to-female ratio. Ectopic kidneys are also prone to traumatic injury because of their abnormal location in the lower abdomen or pelvis.

Ultrasound of the Kidneys

Patient Prep

No patient preparation is needed for a renal sonogram. If the bladder needs to be imaged, it must contain urine and the patient should drink 8–16 oz of fluid about 30 minutes before the examination.

Transducer

The most common transducer to use is a 5–2 MHz curved linear array. A sector/vector transducer may be needed to allow intercostal access as needed (Fig. 9.35). For pediatric patients, especially a newborn, a high-frequency sector array may be used to get between the ribs. If scanning with the patient in the prone position, a curved linear array is preferred.

Breathing Technique

The patient is scanned subcostally in deep inspiration or intercostally with the patient in quiet breathing, full or partial inspiration,

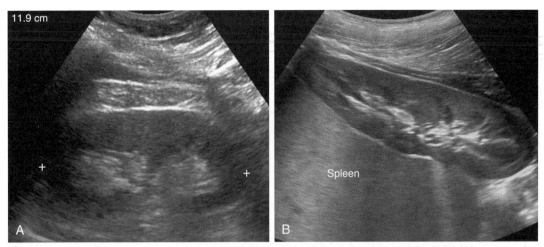

Fig. 9.36 A, The left kidney scanned with the patient in the prone position. **B,** Another example of a left kidney scanned from the prone position that is also visualizing the spleen. (*A,* Courtesy Jeanine and Aubrey Rybynski.)

or expiration. For some patients a combination of techniques may be needed. For example, to see the upper pole of the kidney an intercostal approach with the patient in expiration is used and the mid to lower pole is seen best with the patient in deep inspiration.

Patient Position

Patients are scanned starting in the supine position using the liver and spleen as acoustic windows to obtain the required longitudinal and transverse images. Images will be obtained from an intercostal and/or subcostal approach. If the kidneys are not adequately visualized, right or left posterior oblique positions and right or left lateral decubitus views can be used with scanning performed along the side of the patient or by approaching the kidneys from the patient's back. It may take scanning the patient in a variety of positions to properly evaluate the entire kidney. If the kidneys are still not optimally seen, scanning the kidneys with the patient in the prone position (Fig. 9.36) often can adequately visualize them, especially for length measurements. If the patient cannot lie on their stomach have them roll into a decubitis position and scan with the transducer in their mid back as if scanning them prone.

Technical Tips

In my opinion, kidney ultrasound scans can be easy or a challenge. Do not prejudge image quality based on the size of the patient. Very thin patients may be more difficult to scan, and larger patients may be easier because the excess fat can move the kidney more inferior and can be used as an acoustic window. If you have a unit that can scan in two planes simultaneously, the kidneys are a good organ for using this feature (Fig. 9.37). Scanning the kidneys may involve scanning the patient

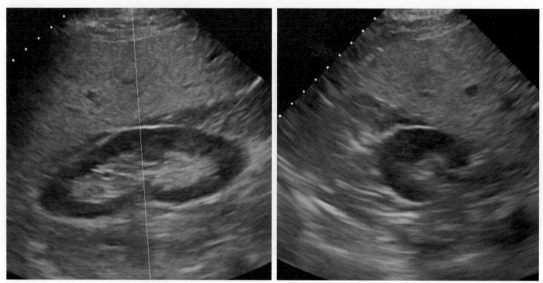

Fig. 9.37 A transducer that can scan in a longitudinal and transverse plane simultaneously. The cursor in the longitudinal plane is where the transverse plane was obtained.

using different breathing techniques, various patient positions, and different transducers. This may require some patience on the part of the patient to perform a complete examination. Renal size is very important for the care of some patients; therefore, make sure that both poles of the kidney are well seen, there is equal cortical thickness, and the kidney is in a true long-axis orientation. Check the measurements of both kidneys and ensure they make sense. If not, repeat the measurements. There are times in which it may be very difficult to see both poles clearly. With these patients, follow the contour of the kidney and imagine where the border should be. Just remember the shape of the kidney, and it can be easy to extrapolate where the end of the kidney should be. It may not be an exact measurement, but should be very close. This is where trying to turn the patient into different positions, including prone, can help. As a sonographer, it is very important to know your machine and how to optimize an image. Look at each image and decide if it needs adjusting. Do not scan with "one size fits all." For example, most machines default to a harmonic setting, and although that may be good for most patients, there will be times when it is best to turn it on and off to see how the harmonic setting affects the image. When you notice that there is a lot of noise in the far field or lack of echoes in the posterior kidney, turn harmonics off to see if that helps. Remember that harmonics is using a higher frequency, which will have increased attenuation (Fig. 9.38).

Renal Required Images

Thorough longitudinal and transverse images should be obtained of each kidney to evaluate for size, contour, echogenicity, and presence or absence of stones, masses, cysts, or hydronephrosis. Images of the liver and right

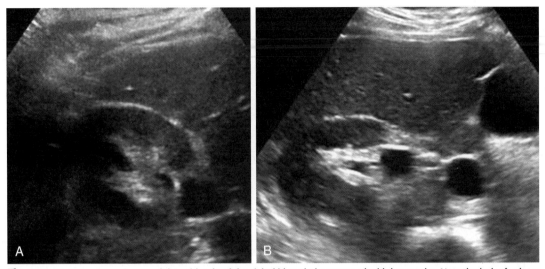

Fig. 9.38 A, A transverse image of the mid-pole of the right kidney being scanned with harmonics. Note the lack of echoes in the posterior aspect of the kidney. **B,** The same patient scanned with harmonics turned off, allowing better penetration of the far field.

kidney and spleen and left kidney should be documented to compare echogenicity. These comparison images need to show both organs on the same image. If this is not possible, the organs need to be compared at the same depth with identical machine settings, that is, TGC, gain, and focal zones. The normal renal cortex should be less echogenic than the normal adjacent liver or spleen. The right kidney may be isoechoic to the liver, which is considered normal. If the kidney cortex is more echogenic than the liver or spleen, this is considered abnormal and medical renal disease is suspected; therefore, it is important to verify that the liver and spleen are normal in echogenicity. For example, if the patient has hepatitis, the kidney will be more echogenic. This is due to the fact that the liver is less echogenic than normal and the overall gain is increased to fill in the echoes of the liver, thus causing the renal echoes to be more echogenic than the liver. However, only the liver is abnormal (Fig. 9.39). The kidneys in a neonate are very echogenic, and the cortex may be as echogenic as the sinus echoes. Around 6 months of age the kidneys should have their normal sonographic appearance and be less echogenic than the liver and spleen. The medullary pyramids are hypoechoic to the cortex. This difference is more pronounced in neonates. When measuring the length of the kidney, it is acceptable to have a rib shadow though the kidney (Fig. 9.40). The goal is to see both ends of the kidney, and the area of the rib shadow would be investigated on another image.

When to Include Bladder Images
If hydronephrosis is detected, the bladder should be scanned to see if it is too full, causing the hydronephrosis. After the bladder is emptied, the kidneys should then be rescanned to evaluate the change in the hydronephrosis, which may disappear.

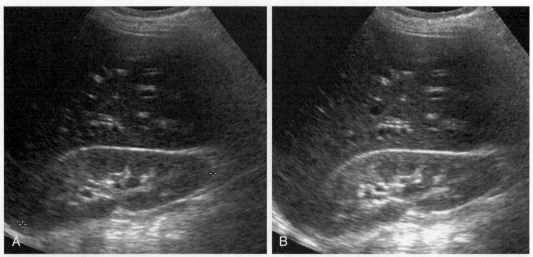

Fig. 9.39 A, A patient with hepatitis. Note how dark the liver is. **B,** The same patient with the overall gain increased to fill in the liver. The kidney is more echogenic than the liver; however, it is not due to medical renal disease because the kidney is normal, but rather to the decreased echogenicity of the liver resulting from inflammation from the hepatitis. This can be confirmed by an image documenting a normal left kidney and spleen relationship.

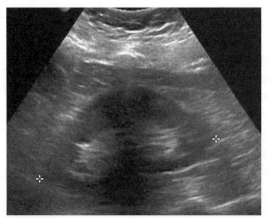

Fig. 9.40 An image of the left kidney with a rib shadow through the middle of the kidney so that both poles can be clearly seen.

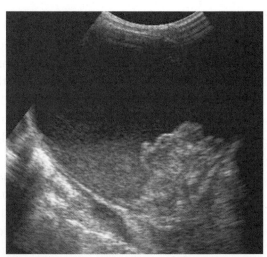

Fig. 9.41 A patient with hematuria. The kidneys only demonstrated medical renal disease, but because of the patient having hematuria, a scan of the bladder was performed. A blood clot was found in the bladder that was probably caused by a recent renal biopsy.

If hematuria is present, longitudinal and transverse images of the bladder should be obtained to evaluate for the presence of stones, clots, tumors, or bladder wall thickening (Fig. 9.41).

If there are kidney stones, color Doppler should be used to evaluate the bladder for ureteral jets. These jets appear as a sudden burst of color and last a few seconds. Normal ureteral jets should occur twice or more per minute and course anteromedially from the trigone, crossing the midline (Fig. 9.42). Weak jets or a constant color

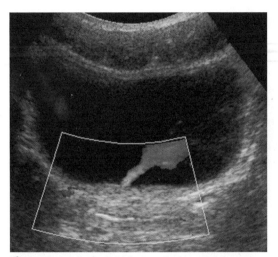

Fig. 9.42 A color Doppler image of a normal right ureter jet.

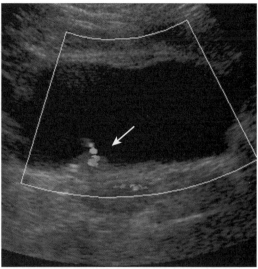

Fig. 9.43 A color Doppler image showing a very weak ureteral jet from a nonobstructed stone *(arrow)* near the ureterovesical junction (VUJ).

that "dribbles" out of the ureteral orifice is suggestive of a nonobstructive stone (Fig. 9.43). If no color is seen, this is suggestive of an obstruction.

When to Include Doppler Images

Some departments might require Doppler information for the following scenarios:

1. The main renal artery and vein at the hilum to assess inflow and outflow in all patients as needed per protocol. Some clinicians just want to know that there is flow to the kidney and flow leaving the kidney (Fig. 9.44).

2. A resistive index (RI) measurement from the segmental or interlobar arteries in patients with hydronephrosis. An increased RI is thought to be due to increased vascular resistance as a result of increases in collecting system pressures.

3. RI measurement from the segmental or interlobar arteries in patients with medical renal disease.

4. RI measurement from the segmental or interlobar arteries in patients with hypertension not caused by renal artery stenosis (Fig. 9.45).

5. A color or power Doppler image showing perfusion in patients with acute kidney injury (AKI) or chronic kidney disease (CKD) looking to evaluate perfusion out to the capsule (Fig. 9.46).

6. A color or power Doppler image showing perfusion in patients with suspected pyelonephritis looking for areas of flow voids that might be caused by early abscess formation (Fig. 9.47).

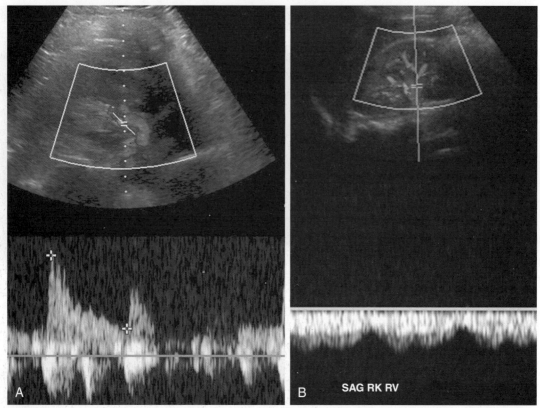

Fig. 9.44 **A,** A normal signal from the main renal artery at the renal hilum. **B,** A normal signal from the main renal vein at the renal hilum.

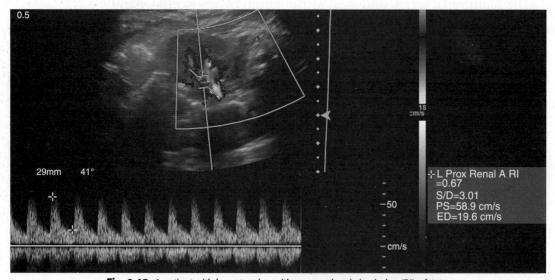

Fig. 9.45 A patient with hypertension with a normal resistive index (RI) of 0.67.

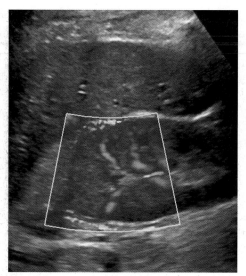

Fig. 9.46 Decreased perfusion of a kidney with acute kidney injury.

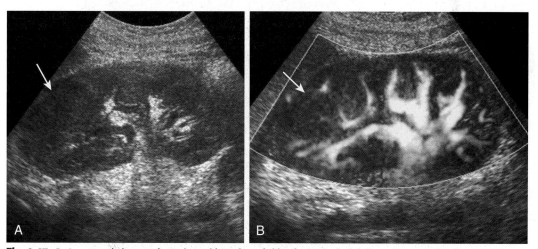

Fig. 9.47 A, A gray-scale image of a patient with pyelonephritis. The *arrow* is pointing to an area of concern. **B,** A power Doppler image shows lack of normal flow compatible with acute focal nephritis.

7. A color or power Doppler image showing perfusion in areas that are suspicious for a renal mass, such as patients with a dromedary hump or fetal lobulations, showing normal perfusion flow or abnormal flow pattern with true masses (Fig. 9.48).
8. Color Doppler can be helpful in identifying small stones because it produces an artifact called the "twinkling" artifact. It is caused by the calcium in the stone (Fig. 9.49). Any uncertain bright echoes should be investigated with color Doppler to see if the twinkling artifact occurs.

The RI is calculated by the ultrasound unit. The equation is peak systole – end diastole/peak systole. The normal kidney should have

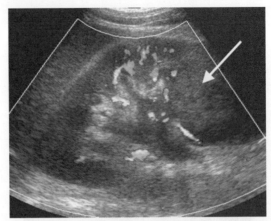

Fig. 9.48 A patient with a renal cell carcinoma in the lower pole. Note the flow around the mass (arrow) but not normal flow in the mass itself. The renal vein is also dilated and filled with echoes compatible with tumor extension into the renal vein.

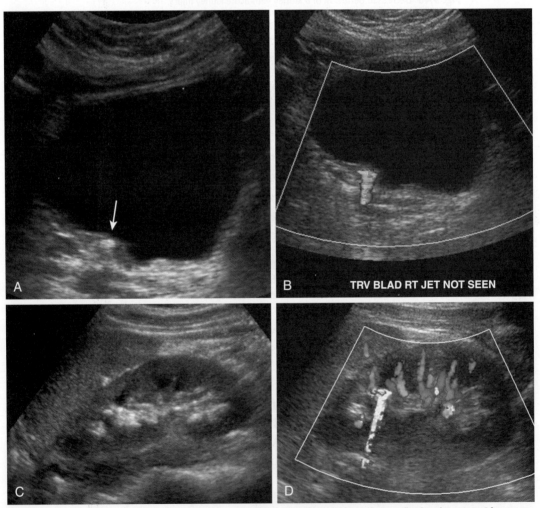

TRV BLAD RT JET NOT SEEN

Fig. 9.49 A, A possible stone (arrow) at the ureterovesical junction. **B,** Twinkle artifact confirming the stone. Of note was a ureteral jet was not seen compatible with complete obstruction. **C,** A kidney with scattered echogenic foci. **D,** The color Doppler twinkling artifact identifies a stone in the upper pole.

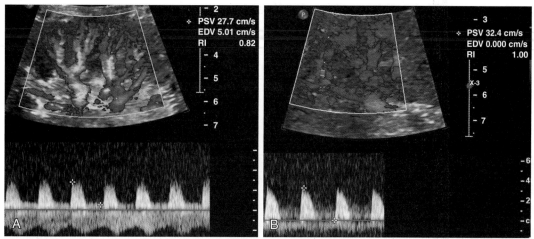

Fig. 9.50 A, The sonographer measured mirror artifact for the end-diastolic value. Note that the intensity of the diastolic flow is similar to that of the venous flow below the baseline. This gave an RI of 0.82. **B,** By observing that the arterial flow totally went away during diastole, the sonographer realized that the flow seen during the diastolic cycle was not arterial flow and that there was no flow at the end of the diastolic cycle; therefore, the correct RI is 1.0.

an RI between 0.6 and 0.7. An RI greater than 0.8 is suggestive of increased vascular pressure, resistance, or compliance inside the kidney. It is not specific for a specific disease. It is important to properly measure the signal. Many sonographers mistake noise and mirror artifact for diastolic flow (Fig. 9.50). Color Doppler is the key to helping determine the RI. If the color is flashing—that is, the arterial flow completely disappears in diastole—the RI is 1. If the arterial flow almost disappears, the RI value will be greater than 0.8. If the arterial flow is preserved and well seen during diastole, the RI is less than 0.7. It is also important to measure at the end of the diastolic cycle, right before the next systolic upstroke, not where the diastolic flow ends.

The required images are a small representation of what a sonographer visualizes during a study. Therefore, the images should be technically accurate to provide the interpreting physician the information to make a correct diagnosis. Any pathologic area must be documented in at least two planes and can be documented on a split screen. Some departments may require a video clip through each kidney.

Right Kidney • Longitudinal Images

1. Long axis of the kidney at midline demonstrating the longest length of the kidney with and without length measurements. Some departments may perform renal volumes and require all three measurements; therefore, the AP measurement will be included with this image.

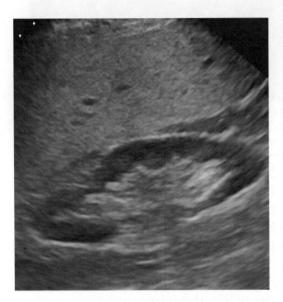 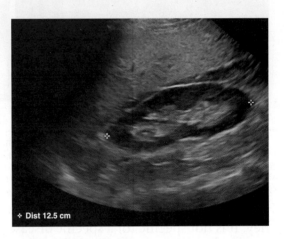

Suggested annotation: **RT KID MID**

2. Long axis of the kidney through the lateral aspect.

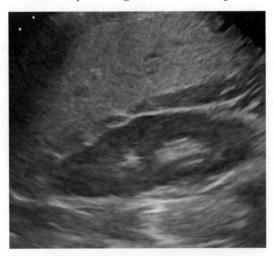

Suggested annotation: **RT KID LAT**

3. Long axis of the kidney through the medial aspect.

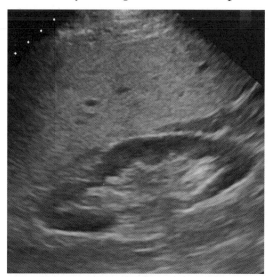

Suggested annotation: **RT KID MED**

4. Long axis of the kidney demonstrating the liver and kidney together for parenchymal comparison.

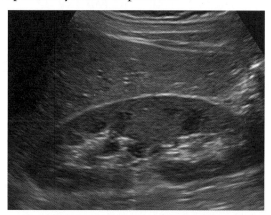

Suggested annotation: **RT KID/LIVER**

Right Kidney • Transverse Images

1. Transverse image of the upper pole of the right kidney.

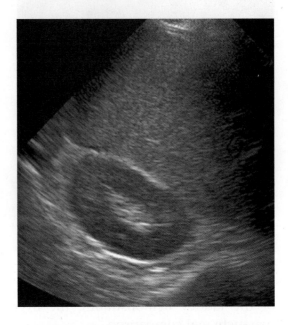

Suggested annotation: **RT KID TRV UP**

2. Transverse image of the mid-pole of the right kidney. If needed, the transverse measurement of the kidney would also be obtained at this level.

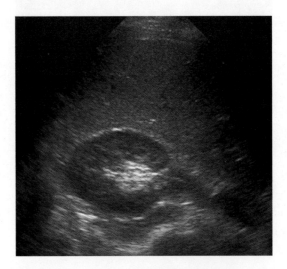

Suggested annotation: **RT KID TRV MID**

3. Transverse image of the lower pole of the right kidney.

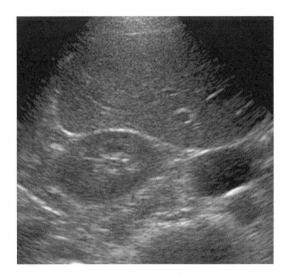

Suggested annotation: **RT KID TRV LOW**

Left Kidney • Longitudinal Images

1. Long axis of the kidney at midline demonstrating the longest length of the kidney with and without length measurements. Some departments may perform renal volumes and require all three measurements; therefore, the AP measurement will be included with this image.

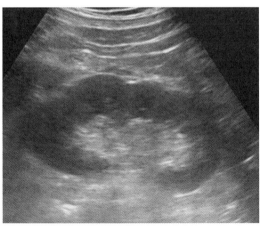

Courtesy Ted Whitten.

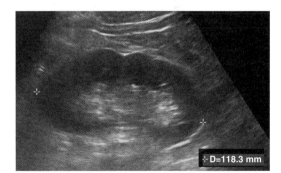

Courtesy Ted Whitten.

Suggested annotation: **LT KID MID**

2. Long axis of the kidney through the lateral aspect.

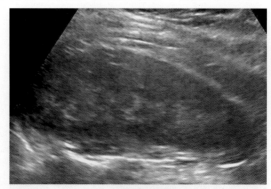

Courtesy Liz Ladrido.

Suggested annotation: **LT KID LAT**

3. Long axis of the kidney through the medial aspect.

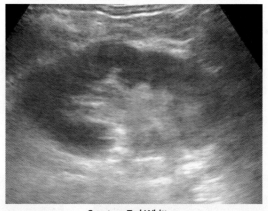

Courtesy Ted Whitten.

Suggested annotation: **LT KID MED**

4. Long axis of the kidney demonstrating the spleen and kidney together for parenchymal comparison.

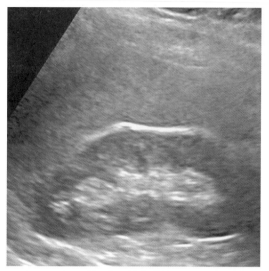

Courtesy Liz Ladrido.

Suggested annotation: **LT KID/SPLEEN**

Left Kidney • Transverse Images

1. Transverse image of the upper pole of the left kidney.

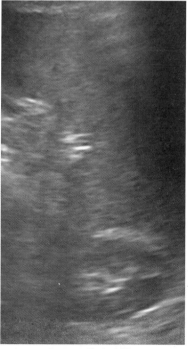

Courtesy Liz Ladrido.

Suggested annotation: **LT KID TRV UP**

2. Transverse image of the mid-pole of the left kidney. If needed, the transverse measurement of the kidney would also be obtained at this level.

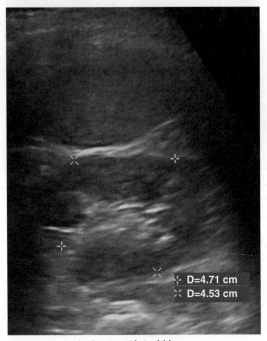

Courtesy Liz Ladrido.

Suggested annotation: **LT KID TRV MID**

3. Transverse image of the lower pole of the left kidney.

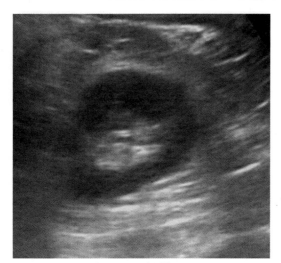

Courtesy Ted Whitten.

Suggested annotation: **LT KID TRV LOW**

Required Images When the Kidneys May Need To Be Evaluated From Other Protocols

When performing a right upper quadrant (RUQ) or liver ultrasound examination, the right kidney will be "in the way" and there will be images of the right kidney included. Some departments may require a dedicated long axis of the right kidney with a length measurement and a transverse image through the mid-pole.

When performing an ultrasound examination of the spleen, the left kidney will be "in the way" and there will be images of the left kidney included. Some departments may require a dedicated long axis of the left kidney with a length measurement and a transverse image through the mid-pole.

If an abnormality is seen in one kidney, images of the contralateral kidney may be required unless a full renal ultrasound examination will be ordered.

If a retroperitoneal, abdominal, or pelvic mass, including uterine fibroids, is discovered, an image of each kidney is obtained to look for hydronephrosis.

Remember that the ureters can be compressed anywhere along their route, causing a blockage.

1. A woman in her third trimester with right flank pain. Ultrasound demonstrated hydronephrosis of the right kidney. The left kidney was normal.

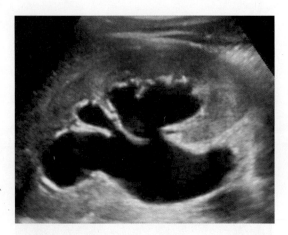

Patients who are pregnant, especially with back or flank pain, may have an image of the kidneys to evaluate for hydronephrosis. Some departments may routinely take an image of each kidney during the third trimester.

Men with an enlarged prostate should have their kidneys evaluated for hydronephrosis.

2. A man with an enlarged prostate gland that had bilateral hydronephrosis.

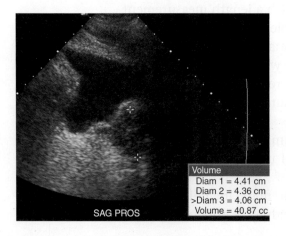

Volume
Diam 1 = 4.41 cm
Diam 2 = 4.36 cm
>Diam 3 = 4.06 cm
Volume = 40.87 cc

SAG PROS

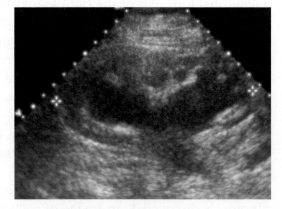

Patients with a AAA or aortic or renal artery dissection should have the length of the kidneys measured and a color or power Doppler perfusion shot to demonstrate that the arterial disease is not affecting flow to the kidney. For patients who have a dissection, a small video clip works best to document perfusion and the flap. If unable to record a video clip, take two or three images during different parts of the cardiac cycle or observe the flow and document when it is abnormal.

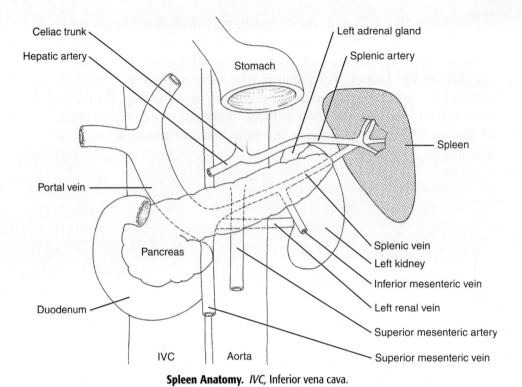

Spleen Anatomy. *IVC,* Inferior vena cava.

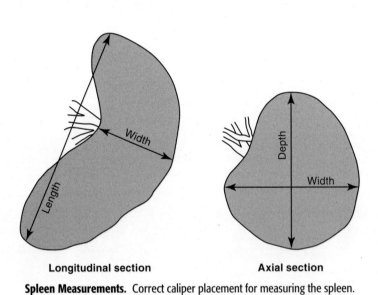

Longitudinal section   **Axial section**

Spleen Measurements. Correct caliper placement for measuring the spleen.

CHAPTER 10

Spleen Scanning Protocol

M. Robert DeJong

Keywords

Accessory spleen	Portal vein
Asplenia	Splenic artery
Infarct	Splenic hilum
Intraperitoneal	Splenic vein
Lymphatic tissue	

Objectives

At the end of this chapter, you will be able to:

- Define the keywords.
- Describe the sonographic appearance of the spleen.
- Describe the transducer options for scanning the spleen.
- List the suggested patient positions when scanning the spleen.
- List normal variants of the spleen.
- Explain the order and exact locations to take representative images of the spleen.

Overview

Splenic ultrasounds are usually performed in the radiology department. A dedicated ultrasound of the spleen is not commonly ordered, with the most common reason being to evaluate the size of the spleen (Fig. 10.1). The spleen is the organ most commonly injured in blunt abdominal trauma (Fig. 10.2), and these patients are usually referred for a computed tomography (CT) scan. Masses in the spleen are rare, and metastases are uncommon and usually occur by hematogenous spread. The spleen is rarely the primary site of disease but is often affected by systemic disease processes such as sickle cell disease, mononucleosis, and portal hypertension. Therefore, the spleen might be included in evaluations of other organs, especially if a pathologic condition is found that could have an impact on the spleen.

Anatomy

The spleen is a very vascular organ and is the largest single mass of lymphoid tissue. It is located in the left hypochondrium, posterolateral to the stomach, lateral to the tail of the pancreas, posterior to the diaphragm, and anterior to the left kidney. It does not extend

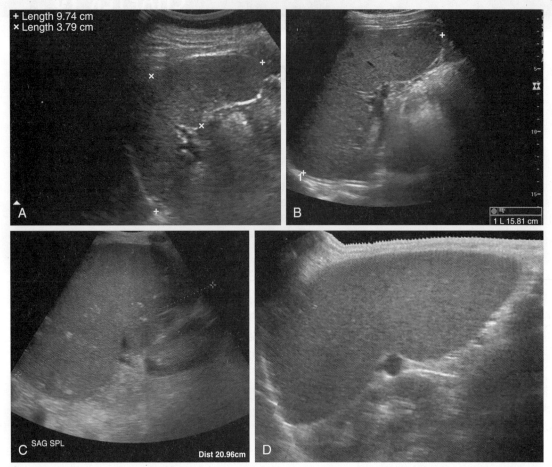

Fig. 10.1 A, An image of a normal spleen measuring the length and anteroposterior dimensions. **B,** The length is being measured on a slightly enlarged spleen. **C,** The spleen is enlarged and cannot fit inside the sector. The inferior tip is estimated. **D,** A very enlarged spleen using the extended field of view feature. The spleen measured almost 26 cm. *SAG SPL,* Sagittal spleen. (Image Courtesy Jeanine and Aubrey Rybynski.)

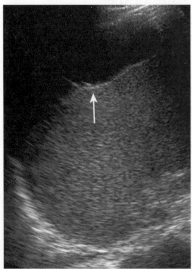

Fig. 10.2 A subcapsular hematoma in a patient who was in an automobile accident. The *arrow* is pointing to the hematoma.

past the left costal margin and cannot normally be palpated on clinical examination unless it is enlarged. It is an **intraperitoneal** organ, surrounded by peritoneum except at the hilum, where the splenic vessels enter and exit. The spleen is covered by a weak capsule that protects the organ and allows it to expand in size as needed.

The spleen has a convex superior surface and a concave inferior surface and can be anatomically divided into two regions. The diaphragmatic surface is in contact with the diaphragm and the ribcage, and the visceral surface is in contact with the abdominal organs, including the tail of the pancreas, stomach, splenic flexure, and left kidney. The shape of the spleen is variable, but it is typically described as crescent or ovoid and measures approximately 12 to 13 cm in length and 6 to 7 cm wide. A good way to remember the dimensions of the spleen is the 1 × 3 × 5 × 7 × 9 × 11 rule, as follows:

- The spleen measures approximately 1 × 3 × 5 inches (about 2 × 7 × 12 cm).
- It weighs approximately 7 oz (about 200 g).
- It is located between the 9th and 11th ribs.

The spleen is a highly vascular organ and receives its blood from the **splenic artery**, which is a branch of the celiac trunk. It runs superior to the body and tail of the pancreas to enter the **splenic hilum**, where it divides into five branches. These arterial branches do not anastomose with each other (Fig. 10.3).

The **splenic vein** is formed by the tributaries of the spleen as it exits the spleen at the splenic hilum. The inferior mesenteric vein empties into the splenic vein. The splenic vein also receives blood from the

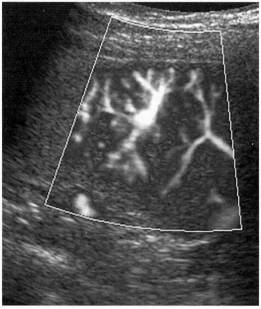

Fig. 10.3 A power Doppler image of the spleen demonstrating normal vascularity. Notice how the intrasplenic arteries do not communicate with one another.

pancreas, stomach, and large intestine. The splenic vein runs along the posterior surface of the pancreas (Fig. 10.4) and joins the superior mesenteric vein behind the neck of the pancreas to form the **portal vein**.

Physiology

The spleen is composed of white and red pulp. The white pulp consists of **lymphatic tissue**, which contains malpighian corpuscles, to produce lymphocytes. The red pulp consists of splenic cords and sinuses that are lined with epithelial cells and are responsible for the destruction of degenerating red blood cells, called phagocytosis. The function of the spleen can be divided into its reticuloendothelial and organ functions. The reticuloendothelial functions include the production of lymphocytes and the storage of iron, and the organ functions include the maturation, storage, and removal of erythrocytes and holding a reserve of blood. The spleen is not essential to life and can be removed if needed.

Sonographic Appearance

Sonographically, the spleen should have a homogeneous medium gray level echo texture. It should be more echogenic than the left kidney and liver (Fig. 10.5). Longitudinal, coronal, and transverse views are obtained to determine size, echo texture, and presence or absence of pathologic conditions. Occasionally, small, bright reflections may be visualized throughout the spleen that represent calcified granulomas (Fig. 10.6). Color or power Doppler will show the vascularity of the spleen (Fig. 10.7). Because the intrasplenic

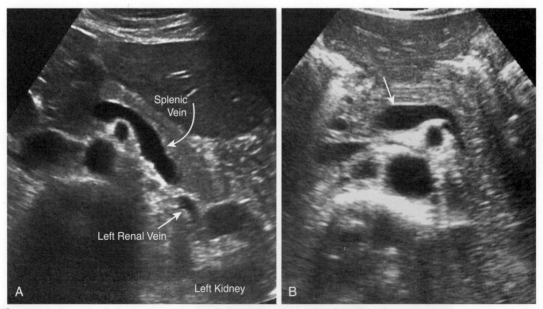

Fig. 10.4 A, The *curved arrow* is pointing to the splenic vein. The *straight arrow* is pointing to the left renal vein. Note how close they are. **B,** The *arrow* is pointing to the portal confluence.

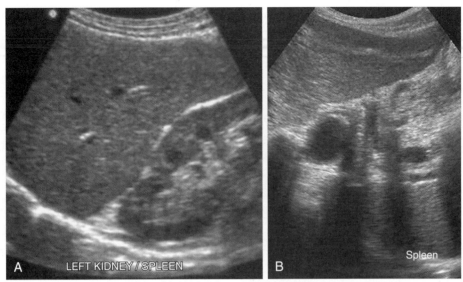

Fig. 10.5 A, Image of the normal relationship of the echogenicity between the spleen and the left kidney. The spleen should be more echogenic than the renal cortex. The renal sinus is the most echogenic structure in the abdomen. **B,** Image of the normal relationship of the echogenicity between the spleen and the liver. The spleen should be more echogenic than the liver.

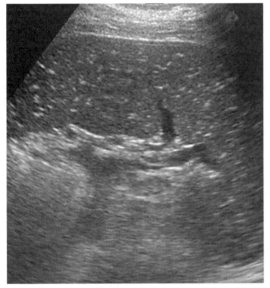

Fig. 10.6 An image of a patient with small echogenic foci scattered throughout the spleen compatible with granulomas from tuberculosis bacterial infection.

arteries do not anastomose with each other (Fig. 10.8), an **infarct** of the spleen will occur with occlusion of a small intrasplenic artery (Fig. 10.9). This may be caused by tumor embolization, leukemia, lymphoma, and bacterial endocarditis. Sonographically, an infarct appears as a wedge-shaped hypoechoic area in the periphery of the spleen (Fig. 10.10) and can be an incidental finding.

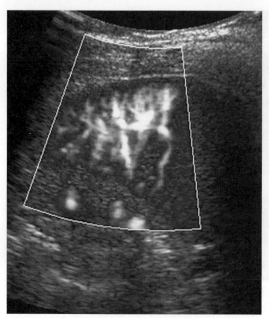

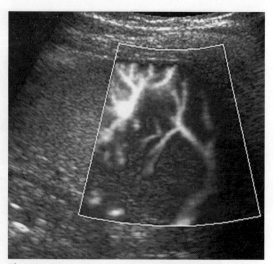

Fig. 10.8 Power Doppler image of the spleen showing normal branching patterns.

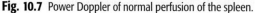

Fig. 10.7 Power Doppler of normal perfusion of the spleen.

Normal Variants

Congenital anomalies of the spleen include but are not limited to shape variations, wandering spleen, polysplenia, **asplenia**, and an accessory spleen, which can be found in about 10% to 15% of the population. An **accessory spleen** is usually located at the splenic hilum and measures less than 1 cm in diameter (Fig. 10.11). It does not cause health problems and is found incidentally on imaging examinations.

Ultrasound of the Spleen

Patient Prep

No patient preparation is needed for a sonogram of the spleen. If the indication is trauma, the patient should be prioritized.

Transducer

The most common transducer used is a 5–2 MHz curved linear array. A sector/vector transducer may be needed to allow intercostal access. For pediatric patients a high-frequency sector array may be needed to image between the ribs.

Breathing Technique

The patient is scanned using an intercostal approach with the patient breathing quietly or in expiration. In some patients the spleen may be adequately seen with the patient in deep inspiration.

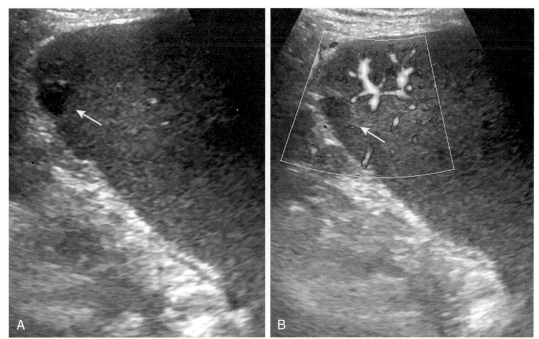

Fig. 10.9 A, The *arrow* is pointing to a small, hypoechoic, triangular area compatible with a splenic infarct. This patient had leukemia. **B,** In the same patient power Doppler demonstrates an absence of flow in the area of the infarct. Compare this flow pattern with that in Fig. 10.7.

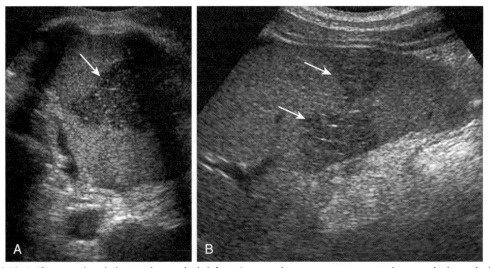

Fig. 10.10   A, The *arrow* is pointing to a large splenic infarct. Because there are no anastomoses between the intrasplenic vessels, the emboli lodged early in the branch, shutting off flow to the spleen from that point to the edge of the spleen. Look at Fig. 10.8 and imagine the embolus is where the vessel touches the *left side of the color box.* All flow from that point on is blocked, causing the tissue to die. That is why the infarcts are triangular, with the base of the triangle along the edge of the spleen. **B,** In this patient the *arrows* are pointing to two splenic infarcts. Patients may have multiple infarcts. Patients with sickle cell disease will have multiple infarcts that can completely infarct the spleen so that the spleen is not seen.

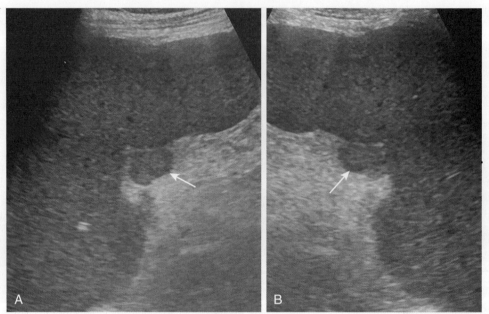

Fig. 10.11 A, A sagittal image of the spleen. The *arrow* is pointing to an accessory spleen. **B,** A transverse image of the same patient in *A* with the *arrow* pointing to an accessory spleen. Note how the accessory spleen has the same echogenicity as the spleen.

Patient Position

Patients are scanned in the supine position with images obtained from an intercostal approach. If the spleen is enlarged, scanning can be from a subcostal approach. If the spleen is not adequately visualized, the patient can be positioned into a left posterior oblique or a right lateral decubitus (RLD) position. Some departments prefer to use the side of the patient that is up so RLD becomes left side up (LSU).

Technical Tips

If a curved linear array transducer is used to evaluate the spleen, care should be taken to evaluate the areas of the spleen obscured by the rib shadow. With the variation in splenic shape, the sonographer needs to pay attention to measuring the spleen correctly.

Spleen Required Images

The required images are a small representation of what a sonographer visualizes during a study. Therefore, the images should be technically accurate to provide the interpreting physician the information to make a correct diagnosis. Any pathologic findings must be documented in at least two planes and can be documented on a split screen. Some departments may require a video clip.

The spleen is small, so not many images are needed to document the entire spleen. Representative images of the spleen should be obtained in longitudinal and transverse planes. An image of the long axis of the spleen is obtained with and without a measurement, and an image that compares the echogenicity of the spleen and left kidney is also obtained. To make sure that there is not a pleural effusion or subdiaphragmatic abscess, an image with the left hemidiaphragm is required. If a splenic volume measurement is needed, an image with the spleen in its widest diameter is obtained with measurements.

The patient should be in a position that allows good visualization of the spleen. The sonographer should pay attention to scan with the patient positioned ergonomically. Some departments may require the patient position in which the images were obtained if the patient was not supine: for example, LSU or RLD SPLEEN LONG AXIS.

Spleen • Longitudinal Images

1. Long-axis image of the spleen with the longest length with and without measurements.

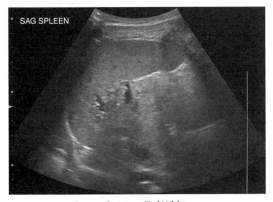

Image Courtesy Ted Whitten.

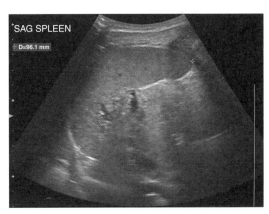

Image Courtesy Ted Whitten.

Suggested annotation: **SPLEEN LONG**

2. Image of spleen and left kidney.

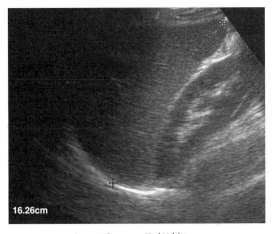

Image Courtesy Ted Whitten.

Suggested annotation: **SPLEEN/LT KID**

3. Additional longitudinal images of the spleen as needed.

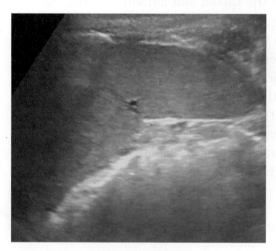

Image Courtesy Ted Whitten.

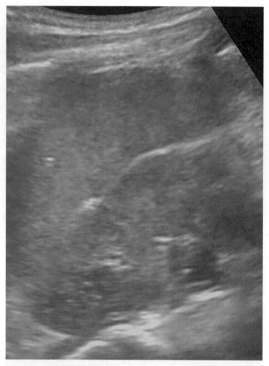

Image Courtesy Ted Whitten.

Suggested annotation: **SPLEEN LONG**

Spleen • Transverse Images

1. Transverse image at the greatest overall dimension with and without a measurement.

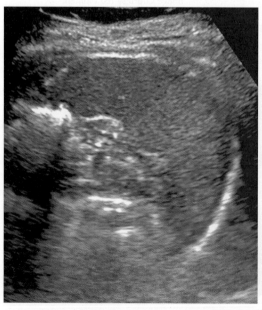

Image Courtesy Jeanine and Aubrey Rybynski.

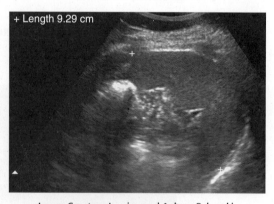

Image Courtesy Jeanine and Aubrey Rybynski.

Suggested annotation: **SPLEEN TRV**

2. If a volume measurement is needed, thickness is measured at the shortest distance between the hilum and the outer surface of the spleen.

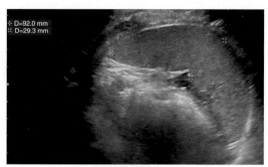

Image Courtesy Ted Whitten.

NOTE: The formula for a prolate ellipsoid, length × width × depth × 0.523, is used to find splenic volume.

3. Additional transverse images as required.

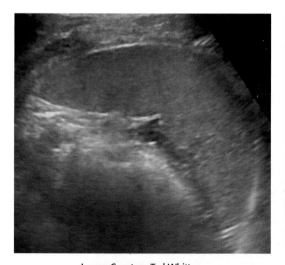

Image Courtesy Ted Whitten.

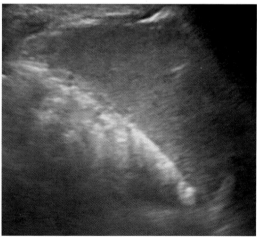

Image Courtesy Ted Whitten.

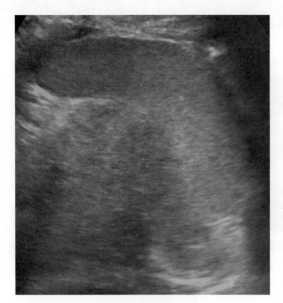

Image Courtesy Ted Whitten.

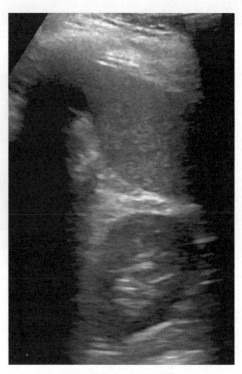

Image Courtesy Liz Ladrido.

Suggested annotation: **SPLEEN TRV**

Required Images When the Spleen Is Part of Another Study

Typically, images of the spleen are needed to evaluate for the size of the spleen; therefore, long-axis and transverse images for size are obtained.

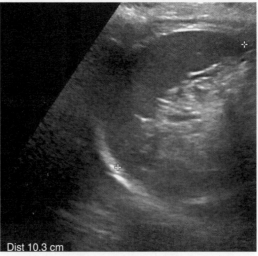

Image Courtesy Liz Ladrido.

Suggested annotation: **SPLEEN LONG**

CHAPTER 11

Image Protocols for Full and Limited Studies of the Abdomen

M. Robert De Jong

Keywords

Ascites	Limited
CPT code	Ordering physician
Complete	RUQ

Objectives

At the end of this chapter, you will be able to:

- Define the keywords.
- Discuss the difference in image requirements between a complete and limited abdominal ultrasound examination.
- List the CPT codes used for a complete and limited abdominal ultrasound examination.
- List the organs and structures that are required to bill for a complete abdominal ultrasound study.
- Discuss how to document when a required structure cannot be seen.

Overview

For an abdominal ultrasound there is the choice of a **complete** abdominal ultrasound or a **limited** abdominal ultrasound. As discussed in Chapter 1, the elements of a complete abdominal ultrasound are defined in the Current Procedural Terminology (CPT) code book. **CPT codes** are universal 5-digit codes that are sent by the billing department to the insurance company for payment. No matter where you work, the same code is sent by your billing department to the insurance company. To bill for a complete abdominal ultrasound, CPT 76700, the following organs need to be documented: the liver, gallbladder, common bile duct, pancreas, spleen, kidneys, upper abdominal aorta, and inferior vena cava. If particular elements cannot be visualized, the reason should be documented: for example, an image of the area of the pancreas showing that the pancreas is obscured by gas. If an organ is missing because of surgery or a congenital anomaly, that should be noted on the image where the organ should be. For example, a patient who had a splenectomy would have an image of the area of the spleen showing the left kidney with the image notated "spleen surgically removed." A complete abdominal ultrasound examination is used as a survey and is not organ specific. Some reasons to perform a complete study include abdominal trauma, focal or diffuse abdominal pain, or to evaluate for metastatic disease. For a pediatric patient this code would be used to look for congenital abnormalities.

Any ultrasound examination that does not require all of the previously mentioned organs, such as images of the spleen or left kidney, will be billed as a limited abdominal examination, with CPT code 76705. These examinations are more organ or quadrant driven, such as to evaluate for right upper quadrant (**RUQ**) pain, spleen size, or to look for **ascites**. Looking for abdominal lymph nodes would use the retroperitoneal code 76770 for a complete study as defined by the CPT book or 76775 for a limited study. Lymph nodes are found in the retroperitoneum.

Ordering physicians may not understand the difference in the various abdominal sonographic examinations. The ordering list may include Complete or Full Abdomen or just Abdomen, Gallbladder, Limited Abdomen, Liver, LUQ, and RUQ. Because the examinations are usually listed alphabetically, the physician will see abdomen first and typically stop there and order a complete abdominal examination with the reason for the study being RUQ pain or to rule out gallstones. A full abdominal study is probably not needed. A call to the ordering physician for clarification is a good teaching moment. To help the physician understand the difference, inquire if the spleen and left kidney need to be imaged. If the response is no, ask if the examination could be changed to a RUQ or gallbladder examination, explaining the difference. In some departments the sonographer can change the order and make a note in the appropriate section stating that the change was approved by the ordering physician, and add the physician's name.

Ultrasound of the Abdomen: Complete and Limited

The following information is more applicable for a complete abdominal examination. Information for a limited abdominal examination can be found in organ-specific chapters.

Patient Prep

Patients should be fasting (nothing by mouth [NPO]), for at least 6 to 8 hours before the examination to reduce bowel gas and allow visualization of the biliary system and gallbladder, especially for limited studies that are focused on the liver and biliary system. Patients being scanned after trauma do not need to be prepped.

Transducer

A 3.5–5 MHz curved linear array transducer is preferred. A sector/vector array transducer with lower frequencies in the 1–3 MHz range may be needed in obese patients, whereas a higher-frequency transducer may be used in thin or pediatric patients.

Breathing Technique

Scanning is performed with the patient holding their breath in a deep inspiration, in expiration, or in suspended or quiet respiration, depending on the organ or area being evaluated.

Patient Position

Typically, the patient will be scanned in a supine position unless a pathologic area is found that may require the patient to be turned to a different position. Most of the scanning will be subcostal and in the abdominal area. Some intercostal scanning may be needed to see the spleen.

Technical Tips

A complete abdominal study does not require the organs to be documented as thoroughly as for a dedicated organ-specific study. For example, one longitudinal image of the kidney with its length measured and one transverse image through the mid-pole is typically all that is required. The spleen is another example with just a longitudinal and transverse image. Some departments might require the length to be measured. Unless a pathologic condition is discovered, the patient may not need to be turned into a right-side-up position to evaluate the gallbladder. The sonographer should follow the protocol as outlined by the department. When evaluating for ascites, images should be obtained as follows: sagittal and transverse at Morison's pouch, transverse right mid-quadrant at the level of the umbilicus, transverse right lower quadrant, sagittal and transverse midline pelvis at the cul-de-sac, transverse left lower quadrant, transverse left mid-quadrant at the level of the umbilicus, and the interface between the spleen and left kidney. Transverse images are preferred because if there is a small amount of fluid, it will be seen in the most dependent portion, and sagittal images along the flank may not demonstrate any fluid.

I would perform an ascites search starting with the transducer orientated in a sagittal plane to obtain an image of Morison's pouch. Remember, this is the most dependent portion of the upper abdomen. Then I would turn the transducer to a transverse plane and scan from the kidney to the symphysis pubis, documenting mid and lower quadrants. At this point I would turn the transducer to a longitudinal plane and scan from side to side documenting the midline pelvic area.

Then it would be back to a transverse plane, documenting the midline, and next scanning up the left flank to the level of the spleen, again documenting the mid and lower quadrants. Finally, a longitudinal image would be done showing the spleen and left kidney. In the case of a moderate amount or more of ascites, more images would be needed to document the extent of the fluid.

Required Images*

Complete Abdomen Views
Complete Abdomen • Longitudinal Images
1. Midline image including proximal aorta
   Suggested Annotation: ML or PROX AORTA

> **NOTE:** Some departments may require the entire aorta imaged on patients older than 60 years to ensure there is no unsuspected abdominal aortic aneurysm.

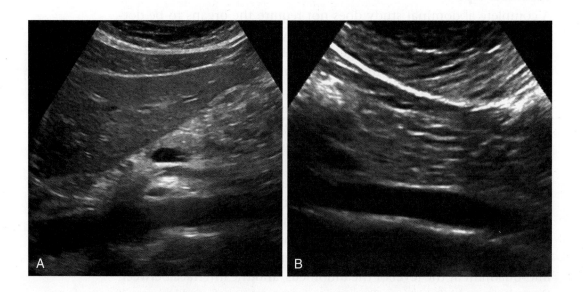

Suggested Annotation: **DIST AORTA**

*All images are courtesy of Liz Ladrido.

2. One or two images of the left lobe of the liver

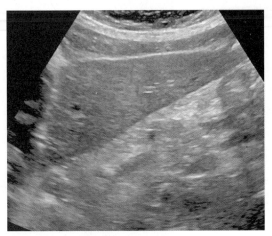

Suggested Annotation: **SAG LT LIVER**

3. An image of intrahepatic portion of the inferior vena cava (IVC).

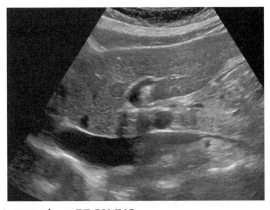

Suggested Annotation: **PROX IVC**

4. Five or six images of the right lobe of the liver.

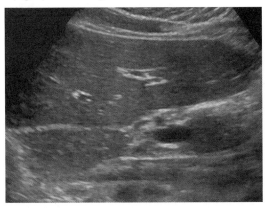

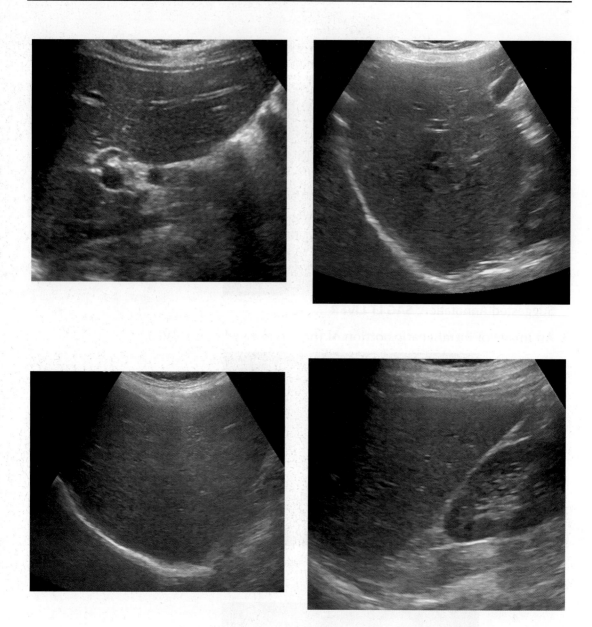

Suggested Annotation: **SAG RT LIVER**

5. An image of right kidney with length measured.

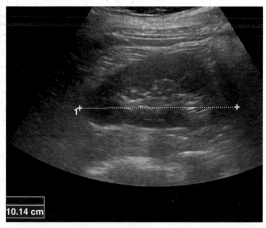

10.14 cm

Suggested Annotation: **SAG RT KID**

6. An image of the right diaphragm and pleural space to look for a hematoma, pleural effusion, or a subdiaphragmatic abscess.

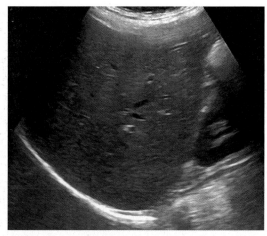

Suggested Annotation: **SAG RT DIAPHRAGM**

7. Two or three images of the gallbladder.

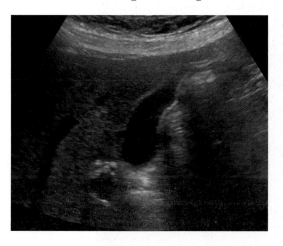
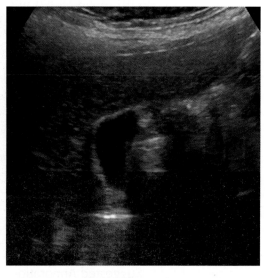

Suggested Annotation: **SAG GB**

8. An image of the common bile duct (CBD) with measurement.

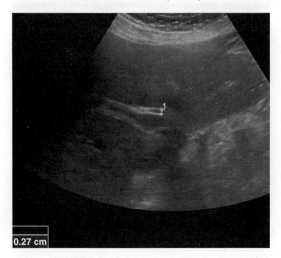

Suggested Annotation: **CBD**

9. Sagittal image of the spleen.

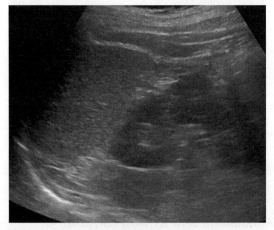

Suggested Annotation: **SAG SPLEEN**

10. An image of left kidney with length measured.

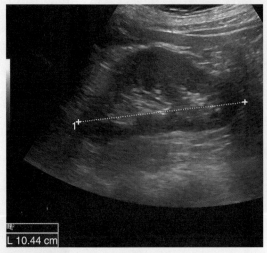

Suggested Annotation: **SAG LT KID**

11. An image of the left diaphragm and pleural space to look for a hematoma or a pleural effusion.

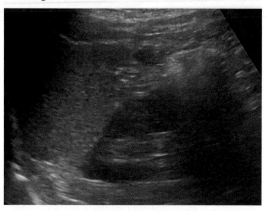

Suggested Annotation: **SAG LT DIAPHRAGM**

Complete Abdomen • Transverse Images

1. One or two images of the pancreas.

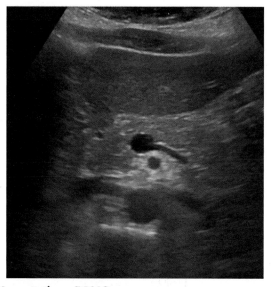

Suggested Annotation: **PANC**

2. One or two images of the left lobe of the liver.

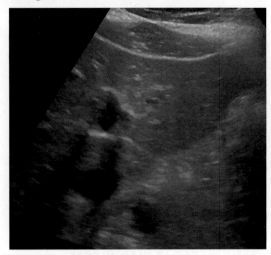

Suggested Annotation: TRV LT LIV

3.   Five or six images of the right lobe of the liver from dome to kidney, including an image of the proximal great vessels.

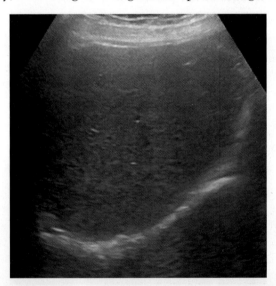

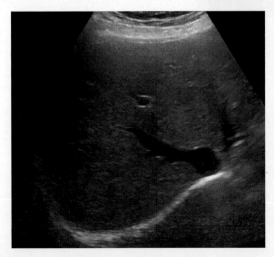

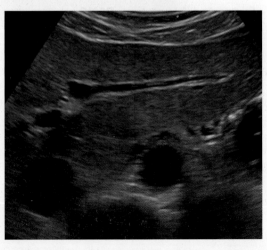

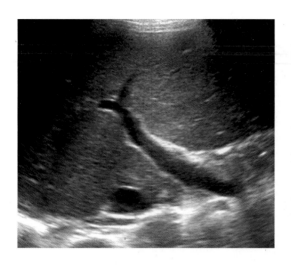
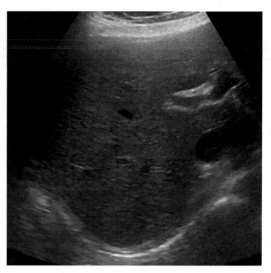

Suggested Annotation: **TRV RT LIVER**

NOTE: Some departments may require a transverse image of the distal aorta in patients older than 60 years to ensure that there is no unsuspected abdominal aortic aneurysm.

Suggested Annotation: **TRV DST AO**

4. Two or three images of the gallbladder.

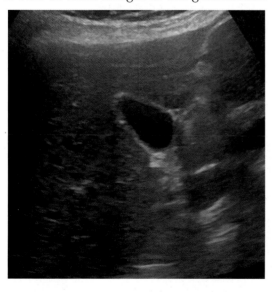
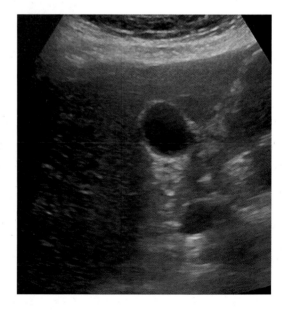

Suggested Annotation: **TRV GB**

5. Transverse image of the mid-pole of right kidney.

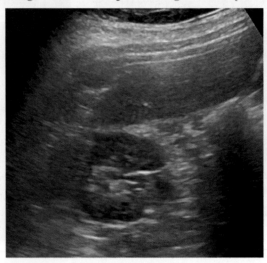

Suggested Annotation: **TRV RT KID MID**

6. Transverse image of the spleen.

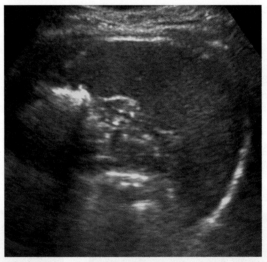

Suggested Annotation: **TRV SPLEEN**

7.   Transverse image of the mid-pole of left kidney.

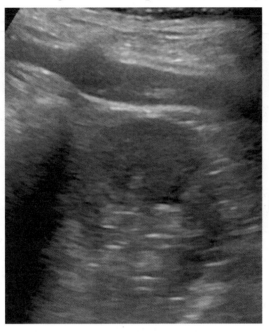

Suggested Annotation: **TRV LT KID MID**

The most common limited abdominal examination is the RUQ.

Complete Abdomen • Longitudinal Images
1. Midline image including proximal aorta.

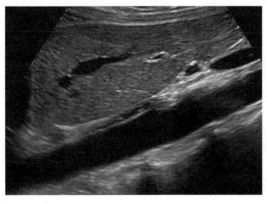

Suggested Annotation: **ML** or **PROX AORTA**

2. Two or three images of the left lobe of the liver depending on its size.

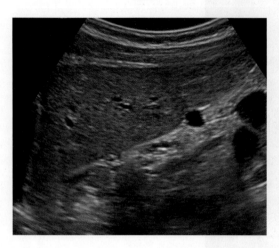 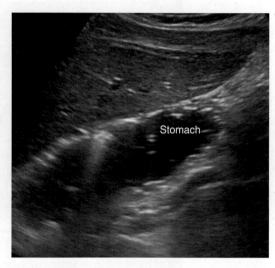

Suggested Annotation: **SAG LT LIVER**

3. Four or five images of the right lobe of the liver from the IVC to the right kidney with liver length measured.

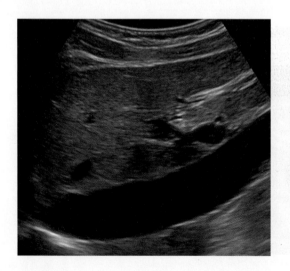 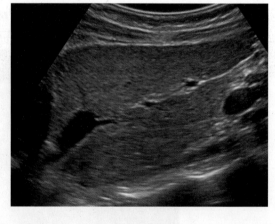

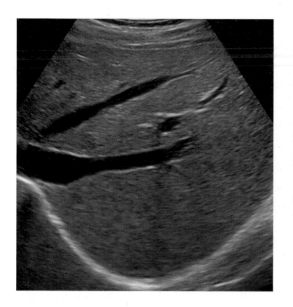
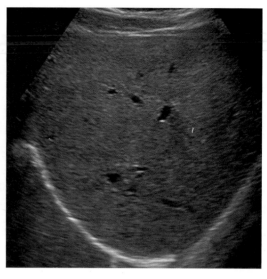

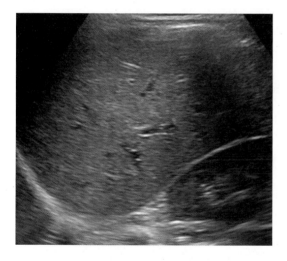
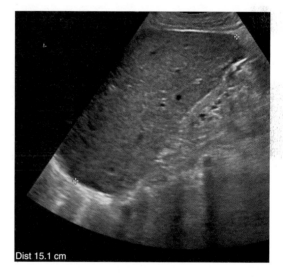

Suggested Annotation: **SAG RT LIVER**

4. An image of right kidney with length measured.

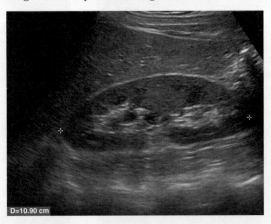

Suggested Annotation: SAG RT KID

5. Three to five images of the gallbladder depending on its size. Some departments may want the length of the gallbladder measured.

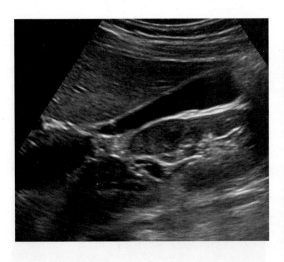

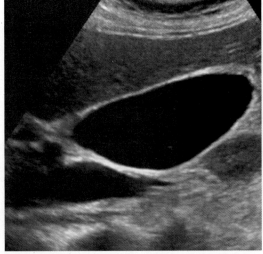

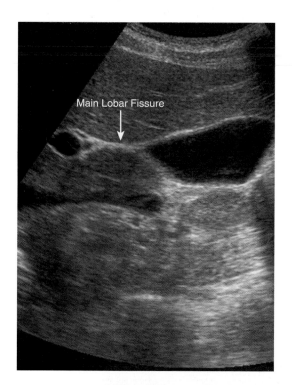

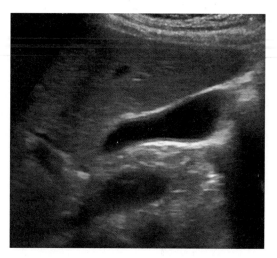

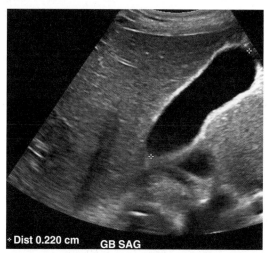

Suggested Annotation: SAG GB

6. An image of the CBD with and without measurement. Some departments might turn on color Doppler to verify that it is the CBD and not a vascular structure.

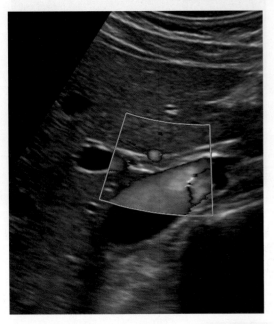
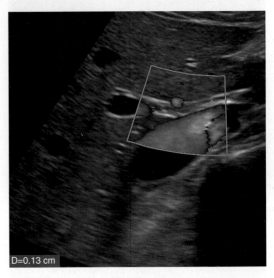

Suggested Annotation: **CBD**

7. An image of the CBD going to the head of the pancreas.

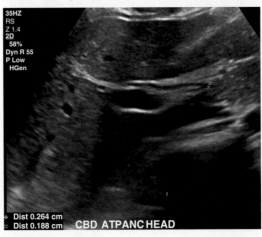

Suggested Annotation: **CBD**

Complete Abdomen • Transverse Images

1. One or two images of the pancreas.

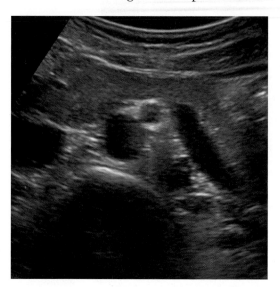 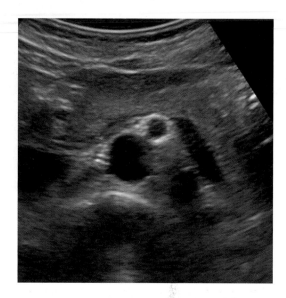

Suggested Annotation: **PANC**

2. An image of the CBD at the head of the pancreas.

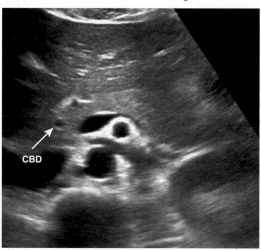

Suggested Annotation: **CBD** at **PANC HEAD**

3. One or two images of the left lobe of the liver.

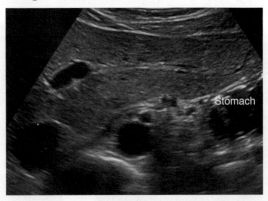

Suggested Annotation: **TRV LT LIV**

4. Four to six images of the right lobe of the liver from dome to mid or lower pole of kidney depending on its size.

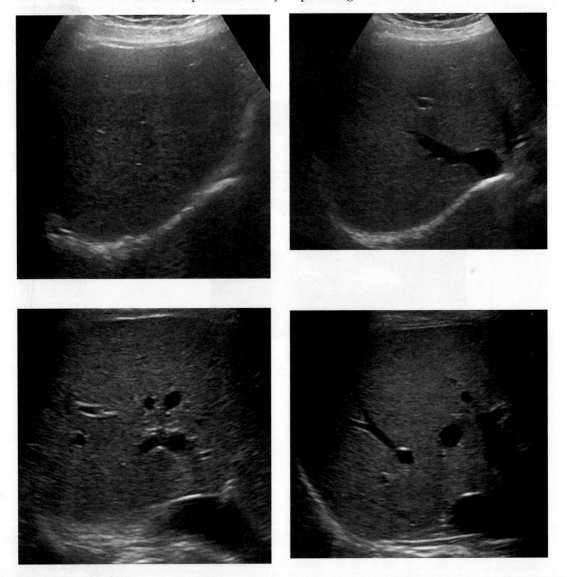

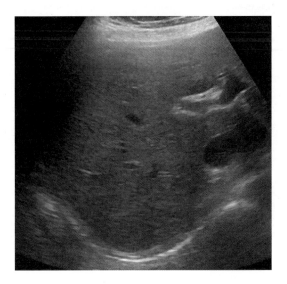

Suggested Annotation: **TRV RT LIVER**

5. Three to six images of the gallbladder depending on its size.

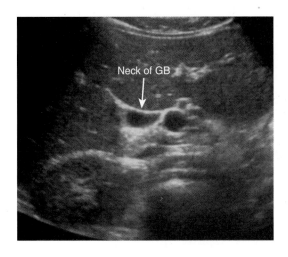

Neck of GB

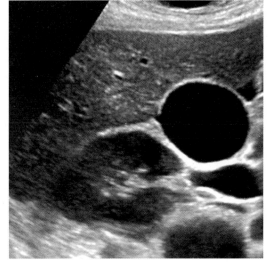

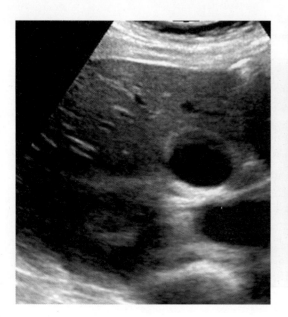 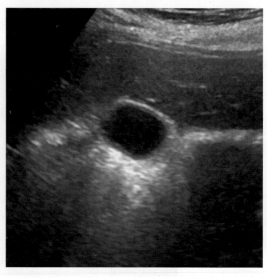

Suggested Annotation: **TRV GB**

6. An image of the gallbladder wall measured.

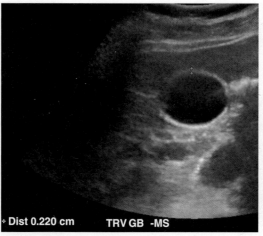

Suggested Annotation: **GB WALL**

7. An image documenting the response to Murphy's sign (MS).

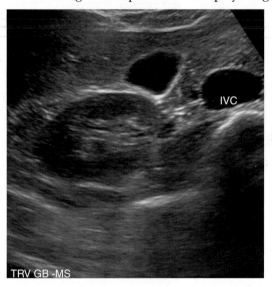

   Suggested Annotation: **+ MS** or **– MS**

8. Transverse image of the mid-pole of right kidney.

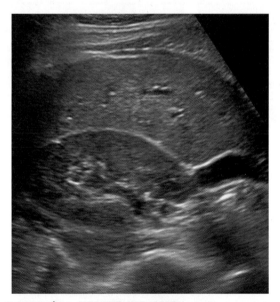

   Suggested Annotation: **TRV RT KID MID**

Left Lateral Decubitus (RSU) Views
RSU • Transverse Images

1. Three to six images of the gallbladder depending on its size.

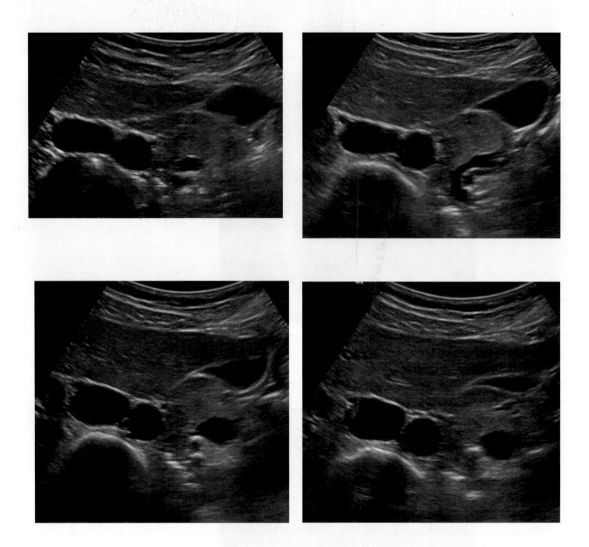

Suggested Annotation: **RSU TRV GB**

2. Some departments may want the gallbladder wall measured again.

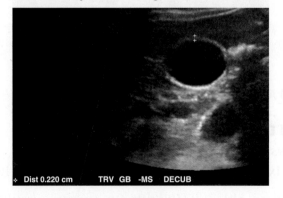

Suggested Annotation: **RSU GB WALL**

3. Some departments may want the response to MS documented again.

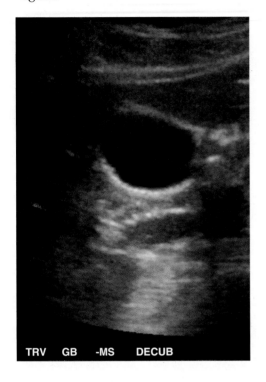 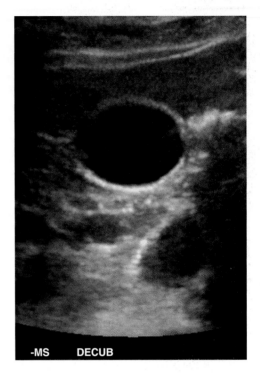

Suggested Annotation: **RSU + MS** or **RSU − MS**

RSU • Longitudinal Images

1. Three to five images of the gallbladder depending on its size.

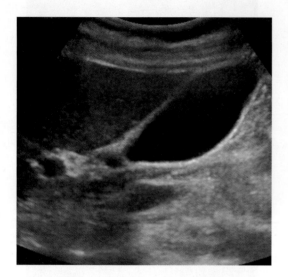

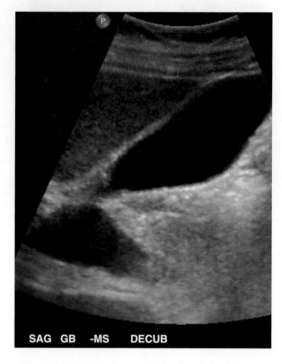

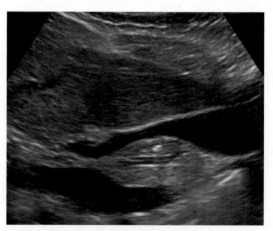

Suggested Annotation: **RSU SAG GB**

2.   An image of the CBD with and without measurement.

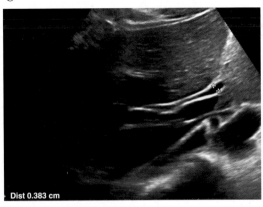

Dist 0.383 cm

Suggested Annotation: **RSU CBD**

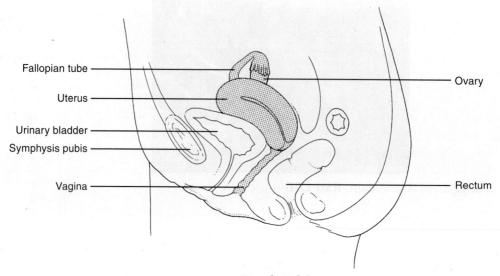

Female Pelvis.

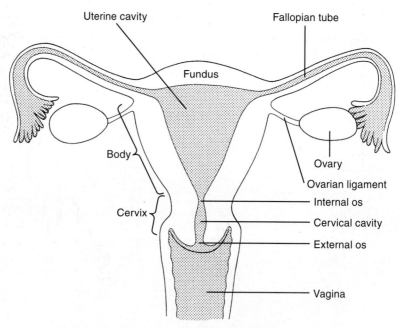

Anatomy of Uterus, Uterine Tubes, Ovaries, and Vagina

CHAPTER 12

Female Pelvis Scanning Protocol

Tricia Turner

Keywords

Adnexa
Anteflexed
Anteverted
Bicornate uterus
Cervix
Corpus luteum
Didelphic uterus
Endocervical canal
Endometrial canal
Endometrial cavity
Endometrial stripe
Endometrium
External os
Fallopian tubes
Follicle-stimulating hormone (FSH)
Follicles
Fundus
Internal os
Luteinizing hormone (LH)
Menstrual cycle
Myometrium
Ovaries
Perimetrium
Primary ovarian follicles
Proliferative phase
Retroflexed
Retroverted
Secondary ovarian follicles
Secretory phase
Urinary bladder
Uterine canal
Uterine cavity
Uterine cornua
Uterine isthmus
Uterus
Vagina
Vaginal canal

Objectives

At the end of this chapter, you will be able to:

- Define the keywords.
- Distinguish the sonographic appearance of the structures in the female pelvis and the terms used to describe them.
- Discuss the transducer options for scanning the female pelvis.
- List the suggested and optional patient positions when scanning the female pelvis.
- Describe patient prep for a female pelvic study.
- Distinguish normal variants of female pelvic structures.
- Discuss the required images for a sonographic examination of the female pelvis.

Overview

Sonographic examinations of the nongravid female pelvis are typically performed in the radiology department or sometimes in the emergency department or gynecologist's office. The main purpose of the examination is to evaluate the uterus, endometrium, cervix, ovaries, and surrounding structures. There are numerous reasons to perform a sonographic examination of the female pelvis, which includes evaluating for vaginal bleeding or discharge, pelvic pain, precocious puberty, abnormal gynecologic examination, determining location of pregnancy, and looking for as well as follow-up of any uterine or ovarian masses. The examination consists of the trans-abdominal (TA) examination and the transvaginal or endovaginal examination. The transvaginal aspect will be discussed in the next chapter. If an early pregnancy is discovered, the sonographer should change the preset to an obstetric preset to ensure the output power is below U.S. Food and Drug Administration guidelines.

Anatomy

The pelvis is the part of the peritoneal cavity extending from the iliac crests superiorly to the pelvic diaphragm inferiorly. The female pelvis consists of the genital tract, which includes the **vagina**, uterus, **fallopian tubes**, and ovaries; the urinary bladder; a portion of the ureters and intestines; pelvic musculature; pelvic ligaments; and peritoneal spaces.

True Pelvis and False Pelvis

The pelvic cavity is divided into the true pelvis and false pelvis by the linea terminalis, which is an imaginary dividing line drawn from the symphysis pubis around to the sacral promontory. The true pelvis is the region deep to the linea terminalis, below the pelvic brim, and contains the reproductive organs. The false pelvis is the area superior to the linea terminalis and inferior to the iliac crests and contains bowel.

Pelvic Regions

The descriptive regions of the pelvic cavity are the right iliac, hypogastric, and left iliac, which are subdivisions of the hypogastrium. The right iliac region contains the cecum of the colon, the appendix, distal end of the right ureter, and the right ovary. The hypogastric region includes the distal end of the ileum, urinary bladder, and the uterus. The left iliac region contains the sigmoid colon, distal end of the left ureter, and the left ovary.

Vagina

The vagina is the most inferior aspect of the genital tract and is located in the midregion of the true pelvis between the **urinary bladder** anteriorly and the rectum posteriorly. The vagina extends from the external genitalia to the cervix of the **uterus** and is a muscular, tubular organ composed of the following three layers: the inner mucosal lining of epithelial cells; the middle thin, smooth muscle wall; and the outer adventitia. The linings of the vagina and uterus enclose a continuous cavity or channel through which the fetus passes at birth. The inner epithelium encloses a centrally located **vaginal canal**, which has an average length of about 9 cm.

Uterus

The uterus is a muscular, hollow organ where the fertilized ovum embeds and the developing embryo and fetus are nourished. The uterus is typically located in the midline of the true pelvis between the urinary bladder anteriorly and the rectum posteriorly. It may also lie just to the right or left of the midline. Its central cavity opens into a fallopian tube bilaterally and into the vaginal cavity inferiorly.

The uterine walls are composed of three layers: the endometrium, myometrium, and perimetrium. The **endometrium** is the inner mucosal layer that encloses the **uterine cavity**; it is also called the **endometrial cavity, endometrial canal**, or **uterine canal**; and is continuous with the vaginal epithelium inferiorly. The thickness of the endometrium varies throughout the menstrual cycle. Just before the onset of menses the maximum anteroposterior (AP) measurement should not exceed 15 mm. After menses it can measure as little as 1 mm in the AP diameter. The endometrium consists of two layers: the superficial functional layer, which increases in size during the **menstrual cycle** and partially sloughs off during menses; and the deep basal layer, which is composed of dense stroma and mucosal glands and is not significantly influenced by the menstrual cycle. The **myometrium** is the middle, smooth muscle layer that forms the bulk of the uterus, and the **perimetrium** is an outer peritoneal thin membrane that completely covers the myometrium (Fig. 12.1).

The uterus is a pear-shaped organ and is divided into four parts: the fundus, body, isthmus, and cervix. The **fundus** is the widest and most superior segment and is continuous with the uterine body. The body or corpus is the largest part of the uterus and is continuous with the uterine cervix. The upper section of the body, the cornua, is where the fallopian tubes penetrate the myometrium. The uterine isthmus is the flexible region of the uterus where the uterine body meets the uterine cervix. Finally, the **cervix** is the lower cylindrical portion of the uterus that projects into the vagina. The cervical portion of the endometrial canal is called the **endocervical canal** and extends 2 to 4 cm from its **internal os** or opening, to its **external os**. The internal os joins the endometrial canal at approximately the same level as the isthmus, whereas the external os projects into the vaginal canal.

The size of the uterus is variable and described in four different ways depending on patient parity and age. The prepubertal maximum size is approximately 2.5 to 3 cm long, 2 cm wide, and 1 cm thick. The cervix comprises a significantly greater proportion of the organ, with a cervix-to-uterus ratio of approximately 2:1. The postpubertal,

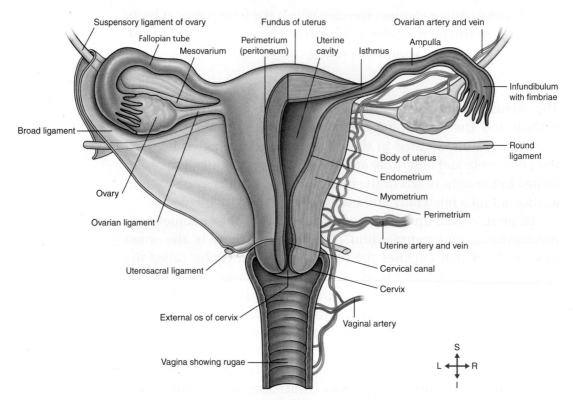

Fig. 12.1 Drawing of the female reproductive organs with all three layers of uterine tissue demonstrated. (From Grant A, Waugh A. *Ross & Wilson Anatomy and Physiology in Health and Illness,* 13th ed. Edinburgh, 2018, Elsevier.)

nulliparous size is usually 7 to 8 cm long, 3 to 5 cm wide, and 3 to 5 cm thick. The multiparous size can measure between 8.5 and 10 cm long, 5 to 6 cm wide, and 4 to 5 cm in AP diameter. The postmenopausal size depends on how many pregnancies the patient had, with the uterus significantly decreasing in size and assuming a prepubertal shape, with the cervix comprising the greater portion of the uterus.

The uterus normally tilts forward, resting on the dome of the bladder. Because of its peritoneal connections and ligaments, there is considerable mobility of the uterus within the true pelvis that allows minimal displacement of the uterus with the filling of the urinary bladder and marked displacement of the uterus during pregnancy. The flexibility of the uterine support structures allows variations in the uterine position that are described in four different ways: anteverted, anteflexed, retroverted, and retroflexed. An **anteverted** position is when the bladder is empty and the vagina and cervix form a 90-degree angle and the body and fundus of the uterus tilts anteriorly at the isthmus toward the pubic bone. An anteverted uterus is the most common position. An **anteflexed** uterus is when the bladder is empty and the vagina and cervix form a 90-degree angle and the body and fundus of the uterus are bent anteriorly at the isthmus toward the pubic bone until the fundus points inferiorly and rests

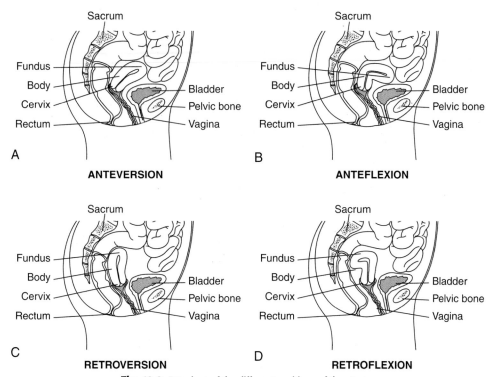

Fig. 12.2 Drawings of the different positions of the uterus.

near the cervix. A **retroverted** uterus is when the bladder is empty and the body and fundus of the uterus tilts posteriorly at the isthmus toward the sacrum until the cervix and vagina are linearly oriented. A **retroflexed** uterus is when the bladder is empty and the body and fundus are bent posteriorly at the isthmus toward the sacrum until the fundus points inferiorly and rests near the cervix. The cervix and vagina are linearly oriented (Fig. 12.2).

Fallopian Tubes

The fallopian tubes are part of the female reproduction organs. They are tortuous, muscular tubes that emerge from the superolateral margins of the uterus at the level of the uterine cornua and then run laterally within the peritoneum along the superior free margin of the broad ligaments until they reach the **ovaries**. Fallopian tubes are responsible for directing the mature ovum from the ovaries to the uterus through gentle peristalsis of its smooth muscle walls. The length of the tube varies from 7 to 12 cm, with the widest diameter approximately 3 to 4 mm. The fallopian tube is divided into four segments: the interstitial, isthmus, ampulla, and infundibulum segments. The interstitial or intramural segment is the narrowest and is enclosed by the uterus. The isthmus is the segment adjacent to the uterine wall and is connected to the interstitial segment. The isthmus is a short, straight, narrow portion of the tube that widens laterally to

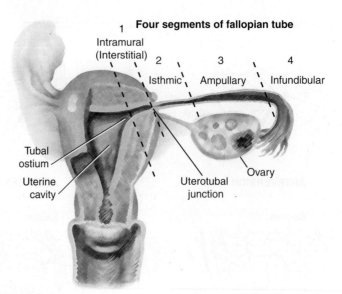

Fig. 12.3 Drawing of the sections of the fallopian tube. (From Mauro MA, Murphy KPJ, Thomson KR Venbrux AC, Morgan RA. *Image-Guided Interventions,* 2nd ed. Philadelphia, 2014, Saunders. 2014.)

form the ampullary and infundibular segments. The ampulla is the coiled and longest segment and is where fertilization usually occurs; the infundibulum is the widest, funnel-shaped end of the tube that opens into the peritoneal cavity adjacent to the ovary. Fringelike extensions of the infundibulum, called fimbria, drape over the ovary and direct the released ovum into the tube (Fig. 12.3).

Ovaries

The ovaries are paired, bilateral, almond-shaped organs of the female reproductive system. The ovaries contain numerous follicles, which are fluid-filled sacs that contain developing eggs, the oocytes. The ovaries are located in the **adnexa**, the peritoneal cavity spaces located posterior to the broad ligaments and lateral to the uterus, within the true pelvis. Each ovary is anterior to a ureter and the internal iliac artery. Finding the ovaries with ultrasound can be challenging because their position can vary and be influenced by the uterine position, bowel activity, and bladder filling. Typically, the ovaries are lateral or posterolateral to the uterus against the pelvic sidewalls in Waldeyer's fossa. Some tips for locating the ovaries are as follows:
- The ovaries are never positioned anterior to the uterus or broad ligaments.
- If the uterus is retroverted, the ovaries tend to lie superolateral, adjacent to the fundus of the uterus.
- When the uterus lies to one side of the midline, the ovary on that side is often displaced from its typical position to lie superior to the fundus of the uterus.
- If the uterus is enlarged, the ovaries can be shifted superolateral.

- After a hysterectomy, the surgical removal of the uterus, the ovaries shift toward midline and superior to the vagina.

The size of the ovaries varies just like the uterus and will depend on the patient's age, phase of the menstrual cycle, and menstrual status. Prepubertal ovaries are relatively large at birth, and between the ages of 2 and 6 the ovarian size remains relatively stable, with a volume of 2.3 cm³ or less. Between the ages of 6 and 7, age-related growth associated with cystic functional changes begins and continues through puberty. Postpubertal ovarian size is approximately 4 to 5 cm long, 3 cm wide, and 2 cm anteroposteriorly. Volume measurements are generally 9.8 cm³ but can range from 6 to 13 cm³, varying with the menstrual cycle. Postmenopausal ovaries are approximately 2 cm long, 1 cm wide, and 0.5 cm anteroposteriorly. Volume measurements are usually 5.8 cm³. It should be noted that ovarian atrophy takes place gradually, and at some point the ovaries may not be visible with ultrasound.

Urinary Bladder

The urinary bladder is a symmetric, hollow, muscular organ. It is part of the urinary system and serves as a reservoir for the urine that is formed in the kidneys. The urinary bladder is fixed inferiorly at its base in the true pelvis, directly posterior to the symphysis pubis and anterior to the uterus and vagina. As the bladder fills with urine, the dome can extend superiorly into the false pelvis. The bladder can hold as much as 16 to 24 oz of urine. The normal distended urinary bladder wall measures 3 mm or less (Fig. 12.4).

A full bladder provides an acoustic window in which to assess the uterus transabdominally as it pushes the bowel superiorly, allowing visualization of the pelvic structures. When performing a transvaginal

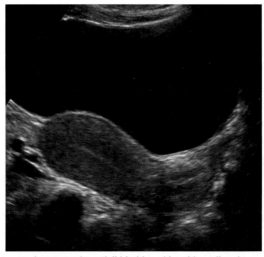

Fig. 12.4 Image demonstrating a full bladder with a thin wall and a normal uterus.

examination, the sonographer needs to have the patient completely empty her bladder because a full bladder may cause acoustic artifacts and push the uterus deeper.

Ureters

The ureters are muscular tubes that are the part of the urinary system and convey the urine from the kidneys to the urinary bladder. The ureters are typically not appreciated sonographically unless a pathologic condition is present. In the true pelvis the ureter runs between the internal iliac artery posteriorly, and the ovary anteriorly, then courses anteromedially to enter the trigone of the urinary bladder just anterior to the vagina. Ureters are clinically significant in the female pelvis because some pelvic pathologic conditions, such as uterine fibroids, can cause obstruction of the ureter and cause hydronephrosis. When pelvic or uterine pathologic findings are present, the sonographer should take a midline shot of each kidney to ensure that there is no hydronephrosis.

Sigmoid and Rectum

The sigmoid colon and rectum are parts of the large intestine and are located within the true pelvis. The sigmoid colon is continuous with the descending colon in the left lower quadrant of the pelvis. It descends toward the rectum in the inferoposterior aspect of the pelvis at the level of the third sacral vertebra. Sonographically the sonographer may appreciate peristalsis of the sigmoid, helping to prove that it is a loop of bowel and not a mass. The rectum is fixed in its position posterior to the vagina. The sonographer should be aware that the rectum can mimic a mass when full. The sonographer may notice either peristalsis or that the mass changes shape while scanning.

Musculature

The pelvic muscles serve as a support and protection for pelvic structures. Muscles tend to be appreciated sonographically as hypoechoic tissue with multiple linear echogenic striations. Bowel may hinder the visualization of muscles. The psoas muscles are paired major muscles on either side of the spine that extend from the lateral aspects of the lower thoracic vertebrae running anterolaterally across the posterior wall of the abdominopelvic cavity to the iliac crests.

The muscles of the false pelvis include the iliopsoas, rectus abdominus, and transverse abdominus. Each psoas muscle joins an iliacus muscle at the level of the iliac crests to form the iliopsoas muscles that travel anteroinferior to insert into the lesser trochanter of the femur. The large pair of rectus abdominus muscles extend from the sixth ribs and xiphoid process of the sternum down to the symphysis pubis. The transverse abdominus muscle forms the anterolateral borders of the abdominopelvic cavity. The muscular sheath surrounding each rectus abdominus muscle fuses with the transverse abdominus muscles to form the tendinous linea alba at the midline.

The muscles of the true pelvis include the obturator internus, piriformis, and pelvic diaphragm. The obturator internus muscles line the lateral walls of the true pelvis. The piriformis muscles are situated in the posterior region of the true pelvis behind the uterus and can be potentially mistaken as enlarged ovaries. The pelvic diaphragm is a group of muscles lining the floor of the true pelvis to support the pelvic organs. The pubococcygeus muscle extends from the pubic bones to the coccyx, encircling the rectum, vagina, and urethra. The iliococcygeus muscles are located lateral to each pubococcygeus muscle. Together these muscles form a hammock across the pelvic floor and are termed the levator ani muscles. Each coccygeus muscle extends from the ischial spine to the sacrum and coccyx, and these are the most posterior muscles of the pelvic diaphragm.

> **NOTE:** To help distinguish between ovaries and muscles, look for the linear fibrous striations within the muscle or for arterial blood flow.

Ligaments

The pelvic ligaments are part of the musculoskeletal system and include the broad, round, cardinal, uterosacral, infundibulopelvic, and ovarian ligaments and provide flexibility and mobility of the pelvic organs. The ligaments of the pelvic structures are typically not appreciated sonographically unless a large amount of free fluid is present. In such cases, the ligaments will appear sonographically echogenic.

The broad ligament extends between the uterine cornu and the ovary (Fig. 12.5). The fallopian tube, round ligament, ovarian ligament, and vascular structures of the uterus and ovaries are positioned between the two layers of the broad ligament. These structures are surrounded by fat and connective tissue called the parametrium. The round ligaments support the uterus and are located just inferior and anterior to the fallopian tubes down to the labia majora. The cardinal ligaments anchor the uterus at the level of the cervix and the vaginal canal to the lateral pelvic wall. The uterosacral ligament stabilizes the uterus from the level of the internal os back to the sacral spine. The infundibular or suspensory ligament attaches the ovary to that lateral pelvic wall, and the ovarian ligaments anchors the ovary to the **uterine cornua**.

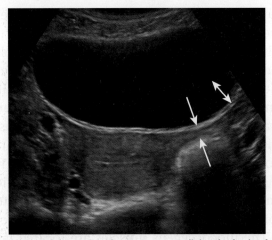

Fig. 12.5 Transverse image of the uterus. The *arrows* are outlining the fascia of the broad ligament, which extends from the uterine cornu to the ovary. The *double-headed arrow* is pointing to the left ovary.

Pelvic Spaces

The three pelvic peritoneal spaces located in the pelvis are the anterior cul-de-sac, the posterior cul-de-sac, and the space of Retzius. The anterior cul-de-sac, or the vesicouterine pouch, is a shallow peritoneal space located between the anterior wall of the uterus and the posterior border of the urinary bladder. This space all but disappears as the urinary bladder fills with urine. The posterior cul-de-sac, or the pouch of Douglas, is the most posterior and dependent portion of the peritoneum. It is located between the rectum and the uterus. The space of Retzius, or prevesical or retropubic space, is a fascial space between the anterior bladder wall and pubic symphysis. It is important to be able to identify these areas to determine the location of any fluid collections or other pathologic condition.

Physiology

Between puberty and menopause, the female reproductive system undergoes monthly cyclical changes referred to as the menstrual cycle. The pituitary gland, which is located in the brain and oversees all hormonal activity, along with the ovaries, secrete hormones that control changes in the ovaries and the uterine endometrium throughout the menstrual cycle. By the onset of menses, each ovary has thousands of undeveloped **follicles** that contain a single primary oocyte. The menstrual cycle is divided into four phases termed the menstrual phase, follicular phase, ovulation phase, and luteal phase, which usually follow a 28-day course. During the ovarian follicular phase, days 1 to 14 of the menstrual cycle, the pituitary gland releases **follicle-stimulating hormone** (FSH) to initiate the development of several **primary ovarian follicles**. As each primary follicle grows, its oocyte reaches a mature size called the ovum. At this stage of development, the ovum and surrounding structures are referred to as **secondary ovarian follicles**. Menses generally occurs during days 1 to 5 of the menstrual cycle. The thickened, functional layer of the endometrium is shed when fertilization of an ovum does not occur. At the end of menses, the endometrium is fairly thin. After menses, the endometrium goes into the **proliferative phase** that lasts until day 14 of the menstrual cycle. During the proliferative phase, the ovarian follicles contain cells that begin to release the hormone estrogen, which initiates thickening and swelling of the endometrium in preparation for implantation of a fertilized ovum. At this point, the endometrium takes on a trilaminar appearance, which is three distinct echogenic lines. On day 14 of the menstrual cycle ovulation usually occurs. Although many follicles develop, only one matures completely and will release a mature ovum at ovulation. When the follicle ruptures and the mature ovum is expelled into the peritoneal cavity, the fimbria of the fallopian tube sweep the released egg into the infundibulum. After ovulation, the ruptured follicle fills with blood and is called the corpus luteum. This begins the ovarian luteal phase and the endometrial **secretory phase** of the menstrual cycle, which occur from days 15 to 28. The **corpus luteum** transforms into an endocrine gland and secretes the hormone progesterone, which promotes glandular secretions of the uterine endometrium, further preparing it for implantation by a fertilized ovum. Simultaneously, throughout the menstrual cycle, **luteinizing hormone** (LH) has been released by the pituitary gland to stimulate the ovaries to secrete estrogen and progesterone. The concentration of estrogen and progesterone promotes continued thickening and swelling of the endometrium. The maximum AP diameter of the endometrium during this secretory phase is 15 mm. In addition, exocrine glands of the endometrial lining produce glycogen-rich mucus to help prepare a suitable environment for implantation. The corpus luteum depends on LH to continue to produce progesterone, but ironically, progesterone levels inhibit LH production. Consequently, the corpus luteum regresses and only a fibrous tissue mass, called the corpus albicans, remains in the ovary. In the absence of fertilization, estrogen and progesterone levels diminish, and a new menstrual cycle starts on day 1 with menses of the endometrium and the beginning of the ovarian follicular phase.

Sonographic Appearance
Urinary System

The urinary bladder cavity is not seen if it is empty; however, when distended with urine, it appears anechoic with bright, reflective walls (see Fig. 12.4). The ureters are not routinely identified sonographically unless they are dilated from an obstruction.

Pelvic Spaces

It is normal to visualize a small amount of free fluid in the posterior cul-de-sac. Any fluid found in the anterior cul-de-sac or lateral pelvic recesses or a large collection of fluid in the posterior cul-de-sac is considered abnormal. The space of Retzius is not seen sonographically unless the urinary bladder appears to be displaced posteriorly. This is a characteristic feature of masses in the space of Retzius, as other pelvic masses typically displace the bladder anteriorly or inferiorly.

Reproductive Organs

The fallopian tubes are not routinely identified sonographically unless they become outlined by free intraperitoneal fluid or are abnormal, for example, by a tubo-ovarian abscess.

Because the uterus and vagina are vertically orientated in the body, their longitudinal and long-axis views are seen in TA, sagittal scanning planes. The sonographic appearance of the uterine endometrium is altered by menstrual cycle, changes. The intermediate layer of the myometrium and the bulk of the normal uterus exhibit a low-gray, homogeneous texture (Fig. 12.6). The only notable sonographic characteristic of the outer perimetrium layer of the uterus is its smooth contour; otherwise it is indistinguishable from the myometrium.

The central, linear, opposing surfaces of the endometrium that form the endometrial canal present sonographically as a bright, thin, midline strip and is referred to as the **endometrial stripe** (Fig. 12.7). As the thickness of the endometrium changes cyclically with the menstrual cycle, so does its sonographic appearance. In the menstrual phase the endometrium appears thin and bright as the superficial layer is sloughed off. During the early proliferative phase, days 5 to 9, the endometrium appears as a thin, bright line that normally measures 4 to 8 mm. In the later proliferative phase, days 10 to 14, just before ovulation, the functional zone becomes thicker because of increased levels of estrogen, and the endometrium exhibits a multilayered appearance. The bright stripe of the endometrial canal is surrounded by the thick functional zone, which appears hypoechoic relative to the bright basal layer that is surrounded by the hypoechoic inner layer of the myometrium. At this stage, the endometrium will normally measure 6 to 10 mm. During the secretory phase, days 15 to 28, the endometrium normally measures 7 to 15 mm as the functional zone becomes even thicker and edematous as a result of increased levels of progesterone and the secretion of a glycogen-rich mucus, which together cause the functional zone to appear brighter and become isoechoic to the basal layer and canal (Fig. 12.8).

The ovaries appear as mid-gray to low-level gray and are homogeneous except for the interruption of the small, anechoic follicles, which are a common finding during reproductive years. These ovarian follicles will vary in size and number (Fig. 12.9).

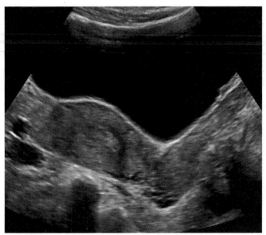

Fig. 12.6 Longitudinal image of the uterus and vagina. Note how the central endometrium looks thick and appears to be in the secretory phase (days 15–28) of the menstrual cycle, during which the basal layer, functional zone, and canal become isoechoic. The vagina appears tubular, its muscular walls are isoechoic to and continuous with the uterine myometrium. The bright stripe representing the centrally located endocervical and endovaginal canals is well delineated. Note the small amount of anechoic free fluid in the posterior cul-de-sac. Note how the normal bladder wall appears thin, smooth, and bright.

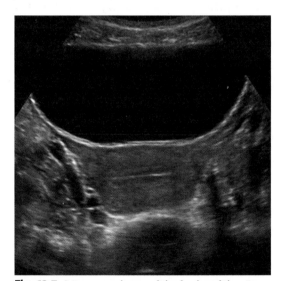

Fig. 12.7 A transverse image of the fundus of the uterus. In this image all of the myometrial layers are distinguishable. Note how the outer and inner fibrous layers appear hypoechoic compared with the low-gray appearance of the intermediate layer. The inner layer has been described as a trilaminar with three distinctive echogenic lines representing the proliferative phase of the endometrium.

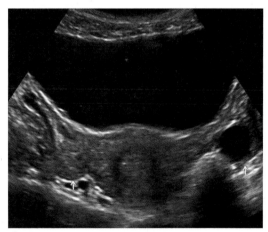

Fig. 12.8 A transverse image of the fundus of the uterus in the secretory phase, days 15 to 28. Arrows point to ovaries.

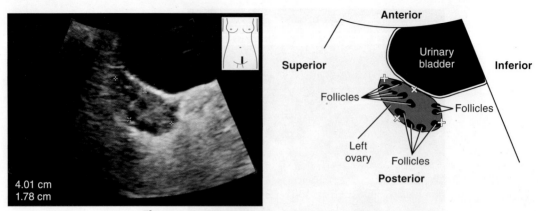

Fig. 12.9 A longitudinal image of the follicles in the ovary.

Normal Variants

Most uterine abnormalities are due to a müllerian duct anomaly, and there are usually associated renal abnormalities as well. The sonographer should obtain a longitudinal image of each kidney to document the presence of each kidney, as renal agenesis is a common associated finding. These uterine abnormalities are best demonstrated on a transvaginal sonogram, usually with three-dimensional images.

A **didelphys uterus** results from complete failure of müllerian duct fusion, and each duct develops fully, with duplication of the uterine horns, cervix, and proximal vagina and with no communication between them. The sonographic appearance is the same as that of the normal uterus, cervix, and vagina, but the anatomy is duplicated and may occur in any uterine position or location.

A **bicornate uterus** is a uterine duplication abnormality resulting in a uterus divided into two horns. It occurs when the upper portions of the paramesonephric ducts do not fuse, but the distal portions that develop into the lower uterine segment, cervix, and upper vagina fuse normally. There may be some communication between the two cavities, usually at the **uterine isthmus**. There may be two cervices, called a bicornuate-bicollis, or just one cervix called a bicornuate-unicollis. The uterus is heart-shaped on transverse images, and the uterine horns are widely divergent with a fundal cleft that is typically more than 1 cm deep. The sonographic appearance is the same as that of the normal uterus, cervix, and vagina, with two divergent uterine horns and endometrial cavities seen. The sonographer should try to determine if there are one or two cervixes.

A septate uterus is the most common uterine anomaly. There is a normal convex external fundal contour that helps to differentiate between a didelphys and bicornuate uterus, because both of these anomalies will have fundal clefts. There is also interruption of the myometrium by a septum at the fundus that is less echogenic than the myometrium. It is caused by the failure of the resorption of the uterovaginal septum, resulting in the appearance of two separate endometrial canals.

Ultrasound of the Female Pelvis

Patient Prep
For a TA sonogram, the patient should have a full urinary bladder. This moves bowel out of the way and serves as an acoustic window for visualizing the pelvic structures. One hour before the examination the patient should drink 30–40 oz of fluid, which does not have to be water. The patient should be finished drinking the fluid within 30 minutes of the appointment time. The patient should be instructed not to void until after the sonogram. An overfilled bladder can actually push the pelvic organs out of view. If this occurs, have the patient partially void. TA sonograms are performed on pediatric patients and those women who do not want a vaginal sonogram. It is more common for the patient to be scheduled for a transvaginal ultrasound. With these patients the TA examination is performed with whatever fluid is in their bladder to provide a global view of the pelvic area. The patient will then empty the bladder for the endovaginal examination.

Transducer
A 3.5–5 MHz curved linear array transducer is used. As with all ultrasound examinations, the highest frequency that will allow proper penetration should be used.

Breathing Technique
The study is performed with the patient breathing normally.

Patient Position
The patient is scanned in the supine position.

Technical Tips
Be conscious of the fact that the patient will have a full bladder. Try not to press too hard. If the patient is too uncomfortable, allow her to partially empty her bladder. A very full bladder can cause the pelvic area to be rigid, making scanning difficult. Have the patient partially empty her bladder. The bladder needs only to be full enough to see the fundus of the uterus.

The location and lie of the ovaries are quite variable and can be a challenge to locate. The long axis of the ovary can lie in a longitudinal, transverse, or oblique scanning plane. Ovaries tend to be lateral to the body or fundus of the uterus but may be found tucked in close to the side of the uterus. Other locations include far posterior, lateral, or superior to the uterus. They are usually easier to find on transverse images. When the ovary is found, keep your eye on it while slowly turning the transducer into a longitudinal image. Another tip is to slide the transducer slightly past midline and angle the transducer to the other side. For example, place the transducer on the left side of the body and angle the transducer to the right side to find the right ovary.

For whatever the reason, if the patient can only have a TA examination, make sure that her bladder is full enough to perform the examination. If the bladder is not full enough, have the patient wait another 10 to 20 minutes and then scan again to see if it is properly distended. Try to answer the clinical question. Use different frequencies and harmonics to optimize the resolution of the image. Finally, make every effort to locate the ovaries.

Some laboratories may want the endometrial canal measured in the TA images. If the patient is not having a TV examination, the endometrial canal or stripe can be measured for the appropriate indication, such as vaginal bleeding on a postmenopausal woman. To attempt to obtain an accurate measurement, enlarge the area to be measured. It is best to perform the measurement on the TV examination because the resolution is much better.

To see the long axis of the uterus, cervix, and vagina, place the transducer perpendicularly at the midline of the body, just superior to and against the symphysis pubis. If needed, angle the transducer slightly superiorly—that is, the footprint angled toward the patient's head, to be perpendicular to the endometrial canal with an anteverted uterus. From the midline position the long axis of the vagina and cervix will be visualized and possibly the body and fundus of the uterus, depending on their position. If the body and fundus of the uterus are not seen in the same scanning plane with the vagina and cervix, slowly rotate the transducer until the body and fundus come into view and visually connect to the cervix. Look for the vagina inferiorly, in the area between the anechoic bladder, seen anteriorly, and the rectum, seen posteriorly. If the vagina and cervix are not visualized, tilt the transducer a little to the right and/or left of midline, or slightly angle the transducer inferiorly, or use a combination of both until the vagina and cervix come into view. Adjust the scanning plane until the long axis of the uterus; vagina; and endometrial, endocervical, and vaginal canals are all visualized together (Fig. 12.10). For a retroverted uterus, slide up to the top of the bladder and angle the transducer toward the

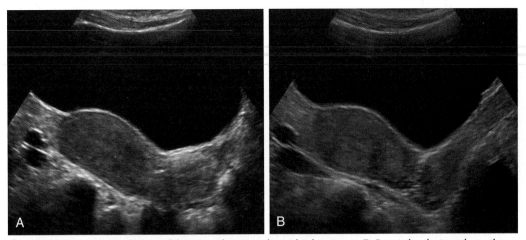

Fig. 12.10 A, A longitudinal image of the uterus; however, the vagina is not seen. **B,** By rotating the transducer, the uterus and vagina are now seen in the same image.

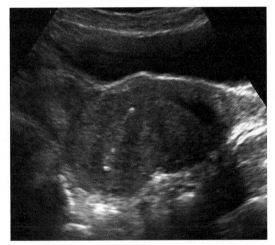

Fig. 12.11 An image of a retroverted uterus.

patient's feet to try and get perpendicular to the endometrial stripe (Fig. 12.11). The transverse images will not look like nice oval shapes on a retroverted uterus, because it is difficult to get perpendicular to the body and fundus.

For transverse images the ultrasound beam needs to be perpendicular to the area being scanned. With an anteverted uterus, place the transducer perpendicular to the floor and obtain a transverse image of the vagina. Keeping the transducer in the same location, start to angle the beam toward the patient's head. The cervix and lower uterine segment can usually be evaluated from this position. To see the fundus, try to keep angling the transducer. If that does not work, place the transducer mid-uterus, perpendicular to the endometrium. Slide the transducer superiorly or angle as needed to evaluate the fundus of the uterus. Continue scanning just past the bladder to ensure that there is no pathologic condition above the bladder.

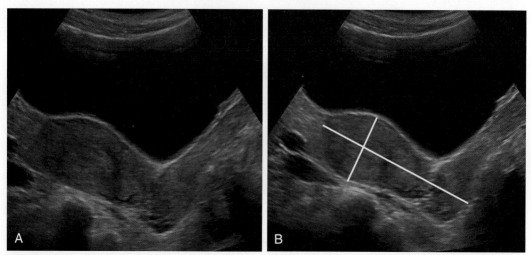

Fig. 12 12 A, A normal longitudinal uterus. **B,** The *two perpendicular lines* show the proper technique for measuring the length and anteroposterior dimensions of the uterus.

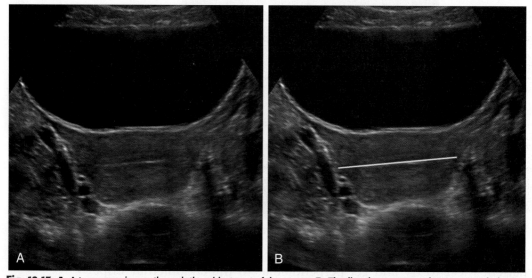

Fig. 12.13 A, A transverse image through the widest part of the uterus. **B,** The *line* demonstrates the proper technique to measure the width of the uterus. Note that the *line* is not straight but has a slight tilt to obtain the true widest measurement.

When measuring the length and AP dimensions of the uterus, measure the length first, and the AP dimension should be perpendicular to the length measurement (Fig. 12.12). When measuring the transverse uterus, the measurement should be with the organ, which will not always be parallel to the floor or transducer (Fig. 12.13).

Measuring the ovaries can be tricky because of their lie in the body. The two measurements should be at right angles to one another. Determine the length of the ovary and perform the length measurement and perform the AP measurement, which will be perpendicular to the length measurement. Determine the lie of the ovary and where the width should be measured. It is rare for the transverse

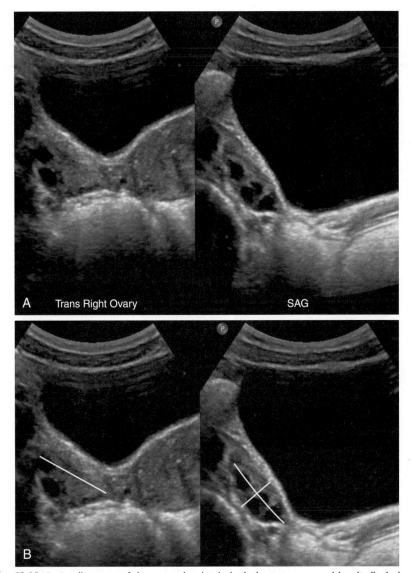

Fig. 12.14 A, A split screen of the ovary showing in both the transverse and longitudinal planes. **B,** The image on the *left* shows how to obtain a proper measurement of the width of this ovary. The sonographer needs to understand how the ovary is positioned to determine the proper width. The *right side* has *two perpendicular lines* showing the proper technique for measuring the length and anteroposterior dimensions of the ovary.

measurement to be parallel to the floor (Fig. 12.14). It is acceptable to use the split-screen approach and have both the longitudinal and transverse images with the measurements together. This is usually done by obtaining the longitudinal first, capturing the image, then turning the transducer 90 degrees to obtain the transverse image, capture the image, and then perform all the measurements.

Doppler

Color and spectral Doppler images are not typically acquired in routine patients, although some departments may require them as part

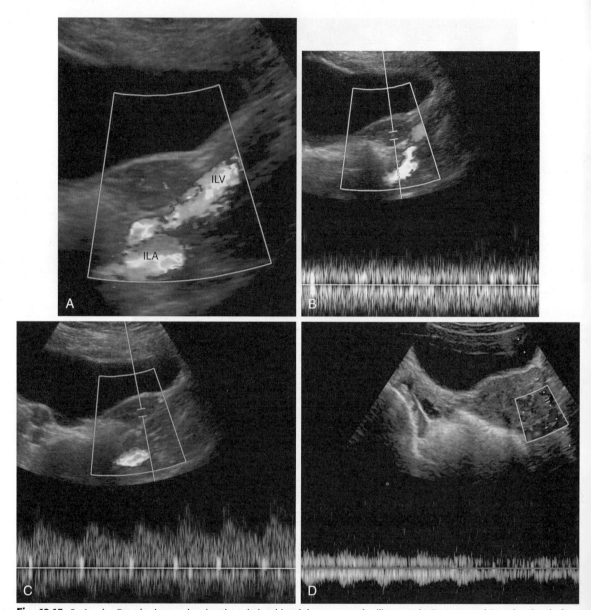

Fig. 12.15 A, A color Doppler image showing the relationship of the ovary to the iliac vessels. **B,** A spectral Doppler signal of an intraovarian vein. The waveform is both *above* and *below* the baseline because the beam is intersecting the vessel at an angle near 90 degrees. The ovarian vessels are typically seen as dots, so determining an angle less than 60 degrees is not possible. **C,** The arterial waveform from the ovulating ovary showing good diastolic flow. **D,** The arterial waveform from the nonovulating ovary showing low flow in both systole and diastole. It can be difficult to stay on the ovary to obtain a spectral Doppler signal that runs across the screen.

of their protocol (Fig. 12.15). Normal arterial waveforms will change with the menstrual cycle. In the follicular phase the velocities will be low. Velocities will increase in the luteal phase. There also may be a difference between sides, with the ovary that is ovulating having more diastolic flow. Because it is almost impossible to angle correctly, measurements are obtained without using angle correction. Postmenopausal women will have low-velocity, high-resistance signals because of low or absent flow during end diastole. When torsion of the ovary is suspected, arterial and venous Doppler images are required of each ovary.

Female Pelvic Required Images

The required images are a small representation of what a sonographer visualizes during a study. Therefore the images should provide the interpreting physician with the most telling and technically accurate information available. Labeling examples used in the chapter are only a suggestion, and you would use the labeling required by the clinical site or your employer.

Uterus • Longitudinal Images

1. Long-axis image of the uterus with the longest length and AP measurements with and without measurements.

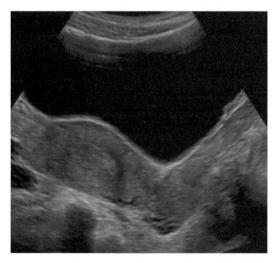 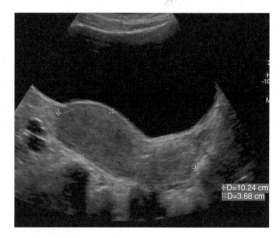

Suggested annotation: **SAG UT or PELVIS SAG ML**

2. Longitudinal image of the right lateral aspect of the uterus.

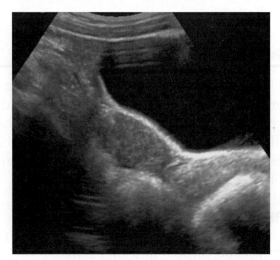

Suggested annotation: **SAG UT RT**

3. Longitudinal image to include the right lateral wall of the bladder and pelvic sidewall.

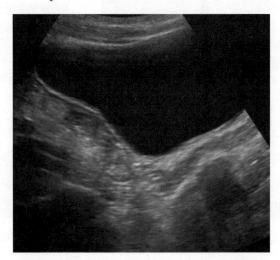

Suggested annotation: **SAG RT ADNEXA**

4. Longitudinal image of the right adnexa past the bladder.

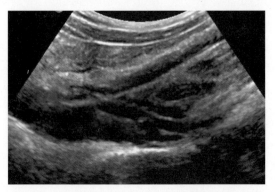

Suggested annotation: **SAG RT ADNEXA**

5. Repeat the image sequence for the left side.

Uterus • Transverse Images

1. Transverse image of the vagina.

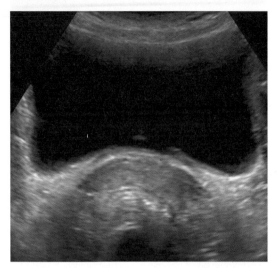

Suggested annotation: **TRV VAG**

2. Transverse image of the cervix.

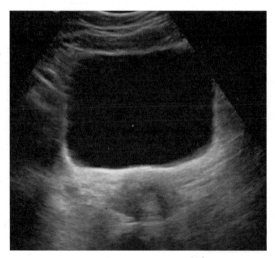

Suggested annotation: **TRV CX**

3.   Transverse image of the uterus body.

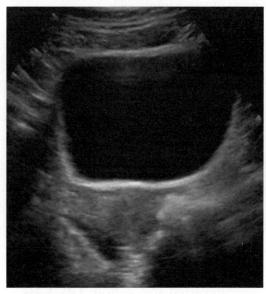

Suggested annotation: **TRV UT BODY**

4.   Transverse image of the uterus fundus with and without the width measured.

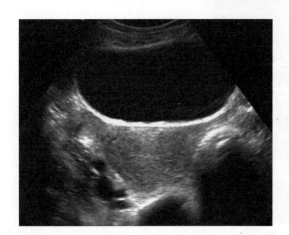 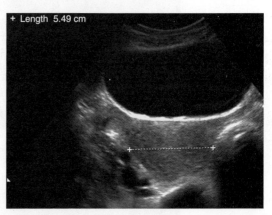

Suggested annotation: **TRV UT FUNDUS**

Ovary • Longitudinal Images

1. Long-axis image of the left ovary with and without measurements of the length and AP dimensions.

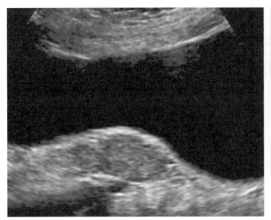 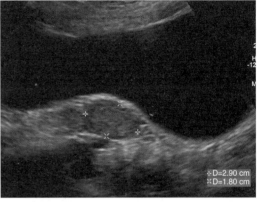

Suggested annotation: **LT OV LONG**

Ovary • Transverse Images

1. Transverse image of the left ovary with and without measurements of the width.

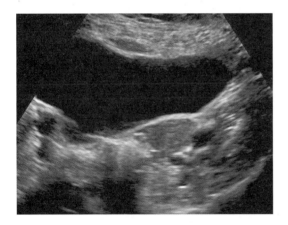 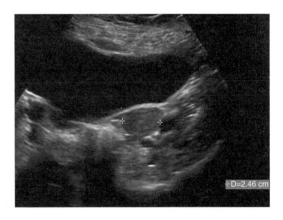

Suggested annotation: **LT OV TRV**
Repeat the images and measurements for the right ovary.

CHAPTER 13

Transvaginal Sonography

Tricia Turner

Keywords

Cervix	Menstrual phase
Chaperone	Ovary
Consent	Perimetrium
Endometrium	Myometrium
Endovaginal	Secretory phase
High-level disinfection	Transvaginal
Internal iliac artery	Uterus

Objectives

At the end of this chapter, you will be able to:

- List the scanning planes and image orientations for transvaginal scanning.
- List the suggested patient position and options for transvaginal scanning.
- Describe the patient prep for transvaginal scanning.
- Discuss how to find the ovaries and uterus.
- Explain the order and locations to take representative images of the female pelvis and its structures.

Overview

Transvaginal ultrasounds on women who are not pregnant can be performed in the radiology department, the emergency department (ED), and the in vitro fertilization (IVF) department. Transvaginal sonography (TVS), sometimes referred to as an **endovaginal** (EV) examination, is an ultrasound performed with the transducer inside the vagina using a specially designed high-frequency transducer called an endovaginal transducer. Sound does not have to travel as deep into the pelvic cavity during a TV examination, so a higher-frequency transducer can be used, and image resolution is much better than the images from a **transabdominal** (TA) examination. TA sonography provides a global view of the pelvic cavity, enabling better depiction of larger pathologic issues, whereas TVS can provide increased detail of the pelvic area and visualize structures not seen on the TA examination. It should be noted that an EV examination might miss structures or pathologic conditions that are above the

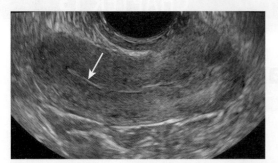

Fig. 13.1 An image of a normal uterus in a postmeno-pausal woman. The *arrow* is pointing to the thin, echogenic endometrium.

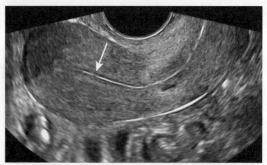

Fig. 13.2 An example of the endometrium in the menstrual phase. The *arrow* is pointing to the normal endometrium.

uterine fundus and have penetration issues in a fibroid uterus. This is why TA and EV examinations are complementary to one another and some laboratories may require that both be performed, except in the case of a short-term follow-up. Because of the effects of bladder distention, there are occasions when there is a difference in orientation between the TA and TV examinations. For example, the uterus may appear anteflexed on the TA examination and retroflexed on the TV examination.

Anatomy and Physiology
Review the female pelvic anatomy and physiology in Chapter 12.

Sonographic Appearance
The **uterus** has three layers, which are from outer to inner the **perimetrium**, **myometrium**, and **endometrium**. The myometrium is the muscular middle layer and is a mid-level gray with homogeneous echogenicity and smooth outer margins. The endometrium is the inner glandular portion, and the sonographic appearance and the thickness of the endometrium will vary with the menstrual cycle. The endometrium will be thin and seen as an echogenic line in postmenopausal women (Fig. 13.1). During the **menstrual phase**, the endometrium is a thin, hyperechoic line (Fig. 13.2). In some patients there may be some fluid compatible with blood in the endometrial cavity. In the proliferative phase, the endometrium starts to thicken and displays the characteristic trilaminar appearance. The first layer is the inner, thin echogenic line, which is caused by the opposed endometrial mucosal surfaces and represents the uterine cavity. The next layer is the hypoechoic functional layer of the endometrium, and the third outer layer is from the basal layer (Fig. 13.3). In the **secretory phase**, the endometrium reaches its thickest measurement and is homogeneously echogenic (Fig. 13.4).

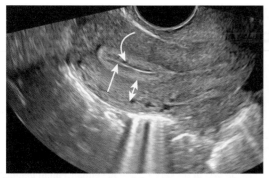

Fig. 13.3 The appearance of the endometrium in the proliferative phase demonstrating the characteristic trilaminar appearance. The *arrow* is pointing to the endometrial canal. The *curved arrow* is pointing to the functional layer. The *double-headed arrow* is pointing to the basal layer.

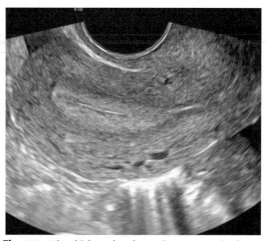

Fig. 13.4 The thickened endometrium as seen in the secretory phase.

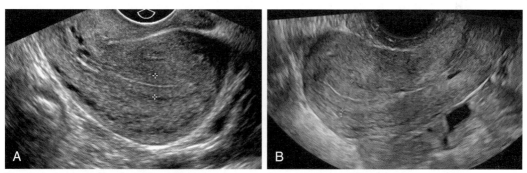

Fig. 13.5 A, Measuring the endometrium in a retroverted uterus in the proliferative phase. B, The endometrium being measured in a patient in the secretory phase.

The thickness of the endometrium is best evaluated and measured with TV ultrasound and is the sum of the two endometrial layers. The endometrium should be measured on the longitudinal image, perpendicular to the long axis of the endometrium, with the cursors placed at the anterior and posterior endometrial-myometrial interfaces where it is the thickest (Fig. 13.5). If fluid is seen in the endometrial cavity, it should be excluded from the measurement and each side measured individually.

The **cervix** is homogeneous and similar in echogenicity to the uterus, with a hypoechoic central canal. On some women a **nabothian cyst**, containing clear fluid, is commonly present in the cervix and typically measures less than 2 cm (Fig. 13.6).

The **ovary** can be variable in shape and position in the pelvis. They can be elliptical or round and typically are heterogenous in appearance because of the follicular cysts present. The ovarian tissue is a midlevel gray with the follicles appearing as small cystic structures (Fig. 13.7). The ovaries will change in their appearance with the menstrual cycle.

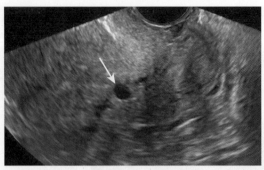

Fig. 13.6 The *arrow* is pointing to a nabothian cyst in the cervix. Note the enhancement behind the cyst.

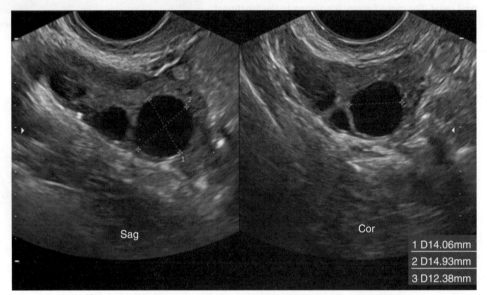

Fig. 13.7 Measuring the dominant follicle. *Cor,* Coronal; *Sag,* sagittal.

The **internal iliac artery** and vein often form the lateral boundary to the ovaries and are a good landmark to find them (Fig. 13.8).

Transvaginal Ultrasound

Patient Prep

Verbal or written **consent** is required depending on the department's policy. If the patient does not speak English, an approved hospital interpreter should be contacted. If the patient is unconscious, a family member must give consent, or two physicians if a family member is unavailable. Explain the details of the examination to put the patient at ease. Inform the patient that the examination may be uncomfortable but is relatively painless, that the inserted transducer may feel like a tampon, and that the examination is necessary because it provides better detail for the physician to help make a diagnosis. If the patient refuses the EV examination, never force the examination on her, but rather have the referring

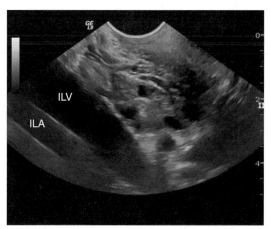

Fig. 13.8 The relationship between the ovary and the internal iliac vessels. *ILA,* Internal iliac artery; *ILV,* internal iliac vein.

physician talk to the patient if available. If the referring physician is not available, try to have the radiologist or sonologist talk to the patient.

The examination *must* be chaperoned by another health care professional. This is primarily for the protection of the sonographer. Female sonographers have been successfully sued for possible misuse of the TV transducer. A family member or a friend cannot be used as a **chaperone**. Depending on the policy, students and front desk workers may be able to chaperone the study. The institution will have a chaperone policy that must be followed. Male chaperones can be acceptable. The chaperone is there to protect you as a sonographer should the patient raise a concern of inappropriate behavior. It may be difficult to prove your innocence if you did not have a chaperone. If found guilty, the hospital may not cover the sonographer under their malpractice policy, and the sonographer also could be terminated. This may lead to having difficulty in being hired by other employers. If there is no chaperone policy in effect, talk to the manager and explain your concern. You could also contact the legal department and ask for a copy of the chaperone policy. It may even be online. This policy is not just for ultrasound but usually covers other types of vaginal examinations such as gynecologic examinations. The initials of the chaperone should be included as a permanent part of the patient records. With current electronic hospital information systems and electronic patient records, this can be incorporated into the fields the sonographer needs to fill out.

Have the patient completely empty her bladder before she gets on the stretcher. The patient, sonographer, or physician may insert the transducer. If the patient is comfortable inserting the transducer, hand her the transducer under the sheet that is covering her pelvic area. When she says it is inserted, reach under the sheet and take the handle. Always inform the patient when you are rotating the transducer between imaging planes.

> **NOTE:** Communication is key. Be sure to completely explain the examination in detail and allow time to answer any questions. Professionalism is very important to keep the patient at ease.

Transducer

Transvaginal examinations are performed with a special transducer that allows insertion into the vagina with a frequency of 8 MHz or higher.

To prepare the transducer, apply gel to the end of the transducer and then cover it with a disposable sheath. Make sure there are no air bubbles at the tip and that the transducer is coated in gel. Small areas of no gel contact with the transducer can cause artifacts and mimic dead crystals. Apply additional gel to the outside of the protective sheath before insertion. If infertility is a consideration, water or non-spermicidal gel should be used for a lubricant.

After the examination, the sheath covering the TV probe should be properly disposed of in the waste receptacle. Some sonographers may drape the transducer over the edge of the trash receptacle while helping the patient off the table. Once the patient has left the room, the transducer disinfection process should begin. With the concerns for hospital-acquired infections, follow the manufacturer's guidelines and the infection prevention department recommendations for cleaning of the TV transducer, including the handle, using a **high-level disinfection** (HLD) method. Studies have shown that viruses and bacteria have infected patients where the transducer was not disinfected properly using HLD, including from the handle, or by not using the proper disinfection products.

Patient Position

Having a gynecologic examining stretcher or a specially designed sonography scanning stretcher that has EV features, such as stirrups and a cutout at the end of the stretcher to easily manipulate the transducer, is optimal. With a gynecologic table, the patient can be positioned with her buttocks at the end of the examining stretcher. If a gynecologic stretcher is not available, use a foam cushion, pillows, or rolled-up sheets to elevate the hips so that transducer positioning is not compromised and can easily be moved without causing the patient discomfort or pain.

Image Orientation

Standard TV scanning uses sagittal and coronal planes from an inferior approach (Fig. 13.9). Proper image orientation is challenging in TV scanning because of the inferior scanning approach and the normal positional variations of the uterus. Proper positioning of the probe in the sagittal plane is confirmed when touching the edge of the probe, which is directed toward the ceiling, anterior of patient, which creates visible motion at the left of the image. From this position, the probe can be rotated 90 degrees counterclockwise to scan in the coronal plane (Fig. 13.10). On newer transducer designs the handle is bent, making orientation easier.

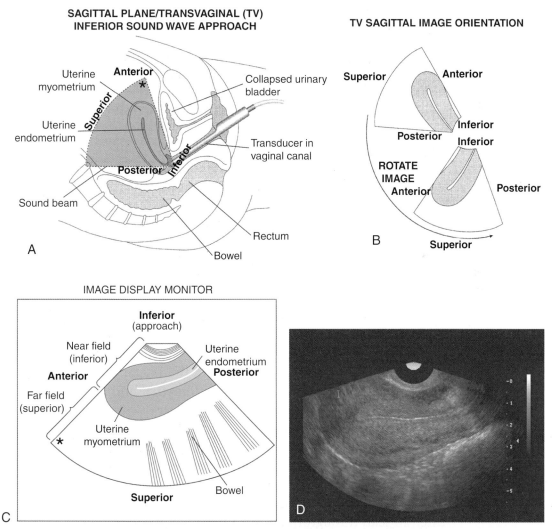

Fig. 13.9 A, An illustration of the scanning orientation in the sagittal plane. **B,** An illustration showing the image orientation in a sagittal plane as seen on the display monitor. **C,** Illustrates a longitudinal section of the uterus in a sagittal plane. The apex of the image on the display monitor corresponds to the anatomy closest to the face of the transducer. In transvaginal (TV) sonography, the near field and left side of the sagittal plane image generally correspond to the inferoposterior region of the true pelvis. The far field and right side of the sagittal plane image generally correspond to the anterosuperior region of the true pelvis. **D,** Image of the uterus from a TV sagittal image that corresponds to the drawing in **C.** Note how the uterus fills the screen, limiting the overall view of the pelvis but providing increased anatomic detail of the uterus and endometrium.

> **NOTE:** The uterus, ovaries, and adnexa are scanned in sections by slightly angling the inserted transducer in different directions.

> **NOTE:** During the TV evaluation, adnexal structures can be brought into view by using one hand to compress the lower abdominal wall while the other hand operates the transducer.

Patient Position

The patient is scanned supine, preferably on a TV ergonomic stretcher or by elevating the patient's hips with rolled up sheets.

Breathing Technique

The examination is performed with the patient in normal breathing.

Technical Tips

1. Begin scanning by slowly lowering the handle toward the floor to view a longitudinal section of the fundus of the uterus (Fig. 13.11). Now move the transducer a little to the right, then to the left, to evaluate its lateral margins. Movements during TV scanning should be small and not too quick so as not to miss anything. Note and evaluate the centrally located endometrial canal. If the bladder contains any urine, it will be seen anteriorly on the left side of the imaging screen.

2. Withdraw the transducer slightly, and slowly lift the handle toward the ceiling to view the body and cervix of the uterus and the posterior cul-de-sac (Fig. 13.12). Now move the transducer a little to the right, then to the left, to evaluate the lateral margins. Note and evaluate the centrally located endometrial and endocervical canals.

3. After evaluating the uterus, evaluate the adnexal regions. Gently reinsert the partially withdrawn transducer. Keep the transducer straight at the midline and lower the handle to relocate the uterine fundus and then the pelvic cavity region superior to the uterus. Now slowly move the transducer handle toward the patient's left thigh to scan through the right adnexa. Return to midline; slowly move the transducer handle toward the patient's right thigh to scan through the left adnexa.

4. Repeat these lateral sweeps through the adnexal regions at the levels of the uterine body and cervix.

5. If the ovaries are seen, obtain images of them. If not, proceed to the coronal images.

NOTE: For a retroverted uterus, the uterine fundus is visualized by lifting the transducer handle toward the ceiling (Fig. 13.13).

6. Following the longitudinal imaging from the sagittal plane, rotate the transducer 90 degrees counterclockwise into the coronal plane. Remember to tell your patient that you are moving the transducer so that the movement does not surprise her.

CORONAL PLANE/TRANSVAGINAL (TV) INFERIOR SOUND WAVE APPROACH

TV CORONAL IMAGE ORIENTATION

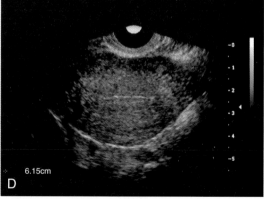

IMAGE DISPLAY MONITOR

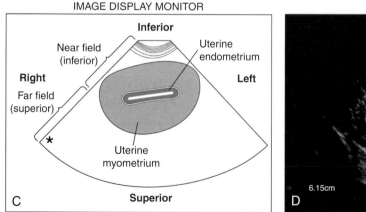

Fig. 13.10 A, An illustration of the transvaginal (TV) transducer position in a coronal plane field of view. When the bladder is empty, the fundus of the typical anteverted uterus tilts forward toward the anterior abdominal wall. Therefore, in TV imaging, the uterus is seen in short axis from a coronal plane. **B,** Depicts the rotation of the image as seen on the display monitor. **C,** Illustrates the uterus in a coronal plane. The apex of the image on the display monitor corresponds to the anatomy closest to the face of the transducer. In TV sonography, the near field and left side of the coronal plane image generally correspond to the inferolateral region of the true pelvis. The far field and right side of the coronal plane image generally correspond to the superolateral region of the true pelvis. **D,** Image of the fundus of the uterus from a TV coronal scanning plane that corresponds to the drawing in **C.** Note how the section of uterus fills the screen, limiting the overall view of the pelvis but providing increased anatomic detail of the uterus.

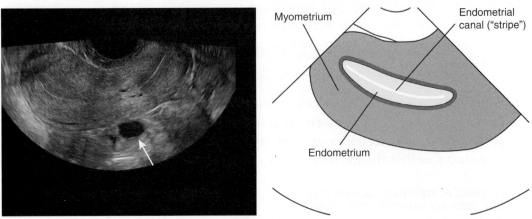

Fig. 13.11 An image and corresponding drawing of a sagittal view of the uterus. The *arrow* is pointing to a cystic area that demonstrated peristalsis compatible with bowel. As you can see the image could be confused with fluid in the cul-de-sac or a cystic lesion. A video clip should be taken to show the peristalsis or another image when the cystic area has changed in appearance.

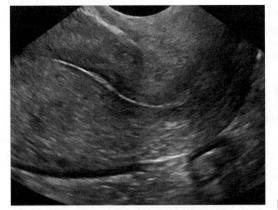

Fig. 13.12 An image of the normal body and cervix of the uterus and the posterior cul-de-sac.

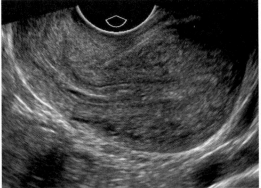

Fig. 13.13 An image of a normal retroverted uterus. The fundus is now closest to the transducer as opposed to far away.

7. Begin scanning by slowly lowering the handle of the inserted transducer toward the floor to evaluate the uterine fundus (Fig. 13.14). If the patient's hips are not elevated enough, this can make it difficult to scan. It may also cause the patient pain or discomfort while you are trying to angle the transducer. If they are on a padded mattress, try pushing with your hand into the padding. If still unable to see the uterus, build up the patient's hips more.

8. Withdraw the transducer slightly and slowly lift the transducer handle toward the ceiling to scan through the uterine body, cervix, and posterior cul-de-sac (Fig. 13.15).

9. After evaluating the uterus, continue the coronal scan through the adnexa. Move the transducer handle toward the floor and relocate the uterine fundus. Now slowly move the transducer handle toward the patient's left thigh to visualize the right adnexa,

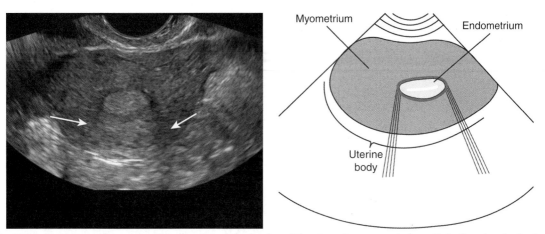

Fig. 13.14 An image and corresponding drawing of the fundus of the uterus in a coronal plane. Note the edge shadowing from the slightly thickened endometrium.

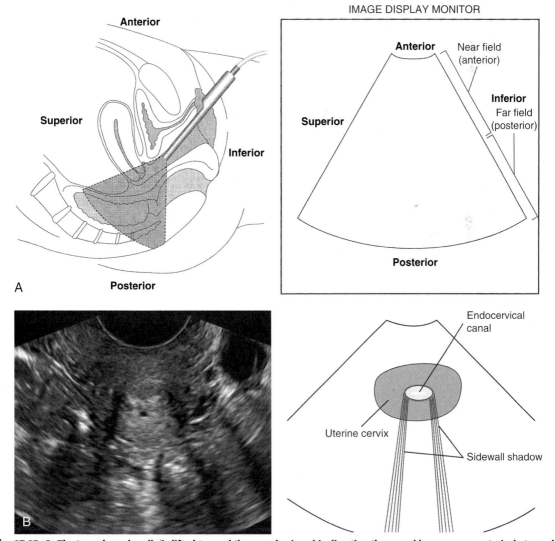

Fig. 13.15 A, The transducer handle is lifted toward the symphysis pubis directing the sound beam more posteriorly to evaluate the cervix. The near and far fields of the transvaginal sagittal plane image now correspond to anterior and posterior regions of the pelvis instead of inferior and superior regions. The left and right sides of the image now correspond more closely to the superior and inferior regions of the pelvis instead of anterior and posterior. **B,** An image and drawing of the transducer in a coronal plane and being angled posteriorly to see the cervix.

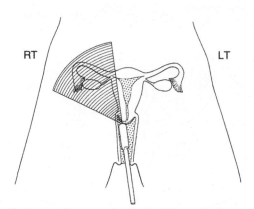

Fig. 13.16 Illustrates the handle being near the patient's left leg to angle the sound beam to visualize the right ovary and adnexa. *LT,* Left; *RT,* right.

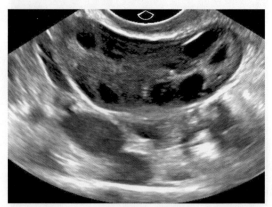

Fig. 13.17 An image of a normal right ovary with multiple follicles.

and very slowly move the transducer handle toward the ceiling to sweep through the area.

10. The ovaries are usually easier seen in the coronal scanning plane.

11. Begin scanning by putting the transducer in a right oblique position. This is done by slowly moving the transducer handle toward the patient's left thigh, which angles the beam toward the right adnexa (Fig. 13.16). Find the ovary by slightly moving the transducer handle up and down (Fig. 13.17). The ovary usually can be seen adjacent to the iliac vessels.

12. When the ovary is located, very slightly move the transducer handle as far up and down as necessary to scan through the ovarian margins.

13. Return the transducer to the midline, then slowly move the handle toward the patient's right thigh to visualize the left adnexa, and slowly move the transducer handle toward the ceiling to sweep through the area (Fig. 13.18)

14. After finishing the coronal images of the ovaries, return to the longitudinal plane by rotating the transducer 90 degrees clockwise while keeping the ovary in view. When possible, try to remember where the other ovary is located so you do not need to return to the coronal plane.

15. Begin scanning by very slightly moving the transducer handle to the right and then to the left to scan through the lateral and medial margins of the ovary (Fig. 13.19). Identify the adjacent iliac vessels, because the ovary will be medial to the iliac vessels.

16. When ready to evaluate the left ovary, move the handle toward the patient's right thigh and repeat the scanning maneuvers used for the right ovary.

17. When measuring the ovaries, if possible, use a split-screen technique. The ovary is typically tilted, so the length and width

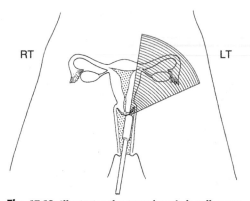

Fig. 13.18 Illustrates the transducer's handle now near the patient's right leg to angle the sound beam to visualize the left ovary and adnexa. *LT,* Left; *RT,* right.

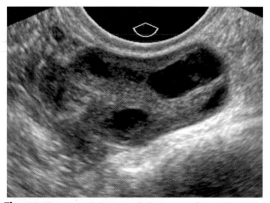

Fig. 13.19 Coronal image of the ovary from Fig. 13.17. Note how the ovary maintains an elliptical shape.

measurements will not always be parallel to the floor. The antero-posterior (AP) measurement should be perpendicular to the length measurement, and the width should be the longest diameter (Fig. 13.20).

Transvaginal Required Images

Uterus • Longitudinal Images

1. Longitudinal midline image showing the long axis of the uterus with and without longitudinal and AP measurements.

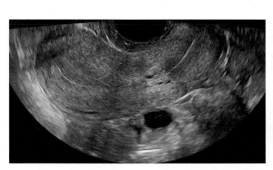
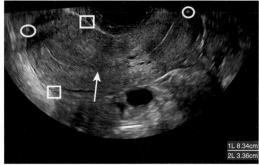

Suggested Annotation: **LONG ML UT**

Note that because of the curvature of the uterus, some units allow a tracing method to obtain an accurate length of the uterus. The *circles* show the cursors for the length, with the *arrow* pointing to where it bends. The *squares* show the cursors for the AP measurement.

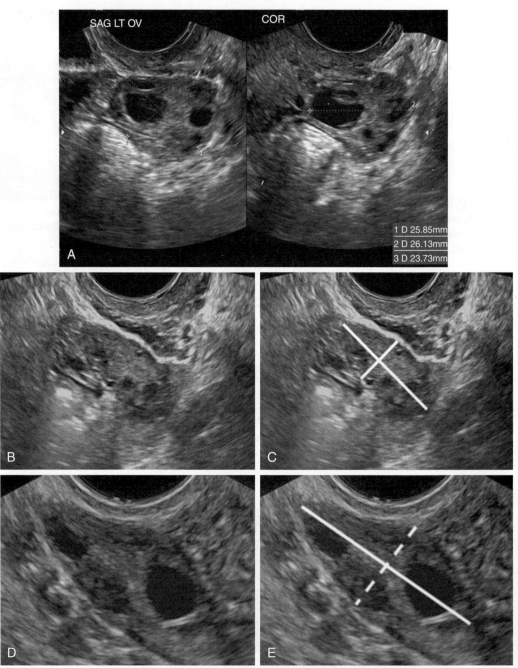

Fig. 13.20 A, An image using the split-screen technique to show sagittal and coronal views of the ovary with measurements. This can make it easy to have all the measurements together for ease of both documenting on a worksheet and dictation by the radiologist. **B,** A sagittal view of a normal ovary. **C,** The same ovary as in Fig. 13.20B. The *lines* demonstrate the proper technique for measuring the ovary. Note that the measurements are perpendicular to one another and form a cross. **D,** A coronal image of a normal ovary. **E,** The same ovary as in Fig. 13.20D showing the proper measurement technique to obtain the width of the ovary. The shape of the ovary and the scanning planes used can make determining the width of the ovary a challenge. Most references suggest using the longest measurement, as seen with the *solid line.* Some sonographers may measure the width as seen with the *dotted line.* Some sonographers measure both ways and let the radiologist decide which measurement to use. If the smaller measurement is close to the AP measurement from the sagittal view, typically the longer measurement will be used.

2. Longitudinal midline image of the endometrium with and without the AP measurement.

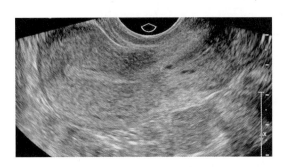 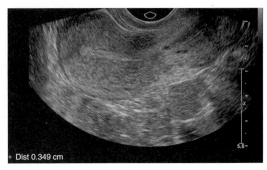

Suggested Annotation: **EMS**

3. Longitudinal image of the uterus fundus to include the fundus of the uterus.

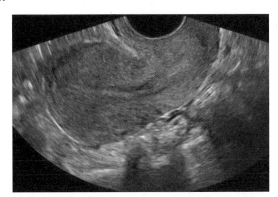

Suggested Annotation: **SAG FUNDUS**

4. Longitudinal image of the lateral border of the uterus. This will be all myometrium.

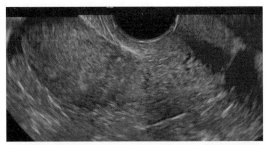

Suggested Annotation: **RT UT or RT LAT UT**

5. Longitudinal image of the uterus body and cervix to include the endometrial cavity.

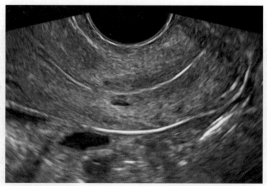

Suggested Annotation: **SAG UT/CX**

Uterus • Coronal Images

1. Coronal image of the cervix.

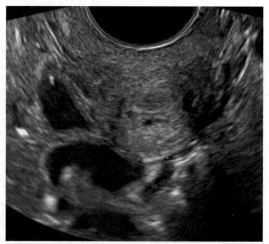

Suggested Annotation: **COR CX**

2. Coronal image of the uterine body.

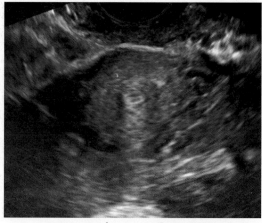

Suggested Annotation: **COR UT**

3. Coronal image of the fundus at the widest area with and without measurements.

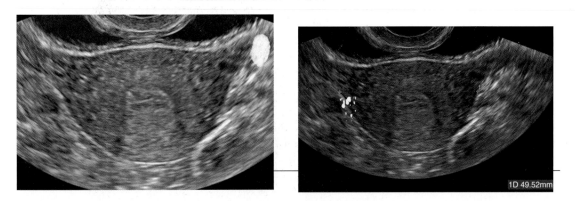

Suggested Annotation: **COR FUND**

4. Coronal image near the top of the uterus at the fundus showing just myometrium.

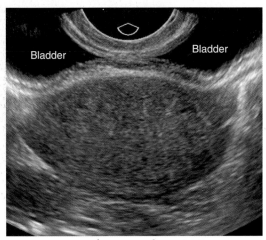

Suggested Annotation: **COR FUND**

Ovary • Longitudinal Images

1. Long-axis image of the right ovary measuring ovarian length and AP dimensions.

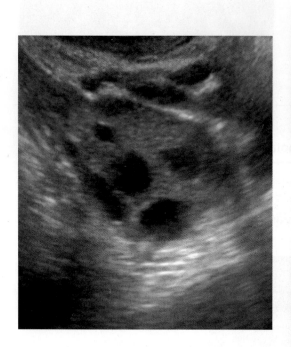
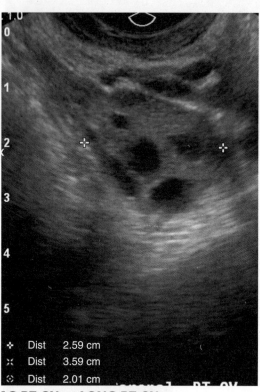

Suggested Annotation: **SAG RT OV or LONG RT OV**

Ovary • Coronal Images

1. Coronal image of the right ovary measuring ovarian width.

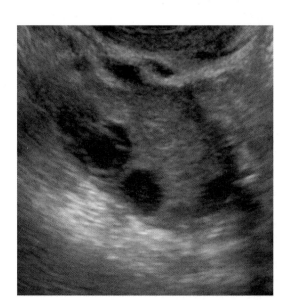 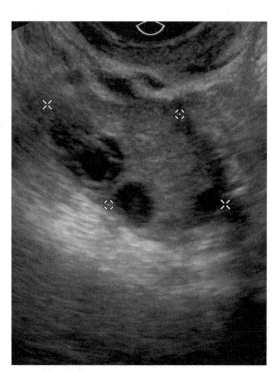

Suggested Annotation: **COR RT OV**

Repeat the longitudinal and coronal images on the left ovary.

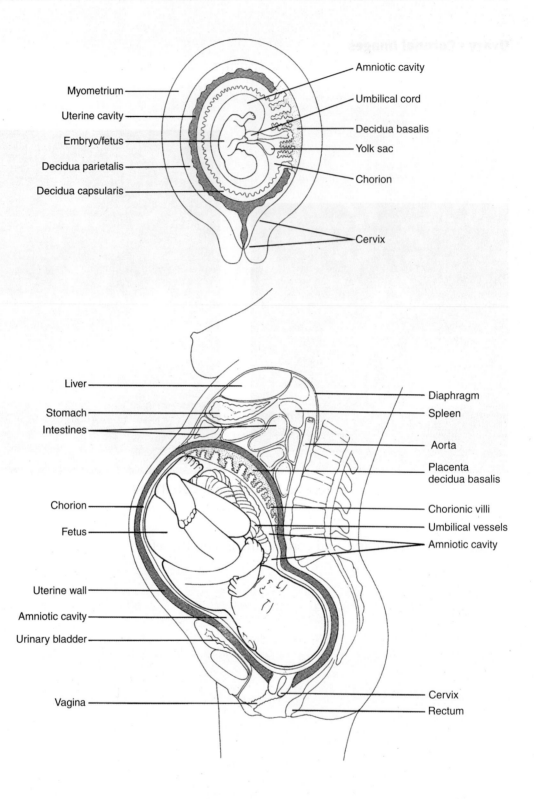

Myometrium

Uterine cavity

Embryo/fetus

Decidua parietalis

Decidua capsularis

Amniotic cavity

Umbilical cord

Decidua basalis

Yolk sac

Chorion

Cervix

Liver

Stomach

Intestines

Chorion

Fetus

Uterine wall

Amniotic cavity

Urinary bladder

Vagina

Diaphragm

Spleen

Aorta

Placenta decidua basalis

Chorionic villi

Umbilical vessels

Amniotic cavity

Cervix

Rectum

CHAPTER 14

Obstetric Scanning Protocol for First, Second, and Third Trimesters

Shannon Trebes

Keywords

Abdominal circumference (AC)	Fetus
Amnion	Foramen ovale
Amniotic cavity	Gestational sac
Amniotic fluid	Gravid
Amniotic membrane	Head circumference (HC)
Basal layer	Mean sac diameter (MSD)
Biparietal diameter (BPD)	Nasal bone
Chorionic membrane	Nuchal translucency
Crown-rump length (CRL)	Placenta
Decidua parietalis	Placental grading
Double bleb sign	Trophoblast
Double sac sign	Umbilical cord
Ectopic pregnancies	Umbilical cord insertion
Embryo	Yolk sac
Femur length (FL)	Zygote

Objectives

At the end of this chapter, you will be able to:

- Define the keywords.
- Define the beginning and end of each trimester.
- List needed fetal measurements for each trimester.
- Discuss anatomic images needed for each trimester.
- Describe the different transducer types and frequencies for scanning during the first, second, and third trimesters of pregnancy.
- List the suggested patient position when scanning during the first, second, and third trimesters of pregnancy.
- Describe the patient prep for the first, second, and third trimesters of pregnancy.

Overview

Obstetric ultrasound is used to evaluate the fetus, placenta, and maternal structures. It is typically performed in a maternal fetal medicine department, obstetrician office, radiology department, or radiology outpatient office. Limited aspects of obstetric ultrasound are performed in the labor and delivery (L + D) department.

Before the examination, a patient history should be taken to include the date of the first day of the patient's last menstrual period, parity, gravidity, pregnancy test results if available, any symptoms, pelvic examination results, history of pelvic surgery, and any known maternal medical conditions. Most sonography departments have standard forms on which this information is recorded or electronic records in which this information has been documented.

Before starting the examination, make sure the obstetric preset is selected on the ultrasound unit to ensure that the proper power levels are used.

Maternal Anatomy and Physiology

The female pelvic organs include the reproductive tract: the uterus, vagina, uterine or fallopian tubes, ovaries, urinary bladder, a portion of the ureters, and the rectosigmoid colon. The osseous or bony pelvis forms the outer boundaries of the female pelvic cavity, and the skeletal muscles that line the pelvic cavity form the inner boundaries. Chapter 12 discusses in detail the anatomy and physiology of the female pelvis and how the menstrual cycle prepares the uterus for implantation by a fertilized ovum.

If fertilization does not occur, hormone levels decrease and the nonimplanted endometrial lining of the uterus is shed during menses. When fertilization occurs, it usually takes place within 1 day of ovulation, around day 15 of the menstrual cycle. Fertilization occurs when the ova and sperm fuse to form a **zygote** or cell mass, normally at the ampulla portion of the fallopian tube. The cell mass repeatedly divides into the morula, which is a cluster of 16 or more cells that leaves the fallopian tube and enters the uterine cavity on day 18 or 19 of the menstrual cycle. On day 20 or 21 of the cycle, the blastocyst starts to implant onto the decidualized or **gravid** uterine endometrium. By day 28, the blastocyst becomes completely imbedded into uterine endometrial tissue, and implantation is complete.

The morula continues to divide and becomes the blastocyst. The outer layer of the blastocyst, the **trophoblast**, will develop into the **chorionic membrane**, the fetal component of the **placenta**.

> **NOTE:** The placenta is an organ that joins the mother and the fetus and allows the transfer of oxygen and nutrients from the mother to the fetus and for waste products to be transferred from the fetus to the mother.

The inner layer of the blastocyst, the embryoblast, or embryonic disk, develops into the **embryo**. The **yolk sac** is a membranous sac attached to the embryo that provides nourishment (Fig. 14.1). The **amnion** contains the fluid that helps cushion, and protect the fetus and the **umbilical cord**, which is a flexible cord, comprising two arteries and one vein, that connects the fetus to the placenta. Embryonic development covers the first 8 weeks of development. At the beginning of the 9th week, the embryo is termed a **fetus.**

Anatomy and Sonographic Appearance During the First Trimester

The first trimester occurs from conception to 13 6/7 weeks gestational age (GA). The blastocyst is too small to be visualized sonographically, but other intrauterine changes can be detected to confirm a pregnancy during the early first trimester. The normal **gestational sac** appears as a small, round or oval, fluid-filled, anechoic chorionic cavity completely surrounded by endometrium (Fig. 14.2).

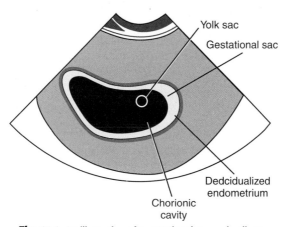

Fig. 14.1 An illustration of a gestational sac and yolk sac.

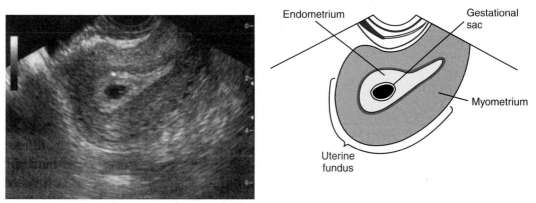

Fig. 14.2 Endovaginal sonogram and illustration of an early gestational sac.

The key sonographic finding in an early intrauterine pregnancy is referred to as the intradecidual sign, which is the fluid-filled gestational sac located at the level of the fundus of the uterus within the endometrium (Fig. 14.3). Note that there should be no displacement or change in size of the endometrial cavity at this early stage. Endovaginal (EV) sonography is usually the best choice for visualizing the gestational sac; however, it can be seen in a transabdominal (TA) approach (Fig. 14.4).

Although the TA examination is generally not the choice for evaluating the intradecidual sign, it can visualize the intrauterine gestational sac as early as 3 to 5 weeks GA when the sac diameter is 2 to 4 mm. At this stage the serum human chorionic gonadotropin (hCG) levels will exceed 1025 mIU/mL. hCG is the hormone secreted by the developing placenta to communicate to the rest of the body that a gestation is present within the uterus. As the gestational sac enlarges, the endometrial walls get thicker and markedly hyperechoic relative to the myometrium.

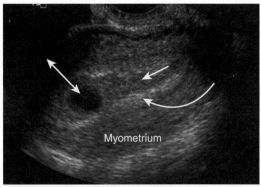

Fig. 14.3 Endovaginal sonogram demonstrating the intradecidual sign. The *arrow* is pointing to the endometrial cavity. The *curved arrow* is pointing to the endometrium. The *double-headed arrow* is pointing to the gestational sac.

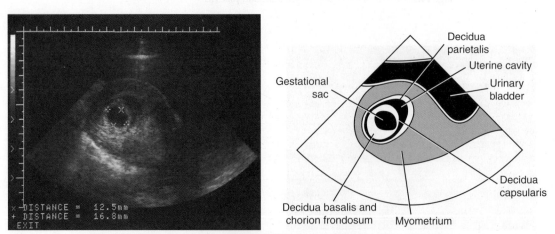

Fig. 14.4 A transabdominal sonogram and drawing of a normal early gestational sac.

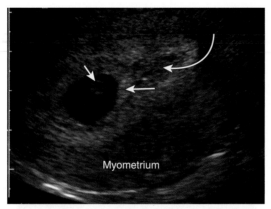

Fig. 14.5 An endovaginal sonogram showing the double sac sign. The *long arrow* is pointing to the decidua basalis and chorion frondosum. The *curved arrow* is pointing to the decidua parietalis. The *short arrow* is pointing to the yolk sac.

Sonographic Appearance and Development During the First Half of the First Trimester

Double Sac Sign

With further growth the gestational sac can take on the distinctive sonographic appearance known as the **double sac sign** (Fig. 14.5). The two bright concentric circles separated by anechoic fluid in the uterine cavity are the decidua basalis and **decidua parietalis**, the layers of the gravid endometrium. Identification of the double sac sign likely represents an intrauterine pregnancy and may be seen before a yolk sac is visualized; however, it does not rule out a pseudogestational sac, which is a collection of fluid or blood in the uterine cavity that can be associated with an **ectopic pregnancy**, a pregnancy that occurs outside the uterus. The presence of a yolk sac, embryo, or both seen within the gestational sac confirms an intrauterine pregnancy.

Yolk Sac

By the end of 4 weeks GA, the primary yolk sac has regressed and is replaced by the secondary yolk sac, which is the first anatomic structure visualized within the gestational sac. The secondary yolk sac provides nutrients to the developing embryo and is the initial site of blood cell development. The sonographic appearance of the yolk sac is a small, round structure with bright, well-defined walls and an anechoic, fluid-filled center. Identification of the yolk sac is variable; however, it can be detected as early as 5 weeks GA with EV transducers and should be visible by 7 weeks GA using a TA approach. A **double bleb sign** is when there is visualization of a gestational sac containing a yolk sac and amniotic sac giving an appearance of two small bubbles. The embryonic disc is located between these two structures. A faint flickering motion seen adjacent to the yolk sac represents the neurologically active heart tissue. From 5 to 10 weeks GA the yolk sac progressively increases to a maximum diameter of 5 to 6 mm (Fig. 14.6). By the end of the first trimester, the yolk sac shrinks and is no longer appreciated sonographically.

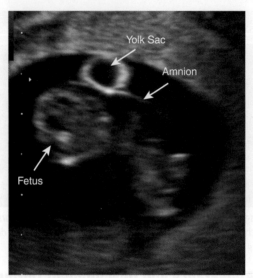

Fig. 14.6 An endovaginal ultrasound showing the yolk sac, fetus, and amnion.

Estimating Gestational Age During the First Half of the First Trimester

Mean Sac Diameter

In the first half of the first trimester, gestational sac size can be used to estimate GA; however, as recommended by The American College of Obstetricians and Gynecologists (ACOG), it should not be used for establishing the due date. The estimated GA based on the gestational sac size can be calculated using the **mean sac diameter** (MSD). The three orthogonal dimensions of the chorionic cavity are added together then divided by 3 to determine the MSD. The length and anteroposterior dimensions can be measured in a long-axis section of the gestational sac, and the width of the sac can be measured at the widest axial section. Note how the bright rim of choriodecidual reaction is not included in the measurement (Fig. 14.7).

Crown-Rump Length

Embryonic development is rapid during 6 to 10 weeks GA. As development continues into the second half of the first trimester, the embryo or fetus can be identified and measured by the **crown-rump length** (CRL). The CRL measurement is the most accurate method for establishing and confirming GA during pregnancy. Before 6 weeks it is not possible to always separate the crown and rump from the embryonic disk length, causing an inaccurate CRL measurement. Between 6 and 8 weeks GA, the embryo's head becomes prominently flexed, making the longest axis for measurement from the neck to the rump. From 8 to 12 weeks GA, the embryo's head extends, making a true crown-rump long axis for measurement (Fig. 14.8).

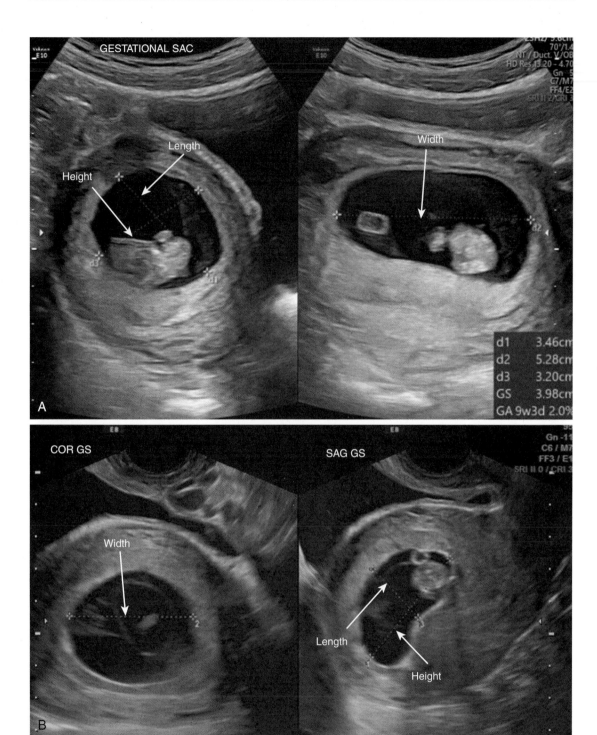

Fig. 14.7 A, Image demonstrating the proper technique to measure the gestational sac from a transabdominal approach. The length and height measurements should be perpendicular to each other. **B,** Image demonstrating the proper technique to measure the gestational sac from an endovaginal approach.

Amniotic Sac

By 6.5 weeks the amniotic membrane and its fluid-filled sac or cavity have enlarged enough to surround the embryo. The thin, reflective **amniotic membrane** encloses the developing echogenic embryo and "bathes" it in the **amniotic fluid** within the amniotic sac. As the trimester progresses,

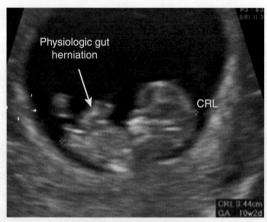

Fig. 14.8 A transabdominal image demonstrating the proper technique to measure the crown-rump length *(CRL)*.

not only do the CRL and amniotic sac diameter increase 1 mm per day but also their measurements are equal. Between 12 weeks and 16 weeks GA, the chorionic cavity will become obliterated when the **amniotic cavity** has enlarged enough for the fusion of the amniotic and chorionic membranes. The yolk sac and embryo retreat from each other but remain connected by the yolk stalk or vitelline duct, which eventually becomes part of the umbilical cord, the three-vessel connection between the embryo/fetus and mother. Also seen during this time is the tail-like appendage that is often identified at the site of the rump.

Sonographic Appearance and Development During the Second Half of the First Trimester

Embryonic Heart

As previously mentioned, the embryonic heart may be detected as early as 5 weeks GA as a flickering motion. Embryonic heart motion should be seen when the CRL measures greater than 7 mm. As the first trimester progresses, the embryonic heart will appear small and pulsatile. The anechoic chambers, echogenic walls, and contour may be discernable by GA weeks 11 or 12.

Skeletal System

The axial and appendicular skeletons form between the sixth and eighth gestational weeks. The bright reflection of the fetal skeleton indicates the degree of mineralization that has taken place within the developing bones. Ultrasound is able to distinguish how ossified portions of the fetal skeleton appear highly echogenic compared with the mid-gray appearance of adjacent cartilaginous structures.

Umbilical Cord

During GA week 8, the embryo assumes a C shape, fetal limb buds start to become visible, placental development begins, and the umbilical cord can be visualized. The cord will appear thick and about as long as

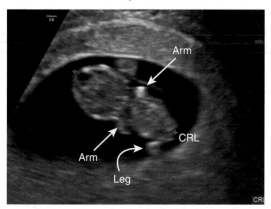

Fig. 14.9 Image of a normal fetus showing the limb buds. *CRL,* Crown-rump length.

the embryo. In short axis it presents as a large, round, anechoic vein with bright walls, flanked by two small, round anechoic arteries with bright walls. A gelatinous tissue, Wharton's jelly, surrounds the three vessels within the cord and prevents it from becoming crushed. The umbilical cord will continue to grow at a rate similar to that of the embryo.

End of the First Trimester

By GA week 10, the limbs are detectable and the head is easily appreciated (Fig. 14.9). It is normal at this time to see normal gut herniation into the base of the umbilical cord. Normal gut herniation should not be seen after GA week 12.

During GA weeks 11 and 12, individual fingers and toes, the anechoic fluid in the stomach and urinary bladder, and the mid-gray, homogeneous liver can be identified. By the end of the first trimester, the oral cavity, including the hard palate and tongue, are consistently identified. The embryonic head and body become proportional, and the embryo has developed into a fetus that assumes a distinct human-like appearance.

Determining Gestational Age During the Second Half of the First Trimester

The ACOG recommends that ultrasound measurements of the embryo or fetus in the first trimester, up to a CRL length of 84 mm, to be the most accurate method for establishing and/or confirming GA. If the pregnancy results from assisted reproductive technology (ART) such as in vitro fertilization, the GA derived from ART should be used to assign the estimated due date. As soon as the patient's last menstrual period date, first accurate ultrasound evaluation, or both are obtained, the estimated GA should be determined and any subsequent change to the estimated due date should be reserved for rare cases.

Sonographic Appearance and Development During the Second (14 0/7 to 27 6/7 Weeks) and Third (28 to 40 Weeks) Trimesters

By GA week 13, the majority of the organs have formed during the first trimester and most are located in their final anatomic positions. During the second and third trimesters, these organs and their associated organ systems become fully developed as other body structures continue to grow and mature. To grow properly and develop normally, the fetus depends on the placenta and umbilical cord for nutrients, oxygen, and removal of metabolic waste products.

Placenta

The early placenta appears medium gray with homogeneous echo texture. It darkens slightly during the second and third trimesters. As the gestation advances, the homogeneous appearance of the placenta may be interrupted by bright, echogenic calcium deposits and/or small anechoic lacunae, which represent maternal venous lakes. Retroplacental and intraplacental arteries may appear anechoic with bright walls. Anechoic tubular structures on the uterine surface of the placenta representing maternal marginal veins that also may be visualized.

Placental Grading

Once popular **placental grading** classifies placenta maturation according to its sonographic appearance. Many departments no longer grade the placenta routinely and only use it when necessary to support a diagnosis such as preeeclampsia. A grade 0 placenta appears normal throughout pregnancy. The chorionic plate, the sac border, remains smooth; the **basal layer**, the uterine border, is free of calcification, and the parenchyma or bulk of the placenta remains medium gray and homogeneous except for anechoic lacunae. With grade I, the chorionic plate shows some subtle indentations, the basal layer becomes hypoechoic or anechoic relative to adjacent structures, and the parenchyma exhibits a few scattered, bright punctate densities or calcifications. These findings are considered normal any time after 34 weeks of development. A grade II placenta presents with medium-sized indentations of the chorionic plate, a few small, linear, bright densities are identified at the basal layer, and the parenchyma contains bright, scattered, "comma-like" densities. These findings are considered normal any time after 36 weeks of development. With grade III, the chorionic plate shows indentations extending as far as the basal layer, dividing the placenta into segments. The basal layer exhibits very long, linear, bright, densities that may, in advanced stages, appear as a bright, unbroken line. The placental parenchyma may contain highly echogenic and anechoic areas. The bright echoes represent large calcifications that may cast acoustic shadows. These findings are considered normal any time after 38 weeks of development (Fig. 14.10).

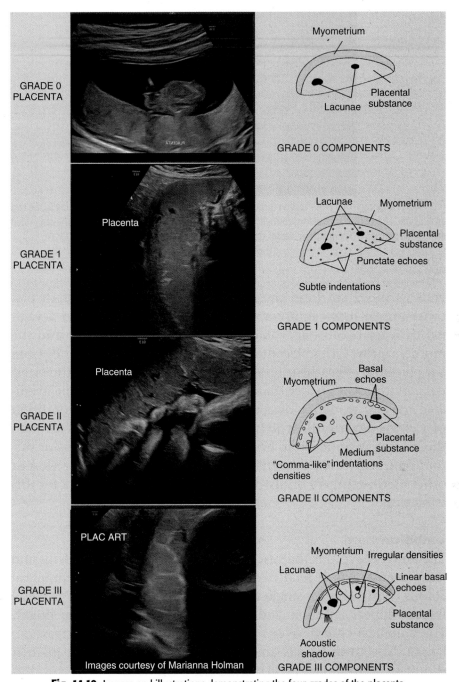

GRADE 0 PLACENTA

Myometrium

Placental substance

Lacunae

GRADE 0 COMPONENTS

GRADE 1 PLACENTA

Placenta

Lacunae   Myometrium

Placental substance

Punctate echoes

Subtle indentations

GRADE 1 COMPONENTS

GRADE II PLACENTA

Placenta

Basal echoes

Myometrium

Placental substance

Medium densities

"Comma-like" indentations

GRADE II COMPONENTS

GRADE III PLACENTA

PLAC ART

Myometrium   Irregular densities

Lacunae

Linear basal echoes

Placental substance

Acoustic shadow

Images courtesy of Marianna Holman   GRADE III COMPONENTS

Fig. 14.10 Images and illustrations demonstrating the four grades of the placenta.

Placenta Location

The location of the placenta is variable within the uterus and may change as the uterus expands to accommodate the growing fetus. Sonographic evaluation of the placenta includes its position relative to the cervical internal os to rule out placenta previa, a condition in which the os is obstructed by overlying and low-lying placenta, a condition in which the inferior margin of the placenta

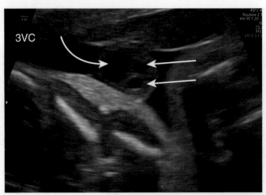

Fig. 14.11 An image of a cross section through the umbilical cord. The *arrows* are pointing to the two arteries and the *curved arrow* to the single vein. When documented during the scan, the suggested annotation would be *3VC* for three-vessel cord.

ends within 2 cm from the internal cervical os. A persistent placenta previa may require a cesarean delivery rather than a vaginal delivery because it would be dangerous for the fetus and the mother. A low-lying placenta can be ruled out if the distance from the placental edge, the inferior margin of the placenta, to the internal cervical os is greater than 2 cm. The placenta should be evaluated for any evidence of accreta spectrum, which is a condition of varying severity in which the placenta grows into or through the uterine myometrium, becoming adherent to the uterus or surrounding structures. Patients with a history of cesarean section or other uterine surgery or instrumentation have a higher risk for this condition.

Umbilical Cord

The umbilical cord is the vascular connection between the fetus and the placenta, where fetal circulation begins. The normal umbilical cord is composed of a single vein flanked by two arteries. The vessel lumens appear anechoic and the surrounding walls appear bright. The umbilical cord develops multiple spiral turns as it increases in length. The three vessels are usually easier to distinguish in their short-axis section (Fig. 14.11).

Umbilical Cord Insertion

After the first trimester, the fetal surface vessels are routinely visualized and can be traced to the site where the vessels merge and penetrate the placental parenchyma. In addition, the **umbilical cord insertion** site where the cord enters the fetus at the umbilicus can be visualized (Fig. 14.12). The umbilical vein runs cephalically to join the fetal portal circulation. The arteries take a caudal course, running on each side of the urinary bladder to meet the iliac arteries.

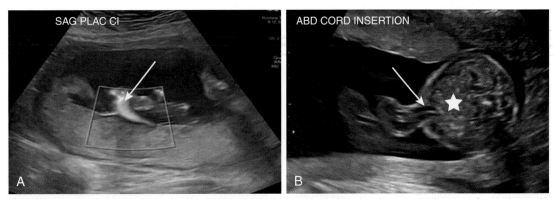

Fig. 14.12 A, The *arrow* is pointing to the umbilical cord where it inserts into the placenta. **B,** The *arrow* is pointing to the umbilical cord where it inserts into the fetus. The *star* is over the fetal small bowel.

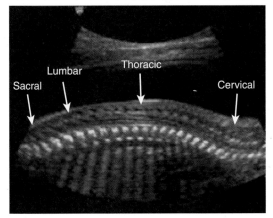

Fig. 14.13 An image of a normal long axis of the spine.

Skeletal System

During the second and third trimesters most of the bones of the skeleton are routinely visualized. The calvaria of the skull appear highly echogenic and prominent. The contour of the normal fetal head should appear smooth and elliptical in shape. Other identifiable bones include the mandible, nasal ridge, orbits, the rib cage in the thorax, and the fetal spine. The vertebrae have a highly reflective appearance, making them easy to recognize. A longitudinal section of the fetal spine can be described as two rows of closely spaced reflectors on each side of the mid-gray to low-gray appearance of the spinal cord. The two rows are roughly parallel, but wider in the cervical and lumbar regions and narrower in the sacral region (Fig. 14.13). The gaps between the vertebral bodies are composed of nonossified margins of adjoining vertebral bodies and the intervertebral disks. In short-axis sections, the vertebral anterior ossification center is seen equidistant from the two posterior ossification centers.

During the early to mid-part of the second trimester, most of the bones of the appendicular skeleton are routinely visualized, which includes the upper and lower extremities. In short-axis sections, they

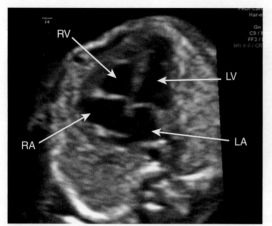

Fig. 14.14 An image of a normal four-chamber view of the heart. The tricuspid valve is between the right ventricular and atrium, and the mitral valve is between the left ventricular and atrium. The *small circle* beneath the left atrium is the thoracic aorta. *LA*, Left atrium; *LV*, left ventricle; *RA*, right atrium; *RV*, right ventricle.

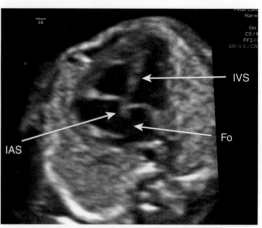

Fig. 14.15 The echogenic structures on either side of the heart are the lungs. *Fo,* Foramen ovale; *IAS,* interatrial septum; *IVS,* interventricular septum.

appear as bright echogenic foci surrounded by low-gray, homogeneous soft tissue. The longitudinal sections of the bones appear linear, bright, and reflective. The femurs especially cast a very prominent shadow. The cartilaginous ends of the bones appear homogeneous and low-gray.

Cardiovascular System
Heart
By 12 weeks GA, the four chambers of the fetal heart can be visualized. The walls of the heart appear mid-gray and hyperechoic relative to the anechoic blood in the chambers. The four chambers should appear relatively symmetric (Fig. 14.14). They are divided by the echogenic atrioventricular septa, which will appear "broken" at the **foramen ovale**, which is a normal opening between the atria allowing blood to move right to left in the fetal heart (Fig. 14.15). The heart is normally visualized on the left side of the thorax.

Blood Vessels
The sonographic appearance of the blood vessels in the fetus appear as they do after birth, bright walls with anechoic blood in the lumens. The superior vena cava, thoracic aorta, and pulmonary artery can be visualized in the upper mediastinum during the second trimester. With advanced GA, the brachiocephalic artery, common carotids, left subclavian, and jugular veins are frequently visualized. The abdominal aorta and inferior vena cava are easy to identify in the posterior portion of the abdomen. The iliac arteries and veins are also often observed. Color Doppler sonography is helpful for resolving small vessel branches such as the celiac axis, superior mesenteric artery, renal arteries, and renal veins.

Respiratory System
Upper Respiratory Tract
Sonography is able to visualize upper respiratory tract structures such as the nose, nasal cavity and septum, and palate. The pharynx, hypopharynx, piriform sinuses, and epiglottis are seen in advanced fetal age and are easily identified because of the anechoic amniotic fluid in portions of the upper tract. The fluid-filled trachea can usually be traced from its distal end to the level of the aortic arch. When the hypopharynx contains amniotic fluid, the larynx can be identified.

Lungs
During the first trimester, the lungs are identified more by the structures adjacent to them such as the heart, ribs, diaphragm, and liver. By the second trimester, however, the lungs become more apparent and appear isoechoic to the mid-gray, homogeneous appearance of the fetal liver. The muscular diaphragm separates the thorax from the abdomen and appears hypoechoic relative to the liver and lungs. As GA advances, the lungs become more echogenic.

Gastrointestinal System
Stomach and Gallbladder
The fetal stomach and gallbladder are readily identified sonographically because they are the only subdiaphragmatic gastrointestinal (GI) system structures normally filled with fluid. The fluid-filled stomach appears anechoic and is easy to identify on the left side of the fetal abdomen. The size of the stomach varies depending on the amount of amniotic fluid swallowed by the fetus. The bile-filled gallbladder appears anechoic and on the right side of the fetal abdomen. The gallbladder may not be visualized after 32 weeks GA. Some experts think that the gallbladder contracts, releasing bile, because of the initiation of gallbladder function.

Liver
The liver is the largest parenchymal organ of the GI system and of the body. It is routinely visualized during the second trimester. It appears mid-gray and homogeneous and occupies the right side and part of the left side of the fetal abdomen. The anechoic umbilical vein is routinely identified coursing through the liver.

Pancreas
The pancreas is another major parenchymal organ of the GI system; it is rarely seen. It may be visualized between the posterior wall of the anechoic fluid-filled stomach and the splenic vein. It appears hyperechoic relative to the fetal liver.

Spleen

Like the fetal liver, the spleen is routinely identified from the second trimester onward. The spleen occupies the left upper quadrant of the fetal abdomen and appears isoechoic to the fetal liver.

Small and Large Bowel

Small bowel loops and large bowel loops can be well distinguished sonographically in the second and third trimesters. The muscle layers of the bowel appear hypoechoic relative to the highly echogenic appearance of the serosa and subserosal linings. By the end of the third trimester it is normal to visualize a small amount of anechoic fluid and bright areas of meconium, fetal waste, within the bowel.

Genitourinary System

Kidneys

The fetal kidneys have been identified sonographically as early as 12 weeks GA. At this stage of renal development, the sonographic appearance of the kidneys can be difficult to differentiate from adjacent structures. However, after 20 weeks GA, the highly echogenic retroperitoneal fat comes to surround the kidneys, making them easier to identify. Normal fetal renal cortex appears mid-gray to low-gray or slightly hypoechoic relative to adjacent structures. Unlike adult kidneys, there is very little fat in the fetal renal sinus, making it virtually indistinguishable from the cortex. This leads to visualization of urine-filled intrarenal structures such as the renal pelvis and infundibula, that are not normally appreciated sonographically in adult kidneys. With advanced GA, the renal sinus can become slightly hyperechoic relative to the cortex, making the kidneys easier to distinguish sonographically. The distinctive elliptical shape and bright renal capsule assist sonographic identification of the longitudinal sections of the fetal kidneys as seen in image (Fig. 14.16).

Urinary Bladder

The urine-filled fetal bladder is easily recognized in the fetal pelvis because of its characteristic anechoic appearance and midline position. Changes in the volume of the urinary bladder can confirm normal fetal renal function. It is important to identify the bladder from cystic pathologic conditions.

Genitalia

Fetal gender can be established from the early second trimester by identifying either the male scrotum or the female labia. The penis and scrotum appear homogeneous with a low-gray to mid-gray shade. It is not uncommon to identify the testes within the scrotum typically after 7 to 8 months GA. The labia have two parts that are sonographically distinguishable, the major labia and minor labia. The major

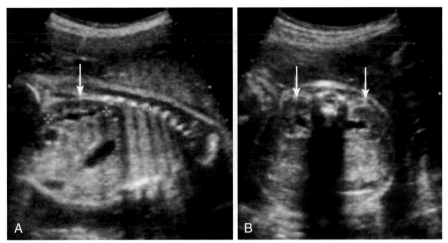

Fig. 14.16 A, An image of the long axis of a fetal kidney. **B,** A transverse image of both kidneys. The *arrows* are pointing to the kidneys. The mild dilatation seen is a normal finding that is typically a transient finding. There is concern if the dilatation is greater than 4 mm.

labia flank the minor. Both appear homogeneous and mid-gray, but the major labia are hyperechoic relative to the minor. The vaginal cleft lies at the midline between the minor labia and appears linear and bright. The labia can be identified sonographically as early as 15 to 16 weeks GA. The sonographer should be certain that they can identify the penis and the scrotum before telling the parents that it is a boy because swollen labia can look similar to the scrotum.

Intracranial Anatomy
Lateral Cerebral Ventricles

By 11 weeks GA, the most prominent intracranial structures visualized are the highly echogenic choroid plexus, easily identified within the body of the lateral ventricles. There is a striking contrast between the appearance of the bright choroid plexus and the anechoic appearance of the ventricles filled with cerebrospinal fluid. The walls of the ventricles appear bright. At this stage, only the ventricular bodies and frontal horns are developed well enough to visualize because the occipital and temporal horns are still rudiments. The outer walls of the lateral ventricles appear as bright linear structures lying the same distance from the interhemispheric fissure. The medial walls of the lateral ventricles are not quite as bright in appearance as the outer ventricular walls. The appearance of the lateral ventricles changes as development continues. The occipital and temporal horns become visible by 18 to 20 weeks GA, and as brain tissue volume increases with normal development, ventricular shape is altered and overall ventricular size decreases. The atria are the sites where the temporal and occipital horns join the body of the lateral ventricles. Ventricular width is normal up to 10 mm. Cerebrospinal fluid flows from the lateral ventricles to the third and fourth ventricles, into the subarachnoid space and then to the dural sinuses, where it is absorbed into the venous bloodstream.

Third Ventricle

The third ventricle lies at the midline of the brain and appears as a highly reflective line parallel to the interhemispheric fissure. Occasionally the third ventricle's cavity fills with cerebrospinal fluid, giving it the appearance of an anechoic, midline slit.

Fourth Ventricle

The fourth ventricle also lies at the midline of the brain, posterior to the third ventricle.

Interhemispheric Fissure and Falx

The interhemispheric fissure visually separates the cerebral hemispheres. The fissure appears as a single, linear, bright structure at the midline of the brain. The falx cerebri, a fold of dura mater, lies within the interhemispheric fissure, and because they are not sonographically distinguishable from one another, the terms are used interchangeably.

Cerebrum

The cerebrum is the largest component of the brain. It is almost completely divided anteroposteriorly into two lateral, symmetric hemispheres by the callosal fissure. It is composed of five lobes, the parietal, temporal, occipital, frontal, and insula, or isle of Reil, which is the only lobe not named for an overlying bone. The normal cerebrum appears homogeneous and is a mid-gray to low-gray shade.

Cerebellum

The cerebellum sits below the cerebrum and superoposterior to most of the brainstem. Like the cerebrum, it is composed of two lateral, symmetric hemispheres. The vermis, a small central lobe relays information between the two hemispheres. The normal cerebellum appears as mid-gray to low-gray with low-level echoes that tend to be hypoechoic relative to the cerebrum. In the posterior portion of the brain, the small, round, cerebellar hemispheres are seen on either side of the homogeneous, mid-gray vermis, which is located at the midline of the brain.

Tentorium Cerebelli

The tent-shaped tentorium cerebelli separates the cerebellum from the more superior structures.

Brainstem

The medulla, pons, midbrain, thalamus, and hypothalamus compose the brainstem, which forms the base of the brain that is continuous with the spinal cord. The components of the brainstem present sonographically as mid-gray homogeneous structures that vary in their echo level intensity depending on the stage of development. The spinal cord is detectable by 15 to 16 weeks GA. Spinal cord neural tissue appears low-gray with low-level echoes. It is easily identified lying between the highly reflective, bony vertebrae.

Thalamus
The thalamus can be identified in the center of an axial section of the temporal lobe of the brain. It is composed of two ovoid-shaped halves that are primarily composed of brain gray matter. Each half lies on either side of and forms a portion of the lateral walls of the third ventricle. Thalami appear mid-gray with medium-level echoes.

Cavum Septum Pellucidi
The cavum septum pellucidi is another anechoic, fluid-filled structure that lies at the midline of the brain. Located superoanterior to the thalamus and third ventricle, it is larger than the third ventricle and subsequently holds more cerebrospinal fluid. It appears as two small, bright parallel lines separated at the midline of the brain by cerebrospinal fluid.

Cerebral Peduncles
The cerebral peduncles are two heart-shaped masses that lie on each side of the midline of the brain. They are similar in shape and texture to the thalami but are smaller and more rounded. Peduncle parenchyma appears mid-gray with medium- to low-level echoes.

Meninges
As the linings of the brain, the pia arachnoid and dura arachnoid, become visible, they can be distinguished by their hyperechoic appearance relative to adjacent structures.

Basilar Artery
The basilar artery can be seen pulsating at the midline of the brain between the anterior portions of the peduncles.

Circle of Willis
The circle of Willis can be seen pulsating at the midline of the brain anterior to the peduncles and can be seen with color Doppler.

Cisterns
Cisterns are varying sizes of enlarged portions of the subarachnoid space, which is the space between the pia mater and arachnoid layer, where cerebrospinal fluid, pia arachnoid, or a combination of both can accumulate. The largest intracranial cistern for cerebrospinal fluid is the cisterna magnum, which should measure less than 10 mm. It is

located in the posterior portion of the brain at the base of the cerebellum and appears anechoic with bright borders. Cisterns filled with pia arachnoid will appear bright.

Fossae

The anterior, middle, and posterior fossae appear anechoic and divided from one another by the highly echogenic appearance of the petrous ridges of the skull posteriorly and the sphenoid bones anteriorly. The posterior fossa contains the cerebellum.

Determining Gestational Age During the Second and Third Trimesters

Second-trimester biometric measurements consist of the **biparietal diameter (BPD)**, **head circumference (HC)**, **femur length (FL)**, and **abdominal circumference (AC)** and should be used once the CRL measures greater than 84 mm. The ACOG has devised guidelines for methods of estimating the due date of a pregnancy. Table 14.1 can be helpful when deciding how to date a pregnancy in instances in which sonographic measurements differ from GA by last monthly period across all gestations.

BPD and Head Circumference

The BPD is a measurement from one parietal bone to the other. The BPD should be measured at the level of the thalami, cavum septi pellucidi, and flax cerebri in an axial view. Neither the lateral cerebral ventricle nor the cerebellar hemispheres should be visible in this scanning plane.

Measurement cursors should be positioned from the outer edge of the proximal skull not including skin, to the inner edge of the distal skull at the widest part of the fetal head and always perpendicular to the falx cerebri.

The HC is an elliptical measurement around the perimeter of the fetal skull from outer to outer skull edge, again not including the skin, at the same level in which the BPD is measured; therefore the BPD and HC can be measured in the same image.

Abdominal Circumference

The AC is an elliptical measurement around the perimeter of the fetal abdomen, including the skin, in a transverse plane at the level where the fetal stomach, spine, and umbilical vein, which should be seen curving into the liver as it joins the portal sinus, are all visible in the same image.

Femur Length Measurement

With the beam insonation perpendicular to the long axis of the femur, calipers should be placed at both cartilaginous ends of the long bones. This guarantees that the plane of section is the long axis. The measurement is confined to the ossified portions and should not include the distal epiphysis.

Table 14.1 Guidelines for Redating Based on Ultrasonography

Gestational Age Range[a]	Method of Measurement	Discrepancy Between Ultrasound Dating and LMP Dating That Supports Redating
≤13 6/7 wk	CRL	
• ≤8 6/7 wk		>5 days
• 9 0/7 wk to 13 6/7 wk		>7 days
14 0/7 wk to 15 6/7 wk	BPD, HC, AC, FL	>7 days
16 0/7 wk to 21 6/7 wk	BPD, HC, AC, FL	>10 days
22 0/7 wk to 27 6/7 wk	BPD, HC, AC, FL	>14 days
28 0/7 wk and beyond,[a,b]	BPD, HC, AC, FL	>21 days

AC, Abdominal circumference; BPD, biparietal diameter; CRL, crown-rump length; FL, femur length; HC, head circumference; LMP, last menstrual period.
[a]Based on LMP.
[b]Because of the risk of redating a small fetus that may be growth restricted, management decisions based on third-trimester ultrasonography alone are especially problematic and need to be guided by careful consideration of the entire clinical picture and close surveillance.
From American College of Obstetricians and Gynecologists. Methods for estimating the due date. Committee opinion No. 700. *Obstet Gynecol* 2017;129:e150–e154.

Obstetric Ultrasound

Transducer
Transabdominal Examinations
For TA examinations a curved linear array probe is typically used. Newer probes have a wide array of megahertz (MHz) ranging from 1 to 9 MHz. Lower frequencies (1–5 MHz) may be used for very large patients. Higher frequencies (3–9 MHz) may be used for thinner patients. In some instances, a higher-frequency probe may still be used for larger patients.

It is not unusual to use different transducers during an obstetric ultrasound examination. For example, if the fetal spine is in the anterior part of the uterus, it may be better evaluated with a higher-frequency transducer.

For transvaginal (TV) examinations a 5–9 MHz EV ultrasound probe should be selected. Every company has its way of describing the transducer. For example, the transducer may be identified as C 9–5 or a 5–9 EV, among other methods. Some transducers may start with the highest frequency and others the lower frequency. Some will have a C for curved and others EV for endovaginal.

Patient Prep
The patient should have a full urinary bladder for a first-trimester ultrasound and a partially full bladder for a second-trimester ultrasound;

after the second trimester, bladder filling is usually unnecessary. The patient should drink 24–32 oz of clear fluid 1 hour before the examination. A full bladder is used in the first trimester to displace the overlying maternal bowel out of the way and serves as a sonic "window" for visualizing pelvic structures. The partially full bladder in the second trimester is used to evaluate cervical length and the lower uterine segment. An overfilled bladder may actually make it difficult to scan the patient and see the fetus and anatomy. If this occurs, have the patient partially void.

The bladder should be empty for a TV examination because a full bladder can push anatomy out of the field of view.

Patient Position

The patient is started in a supine position. To move the fetus into a different position the patient may be rolled into posterior obliques. For a third-trimester examination the patient also could be rolled into a decubitus position if needed to see the fetus. If the patient starts to feel lightheaded, she should be turned onto her side. Once the patient is feeling better, the scan could be continued with the patient on her side, as the cause of the lightheadedness was the fetus lying on the maternal inferior vena cava (IVC). The exam can also continue with the patient in an oblique position, as this will keep the baby off of the IVC.

During the third trimester, if the fetal head is in the lower uterine segment, it may be helpful to elevate the patient's hips with a pillow or foam cushion. If the examination table is adjustable, a Trendelenburg position may help.

Endovaginal Examination

- Verbal consent is required from the patient. Explain the examination in detail, including information such as that it will not hurt the baby, that the inserted transducer feels like a tampon and has been disinfected, and that this allows more detailed pictures. Never force the patient into an EV examination if she does not want it. If possible, have a physician talk to the patient to answer questions and talk about her concerns.
- Another health care employee must be present during the EV examination as a chaperone. The initials of the chaperone must be documented somewhere, such as the patient's electronic record. Performing the examination unchaperoned places you at a very real legal risk and is usually against policy. There have been female sonographers successfully sued. Family members or friends cannot be chaperones.
- Instruct the patient to completely void and get undressed from the waist down before the EV examination. Provide the patient with a sheet or gown to cover herself. Leave the examination room to give the patient privacy during this time.

- If you have an examination table with stirrups, they may be useful during the EV examination.
- Ask permission of the patient before reentering the examination room to ensure she is covered.
- Introduce the chaperone. Assist the patient in getting into the stirrups if available, while dropping the foot of the bed. If no stirrups are available, place a pillow, foam cushion, or sheets under the patient's hips and have her drop her knees to the side.
- Cover the EV probe with a sheath or condom after placing gel inside it and making sure that there are no air bubbles at the tip. Some ultrasound-specific covers come with gel already inside. Apply a liberal amount of gel to the end of the transducer.
- Ask the patient if she wants to insert the probe. If she declines, the sonographer should insert the transducer. Keep the patient covered as much as possible during the examination for modesty.
- After the examination is complete, slowly remove the probe and take off the probe cover, disposing of it properly. The purpose of taking off the cover now is to avoid contaminating other surfaces. Help the patient out of the stirrups or remove the pillow from under her hips. Provide her with something to remove the gel. Instruct the patient to get dressed; leave the room for her privacy.
- When the patient has left the room, disinfect the EV probe with a high-level disinfection technique and product. The examination table and stirrups also should be properly disinfected.

> **NOTE:** For safety precautions regardless of approach, the Thermal Index for soft tissue (TIS) should be monitored for scans performed at less than 10 weeks gestational age including the Doppler aspects of the exam. And the Thermal Index for bone (TIB) should be monitored for scans performed at 10 weeks or greater gestational age. Check the web sites of societies such as the AIUM and ACOG for current recommended values.

Required Images for the First Trimester

Guidelines in this text were established using The American Institute of Ultrasound in Medicine (AIUM) practice parameters. For the most up-to-date parameters, visit the AIUM website.

These protocols are free, and you do not have to be a member to print them. They have been created by multiple societies that perform obstetric ultrasound.

Transabdominal Approach

Scanning planes for some images are determined by position of anatomy.

1. *Uterus (including cervix).* Should be evaluated and documented in two orthogonal planes for the presence and location of a gestational sac or sacs. Any uterine anomalies should be documented. The presence and number of fibroids should be documented, with the largest or the largest fibroid of potential clinical significance measured. These are only recommended labels and the annotations should be those used by the department.

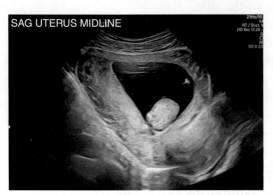

Suggested annotation: **SAG UT ML**

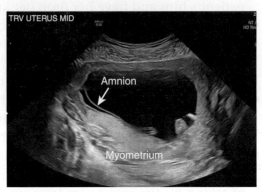

Suggested annotation: **TRV UT MID**

2. *Cul-de-sac.* Should be evaluated for presence or absence of free fluid in the midline long axis of the uterus.

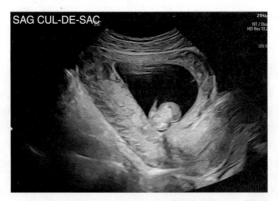

Suggested annotation: **SAG ML or CDS**

3. *Adnexa.* Both right and left adnexae should be evaluated and documented even if the ovaries are not visualized. Document the long and short axis showing pelvic side wall and iliac vessels. Should there be any adnexal pathologic findings, the presence, location, appearance, vascularity, and size of the adnexal mass should be documented. A split-screen technique can be used to document both the sagittal and transverse views on one image. See example. Annotate SAG directly under the sagital image and TRV under the transverse image. For the sake of simplicity only one RT or LT is used for the suggested annotation.

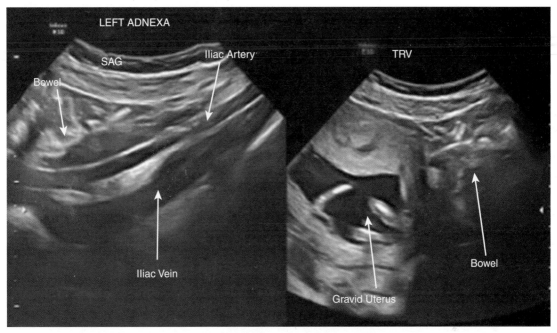

Suggested annotation: **SAG LT   TRV LT ADNEXA**

4. *Ovaries.* If ovaries are visualized, they should be documented and measured in length, width, and height by scanning in their long and short axes. Length and height should be measured in the long axis of the ovary, and width should be measured in the short axis of the ovary. A split-screen technique can be used to document both the sagittal and transverse views on one image.

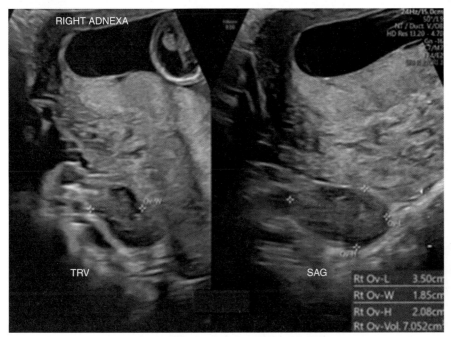

Suggested annotation: **TRV   SAG RT OV**

5. *Gestational sac.* Should be evaluated and measured in the long and short axes with sac diameter measurements. The length and height should be measured in the long axis or sagittal image, and the width should be measured in the short axis or transverse image. Measurements should be from inside wall to inside wall. Carefully evaluate for the presence or absence of a yolk sac or embryo/fetus. If the yolk sac is visualized, this should be documented and labeled as well. Note that depending on how early the gestation is, it may be helpful to magnify the field of view for the gestational sac images. A split-screen technique can be used to document both the sagittal and transverse views on one image. These images demonstrate proper measuring of the gestational sac in an early stage and below in a later stage.

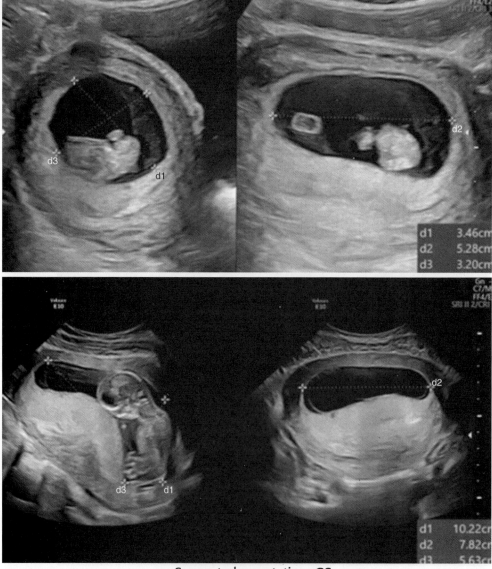

Suggested annotation: **GS**

6. *Yolk sac/amnion.* If present, the yolk sac/amnion should be documented showing the yolk sac adjacent to the amnion.

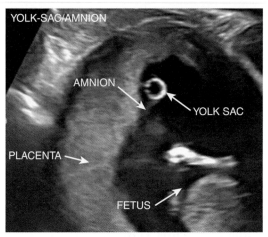

Suggested annotation: **YS/AMNION**

7. *Crown-rump length.* Should be measured when the head and rump can be fully demonstrated while the fetus is in a neutral position or in the early first trimester when the borders of the fetal pole can be well delineated.

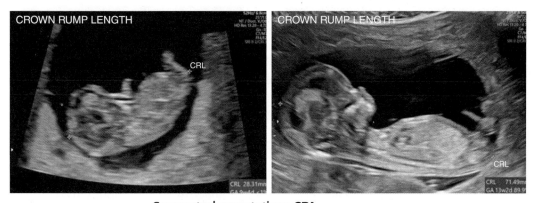

Suggested annotation: **CRL**

8. *Cardiac activity.* Should be documented using M-mode or two-dimensional video clip to capture heart movement. Using M-mode allows the fetal heart rate to be calculated. Each ultrasound unit calculates it differently. Pulsed-wave or color Doppler ultrasound should not be used to document the fetal heart or to let the mother hear the heartbeat because of the increased power levels needed for Doppler.

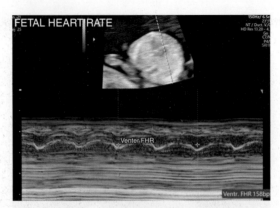

Suggested annotation: **FHM**

Transvaginal Approach

If EV imaging is necessary to better document the pregnancy, pelvic organs, or fetus in the first trimester, the images to be obtained are matched with the guidelines as outlined previously for the TA approach. Box 14.1 contains examples of images from the EV approach.

Box 14.1 Examples of Images From an Endovaginal Approach

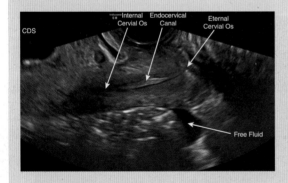

Suggested annotation: **CDS**

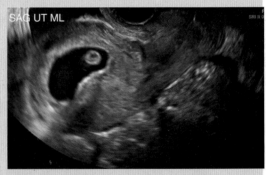

Suggested annotation: **SAG UT**

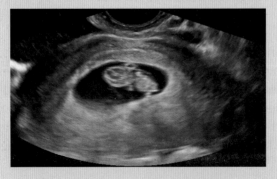

Suggested annotation: **TRV UT**

Box 14.1   Examples of Images From an Endovaginal Approach—cont'd

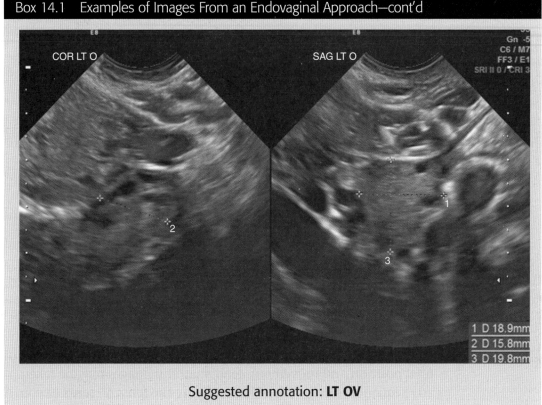

Suggested annotation: **LT OV**

The following fetal anatomy may be documented in the first trimester when the fetus is of sufficient size: the calvarium, abdominal cord insertion, stomach, cardiac axis, bladder, kidneys, presence of limbs, and evaluation of the nuchal region.

Nuchal Translucency

Patients wishing to have a fetal aneuploidy risk assessment may have additional imaging of the **nuchal translucency** and **nasal bone** for first-trimester aneuploidy screening. The sonographer performing the nuchal translucency and nasal bone imaging should be certified. Currently certification is through the Nuchal Translucency Quality Review at https://ntqr.perinatalquality.org/.

Required Images for the Second and Third Trimesters

Guidelines in this text were established using AIUM practice parameters for the standard obstetric evaluation. For the most up-to-date guidelines, visit https://www.aium.org/resources/guidelines.aspx.

Before starting, it is a good idea to know what the fetal presentation is by comparing the long axis of the fetus to the long axis of the uterus. Presentation refers to the fetal part closest to the cervix and includes vertex or cephalic, breech, and transverse (Fig. 14.17).

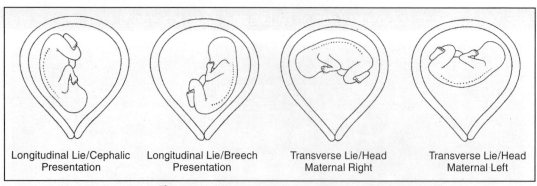

| Longitudinal Lie/Cephalic Presentation | Longitudinal Lie/Breech Presentation | Transverse Lie/Head Maternal Right | Transverse Lie/Head Maternal Left |

Fig. 14.17 Illustrations of the various fetal positions.

Transabdominal Approach

Generally, the nonfetal images are obtained first. Longitudinal and transverse plane images are taken to document the fetal and placenta position and amniotic fluid volume. After those images are obtained, the images needed to determine fetal age and assess the fetal anatomy are obtained. There is no specific order to obtain these images. Typically, the measurements are taken along with the images of the fetal anatomy that is being evaluated. Because of the variability of fetal position and movement, fetal anatomy images may be taken in any sequence. Always take what anatomy the fetus presents to you. A good rule to follow in any ultrasound examination but that especially holds true for fetal imaging is, "Remember you can always get a better image, but you can never get it again." With today's digital storage of images, when a better image is obtained the other one can be deleted.

1. *Lower uterine segment.* In a long axis view, demonstrate the vaginal stripe, cervix and presenting fetal part.

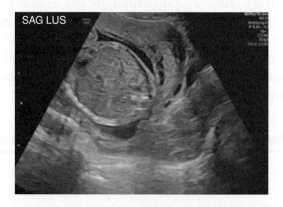

Suggested annotation: **SAG LUS**

2. *Placenta end.* In a long-axis view of the lower uterine segment the inferior margin of the placenta should be clearly seen in relation to the internal cervical os. Some sonographers may annotate the letter *E* to show where the placenta ends.

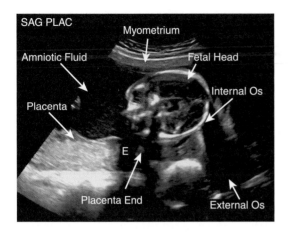

Suggested annotation: **SAG PLAC END**

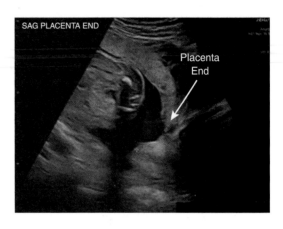

Suggested annotation: **SAG PLAC END**

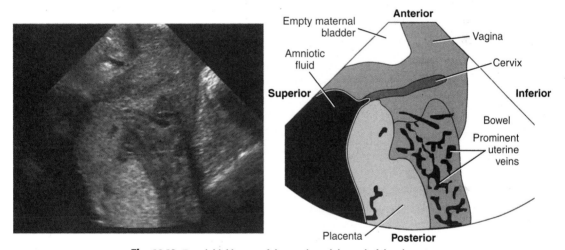

Fig. 14.18 Translabial image of the cervix and the end of the placenta.

An image of the lower uterine segment to include the internal os is required to rule out placenta previa and document the cervix. In cases in which the head of the fetus or the mother's body habitus makes imaging the lower uterine segment difficult, either an EV or translabial image must be obtained. The translabial image is obtained with an empty or nearly empty bladder. The transducer is usually covered with a glove because the transducer is too wide for a standard sheath and placed between the labia. The transducer is angled so that the cervix is nearly perpendicular to the ultrasound beam (Fig. 14.18). In cases in which an accurate assessment of the cervical length is requested, EV ultrasound always should be done if not contraindicated (Fig. 14.19).

3. *Cervix.* In the long-axis view of the lower uterine segment a clear demonstration of the internal and external cervical os along with the endocervical canal should be documented and measured to evaluate for cervical shortening. If cervical shortening is suspected, an EV approach may be used for better visualization. Criteria for an EV cervical evaluation are as follows. The maternal bladder should be empty. The anterior width of the cervix should equal the posterior width to ensure there is no transducer pressure on the cervix. The internal and external cervical os and endocervical canal should be clearly visualized. Calipers should be placed from the internal cervical os to the external cervical os along the endocervical canal. Up to three linear measurements may be performed if the cervix is curved with the measurements added together to determine cervical length. Three cervical length measurements should be obtained over a period of 3 to 5 minutes with the best shortest one reported.

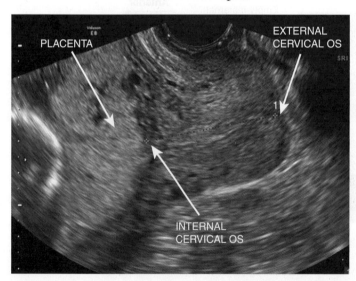

Fig. 14.19 Endovaginal image of the cervix and the end of the placenta. The arrows are also identifying the calipers used to measure the length of the cervix.

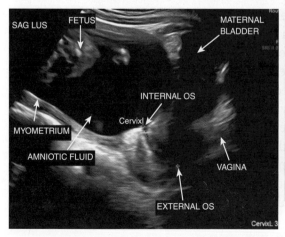

Suggested annotation: **SAG CX**

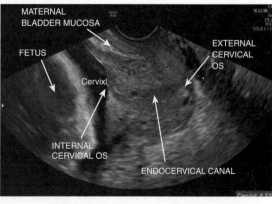

Suggested annotation: **SAG CX**

4. *Placenta and uterus.* In addition to the placenta end image, a long-axis image at the fundus of the uterus containing placenta should be documented to allow for grading and how far fundally the placenta extends. Two other images orthogonal to the long axis should be taken at the right and left lateral margins of the uterus to show any laterality of the placenta and to ensure both the placenta and uterus were surveyed in their entirety. Any uterine or placental pathologic condition should be documented.

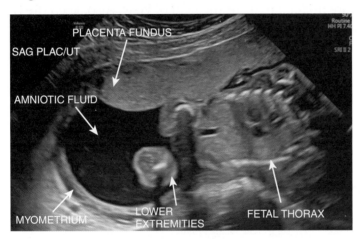

Suggested annotation: **SAG UT/PLAC**

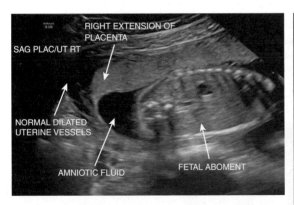

Suggested annotation: **TRV PLAC/UT RT**

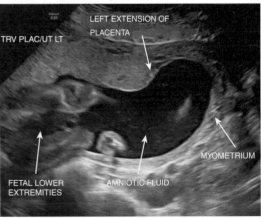

Suggested annotation: **TRV PLAC/UT LT**

5. *Placental cord insertion.* Evaluated in both sagittal and transverse images for normal insertion of the umbilical cord. The umbilical cord should insert more than 2 cm from the edge of the placental margin. If the cord insertion is abnormally positioned in the lower uterine segment, careful examination of the lower uterine segment and internal os should be carried out to look for a vasa previa, which is when fetal vessels are crossing or coming within 2 cm of the internal cervical os (Fig. 14.20). Color Doppler may be used if there are no fetal parts in the field of view. Also, keep the color box limited to the area of concern.

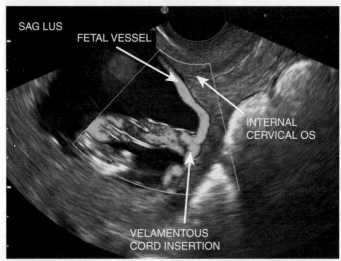

Fig. 14.20 Endovaginal image of a vasa previa. The placental cord insertion was noted to be velamentous, attached to the membranes, and located in the lower uterine segment as seen on the transabdominal examination. Note the fetal vessel that is seen to course over the internal cervical os.

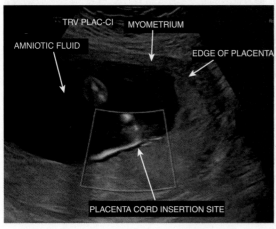

Suggested annotation: **TRV PCI**

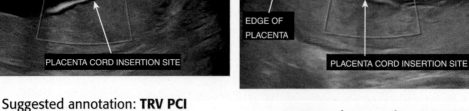

Suggested annotation: **SAG PCI**

6. *Amniotic fluid.* Depending on the GA, the amniotic fluid index (AFI) helps quantify the amount of amniotic fluid. This is determined by obtaining a single maximum vertical pocket *(MVP)* of fluid or four vertical pockets of fluid taken at each quadrant of the uterus to obtain an amniotic fluid index. Each measurement should be from anterior to posterior and free of fetal parts and cord. Color Doppler ultrasound may be used to identify free-floating loops of cord.

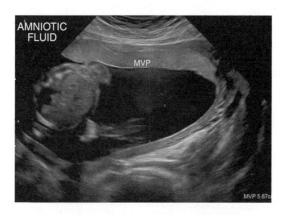

Suggested annotation: **AFI**
Maximum Vertical Pocket: **MVP**

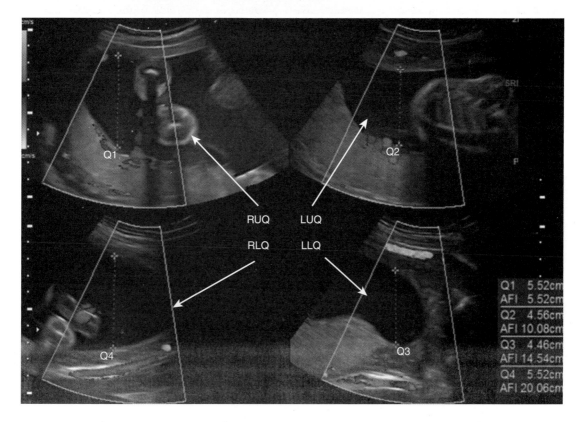

Suggested annotation: **AFI**

7. *Adnexa.* Evaluated in sagittal and transverse views and documented even if ovaries are not visualized as proof adnexal evaluation was performed. Document and measure ovaries if visualized and any adnexal pathologic conditions. Both views can be documented on a split-screen image.

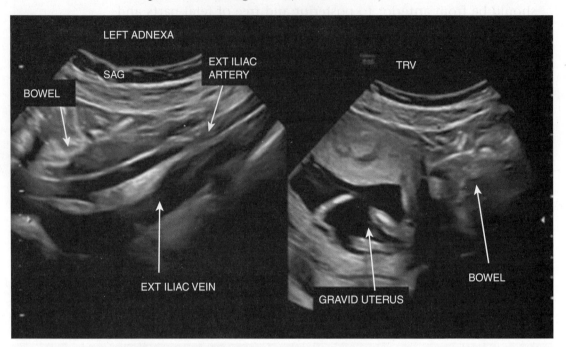

Suggested annotation: **ADNEXA LT**

8. *BPD and HC measurements and landmarks.* As stated before, the BPD and HC should be measured in an axial plane at the level of the cavum septi pellucidi, falx cerebri, and thalami. The BPD is measured from outer to inner skull edge and the HC measured on the outer skull edge.

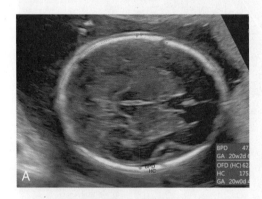

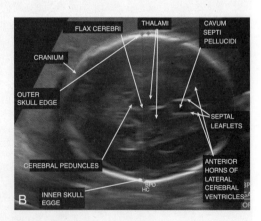

Suggested annotation: **BPD/HC**

9. *AC measurement and landmarks.* As stated previously, the AC should be measured in a transverse plane of the fetal abdomen at the level of the stomach, spine, and umbilical vein as it enters into the liver, about one-third of the way into the abdomen.

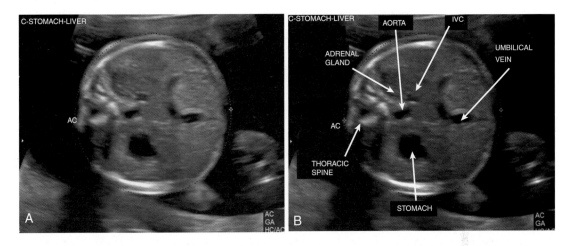

Suggested annotation: **AC**

10. *Femur length and landmarks.* As stated before, the beam insonation should be perpendicular to the long axis of the femur. Calipers should be placed at both cartilaginous ends of the long bones. The measurement is confined to the ossified portions and should not include the distal epiphysis.

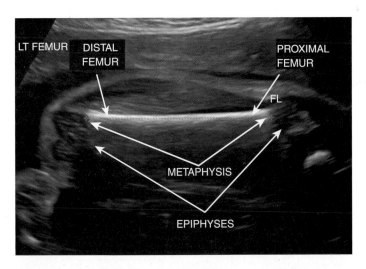

Suggested annotation: **LT FEM ot LT FL**

11. *Lateral cerebral ventricles.* Evaluated for shape, size, and symmetry in an axial transventricular view. The dependent side, the side the fetus is lying on, should be measured. Calipers may be placed at the atrium of the lateral cerebral ventricle just posterior to the choroid plexus from medial to lateral wall following the contour of the ventricle itself. Some institutes may measure the lateral cerebral ventricle diameter using the parieto-occipital sulcus (POS) as a landmark. The nondependent side is typically evaluated for size and symmetry subjectively.

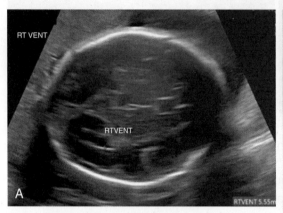

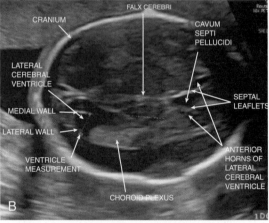

Suggested annotation: **RT VENT**

12. *Choroid plexus.* Evaluated for their symmetry and texture in an axial plane. Choroids should be echogenic and homogeneous.

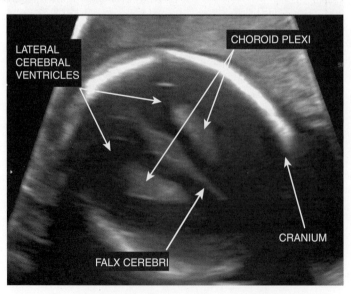

Suggested annotation: **CHOROIDS**

13. *Cerebellum/vermis/cisterna magna/nuchal fold.* Evaluated in an axial transcerebellar plane with the same landmarks as the BPD. The cavum septum pellucidi are seen anteriorly and the cerebellum, vermis, cisterna magna, and nuchal fold are seen posteriorly. Be sure to scan through the cerebellum entirely to evaluate the vermis. The cerebellum, cisterna magna, and nuchal fold should be measured for their size and the vermis evaluated for presence. The cerebellum is measured from one hemisphere to the other. The cisterna magna is measured from the posterior margin of the vermis to the inner occipital skull edge in line with the falx cerebri. The nuchal fold should be measured from the outside of the occipital skull edge to the edge of the skin also in line with the falx cerebri. All three measurements can be done in the same image. The nuchal fold measurement and vermis images are not a requirement for the standard obstetric evaluation but can be measured between 16 to 20 weeks or up to a BPD of 60 mm.

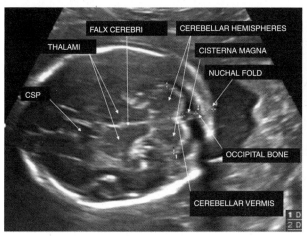
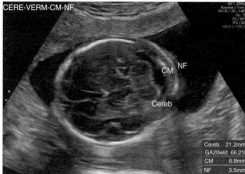

Suggested annotation: **CERE/VERM/CM/NF**

14. *Cavum septi pellucidi (CSP).* Evaluated for presence in an axial transthalamic view and can be easily identified up until 35 weeks of gestation. The cavum is a space in the anterior part of the brain bordered by the septal leaflets. It has the appearance of a "black box." The absence of the CSP could indicate forebrain malformations.

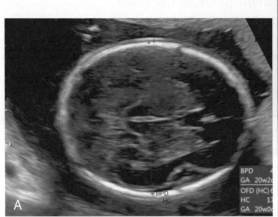 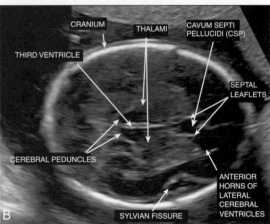

Suggested annotation: **CSP**

15. *Four extremities.* Evaluated for bone length, bone appearance, bone presence, and limb movement in the long axis of the extremity. The proximal long bones, the humerus and femur, should be routinely measured. The two bones in the distal upper, radius and ulna, and lower, tibia and fibula, extremities should be evaluated for their presence. Extremities should be evaluated for normal movement as well.

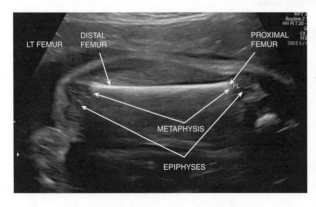 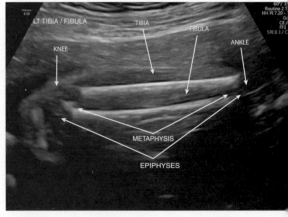

Suggested annotation: **LT FEM**

Suggested annotation: **LT TIB/FIB**

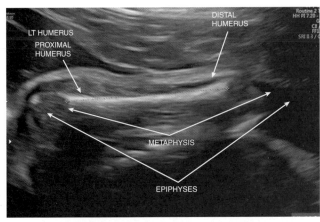

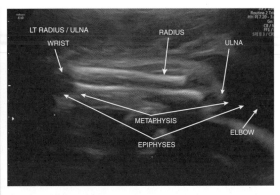

Suggested annotation: **LT RAD/ULN**

Suggested annotation: **LT HUM**

16. *Hands.* Evaluated for presence and position. Digits should be counted, and normal flexion and extension of the fingers and wrists should be observed. The thumb is usually imaged out of plane from the four fingers.

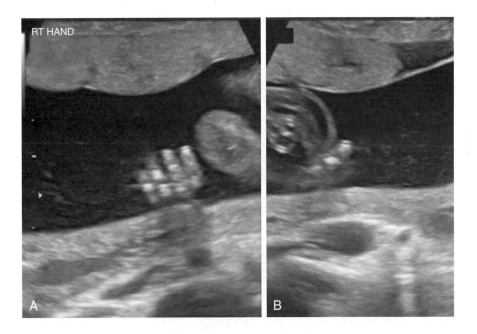

Suggested annotation: **RT HAND. Note image B is of the thumb by the umbilical cord.**

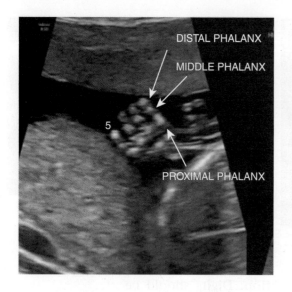

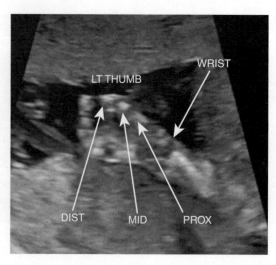

Suggested annotation: **LT Thumb**

Suggested annotation: **LT HAND**

17. *Feet.* Evaluated for presence and position. The plantar surface of the feet should be evaluated to identify digit abnormalities, and the long axis or angle of the feet should be evaluated for clubbing.

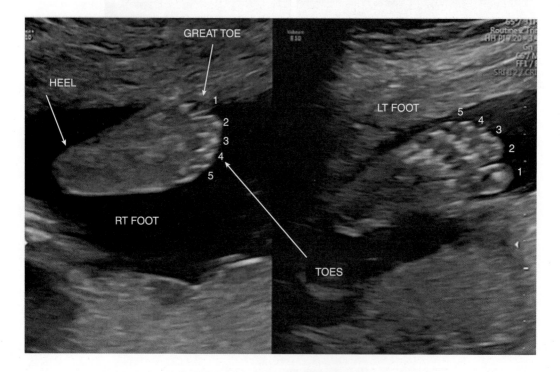

Suggested annotation: **LT/RT FOOT or FEET**

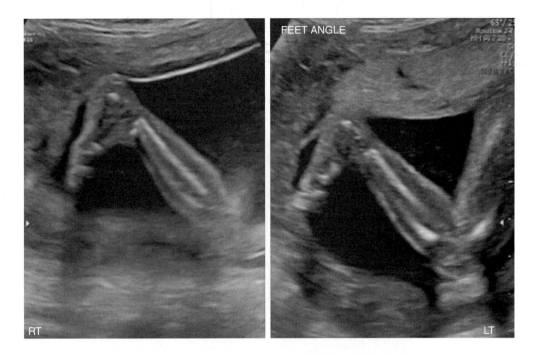

Suggested annotation: **LT/RT FOOT or FEET**

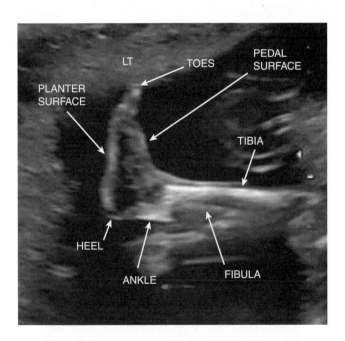

Suggested annotation: **LT FOOT**

18. *Stomach.* Evaluated for position and size in a transverse view of the AC. The stomach should be visualized as a single anechoic bubble on the left side of the fetal abdomen. Variations in stomach size may represent physiologic filling and emptying of the stomach or associated with other congenital anomalies of the GI tract.

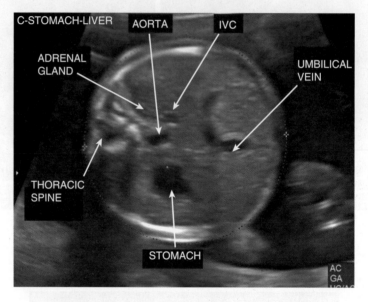

Suggested annotation: **STOMACH or STOM**

19. *Kidneys.* Evaluated for presence, position, size, and echogenicity in transverse and sagittal or coronal planes. The renal arteries can be evaluated in the coronal plane (Fig. 14.21).

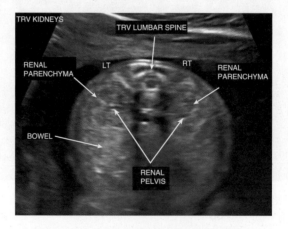

Suggested annotation: **TRV KIDS**

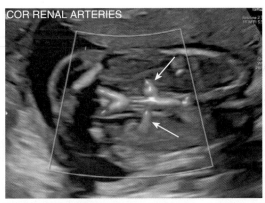

Fig. 14.21 A color Doppler image of the aorta and renal arteries (arrows) scanning the fetus in its coronal plane.

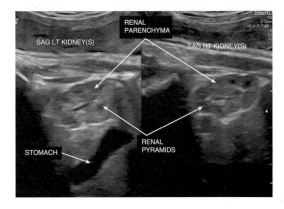

Suggested annotation: **SAG or LONG KIDS**

20. *Urinary bladder.* Evaluate for location and size in both a transverse and sagittal or coronal views. The bladder should be seen in the fetal pelvis.

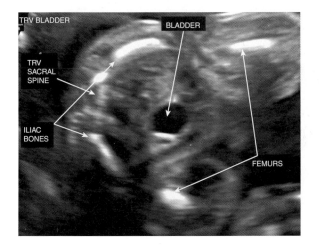

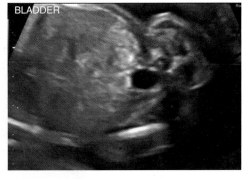

Suggested annotation: **SAG BLAD**

Suggested annotation: **TRV BLAD**

21. *Umbilical cord.* Evaluated for number of vessels in a longitudinal view of the fetal bladder using color Doppler or by counting vessels in a free-floating loop of cord. Cord abnormalities, such as cysts, should be evaluated in real time by following the umbilical cord length from placental insertion to fetal abdominal insertion.

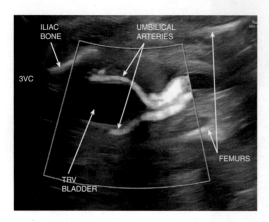

Suggested annotation: **UMB ARTS**

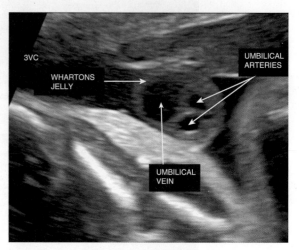

Suggested annotation: **3VC**

22. *Abdominal cord insertion.* Evaluated for abdominal wall defects in a transverse view of the fetal abdomen just superior to the fetal bladder. The umbilical vessels should be seen to traverse the anterior abdominal wall, and the integrity of the skin line on either side of the abdominal cord insertion site should be clearly demonstrated.

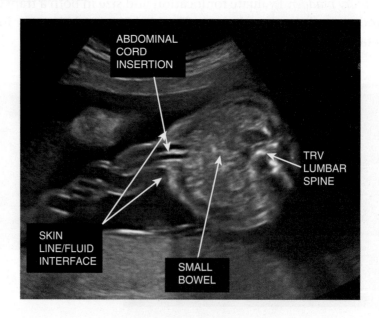

Suggested annotation: **CI**

23. *Upper lip.* Evaluated for clefts in a coronal view demonstrating nostril symmetry of the nose and a smooth intact upper lip.

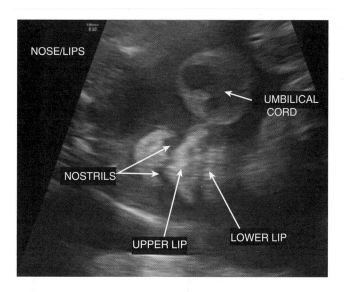

Suggested annotation: **NOSE/LIPS**

24. *Situs.* Evaluated for situs abnormalities in the transverse views of the fetal abdomen and chest. The fetal stomach should be on the left side of the fetal abdomen and apex of the heart pointed toward the left. Fetal presentation should be noted because the reading physician needs to know this to properly identify the right and left side. These images are usually captured side by side in a split screen.

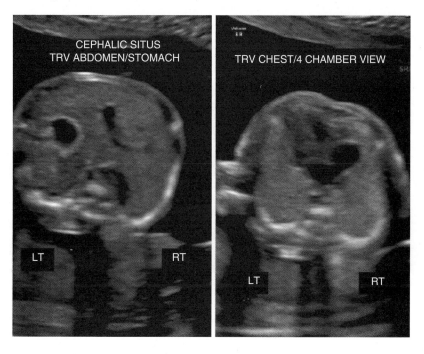

Suggested annotation: **SITUS along with fetal presentation**

25. *Four-chamber heart.* Evaluated for size, position, axis, symmetry, rhythm, and normal arrangement of cardiac anatomy in a transverse view of the fetal chest.

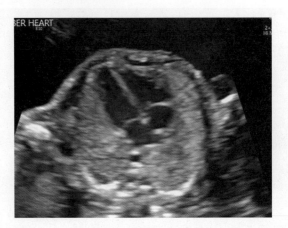

Suggested annotation: **4CH**

26. *Right ventricular outflow tract (RVOT).* Evaluated for size and orientation of the great vessels and normal cardiac anatomy in a short-axis view of the fetal heart. This view also has been referred to as the short-axis view of the outflow tracts. This view demonstrates ventriculoarterial junctions, the right ventricle's connection to the pulmonary artery.

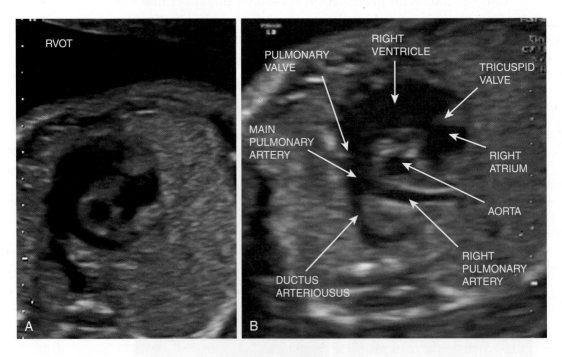

Suggested annotation: **RVOT**

27. *Left ventricular outflow tract (LVOT).* Evaluated for size and orientation of the great vessels and normal cardiac anatomy in a long-axis view of the fetal heart. This view also has been referred to as the five chamber view of the fetal heart. This demonstrates ventriculoarterial junctions, the left ventricle's connection to the aorta. The interventricular septum *(IVS)* should also be evaluated for continuity with the anterior wall of the aorta.

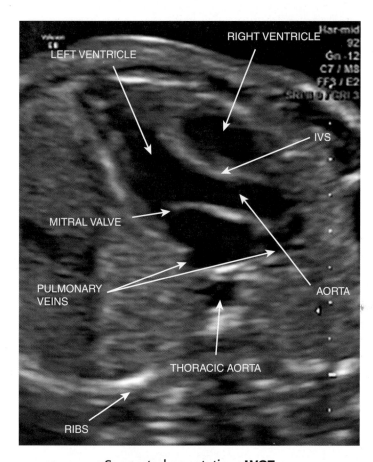

Suggested annotation: **LVOT**

28. *Three vessel view.* Evaluated for vessel number, size, and orientation in a transverse view of the fetal chest just superior to the RVOT. Three vessels of descending size and oblique orientation should be demonstrated in this view starting with the pulmonary artery being the most anterior and largest vessel on the fetal left and ending with the superior vena cava being the most posterior and smallest vessel on the fetal right. The third vessel is the fetal aorta

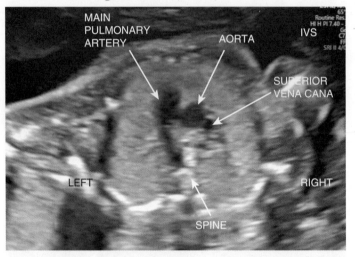

Suggested annotation: **3VV**

29. *Three-vessel trachea view.* Evaluate for vessel number, size, orientation, and aortic arch abnormalities in a transverse view of the fetal chest just superior to the three-vessel view. The ductus arteriosus can been seen to connect with the aorta in addition to other image criteria as noted in the three-vessel view. The aorta should be seen to the right of the trachea.

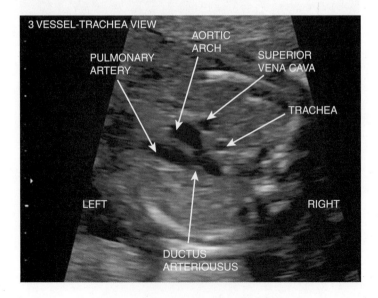

Suggested annotation: **3VTV**

30. *M-mode.* Evaluate for cardiac activity, rhythm, and *FHR* by placing the M-mode cursor through a fetal ventricle and atria to demonstrate a 1:1 ratio of ventricular and atrial contractions. Heart rate is obtained by placing calipers on the waveform from one cardiac cycle to the next. Some machines may be calibrated to measure one, two, or three cycles.

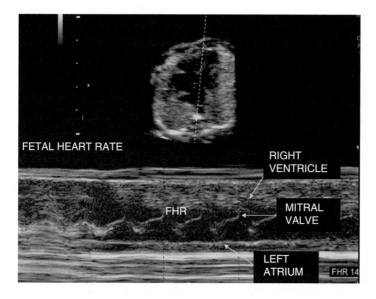

Suggested annotation: **FHR**

Evaluating the Fetal Spine

Locate a long section of the fetal spine and then very slowly twist the transducer first one way, then the other, until the long axis is visualized. As fetal growth progresses, it may not be possible to visualize the long axis of the entire spine in a single view. In those cases, find the longest visible section. Next, very slowly move down along the spine through the sacral end and then slowly back up through the cervical end to the skull. Note that the spine narrows at the sacrum and widens at the skull. Any other deviations seen along the "double line" appearance of the spine may indicate an abnormality.

Relocate the longitudinal cervical section of the fetal spine. Slowly rotate the transducer 90 degrees until a transverse section of the spine comes into view. Look for three small, highly reflective areas of ossification that represent portions of the vertebra. One portion is the centrum or body, and one on each side of the posterior neural arch or transverse processes, that eventually ossify into the laminae. To ensure that each of the seven cervical vertebrae are evaluated, slowly move the transducer until the base of the fetal skull comes into view then back onto the first cervical vertebra. Continue to scan inferiorly through each cervical vertebra until the level of the thoracic vertebra. Keep scanning inferiorly through the thoracic spine until the lumbar spine is seen. Evaluate each lumbar vertebra and then the sacrum until past the sacral margin. Although the entire spine needs to be evaluated, usually just one representative image of the transverse spine at each level is documented unless there is an abnormality.

1. *Cervical spine.* Evaluated for spinal abnormalities and integrity of the skin line in both a transverse and sagittal or coronal plane.

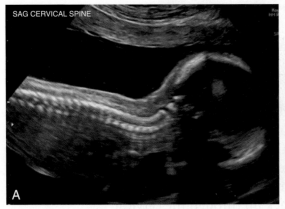

Suggested annotation: **C-SPINE**

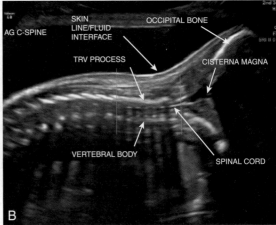

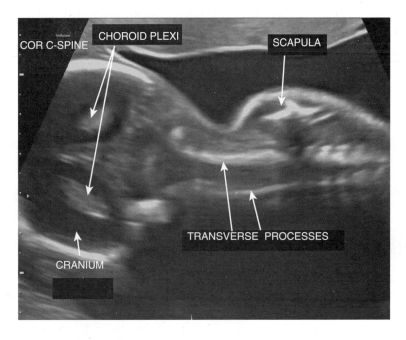

Suggested annotation: **C-SPINE or COR C-SPINE**

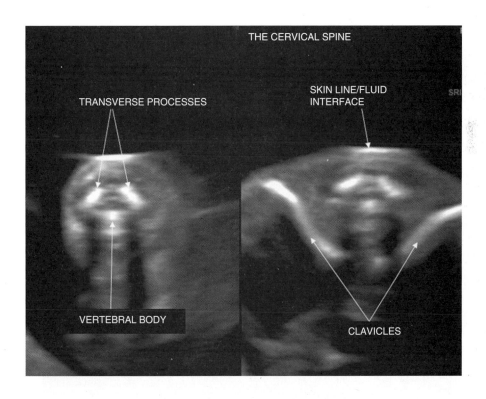

Suggested annotation: **TRV C-SPINE**

2. *Thoracic spine.* Evaluated for spinal abnormalities and integrity of the skin line in both a transverse and sagittal or coronal plane. One or more images may be obtained in the coronal plane to compensate for spine curvature.

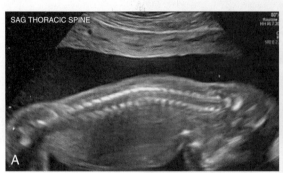

Suggested annotation: **SAG T-SPINE**

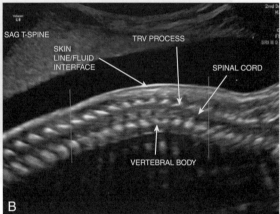

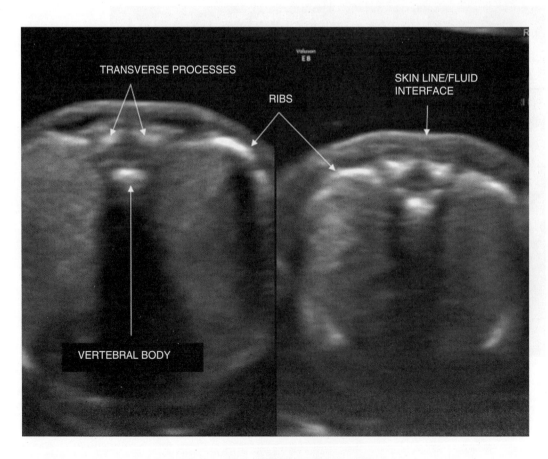

Suggested annotation: **TRV T-SPINE**

3. *Lumbar spine.* Evaluated for spinal abnormalities and integrity of the skin line in both a transverse and sagittal or coronal plane. The lumbar-sacral area is where many spinal defects arise, so careful scanning of this area is important.

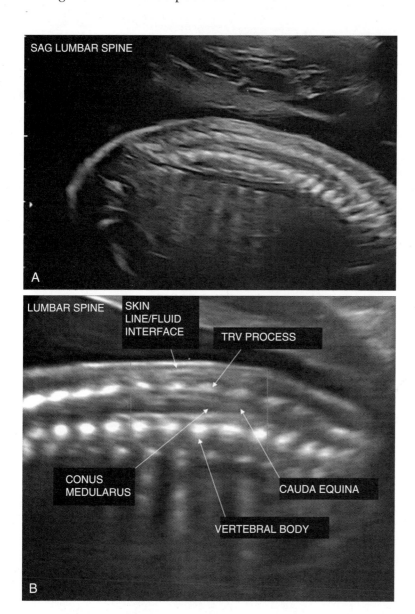

Suggested annotation: **L-SPINE**

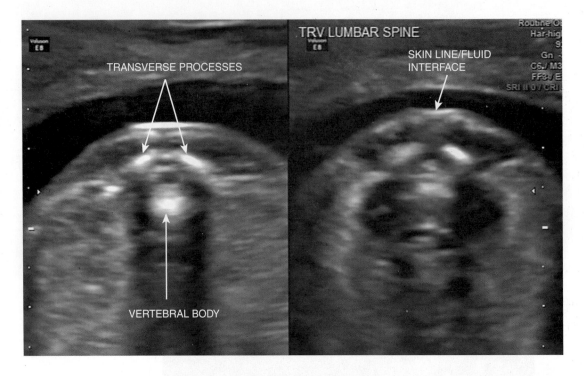

Suggested annotation: **TRV L-SPINE**

4. *Sacral spine.* Evaluated for spinal abnormalities and integrity of the skin line in both a transverse and sagittal or coronal plane.

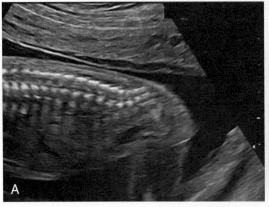

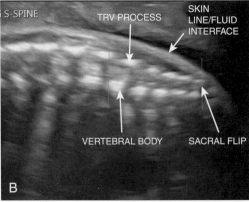

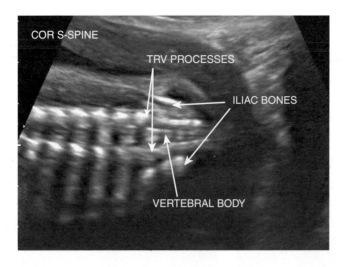

Suggested annotation: **SAG SACRUM or COR SACRUM**

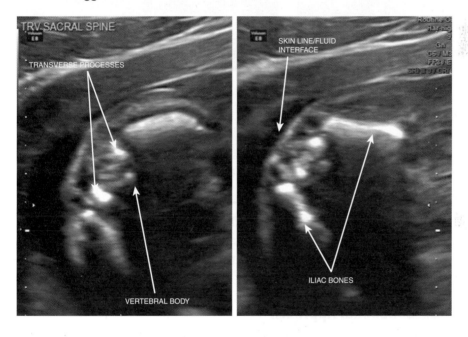

Suggested annotation: **TRV SACRUM**

External Genitalia in Multiple Gestations

The sex of the fetus is sometimes needed to evaluate or confirm chorionicity in twins and higher-order multiples and evaluate for abnormalities of the fetal genitalia. This is not a required standard view.

1. *Genitalia*. Remember that in most fetuses the testicles do not descend into the scrotum until at least 30 weeks GA.

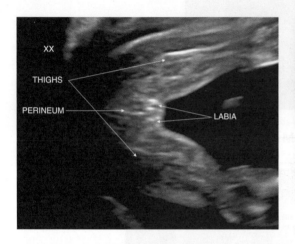

Suggested annotation: **XX**

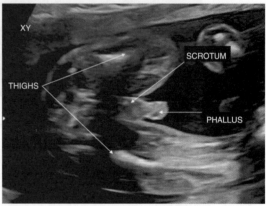

Suggested annotation: **XY**

Required Images for Second and Third Trimester for High Risk

Guidelines in this text were established using The AIUM practice parameters for the detailed fetal anatomic obstetric evaluation. For the most up-to-date guidelines, visit https://www.aium.org/accreditation/accreditation.aspx.

Transabdominal Approach

In addition to the images required for the standard obstetric ultrasound, the following additional images should be obtained for the detailed fetal anatomic survey.

1. *Brain parenchyma*. Evaluated in a coronal transthalamic view to include the cavum septi pellucidi, anterior horns of the lateral ventricles, and surrounding brain parenchyma to look for changes in parenchymal echogenicity and echotexture. The brain parenchyma may be shown in conjunction with other anatomy.

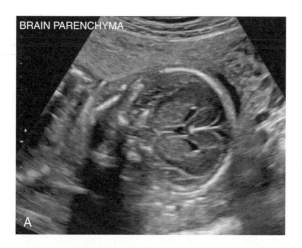

Suggested annotation: **BRAIN PARENCH**

2. *Profile.* Evaluated for abnormalities of the face in the midsagittal plane. The fetal chin should be off of the chest for adequate evaluation of the chin. This is a view that some departments may include in a standard examination.

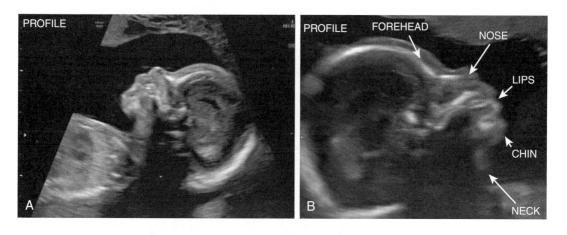

Suggested annotation: **PROF**

3. *Nasal bone (measurement).* Measured in the midsagittal plane on the profile image to evaluate for absence or hypoplasia. *NBL,* nasal bone length.

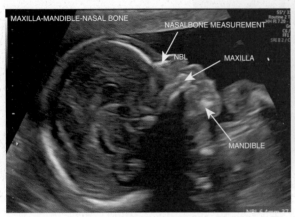

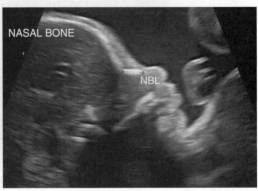

Suggested annotation: **N/B or NBL**

Suggested annotation: **N/B or NBL**

4. *Maxilla.* Evaluated for clefts of the alveolar ridge in the midsagittal plane, profile view, or transverse plane of the alveolar ridge/hard palate.

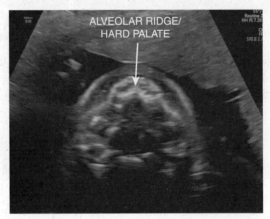

Suggested annotation: **ALV RIDGE/PAL**

5. *Mandible.* Evaluated for micrognathia/retrognathia in either the midsagittal plane profile view or in the transverse plane of the mandible. The nasal bone, maxilla, and mandible can be documented in the profile image as well.

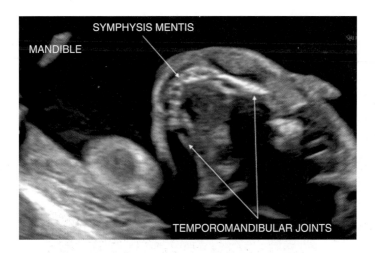

Suggested annotation: **MAND**

6. *Neck.* Evaluated for masses in both the transverse and sagittal planes. A dual screen can be used to document the longitudinal and transverse images together.

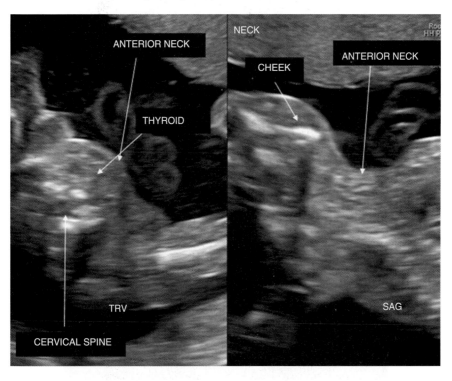

Suggested annotation: **NECK**

7. *Lungs.* Evaluated for lung abnormalities in the four-chamber view of the heart. Demonstrate a normal axis and position of the heart and homogenous echotexture of each lung.

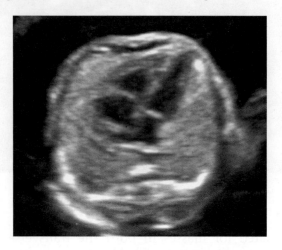

Suggested annotation: **TRV LUNGS**

8. *Diaphragm.* Evaluated for congenital hernia or eversion in the coronal plane demonstrating the stomach in the abdomen and the heart in the chest. In addition, a normal axis and position of the four-chamber view is reassuring.

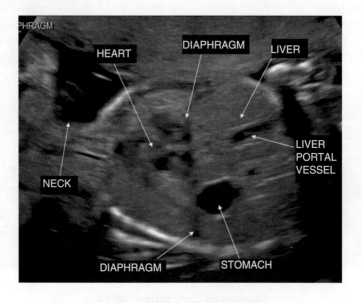

Suggested annotation: **DIAPH**

9. *Aortic arch.* Evaluated for vessel origin, areas of constriction, and lack of continuity in the long parasagittal plane.

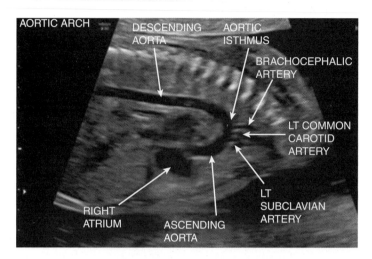

Suggested annotation: **AO ARCH**

10. *Superior and inferior vena cava (SVC and IVC).* Evaluated for normal connections to the right atrium of the IVC inferiorly and the SVC superiorly in the long sagittal view. The IVC should be seen to extend through the fetal liver.

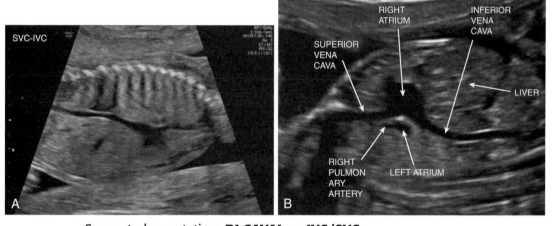

Suggested annotation: **BI CAVAL or IVC/SVC**

11. *Shape and curvature of the spine.* Evaluated for spinal abnormalities in the parasagittal plane along the entire axis of the spine.

Suggested annotation: **SHAPE and CURVE**

Occasionally an EV ultrasound must be done in the second or third trimesters of pregnancy. Typically, but not limited to, the EV approach is reserved for cervical evaluation, placental location evaluation, and to rule out a vasa previa.

Multiple Gestations

Twins have a higher complication rate and should be followed more frequently.

Additional Required Images

Each fetus of a multiple gestation should be imaged as previously described for singleton pregnancies across all trimesters plus the following additional views because they apply to help determine the amnionicity and chorionicity.

The sac separation or dividing membrane should be examined. It is important to determine chorionicity in twins and higher-order multiples as early in the pregnancy as possible because it becomes progressively more difficult to do so with certainty as gestation advances. Monochorionic is when the fetuses share one placenta but have two separate sacs. Monoamniotic is when the fetuses are in the same sac and share the same placenta. With dichorionic pregnancies the fetuses each have a placenta and will have a very thick sac separation in the early first trimester (Fig. 14.22) and will show evidence of intervening placenta tissue called a twin peak sign in the late first and

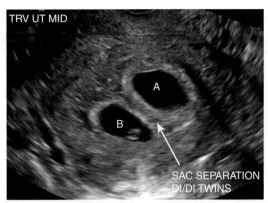

Fig. 14.22 An example of twin sacs in an early pregnancy. The *arrow* is pointing to the thick sac separation in this dichorionic, diamniotic twin pregnancy.

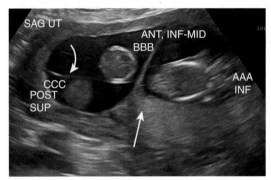

Fig. 14.23 Triamniotic and dichorionic triplets (identified as AAA, BBB, and CCC). The *arrow* is pointing to the twin peak sign. The *curved arrow* is pointing to the sac separation of the monochorionic pair. *AAA INF,* inferior; *ANT, anterior; INF-MID,* inferior mid; *CCC POST SUP,* posterior superior.

early second trimesters (Fig. 14.23). The word "twin" in twin peaks refers to the fact that it deals with twins and not that there are two peaks. Monochorionic pregnancies have a thin sac separation (Fig. 14.24) and clearly no twin peak sign in the first trimester and what has been described as the T-sign, which is the lack of the twin peak, in early second trimesters. The twin peak sign becomes progressively more difficult to visualize as the pregnancy advances (Fig. 14.25). Caution should be taken beyond 16 weeks gestation when using the sac separation as a diagnostic tool for determining chorionicity. No dividing membrane will be seen in monoamniotic pairs. In the late second trimester, it becomes more difficult to determine chorionicity based on the appearance of the sac separation/dividing membrane alone (Fig. 14.26), in which case the number of placentas and gender determination may be helpful.

It is also important to demonstrate the presentation of each fetus. The fetus that is lower in the uterus and closer to the cervix is presumed to be delivered first and should be labeled "A" and the other fetus labeled "B." If there are more than two fetuses, the remaining should be labeled in alphabetical order concurrent with their

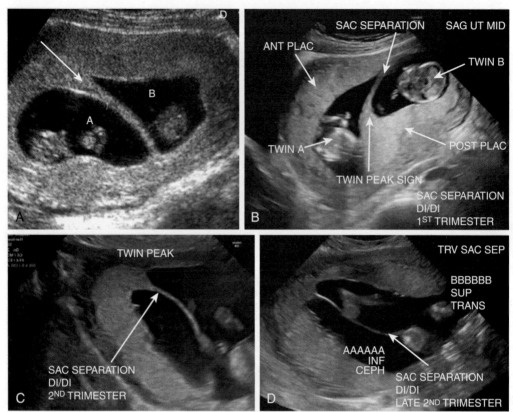

Fig. 14.25 *A,* Images of the same twin pregnancy showing the disappearance of the twin peak sign. Early first trimester. The *arrow* is pointing to the twin peak sign. *B,* Twins in late first trimester showing a prominent twin peak sign. *C,* Twins in early second trimester. Note how the twin peak sign is not as prominent as it was in *B. D,* Twins in late second trimester. Note that the twin peak sign is not seen ANT PLAC, anterior placenta; SAG UT MID, sagittal uterus midline; POST PLAC, posterior placenta; DI/DI, dichorionic, diamniotic. AAAAAA refers to Twin a. INF CEPH, inferior cephalic referring to the fetus is cephalic in position and inferior to fetus B. SEP, separation; SUP TRANS, superior transverse referring to the fetus is in a transverse position and superior to fetus A. BBBBBB refers to twin B..

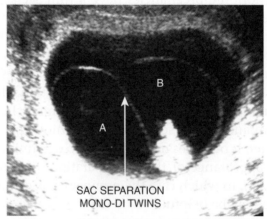

Fig. 14.24 This image is very overgained to be able to see the thin membrane of the sac separation. The sonographer needs to look for these types of subtle findings and adjust the controls, usually the gain, to bring out faint echoes.

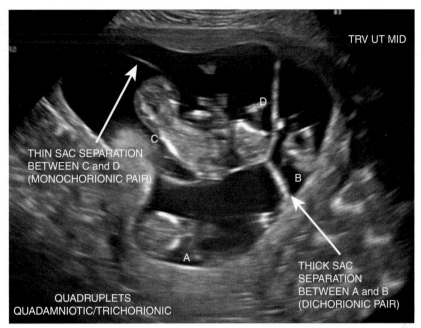

Fig. 14.26 An example of quadruplets that is quadamniotic and trichorionic.

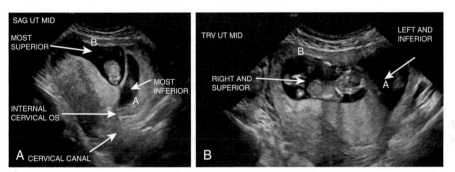

Fig. 14.27 A, Image demonstrating the naming of twins as *A* and *B*. **B,** Image demonstrating the naming of twins as *A* and *B* with laterality. *SAG UT MID,* sagittal uterus midline; *TRV UT MID,* transverse uterus mid.

presumed delivery based on position to the cervix. For instance, if there are four fetuses, the fetus most fundal in the uterus and presumed last to be delivered would be labeled "D." Laterality of each fetus should also be included in the presentation description. This labeling allows individual growth rates to be determined on subsequent follow-ups (Fig. 14.27).

The Biophysical Profile

An examination that is often performed during the late third trimester is the biophysical profile (BPP). This test measures fetal well-being and consists of five parameters. The first part of the test involves a nonstress test. This test is performed in the delivery room or in an obstetrician's office and measures spontaneous heart rate accelerations. This

Table 14.2	Biophysical Profile Scoring	Score (Points)
	Criterion	
Part I		
Nonstress test	2 accelerations of 15 beats/min in 30-min test	2
Part II		
Ultrasound Examination:		
Gross move-ment tone	3 or more discrete body or limb movements in a 30-min examination	2
	1 or more episodes of active extension and flexion of the fetal extremities or opening and closing of the hands in a 30-min examination	2
Respiration	At least 30 s of sustained fetal breathing in 30-min examination	2
Fluid	At least 1 pocket of amniotic fluid measuring greater than 2 cm	2
	Unqualified pass	8 or more
	Maximum total	10

Data from Manning EA, Platt LD, Sipos L. Antenatal fetal evaluation: development of a fetal biophysical profile. *Am J Obstet Gynecol* 1980;136:787–795.

part of the BPP is not performed by the sonographer. The remaining four parameters of the BPP are measured by the sonographer. They are (1) fluid, (2) fetal respiration, (3) fetal tone, and (4) gross body motion. These parameters and scoring of this test are described in Table 14.2.

Required Documentation for a Biophysical Profile

Labeled ciné clips should be taken to document all of the components required of the BPP. Occasionally it is necessary to measure the resistance to blood flow within the umbilical arteries. This measurement is obtained by examining the umbilical cord artery using pulsed wave Doppler. The ratio of the peak systolic flow to the end diastolic flow is calculated and is called the S/D ratio (Fig. 14.28). This number varies with the age of the fetus, and charts are available to determine whether blood flow through the cord is adequate. The ultrasound units will have a calculation package that will perform the calculation; all the sonographer has to do is define peak systolic flow and end diastolic flow. In some cases, the physician may also want to determine whether the blood flow to the placenta from the mother's circulation is adequate, so another Doppler measurement is made of the uterine arteries if possible. The normal uterine signal should be a low-resistance signal with good diastolic flow (Fig. 14.29). The uterine arteries should be assessed for early diastolic notching and increased pulsatility indices (Fig. 14.30), which are abnormal findings.

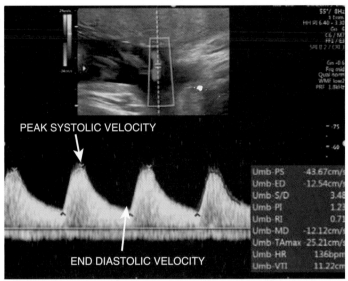

Fig. 14.28 Umbilical artery Doppler measurement of the S/D (systolic/diastolic) ratio. Note how the color Doppler box is very small and just includes the cord. Because this is a ratio, there is no need to perform angle correction.

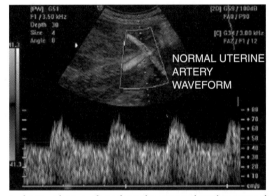

Fig. 14.29 An image of a Doppler waveform from the maternal uterine artery showing a normal low resistance waveform. (From The Fetal Medicine Foundation [2002]. Doppler in obstetrics. Available from https://fetalmedicine.org/var/uploads/Doppler-in-Obstetrics.pdf. Accessed April 16, 2020.)

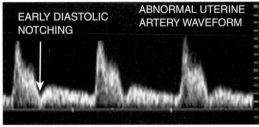

Fig. 14.30 An abnormal high resistance waveform with an early diastolic notch compatible with preeclampsia. (From The Fetal Medicine Foundation [2002]. Doppler in obstetrics. Available from https://fetalmedicine.org/var/uploads/Doppler-in-Obstetrics.pdf. Accessed April 16, 2020.)

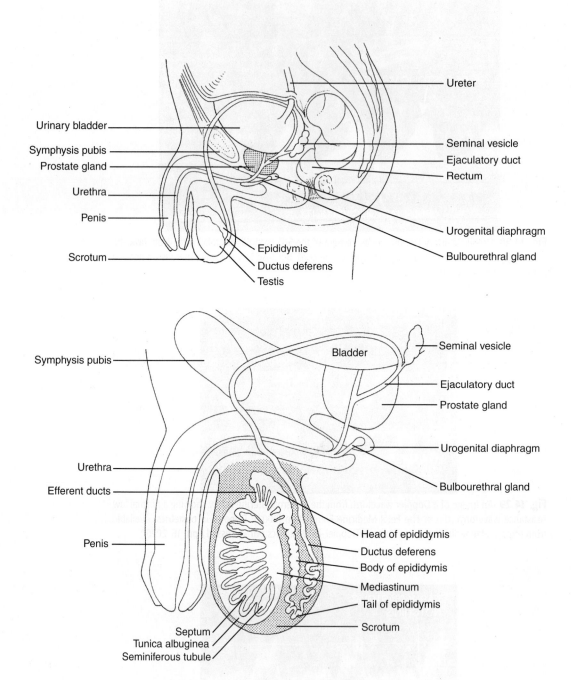

Ureter

Urinary bladder

Symphysis pubis

Prostate gland

Urethra

Penis

Scrotum

Seminal vesicle

Ejaculatory duct

Rectum

Urogenital diaphragm

Bulbourethral gland

Epididymis

Ductus deferens

Testis

Symphysis pubis

Bladder

Seminal vesicle

Ejaculatory duct

Prostate gland

Urogenital diaphragm

Bulbourethral gland

Urethra

Efferent ducts

Penis

Head of epididymis

Ductus deferens

Body of epididymis

Mediastinum

Tail of epididymis

Scrotum

Septum

Tunica albuginea

Seminiferous tubule

CHAPTER 15

Male Pelvis Scanning Protocol for the Prostate Gland, Scrotum, and Penis

M. Robert DeJong

Keywords

Appendix testis
Cavernosal artery
Central gland
Central zone
Corpora cavernosa
Corpus spongiosum
Cremasteric artery
Deep dorsal vein
Deferential artery
Ejaculatory ducts
Epididymis
Mediastinum testis
Neurovascular bundles
Peripheral zone
Priapism
Prostate gland

Prostatic urethra
Rete testis
Scrotum
Seminal vesicles
Seminiferous tubules
Spermatic cord
Spermatogenesis
Testicles
Testosterone
Transitional zone
Tunica albuginea
Tunica vaginalis
Urethra
Vas deferens
Verumontanum

Objectives

At the end of this chapter, you will be able to:

- Define the keywords.
- Discuss the sonographic appearance of the anatomy of the testicles, penis, and prostate.
- Explain the order and locations to take representative images of the prostate gland, scrotum, and penis.
- Name the transducer options for testicular scanning.
- Discuss how to tell the difference sonographically between epididymitis and testicular torsion.
- List the scanning planes and image orientations for endorectal scanning.
- Describe the patient prep for prostate ultrasound studies, including biopsies.
- Discuss the timing of postinjection images for penile Doppler examinations.
- Describe the sonographic difference between low-flow and high-flow priapism.

This chapter will be divided into three parts: scrotum and testicles, prostate, and penis. Sonogram examinations of the male reproductive tract are performed for specific reasons, such as for pain, palpable masses, infertility issues, enlargement, and to evaluate blood flow. These can be very uncomfortable tests for a man because his genitals are exposed; therefore it is important to act in a very professional manner. It is important to explain what you are doing before you touch the patient's penis and scrotum. Some men, especially those under the age of 16, may develop an erection during the course of the examination. With these patients, make sure they are covered and do not react to the erection. An erection may occur because of nerves. Some patients may apologize for having an erection and be embarrassed. If the patient keeps exposing himself, it may be best to find a chaperone. Never put yourself in an uncomfortable situation or create a potential lawsuit.

Sonographic examinations of the male genital system may be performed in a radiology department or in a urology practice. Some urology practices have sonographers performing their ultrasound studies. Unlike endovaginal examinations, there are currently no guidelines for chaperones on any of these studies.

Scrotum and Testicles Protocol

Overview

Common reasons to perform a scrotal/testicular ultrasound include a palpable mass, scrotal swelling, and pain. Acute scrotal pain is an emergent study and should be performed as soon as possible to save the testicle if it is torsed. A man can also be referred for a scrotal ultrasound to evaluate for a varicocele in couples with infertility problems. Testicular cancer is typically discovered in a young age group of between the ages of 15 and 40; however, it has an excellent 5-year survival rate. A rule of thumb is that testicular pathologic conditions are usually malignant whereas extratesticular pathologic conditions are usually of a benign or infectious process.

Anatomy

The **scrotum** is a fibromuscular pouch continuous with the skin of the lower abdomen and is located between the penis and anus. The scrotal wall is a thin layer of skin, and beneath the skin are multiple layers that include from outer to inner; the dartos muscle, external spermatic fascia, cremaster muscles, internal spermatic fascia, and parietal layer of the **tunica vaginalis**. The scrotum hangs outside the body to maintain a slightly lower temperature for the testicles than that of the rest of the body, as required for sperm production. The scrotum is divided into two identical compartments externally by a

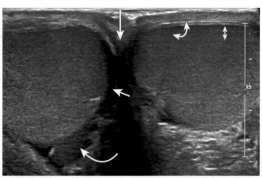

Fig. 15.1 Ultrasound image of a normal scrotum and testicle. The *arrow* is pointing to the median raphe. The *arrowhead* indicates a small amount of normal fluid. The *curved arrow* points to the body of the epididymis. The *curved double-head arrow* indicates the tunica vaginalis. The *double arrow head* points to the tunic albugenia.

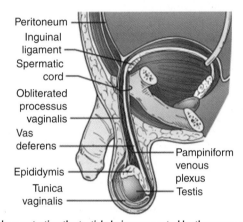

Fig. 15.2 A drawing demonstrating the testicle being supported by the spermatic cord. (From Soni NJ, Kory P, Arntfield R. *Point-of-Care Ultrasound*, 2nd ed. Philadelphia, 2020, Elsevier.)

ridge called the perineal raphe, which connects internally to a muscular partition called the scrotal septum or median raphe. The median raphe is seen as a thin echogenic band with ultrasound. Each side of the scrotum contains a testicle, epididymis, blood vessels, **spermatic cord**, and a small amount of fluid (Fig. 15.1). The normal scrotal wall may vary in thickness from 2 to 8 mm. The purpose of the scrotum is to protect and help regulate the temperature of the testicles for **spermatogenesis**.

The **testicles** are formed in the abdominal cavity and descend through the inguinal canal into the scrotum, usually during the seventh month of gestation. The testicles are ovoid and measure 3 to 5 cm in length and are 3 cm in anteroposterior (AP) and 2 to 4 cm in transverse dimensions and are suspended in the scrotum by the spermatic cord, which contains muscles, vessels, nerves, and ducts that run to and from the testicle (Fig. 15.2). Inferiorly the testicles are anchored to the scrotum by the gubernaculum testis, which is also called the scrotal ligament. Before puberty the testicular volume is less than 5 mL. The average adult testicular volume is approximately 25 mL and will decrease with age.

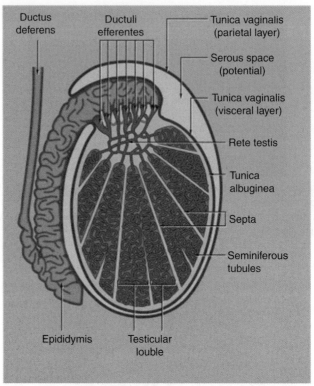

Fig. 15.3 A drawing of internal scrotal and testicle anatomy. The parietal and visceral tunica vaginalis and albuginea are identified. (From Young B, Woodford P, O'Dowd G. *Wheater's Functional Histology*, 6th ed. London, 2013, Churchill Livingstone.)

The testicle is covered by three layers that are, from outer to inner, the tunica vaginalis, tunica albuginea, and tunica vasculosa. The **tunica albuginea** is a fibrous tissue that extends into the testicle and forms the interlobar septa (Fig. 15.3). These septa radiate into the testicle and create 200 to 300 lobules. These lobules converge posteriorly to form the **mediastinum testis**, with the bases of the lobule at the tunica albuginea and the apices at the mediastinum testis. Each lobule contains 3 to 10 convoluted **seminiferous tubules**, where spermatogenesis occurs. The seminiferous tubules empty into the straight tubules, which lead to a network of ducts called the **rete testis**. This network of ducts exits the testis through the mediastinum testis into a series of coiled epididymal efferent ducts. The **epididymis** is located posterolateral to each testicle (Fig. 15.4). The seminiferous tubules are lined by Sertoli cells that function to nourish the developing sperm cells, provide tight junctions to create a blood-testis barrier, and secrete an aqueous secretion to aid with sperm transport. The soft connective tissues surrounding the seminiferous tubules contain interstitial tissue that contains the Leydig cells, which are responsible for **testosterone** production with the help of the hypothalamus and pituitary gland. The testicles are composed of 90% seminiferous tubules, the Sertoli and germ cells, and 10% interstitial tissue, the Leydig cells.

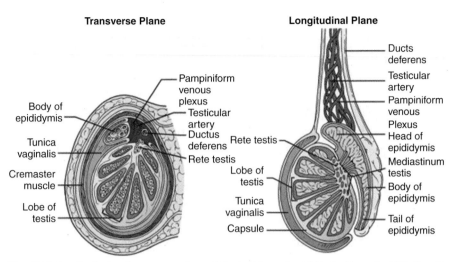

Fig. 15.4 Longitudinal and transverse views of the testicle and epididymis. (From Soni NJ, Kory P, Arntfield R. *Point-of-Care Ultrasound*, 2nd ed. Philadelphia, 2020, Elsevier.)

The second membrane that surrounds the testicle is a double membrane called the tunica vaginalis (see Fig. 15.3). When the testicles descend from the fetal abdomen into the scrotum, through the inguinal canal, they carry a sac of peritoneum with them. This is the tunica vaginalis, which has a parietal layer lining the scrotal wall and a visceral layer covering the testicle and epididymis except at the posterior and superior borders, where the epididymis and spermatic cord are attached to the scrotal wall. It is normal to see a small amount of fluid in this potential space by sonography. It is between the two layers of the tunica vaginalis that bowel can herniate or fluid accumulate, such as a hydrocele.

The tunica vasculosa is formed by vessels and loose connective tissue. It covers the internal surface of the tunica albuginea and the mediastinum testis and provides the nutrient blood supply to the testicular lobules.

The mediastinum testis is an infolding of the tunica albuginea that extends from the top to near the bottom of each testicle and narrows in width as it travels inferiorly. This is why the mediastinum is a bright echo like the tunica albuginea. Numerous septa arise off of it that radiate to the surface of the testicle, dividing it into lobules that house the seminiferous tubules. The mediastinum testis supports the rete testis and is the site of entry for vessels into the testicle and where the ducts exit.

The cremaster muscle covers the testicles and spermatic cord and raises and lowers the testicles to keep them at the proper temperature for spermatogenesis. When the muscle contracts, the spermatic cord is shortened and the testicles are moved closer up toward the body, which provides more warmth to maintain optimal testicular temperature. When the cremasteric muscle relaxes, the testicles are lowered away from the warm body and are able to cool down.

The epididymis is a curved, comma-shaped structure measuring 6 to 7 cm in length but if uncoiled would be 6 to 7 meters. It is formed by the 10 to 15 efferent ductules joining together to form a single convoluted ductule. The epididymis is a tightly coiled tube that stores sperm created by the testicle until they mature, usually in about 60 to 80 days. Its function is to transport sperm and seminal fluid to the **vas deferens**. The epididymal head overhangs the superior pole of the testicle and is isoechoic or slightly hyperechoic to the adjacent testicular tissue.

The epididymis runs along the posterior aspect of the testicle in a craniocaudal fashion and at the lower pole it abruptly turns cephalad to become the vas deferens. It is divided into three parts: the head (globus major), body, and tail (globus minor) (see Fig. 15.4). The head of the epididymis is situated on the superior aspect of the testicle and measures 5 to 12 mm in length. The body of the epididymis is a highly convoluted duct that connects the head to the tail of the epididymis. This is where sperm mature. The tail of the epididymis is continuous with the vas deferens.

The vas deferens is a less convoluted continuation of the epididymis. It joins with the **seminal vesicles** to empty their fluid into the **ejaculatory ducts**; the fluid courses through the prostate and empties into the **prostatic urethra** and finally out of the body during ejaculation.

Two appendages may be seen. The **appendix testis** is located at the anterior-superior aspect of the testicle beneath the epididymis head and represents the blind cranial end of the Müllerian duct remnant. The appendix epididymis is seen as a small protuberance at the superior aspect of the epididymal head and represents the blind cranial end of the Wolffian duct remnant. Neither has any clinical significance except if torsion occurs, because this can cause acute scrotal pain and mimic testicular torsion.

The testicles receive their main arterial blood supply from the testicular artery, which arises from the anterior aspect of the aorta just below the level of the renal arteries (Fig. 15.5). The testicular artery travels through the retroperitoneum and passes through the deep inguinal ring to enter the spermatic cord, where it is surrounded by the veins of the pampiniform plexus. The spermatic cord travels in the inguinal canal to enter the scrotum. Once in the scrotum, the testicular artery gives off a branch to the epididymis before bifurcating into lateral and medial branches. At the posterosuperior aspect of the testicle the testicular artery divides into branches called the capsular arteries. The capsular arteries then pierce the tunica albuginea to run along the surface of the testicle just beneath the tunica albuginea in a layer known as the tunica vasculosa. The capsular arteries then give off the centripetal branches that course between the lobules supplying blood to the testicular parenchyma and converge at the mediastinum. These branches curve into the recurrent rami arteries, which branch off into arterioles. In about 50% of men the transmediastinal artery, a large branch of the testicular artery, enters through the mediastinum and courses through the testicle to supply the capsular arteries. Intratesticular arteries show a low-resistance pattern by Doppler spectrum.

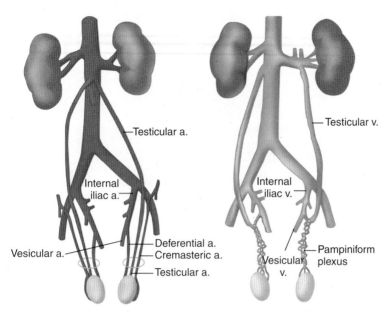

Fig. 15.5 A drawing of the arterial supply and venous drainage of the testicles. The testicular, deferential, and cremasteric arteries are seen. The left testicular vein is shown emptying into the left renal vein. *a*, Artery; *v*, vein. (From Pellerito J, Polack JF. *Introduction to Vascular Ultrasonography*, 7th ed. Philadelphia, 2020, Elsevier.)

Two other arteries supply blood to the scrotum and testicles and also travel in the spermatic cord. The **deferential artery** arises from the inferior vesicle artery and supplies the epididymis and the vas deferens. The **cremasteric artery** arises from the inferior epigastric artery and supplies the scrotal wall and muscles. These arteries tend to have high-resistance waveforms. Both arteries anastomose with the testicular artery.

Blood leaves the testicle through the tunica vasculosa as a number of small veins that combine with those draining the epididymis, to form the pampiniform plexus, which is a major component of the spermatic cord. Once the pampiniform plexus enters the spermatic cord, its branches begin to join until there are about four branches. At the deep inguinal ring the veins continue to join, reducing to one or two larger veins. The veins join to form a single right and left testicular vein. The right testicular vein empties into the inferior vena cava at an acute angle just inferior to the renal veins, and the left testicular vein empties into the left renal vein at a right angle. The testicular veins contain valves to keep blood flowing forward toward the inferior vena cava.

Physiology

The testicles have both an exocrine function, producing sperm, and an endocrine function, producing testosterone. The testicles contain germ cells that differentiate into mature spermatozoa; the Sertoli

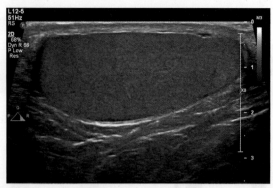

Fig. 15.6 An image of a normal testicle demonstrating homogeneous mid-gray echoes. Note that the scrotal wall is more echogenic than the testicle.

cells, which help nourish the developing sperm cells; and the androgen-producing Leydig cells, which produce testosterone.

A blood barrier exists that separates the seminiferous tubule from the normal circulatory processes of the body. This barrier prevents blood and other body fluids from entering the seminiferous tubules and allows only the secretions from the Sertoli cells to enter the lumen of the seminiferous tubules. These secretions are androgen-binding proteins and are a protein-rich fluid. The blood-testes barrier enables the testicles to maintain a fluid balance that is good for sperm development. The blood-testes barrier also protects the developing sperm from the body's immune system, which would attack the immature sperm.

Sonographic Appearance

The normal testicles are bean or oval shaped, have a mid-gray homogeneous echo texture (Fig. 15.6), and are often compared with the sonographic appearance of the thyroid. The mediastinum testis is seen as a white echogenic line in the posterosuperior portion of the testicle extending in a craniocaudal direction (Fig. 15.7). The epididymal head is an oblong structure located superior and lateral to the testes (Fig. 15.8). It has a coarser echogenicity and is isoechoic or mildly hyperechoic to the testicle and usually demonstrates less vascularity with color Doppler. Spectral Doppler of the epididymal head demonstrates a low-resistance arterial waveform. The tunica albuginea appears as a bright white echogenic structure that surrounds the testicle (Fig. 15.9). The rete testis is seen in about 20% of men as a hypoechoic region near the mediastinum and can appear as multiple small cystic structures. Ectasia of the rete testis is a benign condition caused by partial or complete obstruction of the efferent ductules. The sonographic appearance is an elongated structure of multiple small, cystic structures that replaces the mediastinum with no flow on color Doppler (Fig. 15.10). The appendix testis is seen as an oval structure located

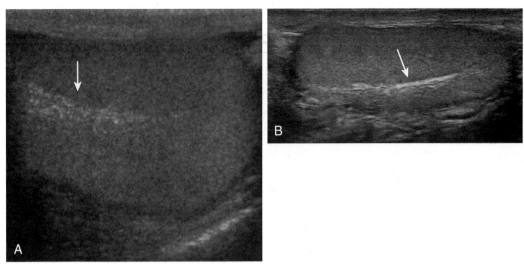

Fig. 15.7 A, The *arrow* is pointing to the mediastinum testis. **B,** The *arrow* is pointing to the mediastinum testis. Note the variations in appearance between the two examples. The mediastinum testis can vary from bright white to a dull white and from a thin line to a wide line.

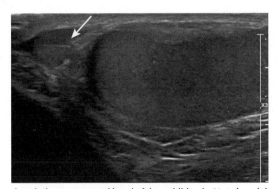

Fig. 15.8 The *arrow* is pointing to a normal head of the epididymis. Note how it is slightly hyperechoic to the testicle.

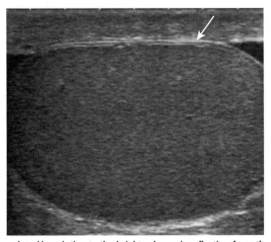

Fig. 15.9 The *arrowhead* is pointing to the bright echogenic reflection from the tunica albuginea.

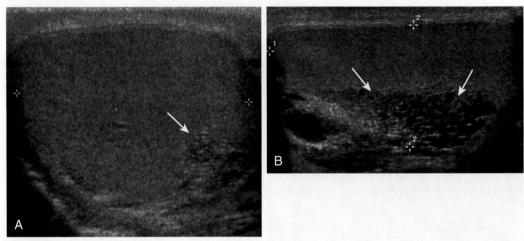

Fig. 15.10 A, The *arrow* is pointing to the normal sonographic appearance of the rete testis. **B,** The *arrows* are pointing to an example of a dilated rete testis.

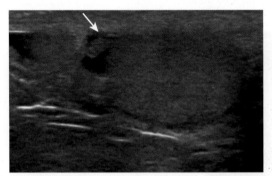

Fig. 15.11 The *arrow* is pointing to the appendix testis seen between the testicle and epididymal head.

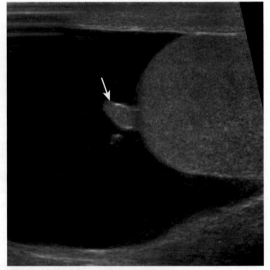

Fig. 15.12 The *arrow* is pointing to the appendix testis in this patient with a large hydrocele.

between the epididymis and testis and is hypoechoic to the testicle (Fig. 15.11). It is usually better visualized when a hydrocele is present (Fig. 15.12). The spermatic cord can be seen in the inguinal canal as a tubular structure just beneath the skin. It appears as an echogenic band in the longitudinal plane, with the cremasteric muscles seen as hypoechoic structures (Fig. 15.13). Color Doppler can aid in finding the spermatic cord by identifying the testicular artery. The scrotal wall is more echogenic than the testicle and measures 2 to 8 mm depending on the contractile state of the cremasteric muscle (Fig. 15.14).

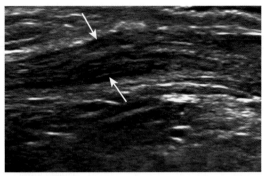

Fig. 15.13 A longitudinal image of the inguinal canal showing the spermatic cord. The *arrows* are pointing to the cremasteric muscles.

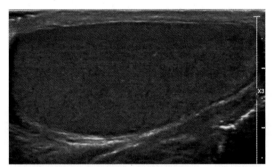

Fig. 15.14 A normal image of the testicle and scrotal wall.

Ultrasound of the Scrotum and Testicles

Patient Prep

There is no patient prep for a scrotal ultrasound examination.

Transducer

A broad-bandwidth 7–15 MHz linear array transducer is used. If the scrotum is swollen, a curved linear array transducer is used to be able to visualize the entire scrotal sac, using the highest frequency possible and, if possible, try to obtain images of the testicle with a high-frequency linear array transducer.

Patient Position

The patient is scanned in the supine position, with the scrotum supported by a rolled-up small towel or a pillowcase. The patient can hold the ends of a pillow case or a towel and pull up gently to hold the testicles in place. The penis is placed on the suprapubic area and covered with a towel (Fig. 15.15). To evaluate small, palpable nodules, the testicle can be held and supported by the sonographer's gloved hand. Superficial nodules may require the use of a standoff pad.

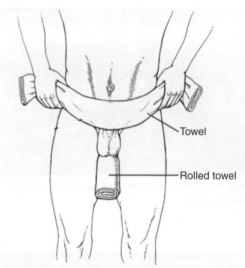

Fig. 15.15 A drawing showing how to prepare the patient for the testicular sonogram. The scrotum is supported by a rolled-up towel, and the penis is placed on the lower abdomen and covered with another towel.

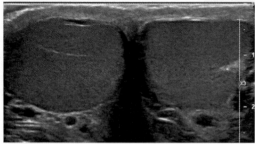

Fig. 15.16 Image showing two normal testicles in a side-by-side comparison. The mediastinum is seen in each testicle. Note that this is not using a split screen technique.

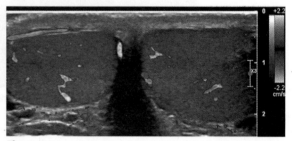

Fig. 15.17 Image showing the color Doppler comparison of two normal testicles. Note the similarity of the perfusion.

Technical Tips

Scans are obtained in the longitudinal and transverse planes. Using a split-screen technique, a transverse scan should be obtained of both testicles at the same level to compare testicular size, echogenicity, and scrotal wall thickness (Fig. 15.16). This technique also should be used to compare blood flow to each testicle (Fig. 15.17).

When performing the color and spectral Doppler aspects of the examination, the wall filters should be set at the lowest setting and the color velocity scale adjusted for a low-flow state (Fig. 15.18). Power Doppler also can be used to evaluate testicular flow because it is more sensitive than color Doppler, especially when testicular torsion is suspected (Fig. 15.19). The different arteries will have different waveforms with the cremasteric and deferential arteries having high-resistance signals (Fig. 15.20), whereas the testicular artery will have a low-resistance signal. (Fig. 15.21). Venous waveforms have a continuous waveform pattern (Fig. 15.22).

Make sure to use warm gel, because cold gel will cause the scrotum to contract, making it difficult to scan the testicles. Also, make sure

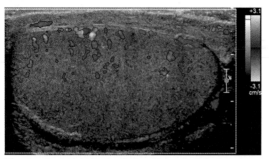

Fig. 15.18 Color Doppler image of a normal testicle showing the color velocity scale at a setting of 3.1 cm/s.

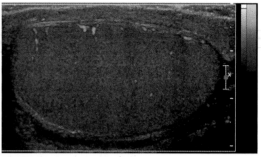

Fig. 15.19 Power Doppler image showing normal testicular flow.

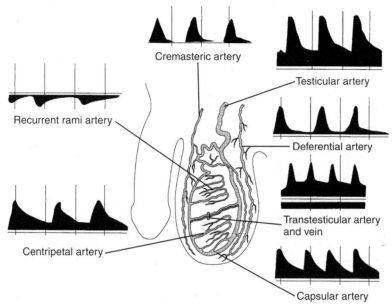

Fig. 15.20 Drawing showing the various flow patterns of the arteries that supply blood to the testicles and scrotum.

the gel is not too hot so as not to burn the patient. Check the gel like checking the temperature for a baby bottle by squirting some on your wrist. Keep the patient covered as much as possible, the curtains pulled, and the door closed to ensure patient privacy.

If there is a palpable mass, holding the testicle with one gloved hand to stabilize the testicle may help to be certain that the area is well seen. Inform the patient why you need to hold his testicle in your hand.

If a testicular mass (Fig. 15.23) is found, look for enlarged lymph nodes in the paraaortic and inferior vena cava area (Fig. 15.24). The lymphatic chain for the testicles follows the testicular veins; therefore, enlarged lymph nodes will be in the paraaortic and paracaval nodes in the region of the renal veins and not in the groin or pelvic area.

Microlithiasis is a condition in which small calcifications develop in the seminiferous tubules and are seen as small echogenic foci scattered throughout the testicle (Fig. 15.25). This is usually an incidental finding. These men may be followed if they have risk factors to develop a testicular mass (Fig. 15.26).

The appendix testis may fall off as a result of torsion and be seen as an echogenic structure casting an acoustic shadow at the bottom of the scrotum (Fig. 15.27).

A cyst in the head of the epididymis can be an incidental finding (Fig. 15.28).

Finally, do not make any comments about the size of the man's genitals. Not only is it very unprofessional, but you never know who can hear you.

Scrotal and Testicular Required Images

The protocol for a scrotal and testicular ultrasound will be guided by the clinical indication. The testicles should be evaluated thoroughly

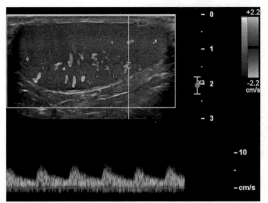

Fig. 15.21 A spectral Doppler tracing of a normal recurrent rami artery.

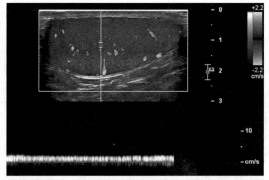

Fig. 15.22 A spectral Doppler tracing of a normal intratesticular vein.

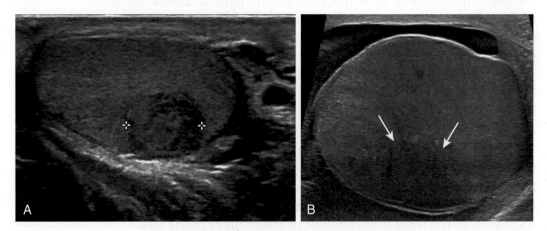

Fig. 15.23 A, An image of a mixed germ cell tumor seen between the calipers. Note that the mass is hypoechoic to the normal testicular parenchyma. **B,** A patient with leukemia. The *arrows* are pointing to the metastatic leukemia. The chemotherapy cannot pass the blood-testis barrier, and therefore the testicle can be a sanctuary site for leukemic cells.

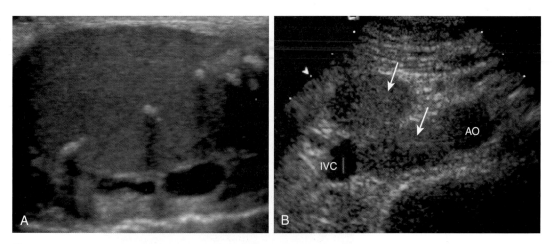

Fig. 15.24 A, A patient with choriocarcinoma showing "burned-out" tumors. These tumors quickly outgrow their blood supply and regress and calcify. Unfortunately, this cancer is not detected by physical examination but is found when metastatic disease appears. It has a very poor prognosis. **B,** The *arrows* are pointing to the enlarged paraaortic lymph nodes in this patient. *AO,* Aorta; *IVC,* inferior vena cava.

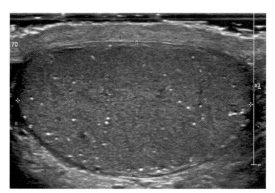

Fig. 15.25 An image of a testicle that has microlithiasis. Note the scattered bright echogenic foci in the parenchyma.

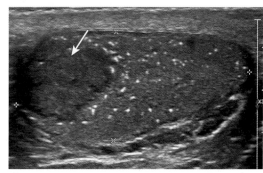

Fig. 15.26 The *arrow* is pointing to a germ cell tumor on this patient with microlithiasis.

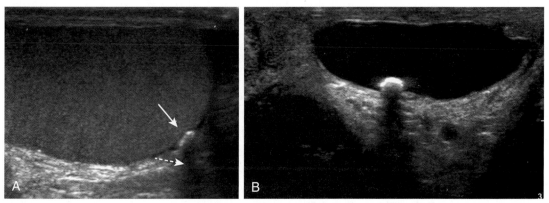

Fig. 15.27 A, The *arrow* is pointing to a "scrotal pearl," which is an appendix testis that has torsed off and calcified. They are mobile and are found at the bottom of the scrotum. The *dashed arrow* is pointing to the acoustic shadow. **B,** A torsed appendix testicle in a patient with a hydrocele casting an acoustic shadow.

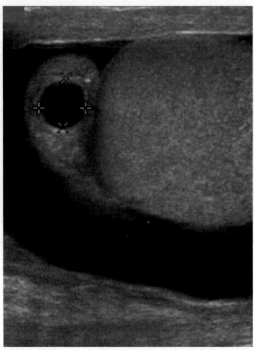

Fig. 15.28 The cursors are measuring an epididymal head cyst. This patient also has a hydrocele.

in both longitudinal and transverse planes. The size, echogenicity, and blood flow of each testis and epididymis should be compared with the contralateral side. If the reason for the examination is a palpable abnormality, that area needs to be scanned and identified as the area of concern or area of palpable mass. If a testicle cannot be found in the scrotum, a search should be made in the inguinal canal (Fig. 15.29). If the reason for the examination is to evaluate for the presence of a varicocele, images with a Valsalva maneuver should be performed (Fig. 15.30, Color Plate 1). If a right-sided only varicocele is found, the abdomen and retroperitoneum should be evaluated for a mass causing the varicocele. An examination for acute scrotal pain is an emergency. After gray-scale images confirm the absence of a testicular mass, the next part of the examination is the Doppler evaluation. Starting with the normal side, color Doppler parameters should be set, and a color perfusion image and a spectral Doppler arterial waveform obtained. Then without changing any controls the side in pain should be evaluated. If there is an increase in color, an infectious process is suspected (Fig. 15.31). If no color is seen, the controls should be further adjusted to try to elicit an arterial signal. Lack of arterial signal is suspicious for a testicular torsion (Fig. 15.32, Color Plates 2 and 3). A color Doppler side-by-side image should be obtained to show the difference in the flow between the two testicles (Fig. 15.33, Color Plates 4 and 5).

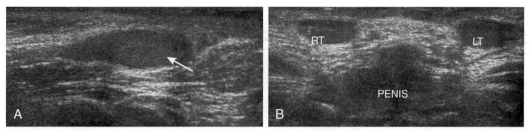

Fig. 15.29 A, A sagittal image through the right inguinal canal on this newborn. The *arrow* is pointing to an undescended testicle. **B,** A transverse image through both inguinal canals on this newborn showing bilateral undescended testicles. *LT,* Left testicle; *RT,* right testicle.

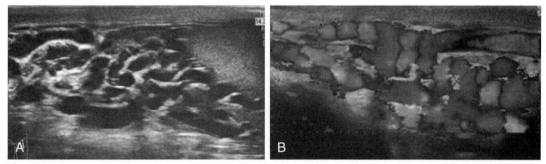

Fig. 15.30 A, An example of a dilated pampiniform plexus superior to the testicle on a patient with a varicocele. **B,** A color Doppler image after having the patient perform a Valsalva maneuver demonstrating the increased flow. See color plate 1.

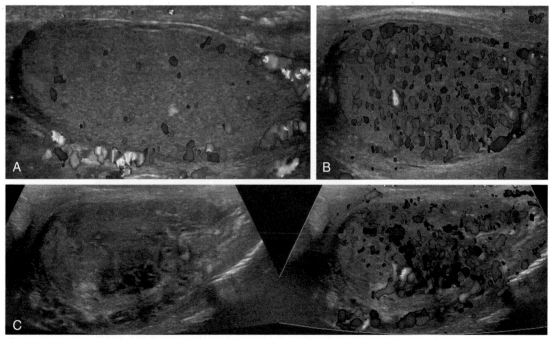

Fig. 15.31 A, A patient with acute left scrotal pain showing normal flow in the right testicle. **B,** The left testicle demonstrates increased flow compatible with orchitis. **C,** Side-by-side images showing an inflamed epididymis.

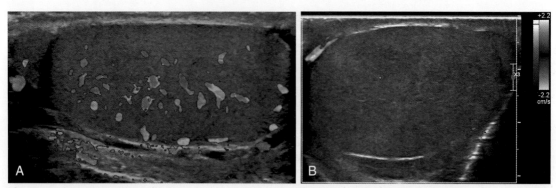

Fig. 15.32 A, A patient with acute left scrotal pain showing normal flow in the right testicle. **B,** A color Doppler image of the left testicle demonstrating no flow compatible with testicular torsion. Some scrotal wall flow is seen, which should not be mistaken for intratesticular flow. See color plates 2 and 3.

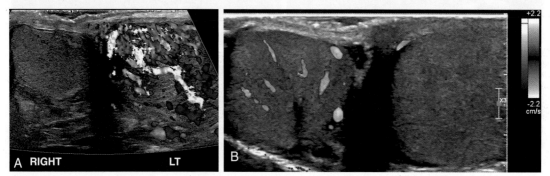

Fig. 15.33 A, A side-by-side image showing the increased flow in the left testicle compatible with orchitis. See color plate 4. **B,** A side-by-side image showing no flow in the left testicle compatible with testicular torsion. See color plate 5.

Scrotum and Testes • Longitudinal Images

1. Longitudinal midline of the testicle with and without length and AP measurements. For simplicity, all images will be marked right.

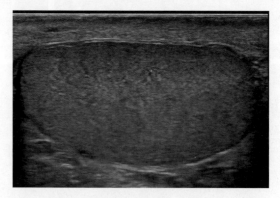

Suggested Annotation: **LONG RT MID**

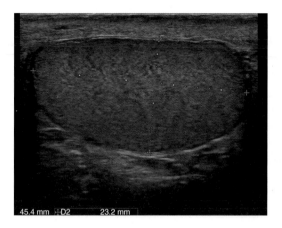

Suggested Annotation: **LONG RT MID**

2. Longitudinal image of the lateral aspect of the testicle.

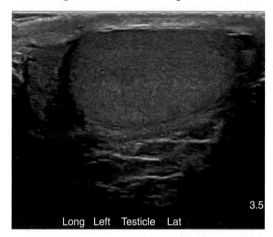

Suggested Annotation: **LONG RT LAT**

3. Longitudinal image of the medial aspect of the testicle.

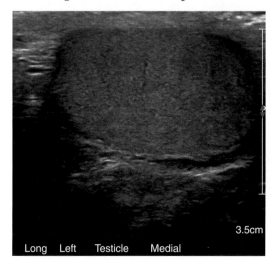

Suggested Annotation: **LONG RT MED**

4. Longitudinal image of head of the epididymis with and without measurement.

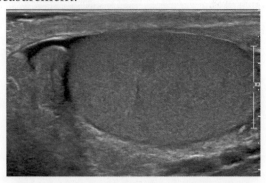

Suggested Annotation: **LONG RT EPI OR EPI HEAD**

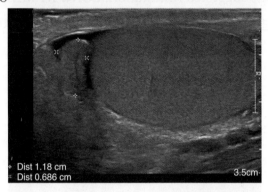

Suggested Annotation: **LONG RT EPI OR EPI HEAD**

5. Longitudinal color Doppler image of the testicle.

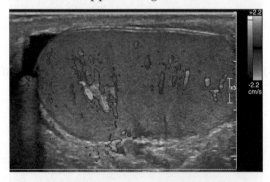

Suggested Annotation: **LONG RT**

Doppler waveforms of the artery and vein are not required except when the indication is for acute scrotal pain. Some laboratories may require them as part of their protocol.

6. Longitudinal spectral Doppler of the testicle arterial signal.

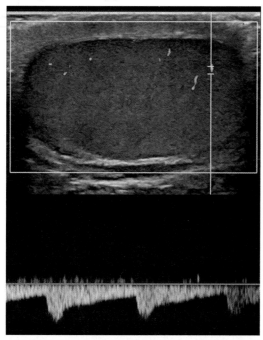

Suggested Annotation: **LONG RT ART**

7. Longitudinal spectral Doppler of the testicle venous signal.

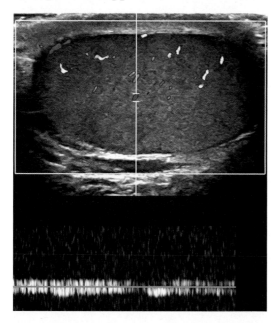

Suggested Annotation: **LONG RT VEIN**

NOTE: It can be possible to have the arterial and venous signal in the same image.

Transverse Images

1. Transverse mid-testicle with and without measurements.

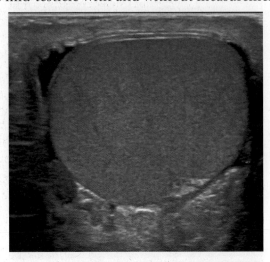

Suggested Annotation: **TRANS OR TRV RT MID**

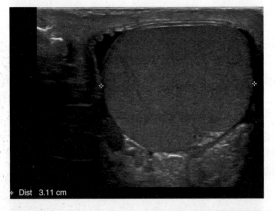

Suggested Annotation: **TRANS OR TRV RT MID**

2. Transverse testicle lower pole.

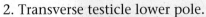

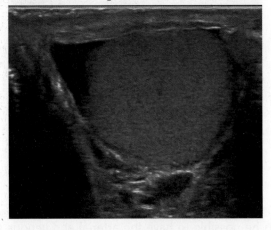

Suggested Annotation: **TRANS OR TRV RT LOW OR LP**

3.   Transverse testicle upper pole.

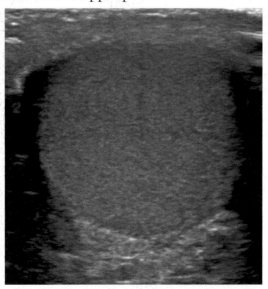

Suggested Annotation: **TRANS OR TRV RT UP**

4. Transverse epididymal head. Not all departments do a measurement.

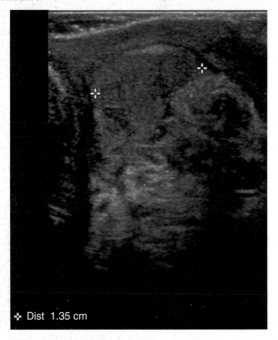

Suggested Annotation: **TRANS OR TRV RT EPI OR EPI HEAD**

5.   Transverse both testicles for comparison gray scale. Annotate RT and LT under the testicle.

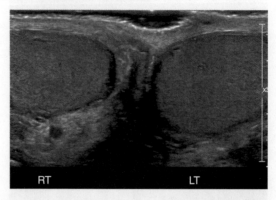

Suggested Annotation: **TRANS OR TRV**

6. Transverse both testicles for comparison gray scale using the trapezoid function to see more of the testicles if needed.

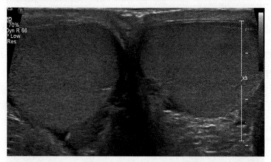

Suggested Annotation: **TRANS OR TRV**

7.   Transverse both testicles for comparison color Doppler.

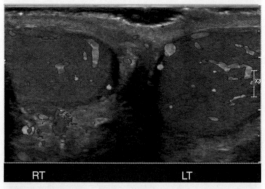

Suggested Annotation: **TRANS OR TRV**

Prostate Gland Protocols

Overview

Prostate ultrasound is performed for specific reasons, with the most common being size, palpable mass, enlarged prostate, and biopsy guidance. Many physicians may do an ultrasound examination with a biopsy to

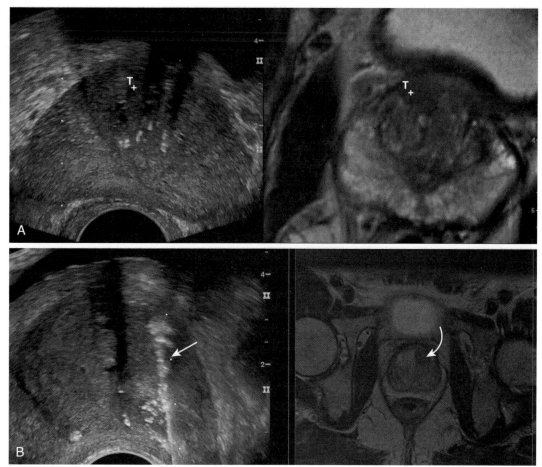

Fig. 15.34 A, An example of prostate ultrasound fusion with MRI. The T+ marker is placed on the MRI side over the suspected lesion and automatically appears on the ultrasound side. This is the area where the biopsy will be performed, which would never have been done using standard blind biopsy techniques. This was the man's fourth biopsy; the other three blind biopsies showed no signs of cancer, yet his prostate-specific antigen level continued to rise. This area was positive for a low-grade prostatic cancer. **B,** A fusion-guided biopsy of another patient with a cancer deep in the left central zone. The *arrow* is pointing to the artifact created by the needle and the curved arrow on the MRI to the area of concern.

follow so as not to subject the man to two probe insertions. Men with elevated prostate-specific antigen (PSA) levels and prior normal biopsy results may have magnetic resonance imaging with biopsy performed of suspicious areas under ultrasound using fusion technology. Fusion technology allows the MRI scan to be uploaded into the ultrasound machine, and through the use of sensors the MRI images will follow the ultrasound images as the patient is scanned, thus pinpointing areas requiring biopsy, including masses in the **central gland** (Fig. 15.34).

There are two methods to evaluate the prostate with ultrasound. The first is a transabdominal (TA) technique using the bladder as an acoustic window (Fig. 15.35). The second method is examining the prostate through the rectum, usually called a TRUS, pronounced truss, for transrectal (TR) ultrasound (Fig. 15.36). The majority of prostate ultrasound examinations, including fusion biopsies, are performed by the urologist in the office. Some radiology practices still perform prostate examinations and biopsies, whereas others may perform only endorectal prostate examinations on patients with prostatitis or a suspected prostate abscess, because these men will have been admitted to the hospital for treatment. The radiology department may also perform TA studies for prostate size and postvoid residual (PVR).

Anatomy

The **prostate gland** is an exocrine gland and is part of the male reproductive system. It is situated anterior to the rectum, inferior to the bladder, and the **urethra** runs through the center of the gland. It is described as chestnut in shape and the size of a walnut and is enveloped in a fibrous capsule. The prostate does not have a true capsule; however, a smooth and regular echogenic border can be seen around the prostate-fat interface that has been termed the prostatic capsule. The superior part is called the base and is in contact with the bladder, and the inferior end is called the apex and is close to the base of the penis. It measures approximately 4 × 3 × 4 cm and weighs between 16 and 25 g.

Under the zonal concept of anatomy, described by Dr. John McNeal, the prostate is divided into three glandular zones, the peripheral, central, and transitional zones; and one nonglandular zone, the anterior fibromuscular stroma (Fig. 15.37).

The **peripheral zone** is located posteriorly and laterally to the distal prostatic urethra and makes up most of the apex (Fig. 15.38). This zone is thin at the base and becomes larger as it approaches the apex. In a normal prostate it is the largest zone. It constitutes 70% of the glandular tissue, and approximately 70% of prostatic cancer originates from this zone. This is the area that is palpated on a digital rectal examination (DRE) and is also the area most commonly affected by prostatitis (Fig. 15.39).

The **central zone** surrounds the ejaculatory ducts (Fig. 15.40). It extends from the base to the level of the **verumontanum**, which is where the ejaculatory ducts empty into the urethra. There is no central

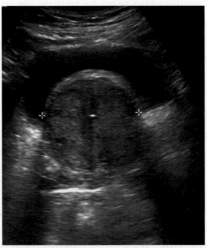

Fig. 15.35 Transverse transabdominal image of an enlarged prostate compatible with benign prostatic hyperplasia.

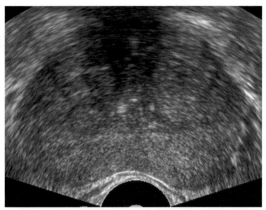

Fig. 15.36 Transrectal image of a patient with very mild benign prostatic hyperplasia. The acoustic shadow is caused by the urethra and is called the Eiffel Tower sign.

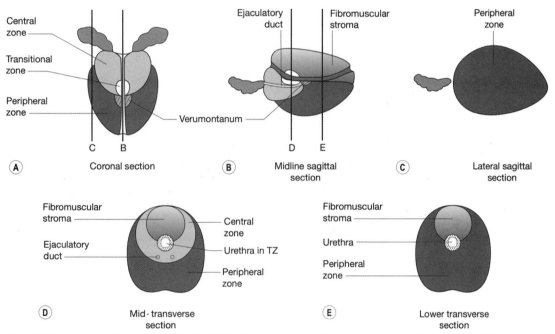

Fig. 15.37 A drawing of the prostate using Dr. McNeal's zonal anatomy. **A,** A transverse view of the prostate with lines *B* and *C* representing the location for sagittal images **B** and **C. B,** A sagittal view of the prostate with lines *D* and *E* representing the location for transverse images **D** and **E.** (From Ryan S, McNicholas M, Eustace S. *Anatomy for Diagnostic Imaging,* 3rd ed. Edinburgh, 2011, Saunders.)

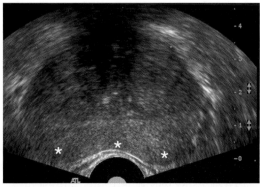

Fig. 15.38 Transrectal image of the prostate. The stars are in the peripheral zone (PZ). The hypoechoic area above the PZ is the central gland.

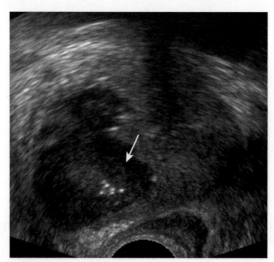

Fig. 15.39 The *arrow* is pointing to a prostatic abscess in the peripheral zone.

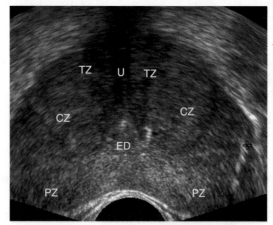

Fig. 15.40 The sonographic anatomy of the prostate gland. This image demonstrates the Eiffel Tower sign, which is created by periurethral calcifications creating an acoustic shadow. *CZ,* Central zone; *ED,* ejaculatory ducts *(two small circles); PZ,* peripheral zone; *TZ,* transitional zone; *U,* urethra.

zone distal to the verumontanum. It constitutes 20% of the glandular tissue, and approximately 10% of prostatic cancer originates from this zone.

The **transitional zone** is a bilobed area located on both sides of the urethra (Fig. 15.41) and ends at the verumontanum. This zone contains a mixture of glandular tissue and stromal elements and is separated from the peripheral zone by the surgical capsule. In a normal prostate it is the smallest zone. It constitutes 5% of the glandular tissue, and approximately 20% of prostatic cancer originate from this zone. Prostate enlargement called benign prostatic hyperplasia (BPH), sometimes referred to as benign prostatic hypertrophy, arises from this zone. The BPH nodules can obstruct the flow of urine, causing a bladder outlet obstruction.

> **NOTE:** The term *central gland* has been used to denote the central zone and transition zone because it can be difficult to see each lobe separately (Fig. 15.42), especially when BPH is present.

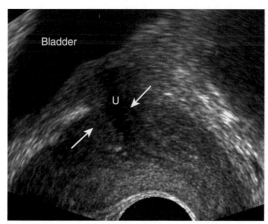

Fig. 15.41 The *arrows* are pointing to the area of the prostatic urethra *(U)*.

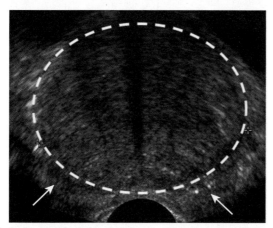

Fig. 15.42 The *dashed oval* defines the central zone. The *arrows* are pointing to the compressed peripheral zone in this patient with BPH.

The anterior fibromuscular stroma is composed of smooth muscle and forms the anterior surface of the gland. This area is relatively free of disease.

The prostate also can be divided into four lobes, although zonal anatomy is used in ultrasound. You might hear a urologist talk about lobes, especially the median lobe, as BPH affects the median lobe. The anterior lobe is the anterior portion of the prostate lying in front of the urethra. It is the nonglandular tissue of the fibromuscular stroma.

The median lobe is cone shaped and is between the two ejaculatory ducts and the urethra. BPH affects the median lobe and is the part of the prostate that extends into the bladder.

The right and left lateral lobes form the majority of the prostate and are continuous along the posterior border. They are separated by the urethra.

The posterior lobe is the posteromedial aspect of the lateral lobes that can be palpated through the rectum during a DRE.

The seminal vesicles lie superior to the prostate under the base of the bladder and are approximately 6 cm in length. The vas deferens are medial to the seminal vesicles and appear more vertical as they join the seminal vesicles (Fig. 15.43) to become the ejaculatory duct

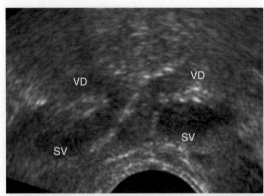

Fig. 15.43 The vas deferens *(VD)* and the seminal vesicles *(SV)* joining together and creating the letter X.

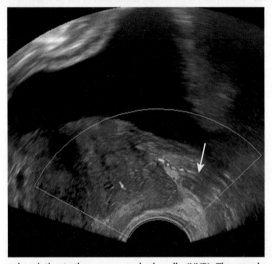

Fig. 15.44 The *arrow* is pointing to the neurovascular bundle (NVB). The vessels of NVB are seen with color Doppler, which helps to identify it. The NVB runs along the side of the prostate gland.

before entering the prostate. Together they form an X-like shape on sonography. The ejaculatory duct passes through the prostate tissue to empty into the urethra.

The prostate receives blood from the inferior vesical artery, which is a branch of the internal iliac artery. It subdivides into the urethral branches, which supply blood to the urethra and the deep parts of the gland, and the capsular branches, which supply blood to the peripheral aspects of the prostate.

The prostatic venous plexus drains the prostate. It joins with the **deep dorsal vein** of the penis to drain into the inferior vesical vein, which finally empties into the internal iliac vein.

Two **neurovascular bundles** (NVBs) travel along the side of the prostate gland. These can be identified with ultrasound as an echogenic area seen at 5 and 7 o'clock (Fig. 15.44). They can be verified with color Doppler by the presence of a small artery and vein. The NVBs are located to give a periprostatic block for a prostate biopsy to help reduce pain during the procedure.

Physiology

The function of the prostate is to secrete a slightly alkaline, milky white fluid to enhance the mobility of the sperm. It contributes roughly 30% to the volume of the semen, with the other 70% being spermatozoa and seminal vesicle fluid. The prostate releases its secretions into the urethra as a result of smooth muscle contractions during ejaculation.

Sonographic Appearance

The sonographic appearance of the normal prostate from a TA approach is round or oval and has a homogeneous low-level gray echogenicity (Fig. 15.45). In a man with BPH the prostate may be circular or irregular in shape and may still be homogeneous or have a heterogeneous texture (Fig. 15.46). On the TA approach the internal anatomy of the prostate cannot be appreciated, although the seminal vesicles may sometimes be seen with a TA approach.

The normal prostate gland should appear symmetric with a smooth contour and well-defined margins in a TR approach. The peripheral zone appears homogeneous with mid-gray echoes and is more hyperechoic than the central gland (Fig. 15.47). The central gland is usually heterogenous from BPH and may have some calcifications (Fig. 15.48). The central and transition zones of the prostate are not normally seen as two separate zones (Fig. 15.49), especially as the prostate enlarges.

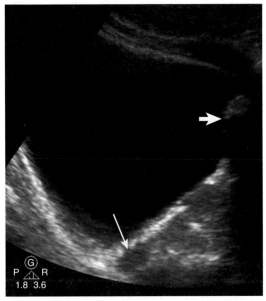

Fig. 15.45 Transabdominal image of the prostate. The *arrow* is pointing to the seminal vesicle. A calcification can be seen in the prostate. The *arrowhead* is pointing to the acoustic shadow from the symphysis pubis.

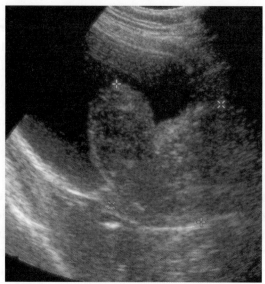

Fig. 15.46 Transabdominal image showing an enlarged median lobe protruding into the bladder. This prostate was 86 g.

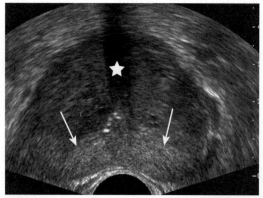

Fig. 15.47 The *arrows* are pointing to the peripheral zone. The *star* is on the Eiffel Tower sign, caused by the small calcifications.

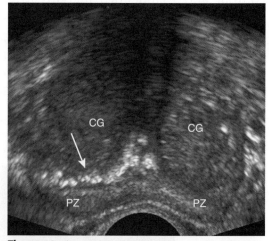

Fig. 15.48 The *arrow* is pointing to an area of calcifications called corpora amylacea that outline the surgical capsule that demarcates the border between the central gland and peripheral zone. *CG,* Central gland; *PZ,* peripheral zone.

The seminal vesicles are seen as ovoid structures with low-level echoes, just superior to the prostate gland, on transverse images (Fig. 15.50). They appear hypoechoic relative to the prostate gland and should appear symmetric in size, shape, and echogenicity. They are seen in their long axis on transverse plane scans. The vas deferens are medial to and have an echo texture similar to that of the seminal vesicles (Fig. 15.51). The ejaculatory duct when seen will appear as double lines on a sagittal scan coursing from the seminal vesicle to the urethra (Fig. 15.52).

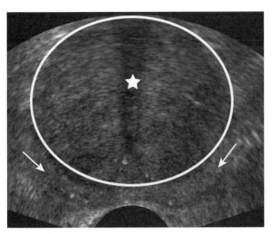

Fig. 15.49 The *circle* outlines the central gland. The *arrows* are pointing to the peripheral zone. The *star* is on the Eiffel Tower artifact.

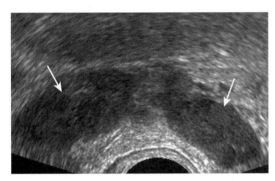

Fig. 15.50 The *arrows* are pointing to normal seminal vesicles which are similar in size, shape, and echogenicity.

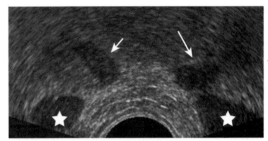

Fig. 15.51 The *arrows* are pointing to the vas deferens as they approach the seminal vesicles *(stars)*.

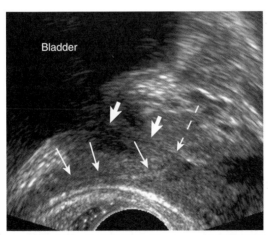

Fig. 15.52 Sagittal image of the prostate gland at midline. The *arrows* are pointing to the ejaculatory duct and the *arrowheads* to the urethra. The *dashed arrow* is pointing to the area of the verumontanum, which is the area that marks where the prostatic urethra ends and the membranous urethra begins, the urethra segment between the prostatic and penile segments. The ejaculatory ducts drain posteriorly in the urethra at the verumontanum.

Ultrasound of the Prostate: Transabdominal Approach

A TA examination is performed to determine prostate size and weight and evaluate the PVR.

Patient Prep

The TA examination is performed with the patient in the supine position and having a full bladder. The patient is instructed to drink 16 to 24 oz of fluid 1 hour before the study and to not void until instructed to do so. For just determining prostate size the bladder only needs to be full enough to see the prostate. However, because the PVR is usually important in these patients, the bladder should be full enough to determine the PVR.

Transducer

For a TA examination a 3.5–5 MHz curved linear array probe is used.

Patient Position

The patient is scanned in a supine position.

Technical Tips

To visualize the prostate gland, the transducer is placed at the top of the bladder and angled beneath the pubic bone, because the prostate gland lies posterior to the symphysis pubis. Transversely, the transducer should be angled caudally 30 to 45 degrees under the pubic bone. It may be necessary to push the transducer under the pubic bone for good visualization of the prostate. Be sure to warn the patient that you will be pushing on their bladder and why.

In the longitudinal plane the gland is measured in the length and height (AP) dimensions (Fig. 15.53), and the width is measured in the transverse plane (Fig. 15.54). The machine will do the calculations when volume is chosen (Fig. 15.55). The calculated results will be in cubic centimeters (cc); however, because the specific gravity of prostate tissue is nearly 1, the cubic centimeters can be converted into grams (g), which urologists prefer because they determine the weight of the prostate gland when performing a DRE and not its size.

When a PVR is required, the bladder needs to be full, and three measurements of the bladder are obtained: length, AP, and width, to calculate the bladder volume (Fig. 15.56). The patient should then be directed to empty their bladder as much as possible and the same measurements repeated, thereby obtaining the PVR. If the bladder is very full, instruct the patient to empty the bladder as much as possible, like he would do at home. Some men may feel under pressure

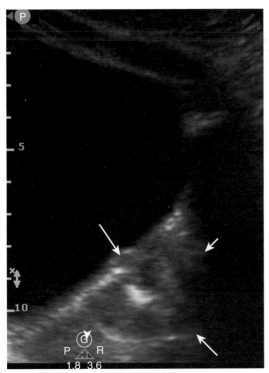

Fig. 15.53 An image demonstrating how to measure the length *(arrows)* and the anteroposterior dimensions *(arrowheads)* of the prostate from a transabdominal approach. These two measurements should be perpendicular to one another. A calcification is seen.

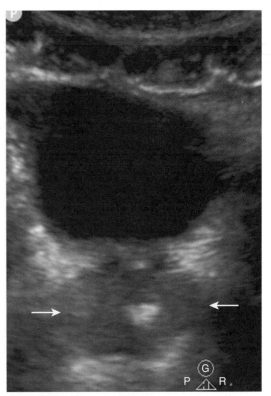

Fig. 15.54 An image demonstrating how to measure the width *(arrows)* of the prostate from a transabdominal approach.

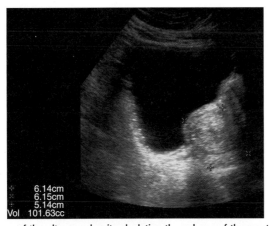

Fig. 15.55 An image of the ultrasound unit calculating the volume of the prostate from a transabdominal approach. Remember that 101 cc corresponds to a prostatic weight of 101 g.

to void quickly so as not to hold up the room. Explain the purpose of having patients empty their bladder as they usually would. Let them know that you understand that this may take some time (Fig. 15.57).

If BPH is present, some departments may require a longitudinal image of each kidney to evaluate for hydronephrosis, similar to for a woman with large uterine fibroids (Fig. 15.58).

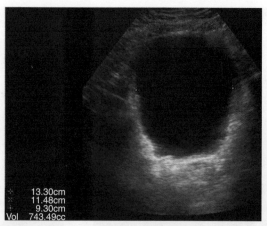

Fig. 15.56 This image shows the volume of the bladder, which measured 743 cc.

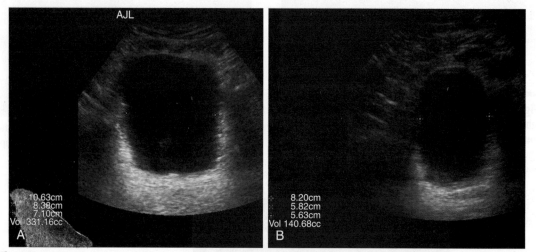

Fig. 15.57 A, Same patient as in Fig. 15.56 measuring a postvoid residual (PVR) of 331 cc. **B,** A second PVR measured 140 cc.

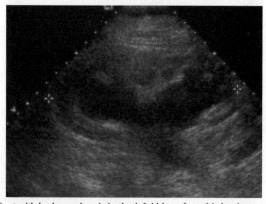

Fig. 15.58 A patient with hydronephrosis in the left kidney from his benign prostatic hyperplasia.

Transabdominal Prostate Required Images

Transabdominal Prostate • Longitudinal Images

Because it is not possible to see detail in the prostate gland, these examinations have few images. The AP measurement should be perpendicular to the length measurement. Even though the cursors do not cover anatomy, some departments may require an image without the calipers.

1. Longitudinal of the prostate with length and AP measurements.

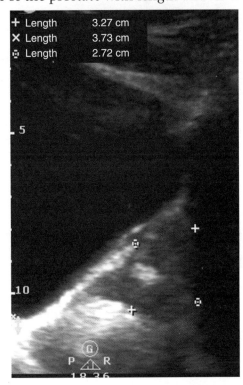

Suggested Annotation: **SAG PROS**

Because there is no guarantee that this image will be at the midline, the word LONG for long axis or SAG for sagittal is a better description.

2. Longitudinal image of the bladder with length and AP measurements.

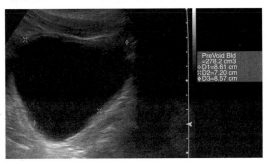

Suggested Annotation: **PREVOID SAG BLAD**. Some laboratories may just annotate SAG BLAD

Transabdominal Prostate • Transverse Images

1. Transverse prostate with width measurement.

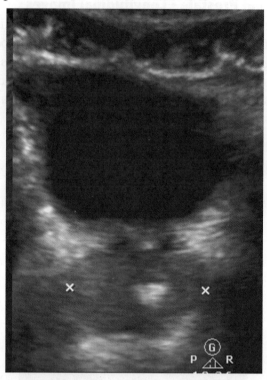

Suggested Annotation: **TRANS OR TRV PROS**

2. Transverse image of the bladder with width measurement.

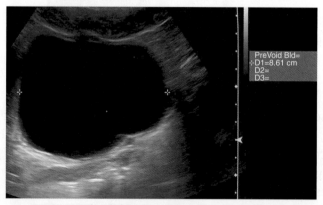

Suggested Annotation: **PREVOID TRANS OR TRV BLAD**, or simply **TRANS OR TRV BLAD**

Transabdominal Prostate • Postvoid Images

1. Longitudinal image of the bladder with length and AP measurements.

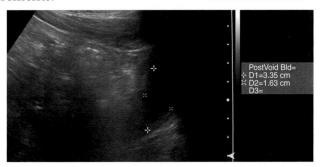

PostVoid Bld=
D1=3.35 cm
D2=1.63 cm
D3=

Suggested Annotation: **POST VOID OR PV SAG BLAD**

2. Transverse image of the bladder with width measurement.

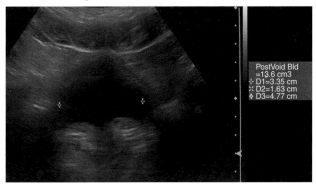

PostVoid Bld
=13.6 cm3
D1=3.35 cm
D2=1.63 cm
D3=4.77 cm

Suggested Annotation: **POST VOID OR PV TRANS OR TRV BLAD**

Ultrasound of the Prostate: Transrectal and Endorectal Approach

A TRUS is performed to evaluate the prostate when increased detail and resolution are needed, such as for cancer, prostatitis, and potential causes for male infertility, among other reasons (Figs. 15.59 to 15.61)

Patient Prep

Some departments may have the patients use a suppository or take an enema before the examination to ensure that the rectum is empty before scanning. The bladder should be emptied, although a small amount of urine in the bladder can be helpful in finding the urethra on sagittal images.

Transducer

Transrectal or endorectal transducers include biplane or now more commonly end fire technologies. The transducer frequency should be a minimum of 5 MHz, with frequencies of 5 to 10 MHz preferred for optimal resolution.

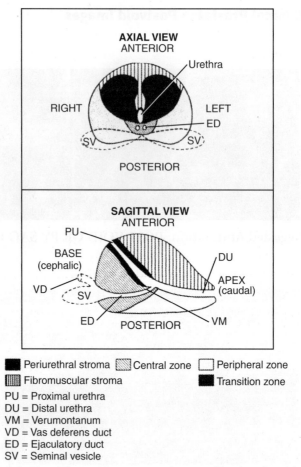

AXIAL VIEW
ANTERIOR

Urethra

RIGHT LEFT

ED

SV SV

POSTERIOR

SAGITTAL VIEW
ANTERIOR

PU

BASE
(cephalic)

DU

VD APEX
(caudal)

SV

ED VM

POSTERIOR

■ Periurethral stroma ▨ Central zone ☐ Peripheral zone
▥ Fibromuscular stroma ■ Transition zone

PU = Proximal urethra
DU = Distal urethra
VM = Verumontanum
VD = Vas deferens duct
ED = Ejaculatory duct
SV = Seminal vesicle

Fig. 15.59 A drawing of the prostate anatomy and sonographic orientation of the images.

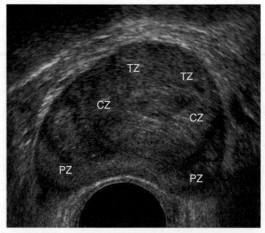

Fig. 15.60 McNeal's zones of the prostate as seen on a transrectal ultrasound. *CZ,* Central zone; *PZ,* peripheral zone; *TZ,* transitional zone.

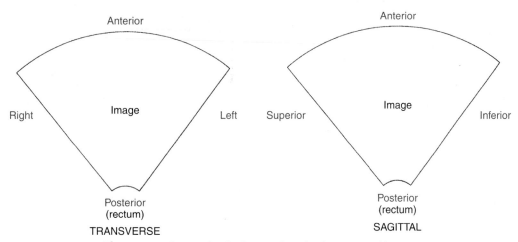

Fig. 15.61 A diagram showing image orientation for transrectal images.

Patient Position

The patient is scanned in right-side-up, left lateral decubitus position, with the knees tucked up to the chest. The patient can move the right leg so that it is in front of the left leg for comfort and to give easier access to the rectum.

Technical Tips

When evaluating the prostate for cancer, the sonographer should optimize the peripheral zone because this is the zone of the prostate where ultrasound can identify any lesions.

The examination should be fully explained to the patient and any questions answered.

Inspect the anus and perineal area before introducing the transducer, looking for anything that may interfere with insertion, such as hemorrhoids. Some departments may perform a quick preliminary DRE to make sure there is no obstruction in the rectum.

Place normal gel inside the latex-free probe cover and make sure that there is no air between the probe and the cover because air will cause shadow artifacts or drop out obscuring anatomy.

Use plenty of gel on the outside of the probe cover, preferably sterile gel, to help reduce any possibility of infection and lubricate the transducer to about halfway down the shaft. Reassure patients that most of the probe will be outside the body. When possible, use lidocaine gel or a combination of lidocaine and sterile gel to help numb the area, especially if a biopsy is to follow.

Position the transducer so it will image the prostate in a transverse plane as you insert the transducer. Slowly and gently introduce the transducer into the rectum using a gentle pressure. There will likely be a small amount of resistance at the anal sphincter, and having the patient perform a Valsalva maneuver may help relax the sphincter, making probe insertion a little easier. Insert the probe slowly and stop if it is difficult or causes the patient pain. If it is difficult to insert, place some extra gel on your gloved index finger and insert it into the rectum. This may help relax the sphincter enough to insert the transducer. The rectum is a curved structure, and the transducer should be angled to follow the curve of the rectum and not inserted straight ahead. This may be the cause of the difficulty with insertion or causing the patient pain when trying to force the probe straight and hitting the rectal wall. If it is still difficult or very painful for the patient, have a physician evaluate the patient and insert the transducer. Once through the sphincter, the probe should be easier to manipulate to image the prostate.

Often if the request is to look for prostate cancer, the patient may be scheduled for a prostate biopsy at the same time. A TR prostate biopsy is not a sterile procedure but rather a clean procedure. However, it is treated like a sterile procedure to reduce the chance of infection. Patients for a TR prostate biopsy should be on a broad-spectrum antibiotic at least 1 day before the procedure and 1 day after the procedure, although the course of antibiotics may vary depending on the policy of the department or office. As a sonographer you can witness a consent and initiate the time out.

The transverse scans are performed first to evaluate for gland symmetry, size, shape, and the lateral aspects of the gland. In transverse scans, the scan is started at the level of the seminal vesicles (Fig. 15.62), and the prostate is scanned thoroughly to the apex of the gland by pulling the probe slowly out of the rectum (Fig. 15.63). Make sure that you do not pull it all the way out. On very enlarged glands, the sector angle may be too small to see the entire peripheral zone in one image. In these patients, document the right side of the gland and then rotate the transducer to the left side of the prostate at the same level, to compare symmetry and echo texture. Perform this right and left scanning technique until the entire prostate can be seen in one image. Remember that the peripheral zone is seen best in this view because it is along the bottom and extends up the lateral sides of the prostate. Measure the prostate at the widest width (Fig. 15.64).

Let the patient know that you are going to rotate the transducer so he has time to be prepared for the sensation. Rotate the transducer 90 degrees until the long axis of the prostate is identified (Fig. 15.65). The longitudinal scans view the apex, base, seminal vesicles, and prostatic urethra. Starting at midline, at the area of the prostatic urethra, measure the length and AP dimensions of the prostate (Fig. 15.66). Next, rotate the transducer clockwise evaluating the left side of the gland until the seminal vesicle is seen. Probably only peripheral zone tissue will be seen at this level (Fig. 15.67). Return to

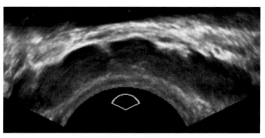

Fig. 15.62 Image of the seminal vesicles. This will be the first transverse image in the transverse images, with the last transverse image obtained from the apex of the prostate.

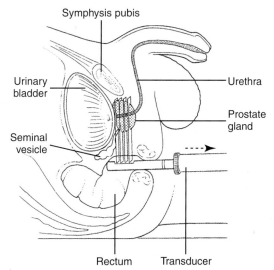

Fig. 15.63 A diagram showing the method to obtain transverse scans by slowly pulling the transducer out of the rectum and observing when the apex has been reached so as not to pull the transducer out of the rectum.

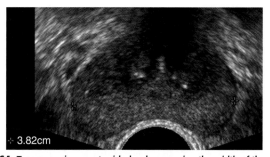

Fig. 15.64 Transverse image at mid-gland measuring the width of the prostate.

the midline and now rotate counterclockwise to evaluate the right side of the gland.

Any suspicious hypoechoic lesions should be documented in two planes (Fig. 15.68). Because prostate cancers can be isoechoic, the sonographer should look for bulges in the capsule of the prostate. Color or power Doppler also can be used to evaluate suspicious areas because

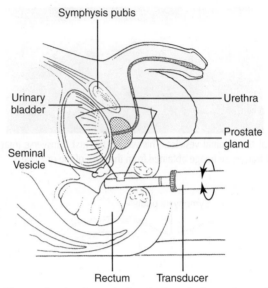

Fig. 15.65 A Diagram showing the method to obtain sagittal scans by rotating the handle.

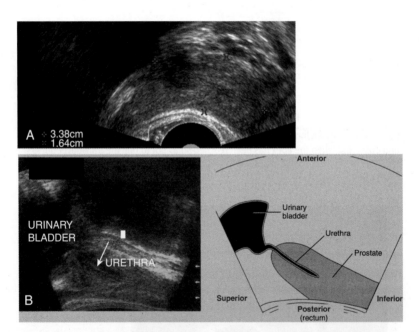

Fig. 15.66 A, Sagittal image at midline showing the proper method to measure the length and anteroposterior dimensions. The measurements should be perpendicular to one another. **B,** An image and drawing of a normal prostate with the *arrow* pointing to the urethra. The echogenic line is the urethra, with the hypoechoic transition zone on either side.

there will be an increase in flow (Fig. 15.69, Color Plate 6). The seminal vesicles should be examined for symmetry when a mass is found, because the cancer can spread through the seminal vesicle (Fig. 15.70).

If a single seminal vesicle is seen, images of the ipsilateral, same-side renal fossa should be obtained to show the presence or absence

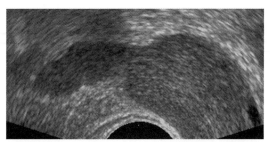

Fig. 15.67 Sagittal image of the seminal vesicle. At this level only peripheral zone tissue is seen.

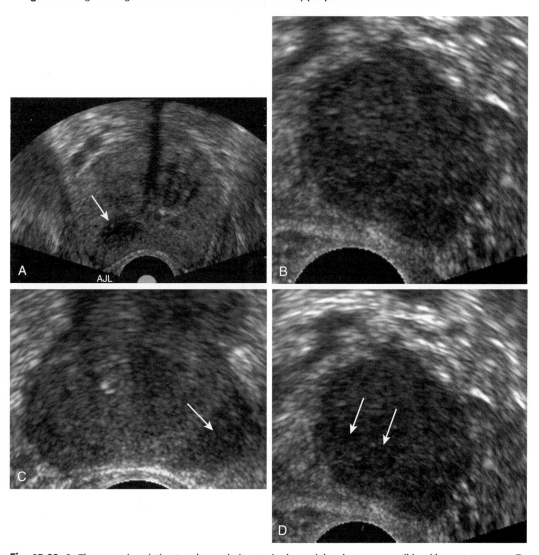

Fig. 15.68 A, The *arrow* is pointing to a hypoechoic area in the peripheral zone compatible with prostate cancer. **B,** Sagittal image very lateral on the *left* showing the peripheral zone. Note how the tissue appears heterogenous. **C,** The *arrow* is pointing to a hypoechoic area very lateral in the left lobe. **D,** By turning the transducer on the hypoechoic area, the *arrows* are pointing to the area missed originally in Fig. 15.63B.

of a kidney (Fig. 15.71). There is a relationship of ipsilateral renal anomalies in patients with seminal vesicle and prostate anomalies.

Patients who have urinary retention from BPH may have some type of procedure to allow urine to pass through the prostate. The result of the procedure can be appreciated with ultrasound (Fig. 15.72).

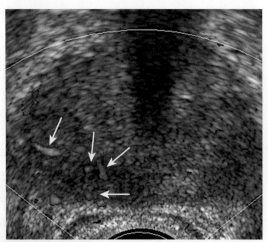

Fig. 15.69 Increased flow with color Doppler in the area of a prostate cancer. The *arrows* are showing the areas of flow. Note that there is no flow seen on the *left* side. See color plate 6.

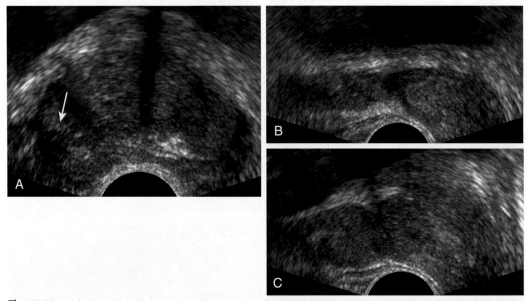

Fig. 15.70 A, The *arrow* is pointing to a prostate cancer in the right lobe. **B,** An image of the normal left seminal vesicle. **C,** Note the difference in appearance of the right seminal vesicle compatible with extension of the prostate cancer.

Men can be the cause of infertility problems in couples about 30% of the time. Men with azoospermia (no sperm in the ejaculate) or oligozoospermia (low sperm count) may have a transrectal ultrasound to rule out an ejaculatory duct cyst (Fig. 15.73) and evaluate the seminal vesicles.

Transducer Disinfection
All TR probes should have high-level disinfection (HLD) and be covered by a disposable sheath or cover before inserting into the rectum. After the examination is finished, the probe cover should be removed

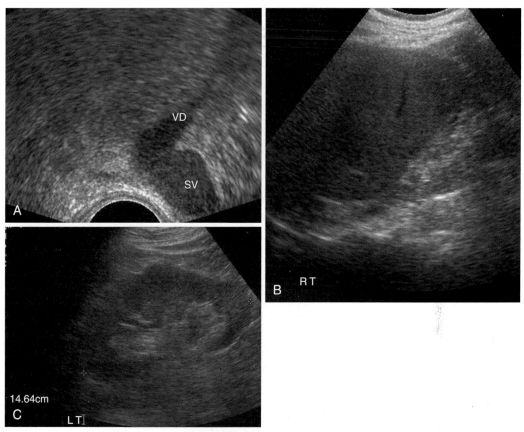

Fig. 15.71 A, A transverse view of the seminal vesicle *(SV)* and vas deferens *(VD)*. Notice that the right SV and VD are missing. **B,** The right renal fossa demonstrating the absence of the right kidney. **C,** The hypertrophied left kidney, which measures 14.64 cm.

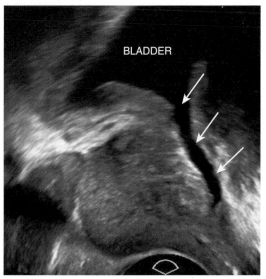

Fig. 15.72 Image of a patient who had a transurethral resection of the prostate (TURP) to alleviate urine retention from benign prostatic hyperplasia. The *arrows* outline the prostatic urethra.

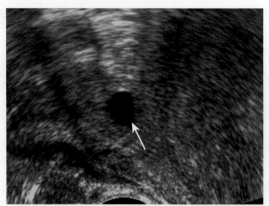

Fig. 15.73 The *arrow* is pointing to an ejaculatory cyst on this man with a low sperm count.

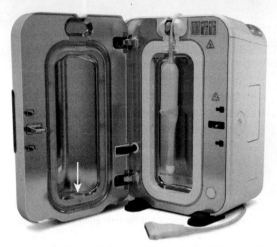

Fig. 15.74 An example of a high-level disinfection (HLD) device. This device, made by Nanosonics, is called Trophon, and uses insonated 35% hydrogen peroxide to achieve HLD. The *arrow* is pointing to the indicator, which will change color to indicate that the disinfection process was successful. This process also disinfects the handle.

and disposed of properly. Any body fluids should be wiped off per manufacturer's guidelines and disinfecting policy. The probe must then undergo HLD as per the manufacturer recommendations and facility guidelines (Fig. 15.74). Remember that the purpose of HLD is to protect the next patient.

Transrectal Prostate Required Images

Transrectal Prostate • Transverse Images

The TR scan is started with the transverse images because this allows comparison of the right and left sides and thorough evaluation of the peripheral zone. It can be easy to miss hypoechoic lesions on the sagittal views.

1. Image of seminal vesicles and vas deferens to compare size, echogenicity, and symmetry.

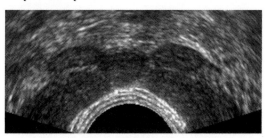

Suggested Annotation: **SV/VD**

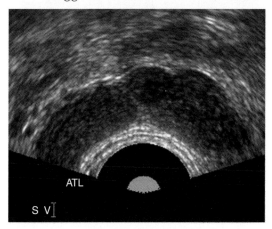

Suggested Annotation: **SV/VD**

2. One to three images of the base depending on the size of the gland.

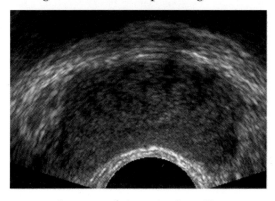

Suggested Annotation: **Base**

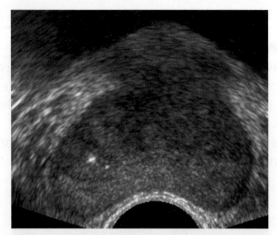

Suggested Annotation: **Base**

3. Three to five images of the midportion with the widest part of the gland measured.

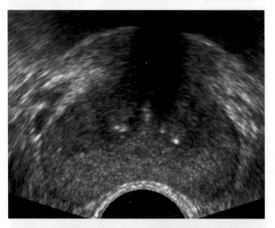

Suggested Annotation: **Mid**

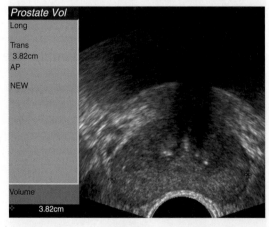

Suggested Annotation: **Mid**

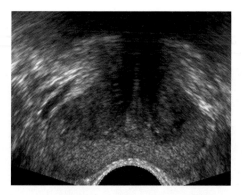

Suggested Annotation: **Mid**

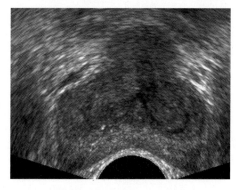

Suggested Annotation: **Mid**

4. Two to three images of the apex.

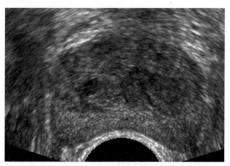

Suggested Annotation: **Apex**

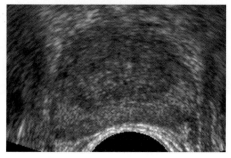

Suggested Annotation: **Apex**

Transrectal Prostate • Longitudinal Images

1. Midline of prostate with and without measurement of the length and AP.

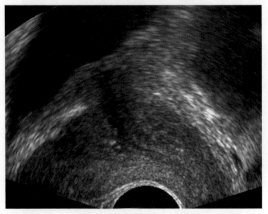

Suggested Annotation: **ML**

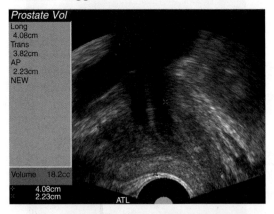

Suggested Annotation: **ML**

2. Two to four images of the left side of the gland.

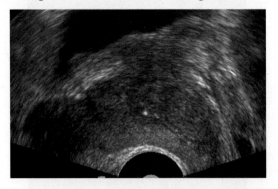

Suggested Annotation: **LT**

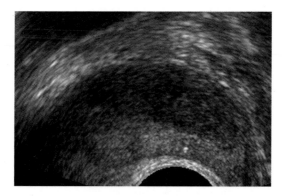

Suggested Annotation: **LT**

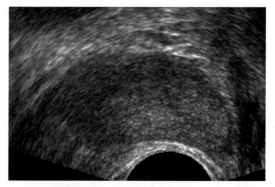

Suggested Annotation: **LT**

3. Image of the left seminal vesicle.

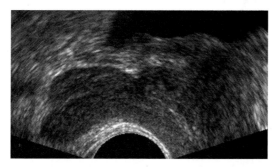

Suggested Annotation: **LT SV**

4. Two to four images of the right side of the gland.

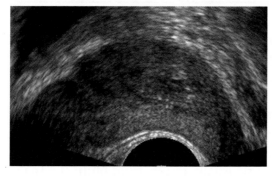

Suggested Annotation: **RT**

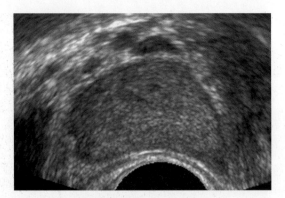

Suggested Annotation: **RT**

3. Image of the right seminal vesicle

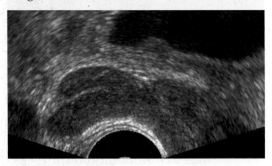

Suggested Annotation: **RT SV**

Penis

The penis has two main functions. When flaccid, it serves to eliminate urine from the body, and when erect, its purpose is to deliver semen into the vagina for fertilization of an egg for reproduction. Penile ultrasound is performed in the urologist's office or in the urology or radiology department. As more urology practices are hiring sonographers, the majority of penile ultrasounds are being performed in the urology office.

Overview

The protocol of images required for a penile ultrasound will depend on the reason for the study. Ultrasound of the penis is typically performed to evaluate for vascular causes of erectile dysfunction (ED). It also can be used to evaluate the penis for other conditions, such as **priapism**, Peyronie's disease, and trauma. Doppler is performed routinely for studies to evaluate for ED and is used when needed in non-ED sonographic examinations. Patients with penile trauma or priapism will usually go to the emergency department to be evaluated. Penile injury usually results from blunt trauma occurring when

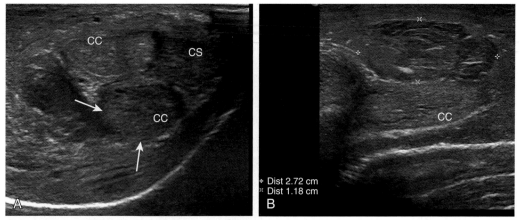

Fig. 15.75 Example of penile trauma with a penile fracture. **A,** A transverse image. The *arrows* are pointing to the ruptured tunica albuginea. **B,** A longitudinal view lateral of the right corpus cavernosa. The calipers are measuring the resulting hematoma. *CC,* Corpus cavernosum; *CS,* corpora spongiosum.

the penis is erect and has sudden lateral bending. A penile fracture occurs when the tunica albuginea is ruptured as it is stretched very thin during an erection. Clinically, penile fracture results in rapid detumescence, pain, swelling, and hematoma. On ultrasound a hematoma may be seen posterior to Buck's fascia and an interruption of the tunica albuginea is identified (Fig. 15.75).

Anatomy

The penis is centrally located on the anterior aspect of the body at the base of the pelvis. It is divided into the root of the penis, which is the internal portion that is not seen, and the body or shaft of the penis, which is the external portion that is seen. The penis is divided into three main sections: the proximal root, the middle body or shaft, and the distal glans or head of the penis (Fig. 15.76). The anatomic position of the penis is with the dorsal side closest to the abdomen and the ventral side continuous with the scrotum and closest to the testicles (Fig. 15.77).

The penis is composed of three cylindrical chambers or corporal bodies that are encased in a sheath called Buck's fascia (Fig. 15.78). The two **corpora cavernosa**, sometimes referred to as erectile bodies, are on the dorsal side and make up the bulk of the penis (Fig. 15.79). These two columns of tissue fill with blood to cause an erection and terminate immediately before the glans penis. The single **corpus spongiosum** is located on the ventral side between the corpora cavernosa and extends from the root to expand and become the glans (Fig. 15.80). Unlike the corpora cavernosa, the corpus spongiosum has constant blood flow during an erection. The distal end of the penis is called the glans, contains the urethral orifice, and has a high concentration of nerve endings, resulting in very sensitive skin. The skin from the shaft extends down over the glans and forms the prepuce or foreskin (see Fig. 15.77). A surgical procedure called

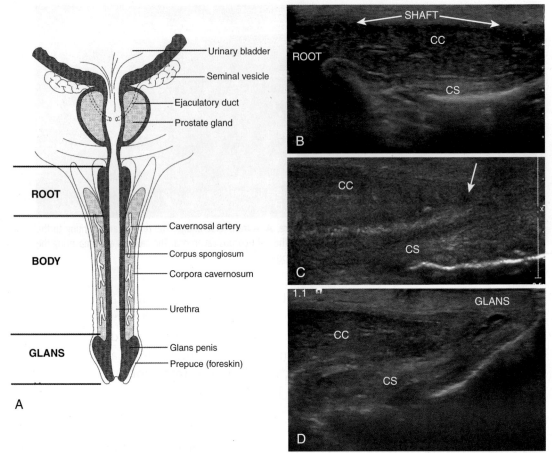

Fig. 15.76 A, A drawing of the anatomy of the penis showing the root, body, and glans. **B,** An ultrasound image of the root and shaft (body) of the penis. The corpus cavernosum *(CC)* is anterior to the corpus spongiosum *(CS)*. **C,** An ultrasound image of the corpora cavernosum with the *arrow* pointing to where it tapers and ends before the glans. **D,** An ultrasound image showing the corpus spongiosum becoming the glans.

circumcision removes the foreskin and is performed for religious or medical reasons.

Connective tissue covers the corpora, with three different layers: the tunica albuginea, Buck's fascia, and dartos or Colles' fascia (Fig. 15.81). The most superficial layer, immediately under the skin, is the dartos or Colles' fascia, which is a smooth muscle layer. The superficial dorsal veins are in the dartos fascia immediately under the skin. Under the dartos layer is Buck's fascia, also known as the deep fascia of the penis, which forms a strong membranous covering that holds all three erectile bodies together, splitting to envelop the corpus spongiosum in a separate compartment from the tunica albuginea. Buck's fascia is immediately posterior to the subcutaneous dorsal vein of the penis. The deep dorsal vein, paired dorsal arteries, and branches of the dorsal nerves are contained within Buck's fascia. Underneath Buck's fascia is a strong fascia called the tunica albuginea. The tunica albuginea is a sheath of strong, dense, fibroelastic tissue that surrounds and separates the dorsal corpora cavernosa from

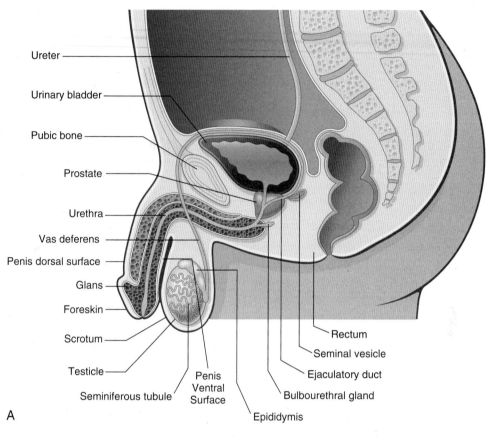

Ureter

Urinary bladder

Pubic bone

Prostate

Urethra

Vas deferens

Penis dorsal surface

Glans

Foreskin

Scrotum

Testicle

Seminiferous tubule

Penis Ventral Surface

Epididymis

Bulbourethral gland

Ejaculatory duct

Seminal vesicle

Rectum

A

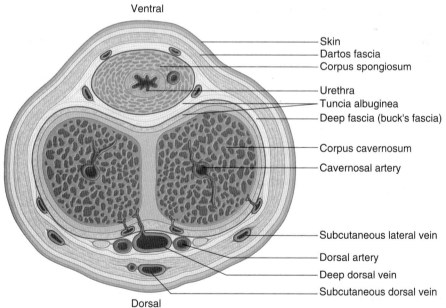

Ventral

Skin
Dartos fascia
Corpus spongiosum

Urethra
Tuncia albuginea
Deep fascia (buck's fascia)

Corpus cavernosum
Cavernosal artery

Subcutaneous lateral vein

Dorsal artery

Deep dorsal vein

Subcutaneous dorsal vein

B   Dorsal

Fig. 15.77 A, A drawing of a side view of the male reproductive organs. The dorsal side of the penis is continuous with the anterior part of the body, and the ventral surface is continuous with the scrotum. (From Chabner D-E. The *Language of Medicine*, 12th ed. St. Louis, 2021, Saunders.) B, A drawing of a cross section through the midshaft of the penis showing the dorsal and ventral surfaces and the internal structures. The layers of the penis are illustrated.

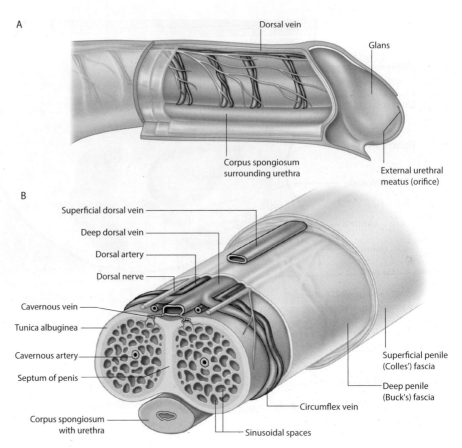

Fig. 15.78 A, A longitudinal drawing of the penis. **B,** A drawing showing the normal anatomy of the penis in a cross-section view. The corpus cavernosum, corpus spongiosum, urethra, and vascular anatomy are very well illustrated. (From Standring S. *Gray's Anatomy*, 41st ed. London, 2016, Elsevier.)

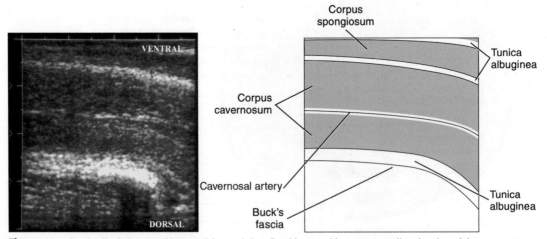

Fig. 15.79 A longitudinal ultrasound image of the penis in a flaccid state with a corresponding drawing of the corpus cavernosum and cavernosal artery.

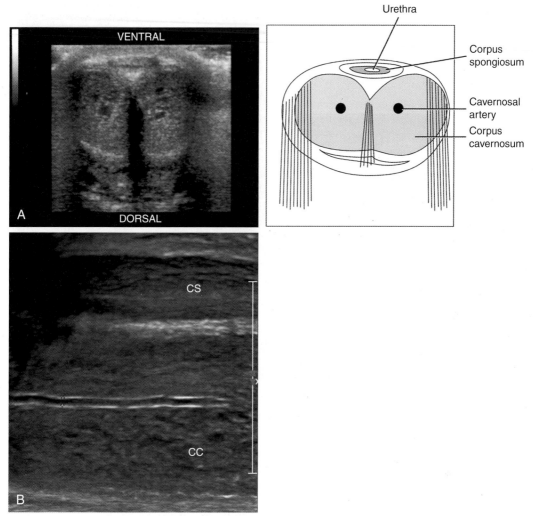

Fig. 15.80 A, A transverse image of the penis with a corresponding drawing showing both corpora cavernosa *(CC)* and the corpus spongiosum *(CS)*. **B,** A longitudinal image of an erect penis with the calipers measuring the cavernosal artery. Note the difference in the appearance between the corpus cavernosum (CC) in this image and the image in Fig. 15.79. With an erection the sinusoids fill with blood and the CCs enlarge. Sonographically the CCs now show a small anechoic or cystic area that represents the dilated sinusoids, giving it a sponge-like appearance.

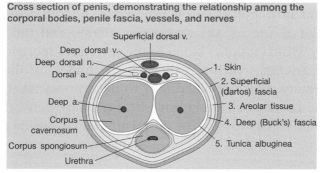

Fig. 15.81 A drawing showing the layers of the penis. Notice how Buck's fascia encircles the corpus spongiosum. *a,* Artery; *n,* nerve; *v,* vein (From Watkin N, Patel P. Diagnosis and management of acquired urethral stricture disease. *Surgery* 2017;35(6): 313–323. Copyright © 2017.)

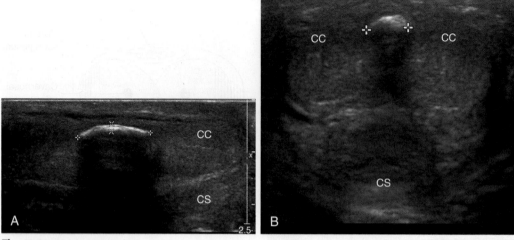

Fig. 15.82 A, A longitudinal image of the penis showing a plaque in the tunica albuginea casting an acoustic shadow. **B,** A transverse image of the plaque compatible with Peyronie's disease. *CC,* Corpus cavernosum; *CS,* corpus spongiosum.

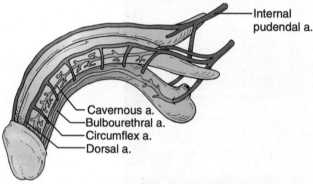

Fig. 15.83 A drawing showing the arterial anatomy of the penis. a, Artery. (From Partin A, Peters C, Kavoussi L, et al. *Campbell Walsh Wein Urology,* 12th ed. Philadelphia, 2021, Elsevier.)

the ventral corpus spongiosum. It is an echogenic structure like the tunica albuginea of the scrotum. Plaques can develop in the tunica albuginea, causing Peyronie's disease (Fig. 15.82).

The arterial blood supply to the penis is from the internal pudendal arteries that originate from the internal iliac arteries (Fig. 15.83). The internal pudendal arteries become the penile arteries, which branch into the dorsal arteries; the cavernous arteries; and the bulbourethral artery, which supplies blood to the cavernous spongiosum. The cavernosal arteries, which run through the middle of the corpora, are the primary source of blood flow to the corpora cavernosa (Fig. 15.84). The **cavernosal artery** ends in a capillary network and the helicine arteries (Fig. 15.85). The dorsal arteries lie outside the tunica

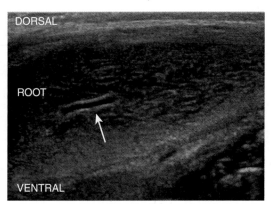

Fig. 15.84 An image of the penis in an erect state. The *arrow* is pointing to the enlarged cavernosal artery.

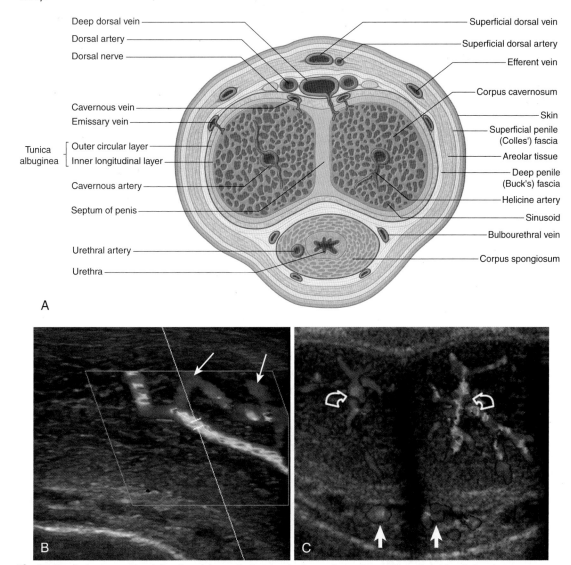

Fig. 15.85 A, A cross-sectional drawing of the penis showing the internal vasculature. (From Standring S. *Gray's anatomy*, 41st edition, London, 2016, Elsevier.) **B,** A longitudinal color Doppler image of an erect penis. The *arrows* are pointing to the helicine arteries. **C,** A transverse color Doppler image of an erect penis. The *open curved arrows* are pointing to the cavernosal arteries. The *solid arrows* are pointing to the dorsal arteries.

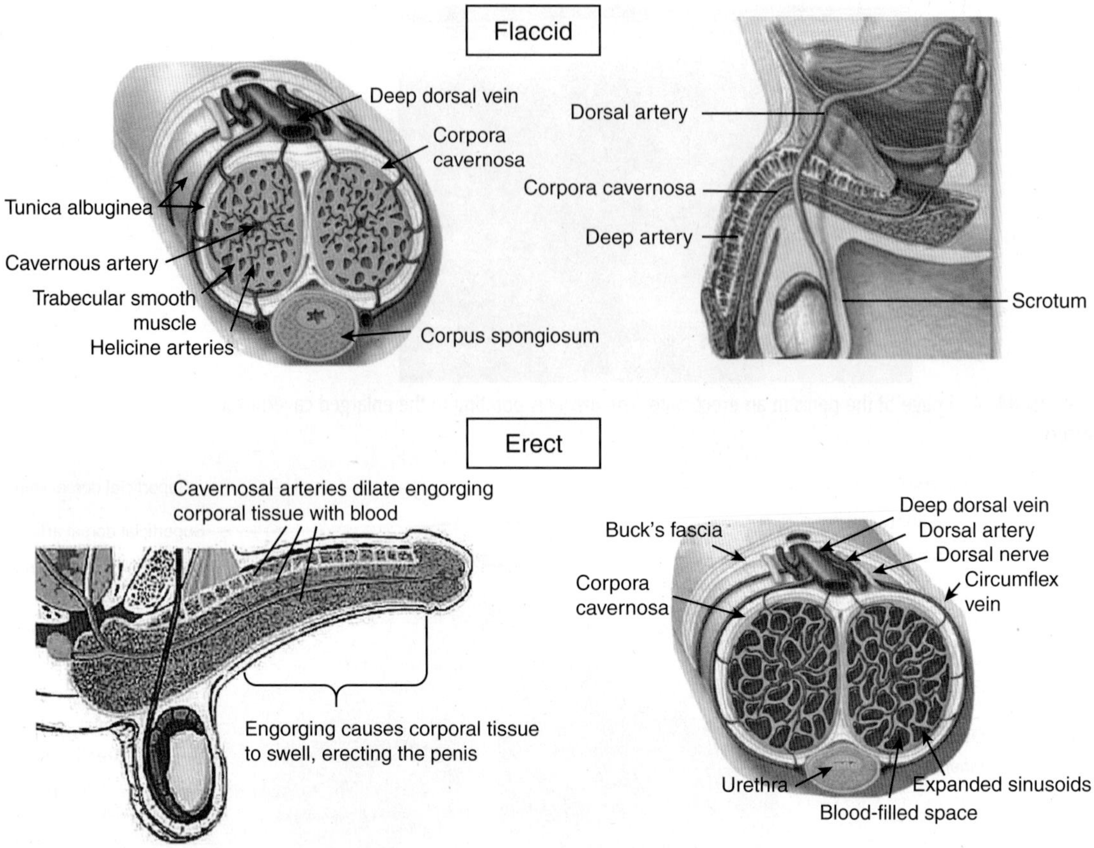

Fig. 15.86 Illustrations of a flaccid and erect penis showing the differences in the corporal tissue and the vasculature. (From Chen L, Shi G-R, Huang D-D, et al. Male sexual dysfunction: A review of literature on its pathologic mechanisms, potential risk factors, and herbal drug intervention. *Biomed Pharmacother* 2019;112:108585. © 2019.)

albuginea and supply blood to the skin and glans of the penis and to the tunica albuginea through its circumflex arteries (Fig. 15.86). During an erection the cavernosal artery is responsible for the tumescence of the corpus cavernosum and the dorsal artery is responsible for the engorgement of the glans penis.

Blood leaves the three corpora of the penis through the emissary veins, which pierce the tunica albuginea. In the proximal portion of the penis, the emissary veins drain into the cavernous vein, which joins the periurethral veins of the urethral bulb to form the internal pudendal veins, which drain into the internal iliac veins. The emissary veins from the distal and middle parts of the penis combine to form circumflex veins, which drain into the deep dorsal vein. The venous drainage of the skin and subcutaneous penile tissue is by superficial veins that join to form the superficial dorsal vein, which drains into the saphenous vein (Fig. 15.87).

Physiology

In the flaccid state there is sufficient arterial flow to meet nutritional needs (Fig. 15.88). Penile erections are the result of vasocongestion, an engorgement of the tissues from arterial blood flowing into the penis.

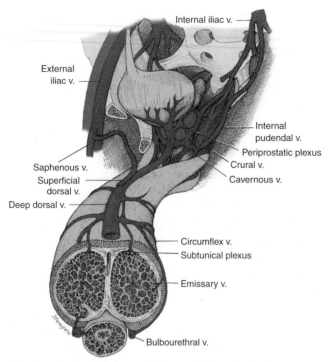

Fig. 15.87 A drawing showing the venous drainage of the penis during detumescence. *v,* Vein. (From Partin A, Peters C, Kavoussi L, et al. *Campbell Walsh Wein Urology,* 12th ed. Philadelphia, 2021, Elsevier.)

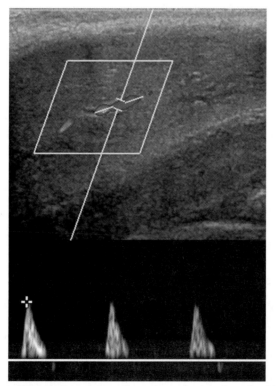

Fig. 15.88 A spectral Doppler signal from the cavernosal artery in a flaccid penis showing a high-resistance signal with a low velocity.

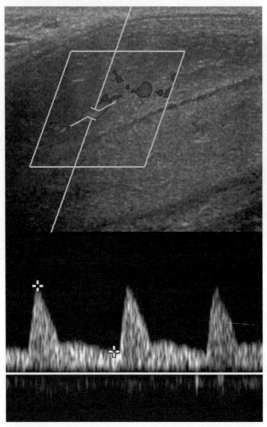

Fig. 15.89 A spectral Doppler signal from the cavernosal artery showing a low-resistance signal that is seen in the filling phase with an increase in the velocity in both systole and diastole.

There are five stages of erection: the latent, tumescent, full erection, rigid erection, and detumescent stages. During sexual arousal, nitric oxide is released from nerve endings near the blood vessels within the corpora cavernosa and spongiosum, which results in relaxation of the cavernous smooth musculature and the smooth muscles of the arteriolar and arterial walls, allowing them to rapidly fill with blood and the sinusoids within the corpora cavernosa to distend. This vasodilation increases the amount of blood that enters the penis, with increased blood flow in both systole and diastole (Fig. 15.89). This rapid increase in blood volume fills the erectile chambers, compressing the emissary veins that drain the sinusoids and decreasing venous drainage of the penis. The tunica albuginea is stretched and compresses the emissary veins, further decreasing venous outflow. This causes intracavernous pressure to increase (Fig. 15.90). The result is that inflow and outflow of blood temporarily ceases, resulting in full rigidity of the penis. The corpus spongiosum and glans react differently during the erection process. Arterial flow increases, but because of the differences in the tunica albuginea, which is thin in the spongiosum and absent in the glans, venous occlusion is less, causing pressures in the spongiosum to be about half of that of the corpora

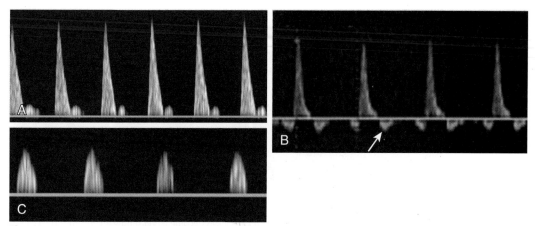

Fig. 15.90 A, A spectral Doppler signal from the cavernosal artery showing a high-resistance signal when the penis is fully erect. The signal looks similar to the flaccid signal; however, the velocity has increased. **B,** The *arrow* is pointing to a reversed flow component that is seen when the penis is fully rigid in the tumescent phase. **C,** In the rigid phase diastolic flow disappears and the velocity decreases.

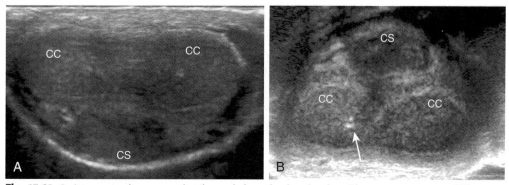

Fig. 15.91 A, A transverse image scanning the penis from the dorsal surface. The corpora cavernosa *(CC)* are on *top* and the corpus spongiosum *(CS)* is on the *bottom*. **B,** A transverse image scanning the penis from the ventral surface. The corpora cavernosa *(CC)* are now on the bottom and the corpus spongiosum *(CS)* is on the top. The *arrow* is pointing to the cavernosal artery.

cavernosa. The deep dorsal vein is compressed between the engorged cavernosa and Buck's fascia, contributing to the rigidity of the glans. After ejaculation or cessation of stimuli, the muscles start to contract, causing the arterial inflow to decrease and the venous blood to leave the penis, allowing the penis to return to its flaccid state.

Sonographic Appearance

The penis can be scanned from a dorsal or ventral approach, which will affect the way the anatomy is seen. On a dorsal approach the corpora cavernosa will be anterior, and on a ventral approach they will be posterior (Fig. 15.91). Remember that the corpora cavernosa are paired structures and the corpora spongiosum is a single structure. The three chambers are best appreciated on a transverse view, in which they have a circular shape.

The corpora cavernosa appears as paired, circular, symmetric homogeneous structures with medium-level echoes. The cavernosal arteries

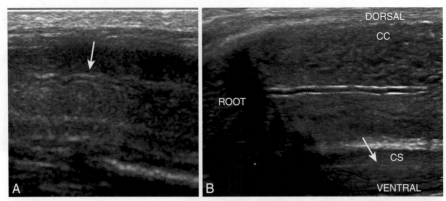

Fig. 15.92 **A,** A longitudinal image of the tortuous cavernosal artery (*arrow*) when the penis is flaccid. **B,** A longitudinal image of the cavernosal artery that has become larger during an erection. The calipers are measuring the diameter of the artery. The *arrow* is pointing to the urethra. *CC,* Corpora cavernosa; *CS,* corpus spongiosum.

can be seen as echogenic parallel lines in a longitudinal plane. When flaccid, the arteries will be small and tortuous. As the penis becomes erect, the arteries become easier to see (Fig. 15.92). On transverse views they are seen as small, pulsating circles located slightly medial in the corpora cavernosa. When erect, the corpora cavernosum enlarge and the sonographic appearance will change to reflect the extra blood now in the corpora. The tissue will have a speckled appearance with small anechoic and cystic spaces representing the dilated sinusoids.

The corpus spongiosum is smaller than the corpora cavernosum with a homogeneous texture that is usually slightly more echogenic than the corpora cavernosa. The corpus spongiosum does not become as erect as the corpora cavernosa, as their veins are located more peripherally, allowing constant outflow of blood, preventing the urethra from being collapsed by the adjacent tissue, which would prevent ejaculation of the semen.

The tunica albuginea is seen as a thin echogenic line that surrounds all three corpora (Fig. 15.93).

Ultrasound of the Penis

Patient Prep
No prep is required.

Transducer
High-frequency broad-bandwidth linear array transducers are used with frequencies from 7–15 MHz.

Patient Position
The patient is placed in the supine position. The penis is scanned from its dorsal or ventral surface for both longitudinal and transverse views. The size of the flaccid penis may determine which surface to

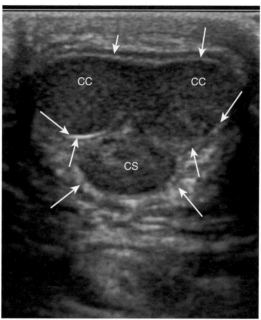

Fig. 15.93 A transverse image through the midshaft of the penis. The *arrows* are pointing to the tunica albuginea. *CC,* Corpora cavernosa; *CS,* corpus spongiosum.

scan. It may be easier to scan the penis from a ventral view when flaccid and from the dorsal surface when erect. There is no wrong way to scan the penis. The images should be obtained with the view that lets you see the needed anatomy.

Technical Tips

When scanning the flaccid penis, all three corpora can be imaged from a single dorsal or ventral approach to the penile shaft. Try not to apply too much pressure when scanning the penis on the ventral side because the urethra can be compressed. One of the main reasons to perform an examination of the penis is a penile Doppler examination to evaluate for vascular causes of ED. The patient will be given an injection near the base of the penis, and images are needed before and after the injection. A physician will perform the injection. This is a very sensitive and potentially embarrassing examination for the patient, and his privacy needs to be maintained. Because the penis will be exposed during the entire examination with the purpose of producing an erection, the sonographer should remain very confident and professional during the examination. Most men will be very nervous about the injection, so try to put their mind at ease and support them during the injection. Explain to the patient the protocol and the length of the examination, letting him know there will be a few minutes between obtaining the images to evaluate the response of the penis to the injection.

A good place to obtain the Doppler signal is the proximal to mid-shaft of the penis because the arteries are bigger here than in the distal shaft by the head of the penis. The cavernosa artery also starts to bend at the root, giving good access to a less than 60-degree Doppler angle.

The Doppler settings on the machine should be optimized for a low flow. Filters should be set at their lowest levels. Both the Doppler and color gain setting are adjusted right before noise is seen. The color velocity scale should be set so that there is no aliasing and the vessel can be identified. As an erection occurs, the settings should be adjusted as needed.

The images required for a penile ultrasound will depend on why the study was ordered. Images should include longitudinal and transverse views of all three corpora. Doppler should be used as needed to help with making the diagnosis. There is a standard protocol for a penile Doppler study for ED, which will be outlined in the next section. Of note, there is not a dedicated non-Doppler penis Current Procedural Terminology (CPT) code, and some laboratories use the scrotal/testicle, 76870, or pelvic limited, 76857, CPT code for billing. There is controversary about using either code because they do not apply to the penis, with maybe pelvic limited being the better choice. CPT code 76857 states: Male: evaluation and measurement of the bladder, evaluation of the prostate and seminal vesicles, and any pelvic pathology. CPT code 76870 is Ultrasound, scrotum and contents. Some laboratories may use 76999, which is used for an unlisted ultrasound examination and may have limited reimbursement. (Note that the CPT code information is discussed so that the sonographer can assist in any billing enquiries and give a knowledgeable answer because this continues to be an uncertainty as to what to bill.) However, most non-ED examinations will require at least a Doppler signal of the cavernosal arteries, and by obtaining a signal of the dorsal vein the penile Doppler code can be used, because all that is required is an inflow and outflow signal. For trauma, Doppler will be needed to ensure that the arteries and veins are still patent. Peyronie's disease is a fibrotic and focal thickening in the tunica albuginea and may cause difficulty in achieving an erection, or painful erections. Many men with Peyronie's disease will also have coexistent ED, with usually veno-occlusive insufficiency as a result of the fibrotic plaques present the reason, although arterial insufficiency or mixed vascular abnormalities may be the cause. Men with Peyronie's disease are usually scheduled for a Doppler ultrasound to evaluate for vascular causes of ED. Color Doppler also can be used to assess perfusion around the area of the plaque, because increased flow is suggestive of active inflammation. A priapism workup is illustrated in the following text.

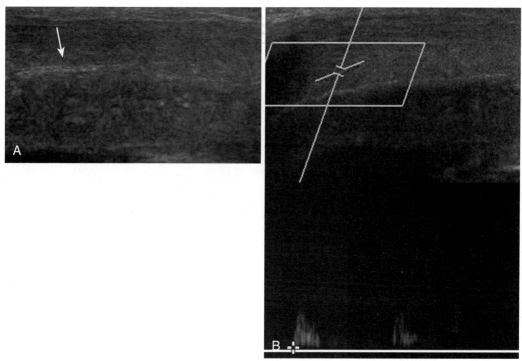

Fig. 15.94 A, The *arrow* is pointing to the cavernosal artery in an erect penis that is small and has no lumen. **B,** There was very weak flow in the artery, and the Doppler signal was a low high-resistance velocity, compatible with a low-flow priapism.

Priapism is a persistent penile erection not associated with sexual excitement lasting longer than 4 hours. It is categorized into low-flow (ischemic) or high-flow (arterial) states. The role of ultrasound is to distinguish between ischemic low-flow priapism and nonischemic high-flow priapism. A third type of priapism is called stuttering priapism and is characterized by recurrent episodes of ischemic priapism.

Venous, or low-flow, priapism is the more common type and results from malfunction of normal penile outflow and is considered a medical emergency, as prolonged obstruction of venous outflow leads to irreversible ischemic changes and permanent ED. A low-flow priapism is painful with a rigid erection. Low-flow priapism usually manifests with a lack of blood flow or with a very high-resistance flow pattern in the cavernosal artery (Fig. 15.94).

High-flow priapism is unregulated penile arterial inflow from a tear in the cavernosal artery resulting in a painless erection. High-flow priapism is commonly a result of pelvic or perineal trauma that results in an arterial fistula between the cavernosal artery and the sinusoids of the corpora cavernosa or a pseudoaneurysm. High-flow priapism typically manifests as a painless, partial erection not associated with sexual desire and is not considered an emergency because it is not associated with pain and permanent ED is unusual. In high-flow priapism, gray-scale imaging will demonstrate an irregular hypoechoic region within the corpora cavernosum. Color and spectral Doppler may demonstrate high blood flow in the cavernosal artery in both

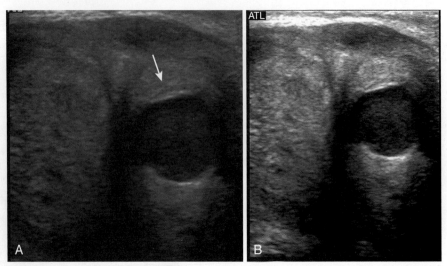

Fig. 15.95 A, A cystic structure *(arrow)* is seen in the left corpus cavernosum in a patient who had penile trauma that represents an arterial-lacunar fistula. **B,** By increasing the overall gain low-level echoes can be seen inside the cystic mass.

systole and diastole, a pseudoaneurysm, or an arterial-cavernous fistula.

Here is an example of images needed for a diagnosis on a patient with priapism. The patient was referred for ultrasound examination for an erection that had lasted almost 6 hours after trauma. The main concern was priapism caused by perineal trauma from a biking mishap. Because the perineum was injured, there was not a concern for a penile fracture. It is important that the sonographer understands the diagnostic images and criteria needed.

The scan was started by having the patient hold the tip of his penis on his abdomen. This allowed access to the ventral portion of the penis. Scanning in the dorsal position would have made it difficult to scan the root of the penis and perineum, which is where the trauma occurred. The scan was started in a transverse plane starting at the base and scanning toward the glans. A cystic area was seen near the base of the penis and was measured in both planes (Fig. 15.95). Longitudinal images of each of the corpora cavernosa were obtained. There were very low-level echoes inside the cystic structure, and by increasing the gain the damaged tissue was appreciated. Color Doppler was turned on and showed flow. Spectral Doppler signals were obtained from each cavernosal artery and the dorsal vein. To see deeper, a curved linear array was used to scan the root, and a vessel was seen leading to the cystic collection (Fig. 15.96). A spectral Doppler signal showed high flow with increased diastolic flow (Fig. 15.97). The increased diastolic flow was due to the fistula created between the cavernosal artery and the lacunae of the corpus cavernosum. The blood from the cavernosal artery bypassed the helicine arteries and went directly to the sinusoids, causing the abnormal

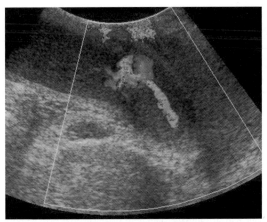

Fig. 15.96 This patient had perineal trauma, and to see deeper, a lower-frequency curved array transducer was used. This allowed the deep aspect of the artery to be seen.

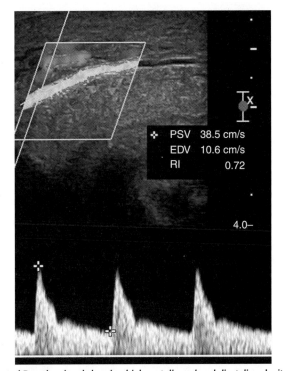

Fig. 15.97 A spectral Doppler signal showing high systolic and end diastolic velocities in the cavernosal artery feeding the arteriovenous fistula.

Doppler signal. Findings were compatible with a posttraumatic high-flow priapism, and the patient was sent for interventional embolization (Fig. 15.98). The images needed are based on what is required to make the diagnosis or show normalcy.

Penile Doppler Required Images

The most common reason to perform a Doppler study of the penis is to evaluate for ED. ED is defined as the inability to obtain or maintain

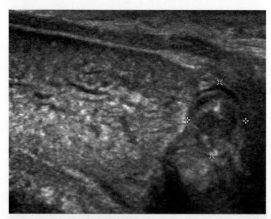

Fig. 15.98 The patient had a traumatic high-flow priapism that was embolized in interventional radiology.

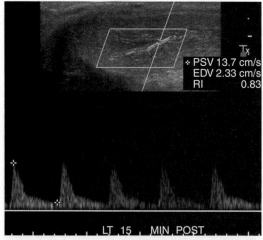

Fig. 15.99 A spectral Doppler waveform of an arteriogenic cause of erectile dysfunction. All the postinjection velocities were less than 25 cm/s.

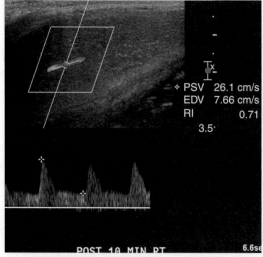

Fig. 15.100 At 15 minutes after injection the systolic flow is greater than 25 cm/s, but the amount of diastolic flow is high, with the end diastolic flow greater than 5 cm/s. Findings are suspicious for a venous cause for erectile dysfunction.

an erection for satisfactory sexual intercourse and can be caused by psychogenic, arteriogenic, venogenic, neurogenic, or a combination of factors. Ultrasound is used to assess whether the cause is arteriogenic or venogenic.

Arteriogenic impotence occurs as a result of stenoses or occlusions that limit blood flow to the corpora cavernosum. If the blood flow is unable to fill the cavernosal sinusoids, tumescence cannot occur, because the draining veins are not occluded and continue to carry blood away from the corpora cavernosa.

Venous incompetence occurs when there is failure of occlusion of the draining veins despite adequate filling of the cavernosal sinusoids. Patients may have partial erections, but rigidity cannot be fully achieved.

Measuring the peak systolic velocity is how the diagnosis of arteriogenic impotence is made. The normal value should be at least greater than 25 cm/s, although some charts use 30 cm/s or 35 cm/s. They all agree that less than 25 cm/s is abnormal (Fig. 15.99). The diameter of the cavernosal artery should increase by 60%. If the peak systolic difference is greater than 10 cm/s, this is an abnormal finding and the artery with the lower peak systolic velocity is considered abnormal.

Patients with a normal arterial inflow but who still have a weak erection may have venous leakage. If a venous leak is present, a decrease or reversal of diastolic flow will not occur. The diagnosis is made when there is persistent diastolic flow in the cavernosal arteries with an end diastolic velocity greater than 5 cm/s (Fig. 15.100).

The deep dorsal vein is not consistently seen in the flaccid phase or in the erection phases. However, it may be seen during detumescence. A prominent deep dorsal vein is commonly seen in venogenic causes of ED (Fig. 15.101).

Preinjection Images

The scan is started with careful transverse images from the base of the penis to the glans looking for pathologic findings, such as calcifications and vascular anomalies (Fig. 15.102). If a pathologic condition is found, the image should be annotated as to its location on the shaft of the penis, such as on the proximal shaft. With the influence of psychological factors on erectile function, the study should be performed in a room that will have no distractions, such as the possibility of people walking into the room unexpectedly, for example, another sonographer looking for a transducer. The procedure should be explained in detail and any questions answered before the examination begins.

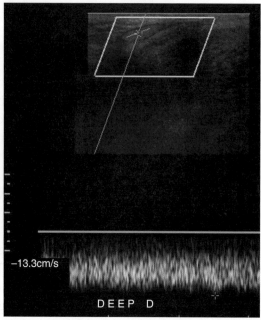

Fig. 15.101 Same patient as in Fig. 15.100. The flow in the deep dorsal vein is well seen, with a velocity of 13.3 cm/s, which confirms the suspicion for a venogenic cause.

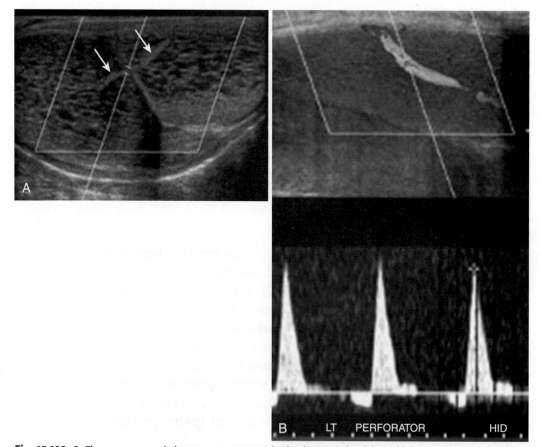

Fig. 15.102 A, The *arrows* are pointing to a cross-communication between the right and left cavernosal arteries. **B,** An example of a communication between the dorsal artery and the cavernosal artery called a dorsal-cavernosal perforator.

1. Transverse images of the flaccid penis preferably from a dorsal approach, which is having the penis point to the patient's feet. Documentation should be at proximal and midshaft and the third obtained in the distal aspect of the shaft just proximal to the glans.

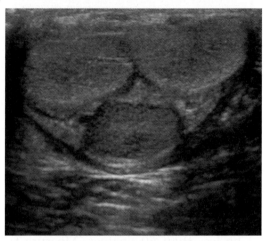

Suggested annotations: **TRV PROX**

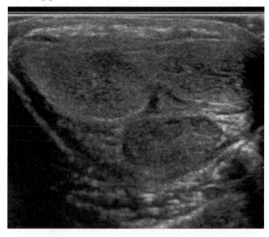

Suggested annotations: **TRV MID**

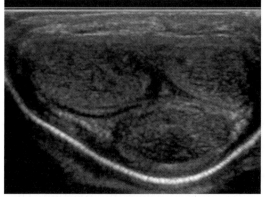

Suggested annotations: **TRV DIST**

2. Longitudinal image of the corpus cavernosum is obtained showing the cavernosal artery with the diameter of the artery measured from inner wall to inner wall. For the suggested annotation, RT will be used.

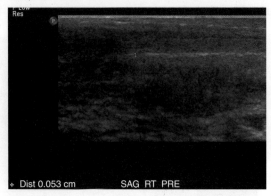

Suggested annotations: **PRE RT**

3. Spectral Doppler signal of the cavernosal artery. The Doppler angle must be less than 60 degrees. Measure the peak systole and end diastole velocities. The machine will usually also display the resistive index (RI). The systolic waveform is damped with a monophasic waveform. There may be a small diastolic component seen.

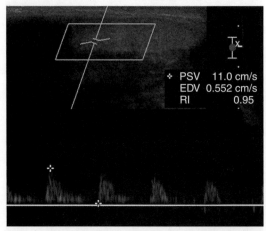

Suggested annotations: **PRE RT**

Doppler waveforms of the cavernosal arteries demonstrate a high-resistance pattern, with low systolic peaks.

4. Repeat for the other side.

Postinjection Images

The gel needs to be removed before the injection. This should be performed by the patient when possible. A consent form is obtained, and the sonographer can be the witness. An erection is then pharmacologically induced by intracavernosal injection with vasoactive medications. The injection is administered into either the right or left corpora cavernosa. The side is unimportant because the drug will diffuse across the septum between the two corpora cavernosa. It is important to note the time of injection. This can be easily documented by taking a blank image or annotating the injection time. Measurement of the diameter of the cavernosal artery and the systolic and diastolic velocities is documented starting 5 minutes after injection and then obtained every 5 minutes for 15 to 20 minutes after injection depending on the protocol being followed. Occasionally, images may need to be obtained after 20 minutes to ensure that the maximal pharmacologic effect has occurred. If after 5 minutes an erection has not yet started or occurred, the physician may give the patient a second injection, which will also need to be documented.

During the latent phase, the diameters of the cavernosal arteries are at their largest diameter and the spectral Doppler signals are a low-resistance signal. During tumescence, the sinusoidal cavities of the corpora cavernosa distend with blood, and the spectral Doppler is a high-resistance signal with a dichrotic notch as diastolic flow starts to decrease. With a full erection the blood flow decreases and the diameters of the cavernosal arteries and maximal systolic velocity should occur and flow reversal is usually seen during diastole. With a rigid erection the diameters of the cavernosal arteries are at their narrowest and the spectral Doppler signal is a low-velocity monophasic signal. The waveform may appear similar to a flaccid waveform, but a dilated artery is seen.

TECHNICAL TIP: Five minutes seems a long time but goes by quickly as you image and perform the measurements on both sides. To ensure that the right and left sides are not mixed up, the sonographer should always start on the same side for both the before- and after-injection images. This will also keep the timing on both sides at appropriate intervals.

After an erection is achieved, the penis should be surveyed to document any arterial anomalies that are now visible. Because timing is critical, this could occur at the end of the examination. The velocities may be documented by the sonographer on a work sheet. The work sheet would have places to document the diameter of the artery, peak systolic velocity, end diastolic velocity, and possibly RI before and every 5 minutes after the injection for the length of the protocol. Note that the right side is imaged first in the following examples, but the left side can be imaged first as well.

1. Image of the right cavernosal artery with the diameter measured at 5 minutes after injection.

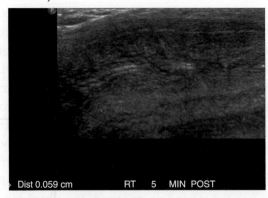

Suggested annotations: **RT 5 MIN POST OR RT 5**

Doppler waveforms of the cavernosal arteries demonstrate a high-resistance pattern, with low systolic peaks.

2. A spectral Doppler image of the right cavernosal artery with peak systole and end diastole measured at 5 minutes after injection.

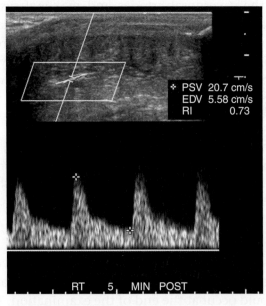

Suggested annotations: **RT 5 MIN POST OR RT 5**

3. Repeat for left side.

4. Image of the right cavernosal artery with the diameter measured at 10 minutes after injection.

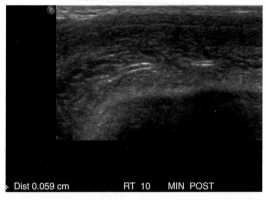

Suggested annotations: **RT 10 MIN POST OR RT 10**

5. A spectral Doppler image of the right cavernosal artery with peak systole and end diastole measured at 10 minutes after injection.

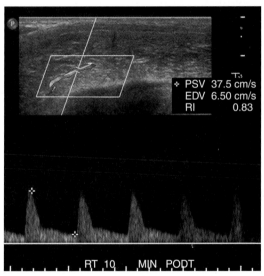

Suggested annotations: **RT10 MIN POST OR RT 10**

6. Image of the right cavernosal artery with the diameter measured at 15 minutes after injection.

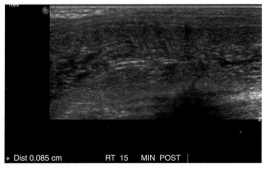

Suggested annotations: **RT 15 MIN POST OR RT 15**

7. A spectral Doppler image of the right cavernosal artery with peak systole and end diastole measured at 15 minutes after injection.

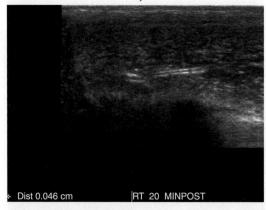

Suggested annotations: **RT 15 MIN POST OR RT 15**

8. Image of the right cavernosal artery with the diameter measured at 20 minutes after injection.

Suggested annotations: **RT 20 MIN POST OR RT 20**

9. A spectral Doppler image of the right cavernosal artery with peak systole and end diastole measured at 20 minutes after injection.

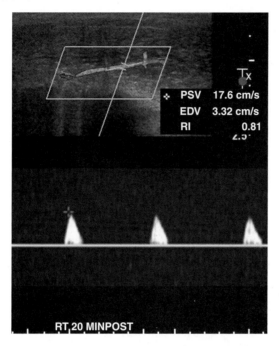

Suggested annotations: **RT 20 MIN POST OR RT 20**

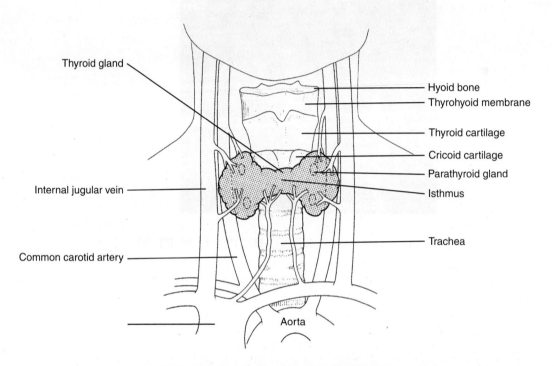

Thyroid gland

Hyoid bone
Thyrohyoid membrane

Thyroid cartilage

Cricoid cartilage

Parathyroid gland

Internal jugular vein

Isthmus

Common carotid artery

Trachea

Aorta

Location and Anatomy of Thyroid and Parathyroid Glands

Suggested Annotation: ML

CHAPTER 16

Thyroid Scanning Protocol

M. Robert DeJong

Keywords

Adenoma
Endocrine gland
Esophagus
Goiter
Graves' disease
Hashimoto's thyroiditis
Hyperthyroidism
Hypothyroidism
Isthmus
Longus colli muscle
Papillary cancer

Pyramidal lobe
Sternocleidomastoid muscle
Strap muscles
Thyroid-stimulating hormone
   (TSH)
Thyrotropin-releasing hormone
   (TRH)
Thyroxine (T4)
Trachea
Triiodothyronine (T3)

Objectives

At the end of this chapter, you will be able to:

- Define the keywords.
- Distinguish the sonographic appearance of the thyroid and the terms used to describe it.
- Discuss laboratory values for the thyroid.
- List the transducer options for scanning the thyroid.
- Explain the patient prep for a thyroid study.
- Explain the order and exact locations to take representative images of the thyroid.
- Describe the nine levels of the neck for neck node mapping.

Overview

The thyroid is the largest **endocrine gland** in the body and is essential for life. It is the only organ that can absorb iodine. Every cell in the body depends on thyroid hormones to function properly. The use of ultrasound to evaluate the thyroid has increased over the years and is now the primary imaging modality to evaluate it. The thyroid is traditionally scanned in the radiology department; however, an increasing number of endocrinologists are purchasing ultrasound equipment and performing their own examinations, usually as they are examining the patient. Ultrasound is being used to scan patients

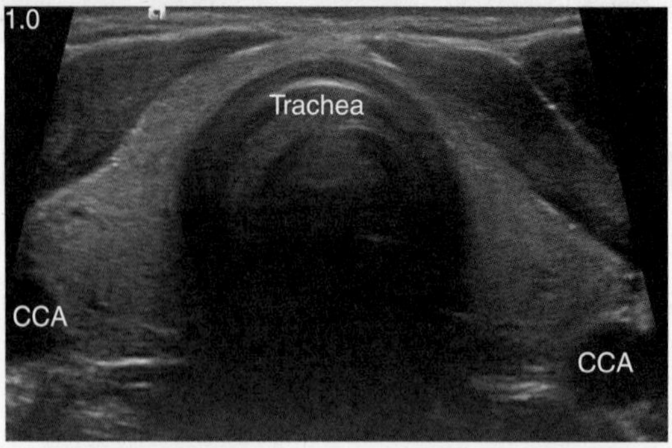

Fig. 16.1 Ultrasound image of the normal thyroid. *CCA,* Common carotid artery.

who have undergone thyroid cancer surgery to evaluate for lymph nodes. This scan is usually called node or neck mapping and is a very meticulous examination to perform. Neck mapping examinations are not performed in every department because of the low reimbursement rate; these scans are currently being reimbursed at the same rate as for a thyroid ultrasound examination, despite the fact that it takes three to five times longer to perform. Ultrasound is used for fine-needle aspiration (FNA) of thyroid nodules because it provides accurate needle localization. These procedures may be performed by a variety of physicians, including radiologists, endocrinologists, and pathologists, with or without a sonographer assisting.

Anatomy

The thyroid is a bilobed structure that consists of the right and left lobes that are connected by the **isthmus**, and normally extends from C5 to T1 vertebra. It is described as butterfly-, H-, or U-shaped and is located inferior to the larynx. Each lobe has a superior and an inferior pole, and they lie lateral to the **trachea** and medial to the carotid arteries and jugular veins. The isthmus drapes over the trachea, where it joins the two lobes in their lower two-thirds, with its superior edge situated just below the cricoid cartilage (Fig. 16.1). The individual lobes usually have a pointed superior pole and a blunted inferior pole that merges medially with the isthmus.

The strap, or infrahyoid muscles, is a group of small, thin muscles below the hyoid bone that include the sternohyoid, omohyoid, thyrohyoid, and sternothyroid muscles. They are seen along the anterior and lateral surface of the gland. The larger **sternocleidomastoid muscle** is more anterolateral to the thyroid, and the **longus colli muscle** is seen posterior and lateral to the gland (Fig. 16.2).

The gland varies in size depending on the patient's height, weight, age, and gender. Each lobe measures 4 to 5 cm in length, 2 to 3 cm in anteroposterior (AP) dimension, and 1.5 to 2 cm in width. The gland weighs 15 to 25 g. The isthmus measures 12 to 15 mm in length (Fig. 16.3). The thyroid is generally asymmetric, with the right lobe larger

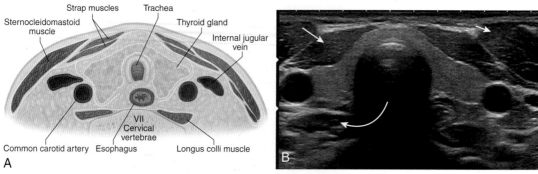

Fig. 16.2 A, Illustration of the relationship of the thyroid and the muscles in the neck. **B,** Ultrasound image of a normal thyroid and surrounding muscles. The *long arrow* is pointing to the strap muscles, the *short arrow* to the sternocleidomastoid muscle, and the *curved arrow* to the longus colli muscle. (*A,* From Rumack C, Levine D. *Diagnostic Ultrasound,* 5th ed. Philadelphia, 2018, Elsevier.)

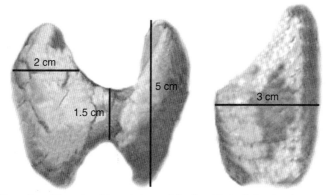

Fig. 16.3 Illustration of frontal and lateral views of the thyroid gland showing the average measurements of the thyroid lobes and the isthmus. The thyroid lobe measures 5 cm in length, 2 cm in width, and 3 cm in anteroposterior dimension. The isthmus measures 1.5 cm. (From Som PM, Curtin HD. *Head and Neck Imaging,* 5th ed. St. Louis, 2011, Mosby.)

than the left lobe, causing it to extend higher and lower in the neck than the left lobe.

Because of shape variations, some departments perform a thyroid volume measurement because this is thought to be more accurate in determining thyroid enlargement and to follow the response to treatment. The formula is based on the prolate ellipse and is Length × Width × Height (thickness) × 0.529 and is performed on each lobe. The ultrasound unit should be able to perform the calculation.

The **pyramidal lobe** is an accessory lobe arising superiorly from the isthmus and lying in front of the thyroid cartilage and extending superiorly as far as the hyoid bone (Fig. 16.4). It can be regularly seen in pediatric patients and will atrophy in adulthood. When present, the pyramidal lobe usually is seen on either side of midline and not directly in the midline. It has been documented in 55% to 65% of cadavers and thyroidectomy specimens.

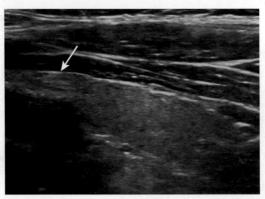

Fig. 16.4 A sagittal image of the thyroid just off of midline on the left side. The *arrow* is pointing to the pyramidal lobe.

The thyroid is highly vascular, with the right lobe normally more vascular than the left. The arterial supply to the thyroid gland consists of two superior and two inferior thyroid arteries. The superior thyroid artery is the first branch off of the external carotid artery. The superior thyroid vein drains into the internal jugular vein. The superior thyroid artery and vein are found at the upper pole of each lobe. The two inferior thyroid arteries arise from the thyrocervical trunk of the subclavian arteries and feed the lower poles of the thyroid. The inferior thyroid artery is located posterior to the lower third of each lobe. The inferior thyroid veins are seen at the lower pole of the thyroid and they drain into the brachiocephalic veins (Fig. 16.5).

Physiology

The thyroid is an endocrine gland, which means it is a ductless gland that secretes hormones directly into the bloodstream. The thyroid has the only cells in the body that can absorb iodine, which is why dietary intake of iodine is so important for the thyroid and therefore our well-being. The thyroid converts the iodine into the hormones **thyroxine** (T4) and **triiodothyronine** (T3). They are so called because T3 contains three atoms of iodine per molecule and T4 contains four atoms of iodine per molecule. These hormones regulate body temperature, heart rate, growth, and how fast the body uses food for energy. T4 accounts for 80% of the thyroid hormones, and T3 is 20% of the hormone but is four times more concentrated than T4. Every cell in the body depends on thyroid hormones for regulation of their metabolism. When the basal metabolic rate drops, the body sends a message to the hypothalamus in the brain to release **thyrotropin-releasing hormone** (TRH), which in turn tells the pituitary gland, located in the base of the brain, to release **thyroid-stimulating hormone** (TSH). TSH then stimulates the thyroid gland to release T3

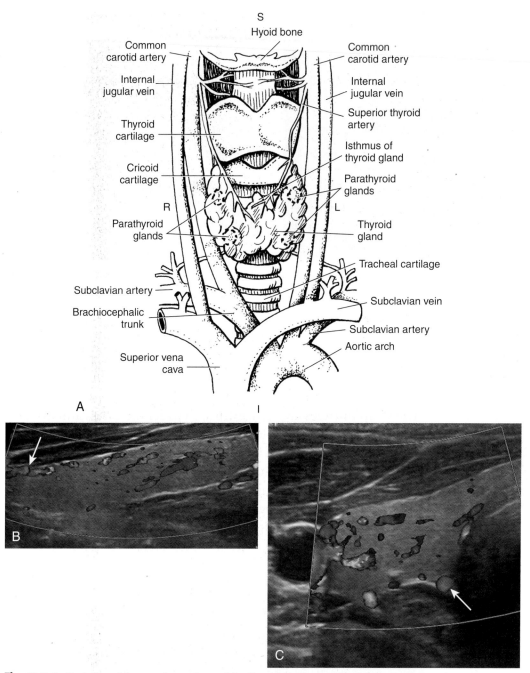

Fig. 16.5 A, Illustration of the vascular anatomy of the thyroid. **B,** The *arrow* is pointing to the superior thyroid artery. **C,** The *arrow* is pointing to the inferior thyroid artery. *L,* Left; *R,* right. (*A,* From Kelley LL, Petersen CM. *Sectional Anatomy for Imaging Professionals,* 4th ed. St. Louis, 2018, Elsevier.)

and T4. Decreased levels of T3 and T4 are associated with **hypothyroidism**, and increased levels are associated with **hyperthyroidism**. Because the thyroid gland is controlled by the pituitary gland and hypothalamus, disorders of these glands can also affect thyroid function. The thyroid also produces the hormone calcitonin, which helps regulate blood calcium levels.

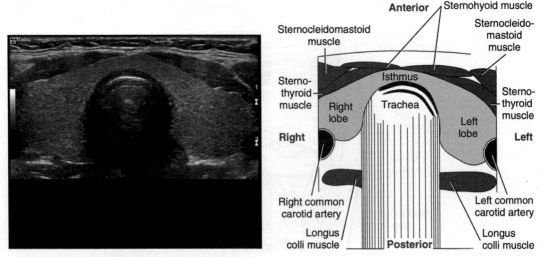

Fig. 16.6 Image and corresponding drawing of the thyroid and surrounding anatomy.

Sonographic Appearance

The normal thyroid parenchyma is a homogeneous, mid-gray echogenicity and is hyperechoic to the adjacent neck muscles (Fig. 16.6). The thyroid capsule is seen as a thin, hyperechoic line that outlines the thyroid lobes (Fig. 16.7).

The **strap muscles** are seen as thin, hypoechoic bands anterior and slightly lateral to the thyroid gland. The sternocleidomastoid muscle is seen as a larger oval band that lies more anterolateral to the thyroid gland. The longus colli muscle is an oval, hypoechoic structure that is located posterior to each thyroid lobe and along the anterior surface of the cervical vertebrae (Fig. 16.8).

The **esophagus** is considered a midline structure but is seen sonographically lateral to the trachea at the posteromedial border of the left lobe. It is recognized by the characteristic sonographic target appearance of bowel in the transverse plane. When the patient swallows, the esophagus will temporarily change shape with the peristaltic movements (Fig. 16.9).

The trachea is seen midline as a curvilinear structure with a ring-down artifact from the air in the trachea (Fig. 16.10).

Sonographic Appearance of Common Pathology

Benign nodules account for the majority of mixed cystic and solid-appearing nodules because colloid appears cystic on sonography. The most common cause of thyroid enlargement is a multinodular **goiter** that can be due to iodine insufficiency. The patient will present with a painless neck mass. These nodules are typically very heterogeneous and can be either solitary or multiple. In addition, there can be diffuse symmetric gland enlargement or a localized nodule in one lobe (Fig. 16.11). In patients with numerous nodules, measurements of all

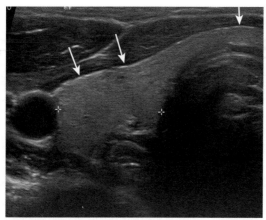

Fig. 16.7 The *arrows* are pointing to the white, echogenic thyroid capsule. The capsule is a specular reflection, so it is seen only when the beam is perpendicular to the capsule. This explains why it is not seen in its entirety.

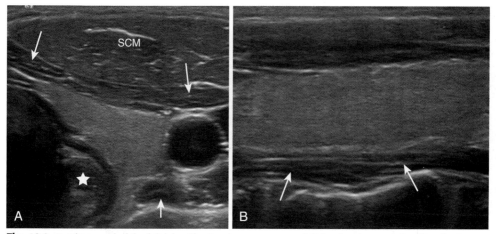

Fig. 16.8 A, Ultrasound of the left lobe. The *two long arrows* are defining the strap muscles. The *short arrow* is pointing to the longus colli muscle. *SCM* is the sternocleidomastoid muscle. The *star* is on the esophagus. **B,** A longitudinal view of the right thyroid lobe. The *arrows* are pointing to the longus colli muscle.

nodules are not necessary and usually the largest nodules or those with suspicious features are measured.

Masses of the thyroid are hypoechoic to the normal thyroid tissue. Most thyroid cancers are usually solid or almost entirely solid; however, some benign nodules, such as **adenomas**, also may be hypoechoic and solid in appearance. Thyroid cancer affects young women more than men, with **papillary cancer** the most common type. Interestingly, less than 25% of thyroid carcinomas occur in men, yet men account for 45% of deaths from thyroid carcinoma. Most men are diagnosed with thyroid cancer over the age of 60 with anaplastic thyroid cancer, which has a very poor prognosis. Thyroid cancer is commonly diagnosed at a younger age than most other adult cancers and sonographically appears as a well-differentiated

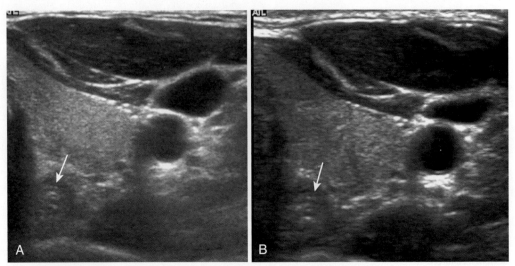

Fig. 16.9 A, The *arrow* is pointing to the esophagus. **B,** Having the patient swallow changes the shape of the esophagus. The tiny white echo in the middle represents air.

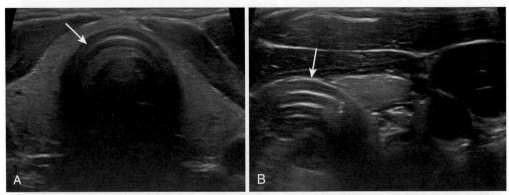

Fig. 16.10 A, The *arrow* is pointing to the trachea. The hypoechoic layer is the tracheal wall. **B,** The *arrow* is pointing to a reverberation artifact caused by the interface between the tracheal wall and air in the tracheal lumen.

hypoechoic mass with punctate nonshadowing microcalcifications, which are seen in about 40% of papillary nodules (Fig. 16.12). Many nodules, particularly benign hyperplastic nodules, contain echogenic foci that are not microcalcifications but instead are caused by colloid, especially if a comet-tail artifact is seen. When a suspicious mass is seen, the neck should be scanned for the presence of enlarged lymph nodes. Remember that most thyroid nodules are not malignant, and suspicious nodules or atypical nodules will have an FNA biopsy (Fig. 16.13). Adenomas are much more common in women than men and are also hypoechoic. If the adenoma ruptures, the mass will enlarge and become very heterogeneous with cystic areas (Fig. 16.14).

Hashimoto's thyroiditis is a type of hypothyroidism. The patient will have low T3 and T4 values and TSH will be elevated. The diffusely enlarged gland will have what are called pseudonodules, which is caused by fibrotic hyperechoic curvilinear bands and the patchy

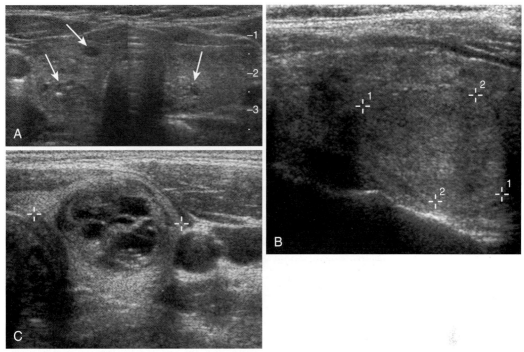

Fig. 16.11 A, A patient with multinodular goiters. The thyroid is being imaged using a split screen with the *arrows* pointing to the nodules. Note the two heterogeneous nodules and the small hypoechoic nodule. **B,** The cursors are measuring a large, homogeneous nodule in a patient with multinodular goiter. **C,** The cursor is measuring a large, complex nodule with cystic areas in a patient with multinodular goiter.

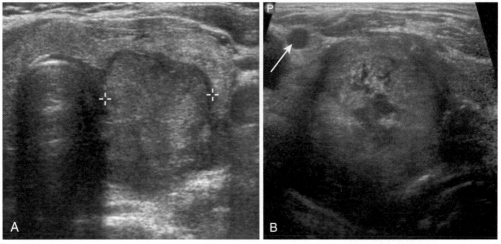

Fig. 16.12 A, The cursors are measuring a papillary carcinoma in the left lobe. Comparing this to the nodule in Fig. 16.11B, this nodule has irregular borders. **B,** An example of an anaplastic carcinoma of the thyroid. These cancers are rapid growing and become large. This cancer is very heterogenic with a necrotic center. The *arrow* is pointing to a metastatic lymph node.

hypoechoic regions (Fig. 16.15, see Color Plate 7). Adjacent cervical lymphadenopathy may be seen in these patients. **Graves' disease** is a type of hyperthyroidism, and the patient will have elevated T3 and T4 values and TSH will be decreased. It can cause the gland to

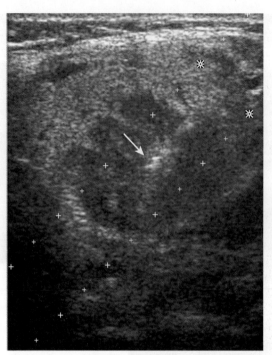

Fig. 16.13 An image of a thyroid fine needle aspiration. The *parallel dotted lines* represent the needle guide pathway. The *arrow* is pointing to a bright reflector that represents the needle tip.

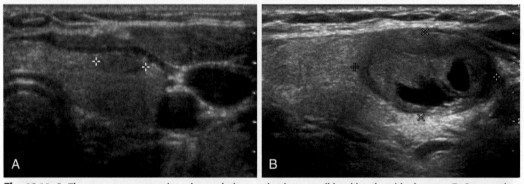

Fig. 16.14 **A,** The cursors are measuring a hypoechoic area that is compatible with a thyroid adenoma. **B,** Same patient at 1-year follow-up. The adenoma had ruptured and is now a complex mass. Biopsy of the solid areas confirmed this to be an adenoma.

enlarge and become hypoechoic and is characterized with increased color Doppler in the gland called "thyroid inferno" (Fig. 16.16, see Color Plate 8).

Ultrasound of the Thyroid

Patient Prep

There is no patient prep.

Transducer

The highest-frequency transducer should be used based on the thickness of the patient's neck. Most patients can be scanned with

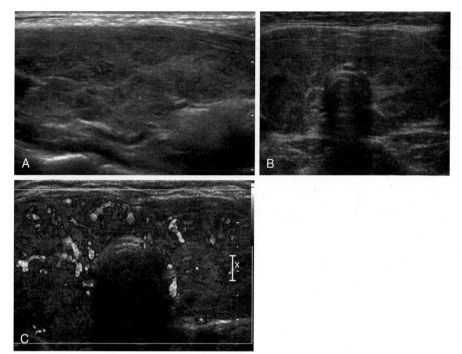

Fig. 16.15 A, The classic appearance of a patient with Hashimoto's thyroiditis. Note how the gland is hypoechoic and has the pseudonodular appearance. **B,** Transverse image showing that the whole gland is enlarged. **C,** An example of the increased vascularity seen with Hashimoto's thyroiditis. See color plate 7.

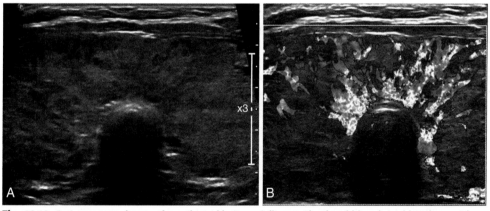

Fig. 16.16 A, A transverse image of a patient with Graves' disease. The thyroid is enlarged but does not have the pseudolobular appearance of the patient in Fig. 16.15B. **B,** A color Doppler image demonstrating the classic "thyroid inferno" that is seen in patients with Graves' disease. See color plate 8.

frequencies of 12–18 MHz. Larger and thicker necks may require using lower frequencies of 7.5–10 MHz. Some very large nodules or masses may require a lower-frequency curved linear array transducer, 2–5 MHz, that is used for abdominal scans (Fig. 16.17).

Patient Position

The patient is scanned with him or her in the supine position. For the best access to the thyroid, a pillow should be placed at the

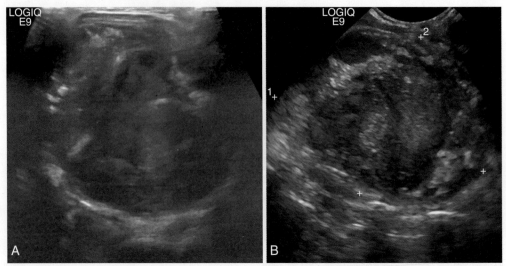

Fig. 16.17 A, A patient with anaplastic thyroid cancer. With the linear array even using the lower frequency, the echoes inside the tumor are not appreciated. **B,** Same patient with an 2–5 MHz curved liner array transducer allowing much better visualization of the tumor.

top of the patient's shoulders so the neck can be hyperextended and the chin raised. If this is uncomfortable for the patient, place a folded sheet or other object under the patient's head for support. Another alternative could be placing a positional sponge or a rolled-up sheet under their shoulders and allow the head to rest on the pillow. If needed, have the patient turn the head slightly to access the neck better.

Breathing Technique

The examination can be performed with the patient in normal or quiet breathing. In some patients, if they breathe too deeply, the thyroid may move with respiration.

Technical Tips

Thyroid sonograms can be perceived as an easy examination, and they may be scanned too quickly without attention to detail. When using high frequencies, especially with harmonics activated, pay attention to the far field. At times the transducer is at its penetration limit, and the far field will be very noisy and there may even be degradation of the image in mid-far field. Consider evaluating the image with harmonics turned off, increasing the acoustic output, or lower the imaging frequency by using the frequency control, which is labeled differently on different manufacturer's units. If the system uses the format in which the frequency choices are classified as resolution (RES), general (GEN), or penetration (PEN),

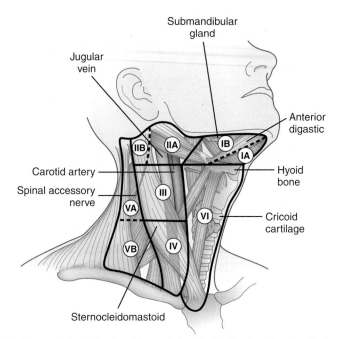

Fig. 16.18 A diagram of the six levels of the neck. In this drawing level VII is at the bottom part of level VI that dips down under the sternum. (From Townsend C, Beauchamp RD, Evers BM, Mattox K. *Sabiston Textbook of Surgery,* 20th ed. Philadelphia, 2017, Elsevier.)

try going down to the next level. For example, if the machine defaults in RES, try GEN. If the machine displays the frequency, cycle down one frequency to see if that improves the image. The goal is to clean up the far field without sacrificing image resolution. When a mass is seen, careful scanning is needed to look for punctate internal microcalcifications, which might indicate a malignancy.

Neck Nodes and Mapping

Ultrasound has an important role in patients with cancer who have undergone thyroidectomy to look for metastatic nodes in the neck. The presence of enlarged lymph nodes does not mean that the thyroid cancer has metastasized. The lymph nodes of the neck are divided into seven levels (Fig. 16.18). The two main areas are the central neck and the lateral neck and are separated by the carotid artery. Most thyroid cancers drain directly into the central level, level VI, whereas cancers in the superior third of the thyroid may drain directly into the lateral level and are called skip metastases. Rarely are the lymph nodes in the submental or submandibular region, level I, involved.

It is important to use the anatomically defined levels for good communication with the surgeon.

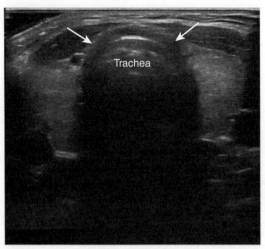

Fig. 16.19 The *arrows* are pointing to the hypoechoic, arch-shaped cricoid cartilage. The lower hypoechoic area is the walls of the trachea.

Neck Levels

- Level I: The *submental and submandibular nodes* are superior to the hyoid bone, anterior to the submandibular gland, and inferior to the mandible. The boundary between levels I and II is the posterior edge of the submandibular gland.
- Levels II, III, and IV are internal jugular nodes and are divided into three groups by the hyoid bone and the inferior border of the cricoid cartilage. The cricoid is seen best on a transverse view because it has an archlike appearance with a posterior white border (Fig. 16.19). It is found superior to the isthmus and between the upper lobes of the thyroid.
- Level II: The *anterior cervical upper internal jugular chain* is from the base of the skull to the inferior border of the hyoid bone, which is near the carotid bifurcation.
- Level III: The *middle internal jugular chain* is between the hyoid bone and the inferior border of the cricoid cartilage.
- Level IV: The *lower internal jugular chain* is below the inferior border of the cricoid cartilage to the clavicle.
- Level V: Nodes in *the spinal accessory chain and transverse cervical and supraclavicular group* are in the posterior triangle of the neck that is bound anteriorly by the posterior border of the sternocleidomastoid muscle and posteriorly by the anterior border of the trapezius muscle, and extends from the union of the sternocleidomastoid and trapezius muscle to the clavicle.
  - Level Va: The superior half that is posterior to levels II and III and is between the base of the skull and the inferior border of the cricoid cartilage.
  - Level Vb: The inferior half that is posterior to level IV and is between the inferior border of the cricoid cartilage and the level of clavicles.

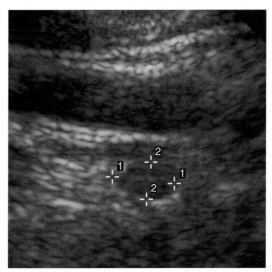

Fig. 16.20 A node in level VII using a high-frequency curved array transducer because it gave better access to see the node.

- Level VI: The *central compartment* is between the suprasternal notch and the hyoid bone and between the carotid arteries.
- Level VII: The *central anterior compartment* is between the carotids and below the manubrium (suprasternal notch). This level is not recognized by all surgeons; some consider it part of level VI.

For neck mapping it is very important to have the patient lie in the position he or she will be in for surgery. This is usually with the patient supine and looking straight ahead. When possible, discuss with the surgeon how the patient will be positioned. Turning the neck may place the node in a different-appearing location if the operative position is supine. This is especially true for nodes near the carotid artery. With the head straight, the node is in level IV; however, when the head is tilted, it now appears that the node is in level VI.

A neck mapping is usually started with the transducer in the transverse plane. Most sonographers have a scanning routine that they follow. A good place to start is level VI because nodes are common here, and then proceed to evaluate level I. Levels II to IV are scanned along the jugular veins and carotid artery from the mandible to the clavicle. Move the transducer lateral to evaluate level V by scanning from the mastoid tip to the clavicle. If level VII is included in the protocol, angle the transducer under the suprasternal notch. Switching to a high-frequency curved linear array transducer, including an endovaginal transducer, may allow for better access under the clavicle (Fig. 16.20). Obtaining video clips of each level can be very helpful to see the node as it comes into and out of the image. Some departments may have the sonographer fill out a worksheet to document the location of the nodes (Fig. 16.21). When

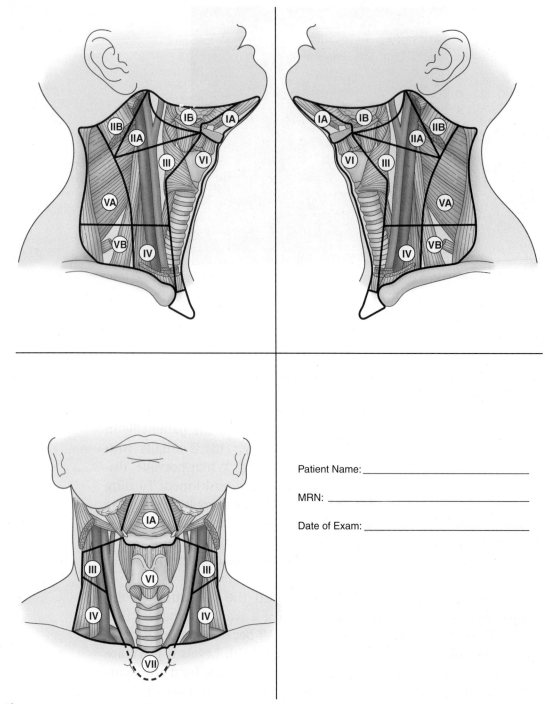

Fig. 16.21 An example of a worksheet to document the locations of any nodes seen in the neck. (Original drawing courtesy Paul Wiernicki, RDMS, RVT, who is an incredible artist and sonographer.)

verified by the radiologist, this may be sent to the surgeon to aid them in surgery.

The specific level of the enlarged node should be documented, and the node measured in three dimensions: length, AP, and width. Features of malignant nodes are usually hypoechoic to surrounding

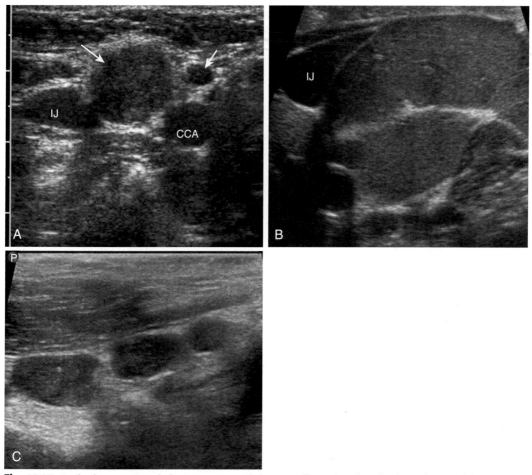

Fig. 16.22 A, The *long arrow* and *short arrow* are pointing to malignant lymph nodes. Note the round, homogenous shape and lack of fatty hilum. The node was lateral to the carotid and posterior to the hyoid, putting it in level III. **B,** Some large nodes seen in the left neck lateral to the carotid and displacing the internal jugular *(IJ)* vein. These nodes were below the cricoid cartilage putting them in level IV. **C,** Three small nodes that were in level III from the anaplastic carcinoma of the patient in Fig. 16.12B. *CCA,* Common carotid artery.

muscles, round, homogeneous, lack an echogenic hilum, called a fatty hilum, have microcalcifications, and peripheral flow is seen on color or power Doppler (Fig. 16.22). It is important to realize that not all malignant nodes will have all of these characteristics. If a fatty hilum is present, the node should be evaluated for cystic degeneration from necrosis, irregular margins, and cortical thickening. Most inflammatory nodes are oval with a fatty hilum that resembles the sonographic appearance of a kidney, and hilar flow can be seen with color or power Doppler in some nodes, especially if greater than 5 mm (Fig. 16.23). Abnormal lymph nodes will have an FNA to evaluate for malignancy.

Thyroid Required Images

The thyroid gland is small and can be seen in its entirety by some transducers, but it is still evaluated by viewing the lobes individually.

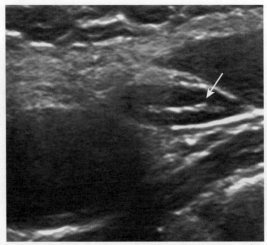

Fig. 16.23 An example of the characteristics of a benign node, oval with a fatty hilum *(arrow)*. Note how they look like a small kidney.

The study usually starts with the transverse images and then the sagittal images, starting on either side. Any nodules should be measured in all three planes—length, width, and AP. If possible, do a side-by-side image with the longitudinal image on one side and the transverse image on the other side.

Thyroid • Transverse Images

1. Transverse image of both lobes at mid-gland.

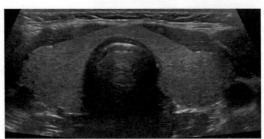

Suggested Annotation: **TRV MID**

2. Transverse image of both lobes at mid-gland with color Doppler.

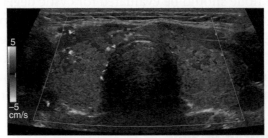

Suggested Annotation: **TRV MID**

3. Transverse image of the isthmus with and without measurement.

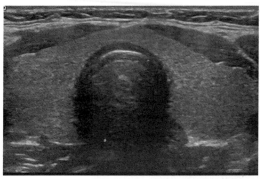 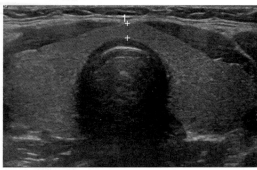

Suggested Annotation: **TRV ISTHMUS**

4. Transverse image of the right lobe at mid-gland with and without width measurement. Use the function to make the beam into a trapezoid format if needed to see the entire gland.

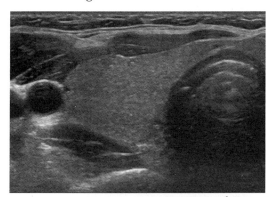 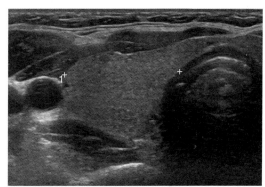

Suggested Annotation: **TRV RT MID**

5. Transverse image of the right lobe at upper pole.

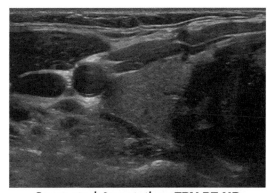

Suggested Annotation: **TRV RT UP**

6. Transverse image of the right lobe at lower pole.

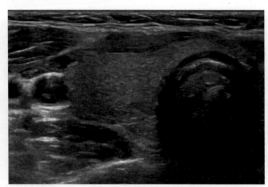

Suggested Annotation: **TRV RT LOW**

7. Repeat for left lobe.

Thyroid • Longitudinal Images

1. Midline of the right lobe with and without measurements of length and AP.

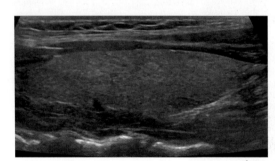 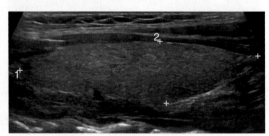

Suggested Annotation: **RT ML**

2. Midline of the right lobe with color Doppler.

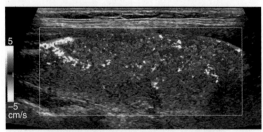

Suggested Annotation: **RT ML**

3. Sagittal of the medial right lobe.

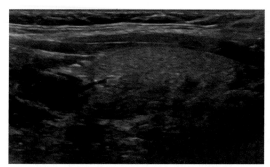

Suggested Annotation: **RT MED**

4. Sagittal of the lateral right lobe.

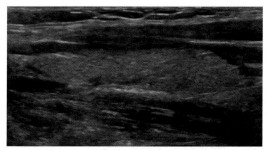

Suggested Annotation: **RT LAT**

5. Repeat for left lobe.

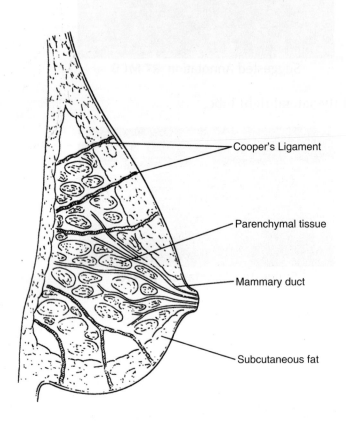

Cooper's Ligament

Parenchymal tissue

Mammary duct

Subcutaneous fat

CHAPTER 17

Breast Scanning Protocol*

Tricia Turner

Keywords

Antiradial plane	Parenchymal elements
Breast	Pectoralis major muscle
Breast parenchyma	Radial scan
Cooper's ligaments	Retromammary layer
Lactiferous ducts	Subcutaneous layer
Mammary layer	

Objectives

At the end of this chapter, you will be able to:

- Define the keywords.
- Distinguish the sonographic appearance of the breast and the terms used to describe it.
- List the transducer options for scanning the breast.
- List the suggested patient position and options when scanning the breast.
- Discuss radial and antiradial scans.

Overview

Breast ultrasounds are usually performed in a breast imaging suite or a women's health center. Some radiology departments may perform breast ultrasound or may perform breast ultrasound for a specific reason, such as a looking for breast abscess, and will not perform studies to evaluate the breast for a mass or cancer.

One out of eight American women will develop breast cancer over the course of their lifetime, with an estimated 277,000 new cases annually with about 42,000 women dying from breast cancer. Breast cancer is the most common type of cancer among women in the United States and is the second leading cause of cancer death after lung cancer. It is estimated that the lifetime risk for a women

*The author wishes to thank Jeanine Rybyinski for providing the sonograms in this chapter.

developing breast cancer is approximately 12%. Ultrasound of the breast plays an important role in the detection and characterization of breast masses.

Breast sonography has become the first choice for imaging palpable masses in women under 30 and for lactating and pregnant women. Breast sonography is not recommended as a screening study to replace mammography. A breast ultrasound is generally performed to determine the composition or characterization of a localized lesion(s), which may or may not be palpable, and to further evaluate mammographic and clinical findings. Additional indications for breast sonography include using it for ultrasound-guided biopsies, evaluating complications associated with breast implants, and women in which mammography is contraindicated, such as patients with inflammation or trauma. In some cases, whole-breast scanning may be recommended for diffuse diseases, such as fibrocystic disease. Recently, breast ultrasound has been recommended for women with dense breasts. On mammography, dense breast tissue appears white, as does breast cancer, making it difficult to identify the breast cancer. With ultrasound, dense tissue is echogenic and breast cancer is hypoechoic, making it easier to identify.

Anatomy

The breast lies anterior to the pectoralis major, serratus, and external oblique muscles. The second and third ribs form the superior border of each breast, and the seventh costal cartilage is the inferior border. The medial border of each breast is the sternum. Laterally the breasts are bound by the margin of the axilla. Breast tissue is supported by **Cooper's ligaments**, which are suspensory ligaments that extend posteriorly from the deep muscle fascia, through the breast, and to the skin. The breast comprises **parenchymal elements** that include the lobes, ducts, and alveoli; and stromal elements, which include connective tissue and fat. The breast is described in terms of three layers, as follows. The first layer is the **subcutaneous layer** of skin and subcutaneous fat lobules. The next layer is the **mammary layer** of 15 to 20 lobes that contain alveoli, multiple glandular tissue lobules, **lactiferous ducts** that drain to the nipple, fat lobules, and connective tissue. The third layer is the **retromammary layer** that includes fat lobules and connective tissue.

Physiology

The breasts, or mammary glands, are exocrine glands whose primary function is the secretion of milk, or lactation. After pregnancy, the breast starts to produce milk, which is drained into the lactiferous ducts, which are ducts in the **breast parenchyma**, to the nipple. Remember that exocrine glands use ducts as opposed to endocrine glands, which use osmosis.

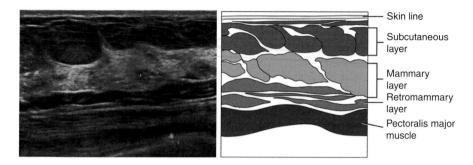

Sonographic Appearance

Sonographically, three layers of the breast are distinguishable, with their normal appearance described as follows:

1. The subcutaneous layer is the most anterior layer, bordered anteriorly by the bright skin line and posteriorly by the mammary layer. This layer is thin and contains subcutaneous fat lobules that appear as low-level echoes with bright margins. Usually fat is echogenic; however, in the breast it is the least echogenic tissue, appearing hypoechoic, with the ducts, glands, and ligaments appearing echogenic.

2. The mammary layer is the middle layer of the breast that contains glandular tissue and is the functioning portion of the breast. This area contains 15 to 20 lobes that contain the milk-producing glands and radiate from the nipple. Fatty tissue is seen between the lobes. Typically, it appears hyperechoic compared with the subcutaneous and retromammary layers because of its mixed parenchymal appearance depending on the amount of fat present. When there is a small amount of fat, it is highly echogenic because of the reflective appearance of the existing connective tissue, collagen, and fibrotic tissue. When fat is present, the appearance includes areas of low-level echoes from fat mixed with areas of high echogenicity from the connective tissue. When visualized, the ducts appear as small anechoic branches running throughout the layer.

3. The retromammary layer is generally hypoechoic relative to the mammary layer and hyperechoic compared with its posterior border, the pectoralis major muscle. The **pectoralis major muscle** is a large chest muscle that is hypoechoic and seen between the retromammary layer and the ribs. The ribs appear sonographically as hyperechoic curved structures with posterior acoustic shadowing and should not be mistaken for a mass (Fig. 17.1).

The sonographic appearance of the breast changes with age. Although all the breast layers are influenced by the age of the woman and the functional state of the breast, the mammary layer shows the greatest changes sonographically. The breasts of young women contain a higher percentage of parenchymal elements and little fat. This causes the mammary layer to be dense and appear highly echogenic

(Fig. 17.2). In older women, the subcutaneous and retromammary layers become more prominent as the mammary layer decreases in size as the parenchymal tissues atrophy and are replaced by fat (Fig. 17.3).

Cooper's ligaments are seen as bright, thin linear lines that appear hyperechoic relative to the adjacent structures (Fig. 17.4).

Normal Variants

A fatty breast is seen when there are increased fatty components throughout the breast resulting from age, parity, and menopause. When fat is present, the sonographic appearance is areas of low-level echoes from fat mixed with areas of high echogenicity from connective tissue surrounding the mammary ducts (Fig. 17.5).

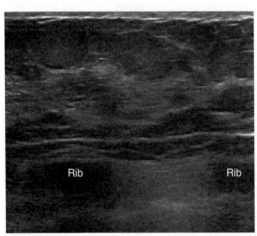

Fig. 17.1 An ultrasound image of a normal breast with the ribs identified.

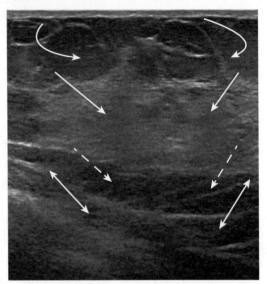

Fig. 17.2 An image of a breast from a young woman. The *curved arrows* are pointing to the subcutaneous layer. The *straight arrows* point to the mammary layer. The *dashed arrows* point to the retromammary layers. The *double-headed arrows* point to the pectoralis major muscle

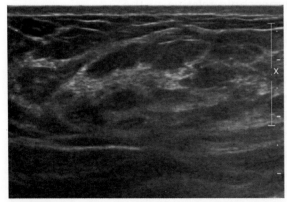

Fig. 17.3 An image of a breast of an older woman. Note that the mammary layer is smaller compared with the breast in Fig. 17.2 and the subcutaneous layer is increased in size.

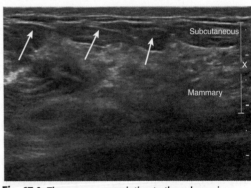

Fig. 17.4 The *arrows* are pointing to the echogenic Copper's ligaments.

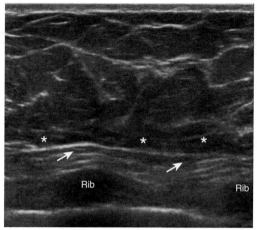

Fig. 17.5 An image of a fatty breast. The *stars* are in the mammary layer and the *arrows* are pointing to the retromammary layer. The pectoralis major muscle is under the *arrows* and above the ribs.

A fibrocystic breast is commonly found in women of childbearing age. In these breasts, fibrous tissue and cystic areas occur throughout the breast, and an increase in the amount of dense connective tissue will cause the breast to appear highly echogenic.

Ultrasound of the Breast

Patient Prep
No patient prep is needed except for the removal of all clothes from the waist up. The patient is given a gown, to be worn with the opening in front to allow access to the breast. This allows the breast not being scanned to be covered.

Transducer
A high-frequency linear array transducer is used with frequencies in the 12–18-MHz range. For the best resolution, the highest frequency that allows for adequate penetration should be used. However, if the overall gain is introducing noise into the image, the frequency is too high and a lower frequency should be used. This is important because excess noise in the image may mask a pathologic condition.

Breathing Technique
Patients can breathe normally during the examination. If respiratory motion is a problem, the patient will need to suspend breathing when capturing the image to reduce any potential blurriness that may occur with movement of the tissue.

Patient Position
When scanning the breast to evaluate a lesion, the patient is supine to minimize the thickness of the portion of the breast being evaluated.

If a mass was seen on mammography and cannot be found on the ultrasound examination with the patient supine, the patient should be scanned in an upright position to mimic the breast position from the mammogram.

When scanning the whole breast, the patient is in the supine position with a wedge or cushion placed under the shoulder of the side of the breast being scanned. The arm of the side being imaged should be placed above the patient's head because this helps even out the breast tissue and give better access to the axillary region. To help level out the breast tissue in the lateral margins, the patient may be placed in a posterior oblique position facing away from the side being scanned, with a wedge or sponge placed under the back or shoulders for support.

Technical Tips

All prior imaging should be reviewed, and the location of potential or known masses or cysts documented for correlation while scanning if needed.

The overall gain should be set so that the fat tissue appears to be medium-level echogenicity. Multiple focal zones should be used for optimal resolution (Fig. 17.6). Using harmonics is the equivalent to using a higher frequency without much loss in penetration, and it also reduces artifacts in the image, especially cystic structures. Edge enhancement and spatial compounding can be used to help improve border visualization. Manufacturers offer many features to help optimize image quality. Knowing the equipment thoroughly and when to apply these features will assist in the diagnostic process. The depth should be set so that all images show the pectoralis muscle at the bottom of the image to ensure that the breast has been imaged to its posterior border (Fig. 17.7).

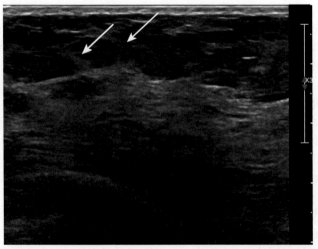

Fig. 17.6 An image of a breast with proper gain settings. The *arrows* are pointing to Copper's ligaments.

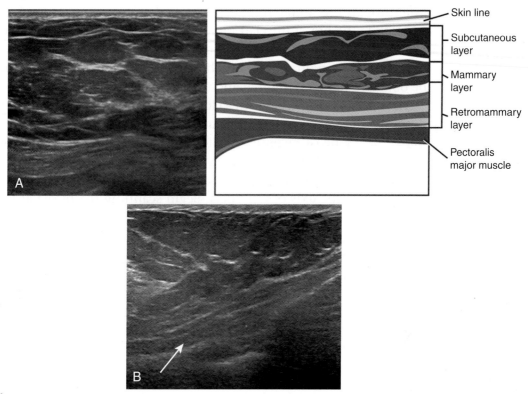

Fig. 17.7 A, An image of a normal breast showing that the pectoralis major muscle is seen and therefore the depth is at a proper setting. **B,** A more medial image of the breast in which mostly subcutaneous tissue is seen. The *arrow* is pointing to the pectoralis major muscle.

Any mass or suspicious area needs to have compression techniques to assess compressibility and mobility. Compressible lesions are usually benign. The transducer may need to be heel-toed to minimize critical angle reflections from the Cooper ligaments, to better visualize duct walls, and to help better visualize the capsule of solid masses.

Using the America College of Radiology Breast Imaging, Reporting and Data System (ACR BI-RADS) recommendations, all masses should be assessed for *shape* (oval, round, or irregular), *orientation* (parallel or not parallel), *margins* (circumscribed or not circumscribed), *echo pattern* (anechoic, hyperechoic, hypoechoic, isoechoic, complex, or heterogeneous), *posterior acoustic features* (none, enhancement, shadowing, or combined pattern), *calcifications* (in mass or outside mass), special characteristics of architectural distortion, ductal changes, skin thickening or retraction, and vascularity, looking for internal flow, vessels in rim, or no vascularity present.

Breast sonography also can be focused to an area of interest. For example, if the woman has a tender breast with a suspicion for an abscess, the examination would consist of only longitudinal and transverse images over the area of pain or tenderness. The images may be annotated as Area of Pain (AOP) and the quadrant of the breast where it is located. The breast is divided into four quadrants using a line through the nipple in both horizontal and vertical planes. This will divide the breast into left upper outer quadrant, left lower outer quadrant, left upper inner quadrant, and left lower inner quadrant (Fig. 17.8). The right will follow the same divisions. Images also can be obtained in a longitudinal and transverse imaging plane

The breast is also scanned in a clock-like manner called radial scanning. If a mass is seen, the transducer is turned 90 degrees to see the mass; this plane of imaging is called antiradial. Transducer orientation is set up so that the breast is viewed in sections from the nipple outward, with the orientation notch near the nipple. This also scans the breast in the axis of the ducts. Begin scanning the breast at the 12-o'clock position and scan around the breast in a clockwise manner, covering all the breast anatomy (see Fig. 17.8). The annotation for a breast mass should include the distance in centimeters it is from the nipple (Fig. 17.9). Remember that 3 o'clock is medial breast tissue on the right and lateral breast tissue on the left; 9 o'clock also will be different, with it being lateral on the right and medial on the left. Do not reverse the numbers for the left breast so that 3 o'clock would correspond to medial breast to be consistent with the right side.

A survey of the breast can be performed to locate any areas of abnormality. With the transducer in a transverse plane, scan the breast starting on the lateral edge, scanning from the top to the bottom of the breast. While at the bottom, move the transducer medially with some overlap of tissue and scan to the top of the breast. Continue scanning in this manner to the medial edge of the breast (Fig. 17.10). With the transducer in a longitudinal plane, examine the breast starting at the top of the breast and scanning medial to

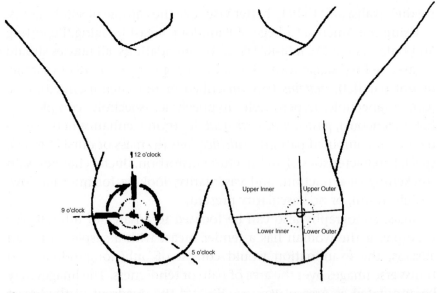

Fig. 17.8 A diagram showing the scanning technique for radial scanning and of the breast divided into quadrants.

lateral. At the end of the "row," move the transducer down and again with some overlap scan back to the medial aspect of the breast. Continue scanning in this manner until the bottom of the breast is reached (Fig. 17.11). This helps plan the documented images by knowing if the breast is normal or if there are suspicious areas. Some sonographers might also do a survey with **radial scans** starting at 12 o'clock and scanning clockwise around the breast until back at the 12 o'clock position (Fig. 17.12). It is important that the sonographer thoroughly evaluates the breast because documentation will be only selected images.

Ultrasound is used to help determine whether a mass is cystic or solid. Breast cysts need to have the ultrasound criteria of a cyst: thin wall, round shape, no internal echoes, and posterior enhancement. If a cyst does not meet these criteria, it is a complex cyst and may need

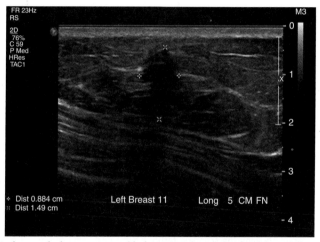

Fig. 17.9 An image of a breast cancer with the annotation stating that it is 5 cm from the nipple.

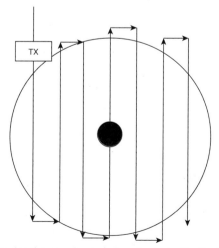

Fig. 17.10 A diagram showing the scanning technique for evaluating the breast in the longitudinal plane. Note that the transducer will be in a transverse orientation.

to be further investigated, including aspiration (Fig. 17.13). Benign masses will compress the surrounding tissue, will have smooth margins with an echogenic capsule, and are hyperechoic. Other sonographic characteristics of a benign mass are posterior enhancement, mobility, and lack of flow inside the mass. Fibroadenomas are a common benign solid mass that are homogeneous, with an oval shape, or have gently lobulated margins (Fig. 17.14). The back wall is seen, and an edge artifact may be seen from the borders of the more circular masses.

Most breast cancers originate in the ducts of the breast, with a smaller percentage originating in the glandular tissue. The majority of

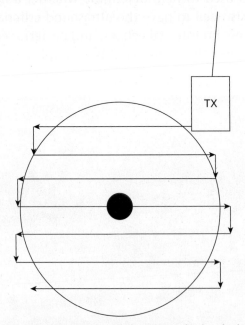

Fig. 17.11 A diagram showing the scanning technique for evaluating the breast in the transverse plane. Note now that the transducer is in a longitudinal orientation.

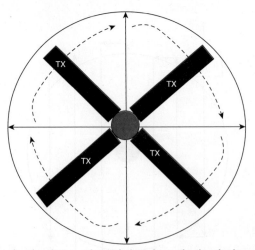

Fig. 17.12 A diagram showing the scanning technique for evaluating the breast in the radial plane. Note that the transducer will be in a longitudinal orientation at 12 o'clock and 6 o'clock and in a transverse orientation at 3 o'clock and 9 o'clock.

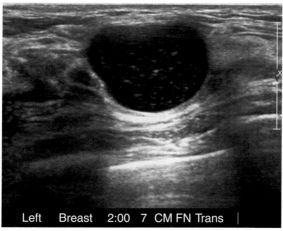

Fig. 17.13 An example of a cyst with some internal echoes. Note the amount of acoustic enhancement under the cyst.

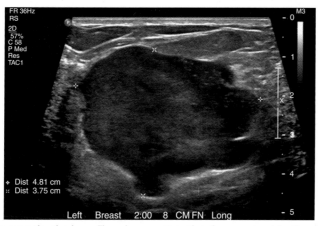

Fig. 17.14 An example of a large fibroadenoma. Note that the mass is wider than taller and has smooth, gently lobulated margins.

breast cancers are located in the upper outer quadrant of the breast. Sonographic characteristics of malignant masses include angular margins, indistinct margins, hypoechoic appearance, microcalcifications, presence of an acoustic shadow, firmly fixed, noncompressible, exhibit ductal extensions, and the masses will be vascular. Malignant lesions are typically described as taller than wider and can grow through the tissue in finger-like extensions called spiculations. The back walls of cancers are usually hard to define (Fig. 17.15). One technique to help define the walls of the mass is called fremitus. Fremitus refers to vibrations transmitted through the body that can be felt or heard with a stethoscope, usually in the chest. When a person speaks, the vocal cords create a vibration that can be passed through the lungs and chest wall. In ultrasound, having the patient hum, preferably in a deep voice, sends these vibrations through normal breast tissue. As they cause the tissue to vibrate, a Doppler shift is created. By using power Doppler, the normal tissue will be color encoded and the abnormal tissue will be void of echoes, allowing the margins of the mass to be identified (Fig. 17.16).

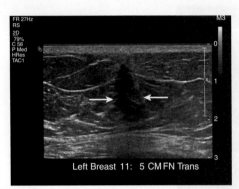

Fig. 17.15 The *arrows* are pointing to a breast carcinoma. Note that the mass is taller than wider, it has no internal echoes, and the posterior border is not well seen.

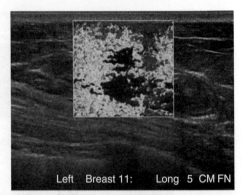

Fig. 17.16 An example of the fremitus technique on the same mass as in Fig. 17.15. Note the lack of color inside the cancer and how the posterior border is better appreciated.

Breast Required Images

The breast should be evaluated using the current ACR recommendations, and the reader is encouraged to visit the ACR website at http://www.ACR.org for the latest information. The following information is from the ACR document entitled *ACR Practice Parameter for the Performance of Whole-Breast Ultrasound for Screening and Staging,* which was updated in 2019. From the ACR practice parameter: A whole-breast handheld ultrasound screening examination should document at minimum each of the four quadrants and the subareolar region. The axilla may be included per facility practice and as per exam indication.

The department may decide how the breast is to be annotated. In the following examples the quadrant method is used.

1. Image of the breast at 12:00 o'clock longitudinal/radial.

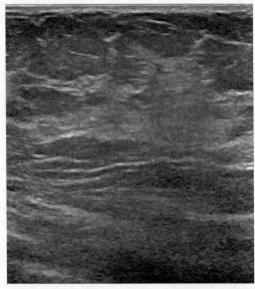

Suggested Annotations: **LT BREAST 12:00 RAD**

2. Image of the breast at 12:00 o'clock antiradial.

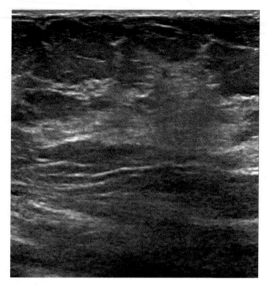

Suggested Annotations: **LT BREAST 12:00 A RAD**

3. Image of the breast in upper inner quadrant radial.

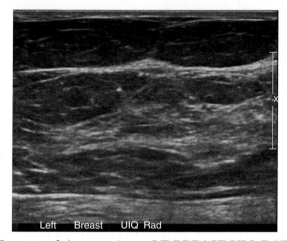

Suggested Annotations: **LT BREAST UIQ RAD**

4. Image of the breast in upper inner quadrant antiradial.

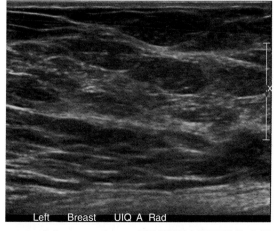

Suggested Annotations: **LT BREAST UIQ A RAD**

5. Image of the breast in lower inner quadrant radial.

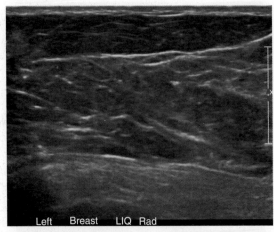

Suggested Annotations: **LT BREAST LIQ RAD**

6. Image of the breast in lower inner quadrant antiradial.

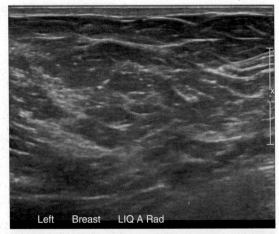

Suggested Annotations: **LT BREAST LIQ A RAD**

7. Image of the breast in lower outer quadrant radial.

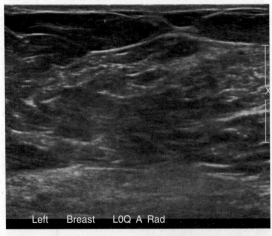

Suggested Annotations: **LT BREAST LOQ RAD**

8. Image of the breast in lower outer quadrant antiradial.

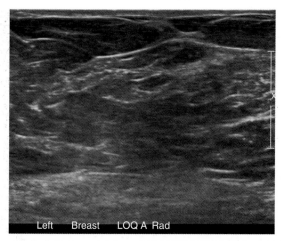

Suggested Annotations: **LT BREAST LOQ A RAD**

9. Image of the breast in upper outer quadrant radial.

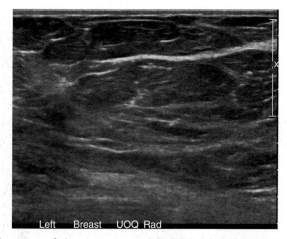

Suggested Annotations: **LT BREAST UOQ RAD**

10. Image of the breast in upper outer quadrant antiradial.

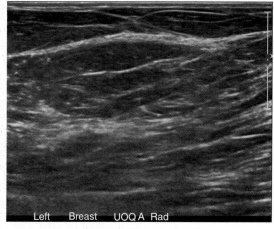

Suggested Annotations: **LT BREAST UOQ A RAD**

11. Image of the retroareolar area.

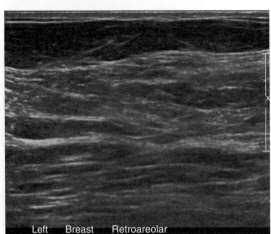

Suggested Annotations: **LT BREAST RETROAREOLAR**

Following is an example using the clock annotation to document the quadrant. For example, instead of lower outer quadrant on the left breast, 4:00 Rad and A Rad could be used.

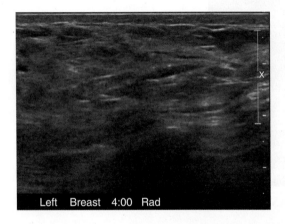 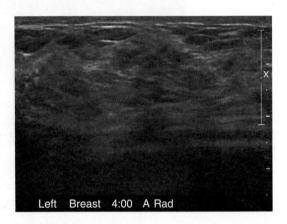

Breast Lesion Required Images

When a localized mass of the breast is to be evaluated, it will need to be scanned in two orthogonal planes. Breast masses may be assessed and documented in radial and antiradial planes, or it may be beneficial to also assess them with longitudinal and transverse planes. Radial scans are important to identify abnormalities along the ductal system.

The location of the mass must be recorded to accompany the required images. The location of the lesion can be documented by one of the following methods:

1. Shown on a diagram of the breast.
2. Specifying the quadrant.
3. Using clock notation and the distance from the nipple. Some laboratories will draw centimeter marks on the transducer for accuracy and consistency.

Images must be taken with and without measurements so that the cursors do not obscure any of the anatomy. When measuring a suspected cancer, include the echogenic halo that surrounds the mass. The longest length should be measured along with the plane from where it was obtained, that is, longitudinal or radial. This is important information for future follow-up to ensure that the same plane is used.

1. Longitudinal or radial plane.

   The scanning plane will be determined by the shape and lie of the mass.

2. An image without measurements and with long axis and anteroposterior direction measured.

   The annotation will depend on the location of the mass. For example, RT 5:00 3 CM FN RAD.

   The annotation should be very descriptive so that the area of the mass can be located as needed.

3. Transverse or antiradial plane

   The scanning plane will be 90 degrees from the longitudinal or radial plane.

4. An image without measurements and an image with width measured.

   The annotation will be the same except for the scanning plane. RT 5:00 3 CM FN ARAD.

HINT Placing the scanning plane last in the annotation makes it easy to backspace and just change the scanning plane.

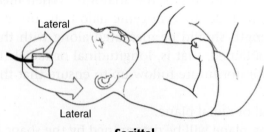

Sagittal

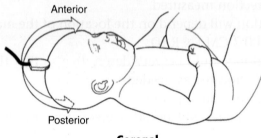

Coronal

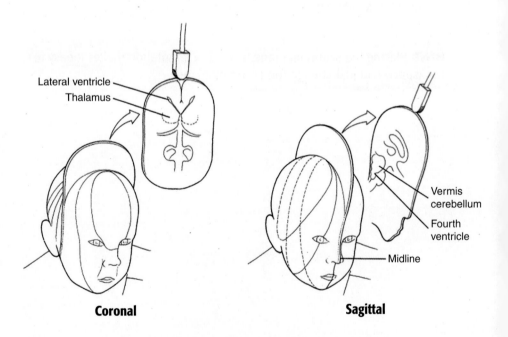

Coronal

Sagittal

CHAPTER 18

Neonatal Brain, Spine, and Hip Scanning Protocols

Ashley Upton; Ted Whitten

Keywords

Acetabulum
Anterior fontanelle
Aqueduct of Sylvius
Barlow maneuver
Brainstem
Cauda equina
Caudate nucleus
Cavum septum pellucidum
Cavum vergae
Cerebellum
Cerebral peduncle
Cerebrospinal fluid (CSF)
Cerebrum
Choroid plexus
Cisterna magna
Conus medullaris
Corpus callosum
Falx cerebri
Femoral head
Filum terminale

Foramen of Magendie
Foramen of Monro
Foramina of Luschka
Germinal matrix
Interhemispheric fissure
Ischium
Labrum
Lateral ventricles
Massa intermedia
Ortolani maneuver
Pubis
Quadrigeminal plate
Sulci
Sylvian fissure
Tentorium
Thalamus
Triradiate cartilage
Vermis
Vertebral bodies

Objectives

At the end of this chapter, you will be able to:
- Define the keywords.
- Distinguish the sonographic appearance of the neonatal or infant brain, spine, and hips and the terms used to describe them.
- Describe the transducer options for scanning the neonatal or infant brain, spine, and hips.
- List the suggested patient positions and options when scanning the neonatal or infant brain, spine, and hips.
- Explain the patient prep for a neonatal or infant brain, spine, and hips studies.
- Discuss the images needed to evaluate the entire neonatal brain.
- Discuss the images needed to evaluate the neonatal spine and spinal canal.
- Discuss the images needed to evaluate the neonatal or infant hips for developmental dysplasia of the hip.

Ultrasound of the Neonate

Pediatric ultrasound is usually performed by the radiology or pediatric radiology department. In some hospitals it may be performed by the PICU and NICU physicians. Ultrasound is the preferred imaging modality for pediatric patients because there is no radiation, usually no need for sedation, and no need for nephrotoxic contrast media. Because ultrasound can be performed as a portable examination, the examinations can be performed in the patient's room for the safety of the patient. Ultrasound also lends itself for follow-up examinations after initial magnetic resonance imaging (MRI) or computed tomography (CT). Another advantage of ultrasound is the ability to evaluate blood flow and observe dynamic motion, something MRI and CT cannot do. To reduce any potential bioeffects, the lowest possible ultrasonic power should be used, following the ALARA (*as low as reasonably achievable*) principle.

When performing portable examinations in the pediatric intensive care unit (PICU) or neonatal intensive care unit (NICU), it is important to work with the staff taking care of the infant. Because babies in the NICU will be in an isolette and have intravenous lines and multiple other lines attached, it is important to be extra careful so as not to accidentally pull out a line. Keeping the baby warm is very important, so scanning should be performed as quickly and efficiently as possible. This will also reduce interfering with the NICU team as they take care of the baby. There may be times when it is very difficult to place the ultrasound unit near the patient, especially with infants or children on extracorporeal membrane oxygenation (ECMO), because these units are quite large. This may require placing the ultrasound machine in an unusual location and for the sonographer to scan in an unusual position, such as facing the patient's feet. There will be times when a second sonographer is needed so one sonographer will perform the examination and the other adjust the controls and capture the images. Performing examinations on the unit can take some patience and understanding of the needs of the other staff as they try to do their job and take care of the patient. One of the most important aspects of performing studies in the NICU or PICU is practicing good infection prevention by properly washing your hands and wearing gowns and masks as required by policies. The transducer should also be cleaned and properly disinfected between patients as you go from patient to patient to reduce the risk of spreading infections. This is actually good practice for all patients. An interesting situation can occur when another person wants to perform an ultrasound at the same time. Although in theory this may sound acceptable because it is two different areas of the body, there is a chance that the sound beams will interfere with one another or echoes from critical angles will interfere with the other transducer, causing degradation of the image. If both units need to use the same wall socket, there is a good chance that both images will suffer image degradation from electrical interference, which also is known as 60-cycle noise.

Neonatal Brain Overview

Intracranial Anatomy and Sonographic Appearance

There are four ventricles in the brain, two lateral ventricles, a third ventricle, and a fourth ventricle.

Lateral Ventricles

The **lateral ventricles** are cerebrospinal fluid–filled cavities within each cerebral hemisphere. **Cerebrospinal fluid** (CSF) is a clear liquid that is predominately produced by the choroid plexus, circulates through the ventricles and subarachnoid spaces, and is reabsorbed by the arachnoid villi. Its main functions are to distribute nutrients and serve as a shock absorber against injury to the brain and spinal cord. Each lateral ventricle is divided segmentally into a frontal horn, body, occipital horn, and temporal horn. The atrium or trigone is the junction of the body and occipital and temporal horns.

The lateral ventricular walls appear echogenic and curvilinear. These slit-like structures lie the same distance from the interhemispheric fissure. The lateral ventricles contain CSF, which appears anechoic, and the choroid plexus, which is echogenic.

Third Ventricle

The third ventricle is a small, teardrop-shaped, midline cavity that lies between the thalami and is connected to the lateral ventricles via the foramen of Monro, which are midline channels that mark the communication between the lateral and third ventricles. The walls are echogenic, and the cavity contains CSF and is anechoic.

Fourth Ventricle

The fourth ventricle is a small, thin, arrowhead-shaped, midline cavity that appears to project into the cerebellum. It is best seen in the transmastoid view and is vaguely seen except when there is massive ventricular dilatation. It is located below and connected to the third ventricle by a small channel called the aqueduct of Sylvius, which is a narrow opening for the passage of CSF. It directs CSF into the subarachnoid space through the **foramen of Magendie** and **foramina of Luschka**, three small holes in the floor of the fourth ventricle. The walls of the fourth ventricle are echogenic. The cavity contains CSF and is anechoic.

Corpus Callosum

The **corpus callosum** is flat, broad nerve fibers between the right and left cerebral hemispheres that form the roof of the lateral ventricles. The parenchyma appears as mid-gray or medium-level echoes.

Cerebrum

The **cerebrum** is the largest part of the brain and is divided into two identical, symmetric right and left hemispheres that communicate through the corpus callosum. They are separated from each other at the midline by a deep groove called the interhemispheric fissure. Each cerebral hemisphere is divided into four lobes, named after the overlying cranial bones: the frontal, parietal, temporal, and occipital lobes. The cerebrum is mid-gray with medium-level echoes.

Cavum Septum Pellucidum

The **cavum septum pellucidum** (CSP) is a fluid-filled cavity that is between the membranes that form the septum pellucidum. It is bounded superiorly and anteriorly by the corpus callosum and inferiorly by the fornix. The **cavum vergae** (CV) is a posterior extension of the CSP, and the two begin to fuse from posterior to anterior starting at approximately 24 weeks gestational age. They have no connection with the ventricles and separate the frontal horns of the lateral ventricles, forming their medial margins at the midline of the brain. By term, the CV is closed and the CSP persists in over 85% of infants. By 3 to 6 months of age, there is closure to form a single septum pellucidum in 85% of patients. In a sagittal plane the CSP appears anechoic and comma-shaped and in a coronal plane is triangular in shape.

Thalamus

The **thalamus** is two large, egg-shaped structures, the thalami, that lie on each side of the third ventricle, forming most of its lateral walls. It is homogeneous and mid-gray with medium-level echoes.

Cerebellum

The **cerebellum** is the second-largest portion of the brain and lies immediately posterior to the fourth ventricle, occupying the majority of the posterior fossa of the skull. It is immediately inferior to the occipital and temporal lobes. The cerebellum is composed of symmetric, bilateral hemispheres that are connected by the **vermis** on its medial portion. The parenchyma of the cerebellum is a mid-gray or medium-level echoes. The central echogenic portion of the cerebellum is the vermis.

Cisterna Magna

The **cisterna magna** is the largest expanded subarachnoid space in the brain. It is located at the base of the cerebellum in the posterior portion of the brain. The cavity contains CSF and appears anechoic.

Massa Intermedia

The **massa intermedia** is a pea-shaped, soft tissue structure that is suspended within the third ventricle and has no known function. It is mid-gray with medium-level echoes and is best seen with ventricular dilatation.

Choroid Plexus

The **choroid plexus** is a network of capillaries and specialized ependymal cells that are found in all four ventricles of the brain. The choroid plexus produces CSF and also provides a toxin barrier to the brain and other central nervous system tissues.

The choroid plexus consists of two curvilinear, highly echogenic structures that arch around the thalami anteriorly from the floor of the body of the lateral ventricle and posteriorly to the tip of the temporal horn. Note that the choroid plexus does not extend into the frontal or occipital horns.

Aqueduct of Sylvius

The **aqueduct of Sylvius** is a midline channel that connects the third and fourth ventricles. It is rarely seen sonographically unless dilated.

Foramen of Monro

The **foramen of Monro** is a narrow, midline channel that connects the third ventricle with each lateral ventricle for the passage of CSF. This is an anechoic area just posterior to the level of the frontal horn of each lateral ventricle.

Brainstem

The **brainstem** is a columnar appearing structure that connects the forebrain and the spinal cord. It consists of the midbrain, pons, and medulla oblongata. The brainstem is mid-gray with medium to low-level echoes.

Intrahemispheric Fissure

The **interhemispheric fissure** is a deep groove or indentation separating the right and left cerebral hemispheres. It contains the **falx cerebri**, which are folds of dura mater, CSF, and some midline branches of the anterior cerebral artery and the posterior cerebral artery. The interhemispheric fissure appears as a thin, linear, echogenic, midline structure.

Cerebral Peduncle

The **cerebral peduncle** is a Y-shaped structure inferior to the thalami and fused at the level of the pons. It is a mid-gray with low-level echoes.

Sulci

The **sulci** are grooves separating the gyri on the surface of the brain. The sulci are echogenic, spider-like fissures separating the gyri or folds of the brain. The premature neonate usually has fewer sulci than a full-term infant.

Dura Mater

The dura mater is a flap that separates the cerebral hemispheres from the other structures in the brain. The dura mater is an echogenic structure that is tent-shaped in a coronal plane.

Sylvian Fissure

The **Sylvian fissure** is a groove separating the frontal and temporal lobes of the brain. It resembles an echogenic Y turned on its side. The middle cerebral artery can be seen pulsating here.

Caudate Nucleus

The **caudate nucleus** is located within the concavity of the lateral angles of each lateral ventricle. The caudate nucleus is mid-gray with medium-level echoes.

Germinal Matrix

The **germinal matrix** is a vascular network located in the region of the caudate nucleus and thalamus called the caudothalamic groove. When visualized, it appears small and echogenic. Note that this is the most common site for a subependymal hemorrhage.

Quadrigeminal Plane

The **quadrigeminal plate** is posterior to the third ventricle. It is an echogenic structure immediately superior to the apex of the **tentorium**, resembling the top of a pine tree.

Ultrasound of the Neonatal Brain

Patient Prep

There is no patient prep.

Transducer

A 10–15 MHz curvilinear or phased array transducer is used, with higher frequencies employed for premature infants less than 32 weeks gestation or less than 1500 g. A linear array transducer of 10 to 15 MHz can be used to evaluate the superior sagittal sinus, extra-axial fluid, and midline and para-midline structures. A lower-frequency phased array transducer may be needed for older infants with an open anterior fontanelle.

Patient Position

Usually the infant is scanned in a supine position with the head facing up. The infant may be in a prone position with the head facing to either side. It can be helpful to place a small cloth or towel under and/or beside the baby's head to help immobilize it during the scan.

Technical Tips

The anterior fontanelle, the soft, unossified membrane-covered space between the sutures of the skull at the top of the head, is used as a window to see the cranial structures. The transducer will be angled or pivoted to see the entire brain. The size of the fontanelle may restrict the amount of angulation and anatomy seen, especially in older infants. The posterior fontanelle can be used as needed.

If the baby has a scalp intravenous line, it may be difficult to obtain a complete study. Discuss with the baby's nurse or physician before attempting **anterior fontanelle** views. Images can be obtained by using the posterior fontanelle, transtemporal, and transmastoid windows.

An ample amount of gel is needed so as not to apply too much transducer pressure when scanning. Coupling gel should be at body temperature.

The baby should be disturbed as little as possible and left inside the isolette. Keeping the baby warm is very important for the infant's well-being. If the baby is in a high-oxygen environment, this should be maintained as much as possible.

Hands are washed and gloves and gowns are worn as per hospital policy. The ultrasound system and the transducers should be carefully wiped down with a cleaning agent before and after the scan.

Pay attention to intracranial symmetry. Always use the highest frequency that allows for proper penetration. A lower-frequency transducer may be needed for older babies or tight fontanelles. Some departments may routinely obtain Doppler signals from the anterior cerebral artery and the superior sagittal sinus.

Required Images

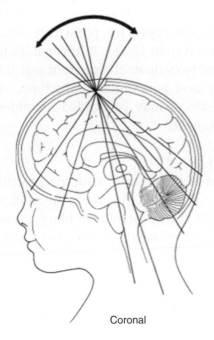

Coronal

Begin with the transducer perpendicular at the anterior fontanelle. The indicator should be toward the patient's right. Angle the transducer toward the face to see the frontal horns and the frontal lobes of the brain. Angle the transducer posteriorly to see the occipital horns and into the occipital lobes of the brain.

Anterior Fontanelle Approach • Coronal Plane

1. An image of the frontal lobes of the brain with the interhemispheric fissure and the orbital ridge.

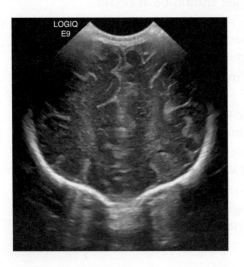

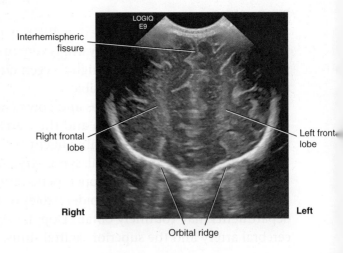

Interhemispheric fissure

Right frontal lobe

Left frontal lobe

Right

Left

Orbital ridge

Suggested annotation: **CORONAL**

2. An image of the frontal horns of the ventricles encompassing the caudate nucleus. Include the germinal matrix adjacent to the ventricles and corpus callosum.

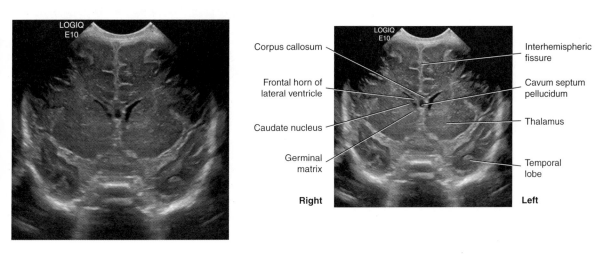

Suggested annotation: **CORONAL**

3. An image of the frontal horns and thalamus including the Sylvian fissures, cavum septum pellucidum, third ventricle, and foramen of Monro.

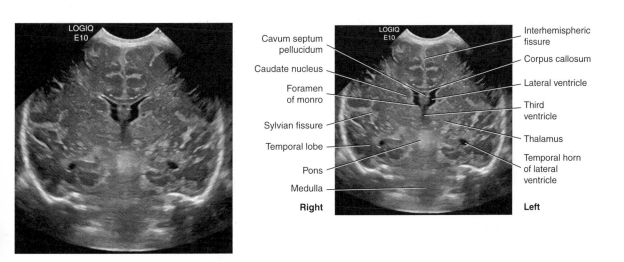

Suggested annotation: **CORONAL**

4. An image of the bodies of the lateral ventricles, thalamus, and Sylvian fissures.

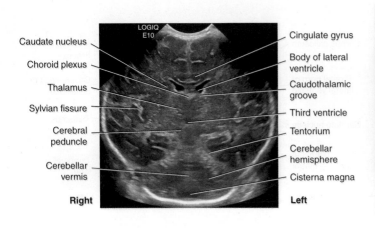

Caudate nucleus
Choroid plexus
Thalamus
Sylvian fissure
Cerebral peduncle
Cerebellar vermis
Right

Cingulate gyrus
Body of lateral ventricle
Caudothalamic groove
Third ventricle
Tentorium
Cerebellar hemisphere
Cisterna magna
Left

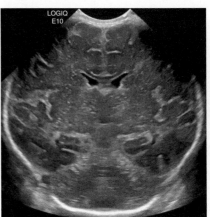

Suggested annotation: **CORONAL**

5. An image of the tentorium, including the Sylvian fissures and the quadrigeminal plate.

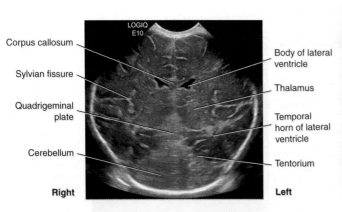

Corpus callosum
Sylvian fissure
Quadrigeminal plate
Cerebellum
Right

Body of lateral ventricle
Thalamus
Temporal horn of lateral ventricle
Tentorium
Left

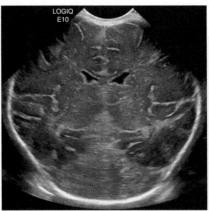

Suggested annotation: **CORONAL**

6. An image of the choroid plexus in the atrium or trigone region.

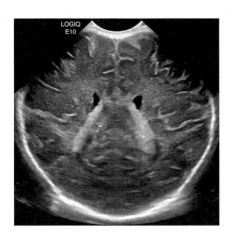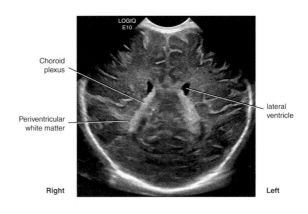

Suggested annotation: **CORONAL**

7. An image of the occipital lobes of the brain.

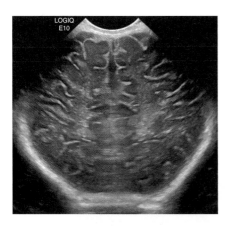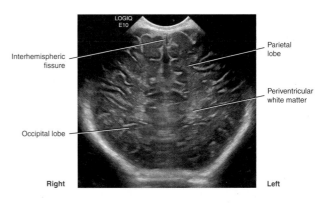

Suggested annotation: **CORONAL**

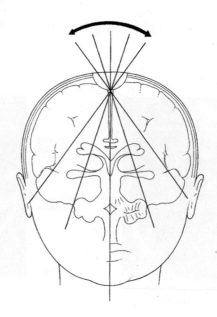

Anterior Fontanelle Approach • Sagittal Plane

1. Begin with the transducer perpendicular at the anterior fontanelle.
2. Angle the transducer laterally toward the right lateral ventricle. The transducer may be slightly oblique to stay truly in long axis to the ventricle and choroid plexus. Scan through the temporal lobe of the brain to the level of the Sylvian fissure.
3. Angle the transducer laterally toward the left lateral ventricle. The transducer may be slightly oblique to stay truly in long axis to the ventricle and choroid plexus. Scan through the temporal lobe of the brain to the level of the Sylvian fissure.

Midline • Sagittal Plane

1. Sagittal midline image of the cavum septum pellucidum, corpus callosum, third ventricle, fourth ventricle, and cerebellum, including the massa intermedia. This image should be perpendicular at the midline.

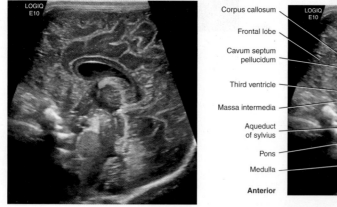

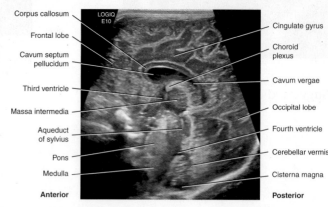

Suggested annotation: **SAG ML**

Right Hemisphere • Sagittal Plane

1. Sagittal image of the right ventricle, germinal matrix, caudothalamic groove, caudate nucleus, thalamus, and choroid plexus. In some patients the frontal horn, body, temporal horn, and occipital horn cannot be imaged in the same plane. Therefore, additional image(s) may be necessary.

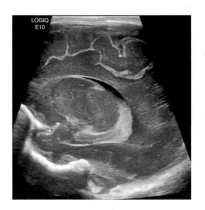 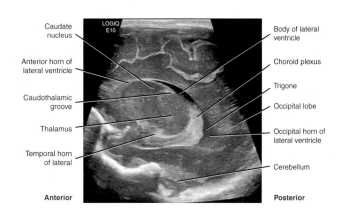

Suggested annotation: **SAG RT**

2. An image of the right temporal lobe of the brain at the level of the Sylvian fissure, including the periventricular white matter.

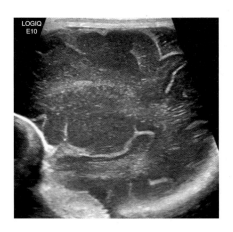 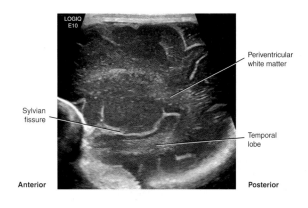

Suggested annotation: **SAG RT**

Left Hemisphere • Sagittal Plane

1. Sagittal image of the left ventricle, germinal matrix, caudothalamic groove, caudate nucleus, thalamus, and choroid plexus. In some cases the frontal horn, body, temporal horn, and occipital horn cannot be imaged in the same plane. Therefore, additional image(s) may be necessary.

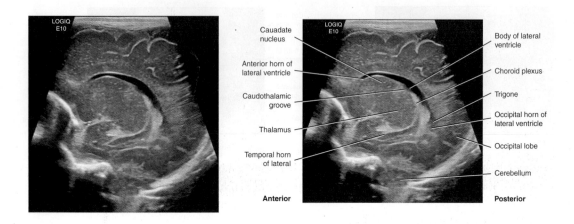

Suggested annotation: **SAG LT**

2. Sagittal image of the left temporal lobe of the brain at the level of the Sylvian fissure, including the periventricular white matter.

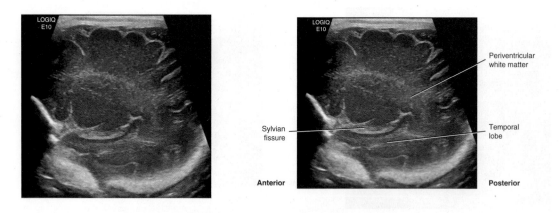

Suggested annotation: **SAG LT**

Additional Images

Alternative axial views through the temporal recess or posterior fontanelle are options to further evaluate the lateral ventricular walls and/or the occipital horns, respectively.

1. Posterior image of the occipital horn of the lateral ventricle and periventricular white matter. View is scanned using the posterior fontanelle.

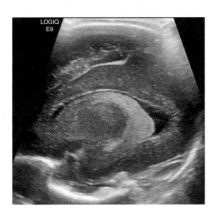 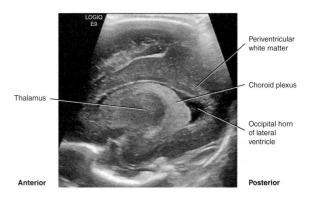

Suggested annotation: **POSTERIOR RT or LT**

2. An axial image of the posterior fossa. Include the cerebellar hemispheres, fourth ventricle, and third ventricle. View is obtained using the mastoid fontanelle.

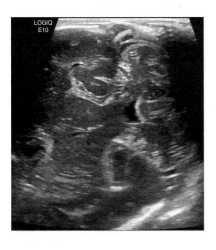 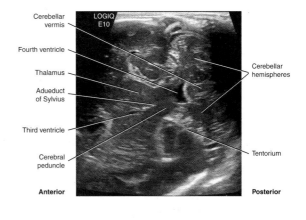

Suggested annotation: **MASTOID RT or LT**

3. Magnified coronal image of the extra-axial fluid space using the anterior fontanelle to include the extra-axial fluid and superior sagittal sinus.

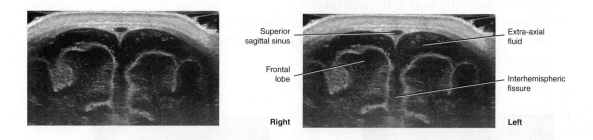

Superior sagittal sinus

Extra-axial fluid

Frontal lobe

Interhemispheric fissure

Right

Left

Suggested annotation: CORONAL

NOTE Use minimal transducer pressure with this view, because pressure can affect measurements of the extra-axial space. Use a high-frequency linear transducer for optimal resolution.

Neonatal and Infant Spine Overview

Scanning of the spinal canal is requested if there is a sacral dimple located above the gluteal crease, skin tags, midline or para-median masses, midline skin discoloration, hair tufts, or hemangiomas. The examination is ordered to evaluate for the presence of a tethered spinal cord or other cord abnormalities, spinal dysraphism, diastematomyelia, or syringomyelia. Scanning should not be performed over open defects or areas of thin skin because there is a risk of infection.

Spinal Anatomy and Sonographic Appearance
Conus Medullaris
The **conus medullaris** is the terminal end of the spinal cord, terminating between T12 and L1 or L2. This tubular, hypoechoic structure with an echogenic linear center is located within the central part of the spinal canal (Fig. 18.1). It gradually tapers down to a tip, where it terminates at the **filum terminale**.

Cauda Equina
The **cauda equina** is a group of nerve roots distal to the conus medullaris that resembles a horse's tail. The cauda equina are thin echogenic linear hair-like structures (see Fig. 18.1) that are seen to freely move with gentle oscillating movements in response to the infant's

cardiac pulsations. They should lie in the dependent portion of the thecal sac.

Filum Terminale

The filum terminale is a fibrous tissue continuation of the conus medullaris with an attachment at the level of the coccyx. It provides a support for the spinal cord.

The filum terminale appears as an echogenic linear structure extending from the tip of the conus medullaris to the level of the coccyx (see Fig. 18.1). It is surrounded by the cauda equina, sometimes making it difficult to separate; however, the filum terminale is more echogenic.

Vertebra

The vertebrae are bony segments that form the spinal column. Each vertebra is made up of an anterior vertebral body and posterior arch. The posterior arch gives rise to the transverse and spinous process. The spine is divided into the 7 cervical vertebrae, 12 thoracic vertebrae, 5 lumbar vertebrae, 5 sacral vertebrae, and the coccyx.

The unossified spine appears hypoechoic, whereas the ossified vertebral components appear echogenic in the near field with posterior shadowing.

Ultrasound of the Neonatal and Infant Spine
Patient Prep

The baby's clothing will have to be removed to allow access to the baby's back and buttocks. Patient prep is geared around the infant's comfort. It is important to remember that infants have difficulty maintaining normal body temperature. The baby should be kept warm

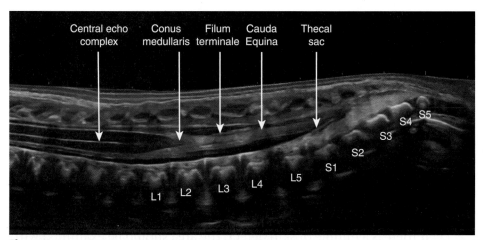

Fig. 18.1 Long axis of the spine and spinal contents. The *arrows* are pointing to a central echo complex and the cauda medullaris, filum terminale, corda equina, and thecal sac. (Courtesy Tara Cielma.)

enough to maintain normal body temperature during the examination, the gel should be warmed, and the room should be kept at a comfortable temperature. It is beneficial for a good examination to have a quiet and still infant. Scanning the baby immediately after feeding or having a pacifier dipped in glucose solution can help keep the baby calm. An infant who is moving and trying to roll over will make for a difficult examination.

Transducer

A high-frequency linear array transducer is needed that allows adequate penetration to fully evaluate the spinal contents. The transducer may be in the 9–18 MHz range.

Patient Position

The baby should be placed in a prone position with a towel or blanket underneath the abdomen and the legs flexed. This is necessary to splay the vertebrae to better visualize the spinal contents. The head should be slightly higher than the feet to better fill the lower CSF space. If needed, the baby can be scanned in a decubitus position with scanning on the back over the spine. If the baby is fussy and will not keep still, consider having the mother lie on the examining table and place the infant on her chest. To protect the mother from gel, place a protective pad between the mother and the child.

Vertebral Body Level

It is important to determine the vertebral body level so the level at which the conus medullaris tip terminates can be determined. A normal conus terminates above L2, and a low conus below the level of L2 is suspicious for a tethered cord. Two methods can be used to determine the **vertebral bodies**. One is to identify the 12th rib as T12 and count down. Another method is to begin counting the sacral vertebral bodies from S5 to the level of S1. The L5-S1 junction can be identified at the inflection point between the more horizontal lumbar vertebrae and the obliquely oriented sacral vertebrae. Some sonographers may do both to verify that they have correctly identified the vertebral bodies. The images should include the numbering of the vertebral bodies adjacent to their structure.

Technical Tips

Because of the association of spinal and renal abnormalities, limited images of both kidneys should be documented.

If there is a dimple or skin defect, the area should be examined with a high-frequency probe to look for a tract between the skin surface and the spinal canal. Minimal pressure should be used so as not to compress and possibly obscure the fistula tract.

A cine loop clip can be used to document abnormal motion of the cord and the corda equina. The cord is normally positioned centrally within the spinal canal, and any deviation from normal should be documented. The vertebral bodies should be evaluated for any abnormalities such as a hemivertebrae.

Required Images
Spine • Sagittal Plane

1. Sagittal midline views of the spine to include the spinal cord, conus medullaris, cauda equina, and numbered vertebrae. The visualized vertebral segments should include the lower thoracic and entire lumbar, sacral, and coccygeal vertebrae.

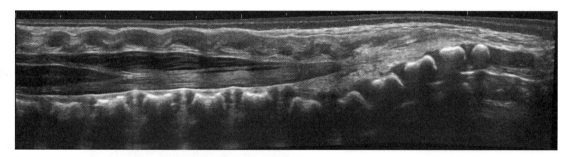

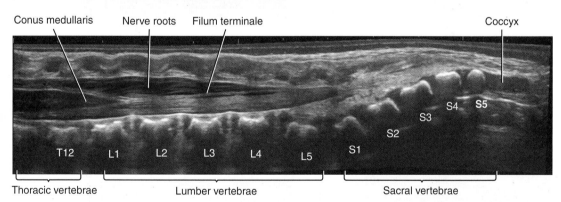

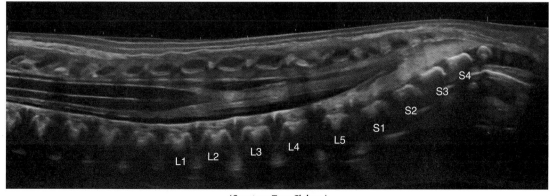

(Courtesy Tara Cielma.)

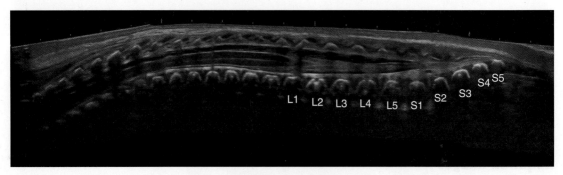

(Courtesy Tara Cielma.)

Suggested annotation: **SAG**

Spine • Transverse Plane

1. Transverse image of the spine, including the spinal cord, transverse processes, and spinous process.

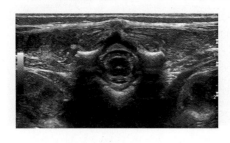 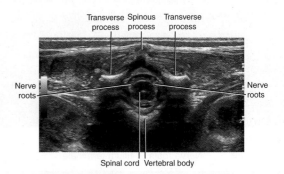

Suggested annotation: **TRANS**

2. Transverse image of the spine, including the conus medullaris and the nerve roots.

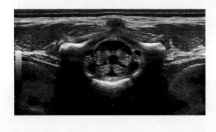 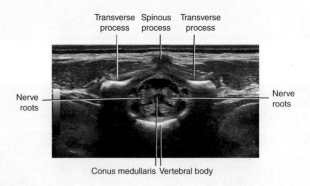

Suggested annotation: **TRANS**

3. Transverse image of the inferior spine, including the cauda equina.

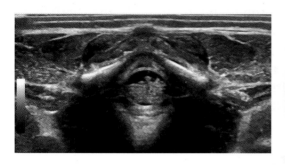
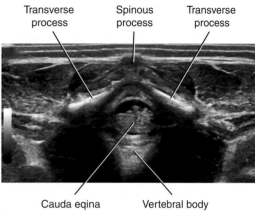

Transverse process · Spinous process · Transverse process

Cauda eqina · Vertebral body

Suggested annotation: **TRANS**

Infant Hip Overview

Developmental dysplasia of the hip (DDH) is one of the most common causes of disability among children. DDH encompasses a variety of pathologic conditions and is a general description that includes dislocation, subluxation, inadequate acetabular development, and morphologically dysplastic hips, among other causes. A normally positioned **femoral head** is covered more than 50% by the **acetabulum**, whereas an infant with DDH will have a shallow acetabulum and decreased coverage of the femoral head.

DDH is more common in girls, Caucasians, and infants with a history of oligohydramnios and affects the left hip more. The ossification centers of the ilium, **ischium**, and **pubis** merge to create the acetabular cup. Ultrasound has the advantage of being able to see the cartilaginous structures, allowing the coverage of the femoral head by the cartilage of the acetabulum and the **labrum** to be evaluated.

With the ability to perform dynamic maneuvers, ultrasound is the test of choice to evaluate an infant for DDH. Some of the indications to perform a study include a frank breech birth, especially if the neonate is female; findings are abnormal or equivocal of hip instability on physical examination; a click sound is heard; findings are positive for the Ortolani or **Barlow maneuver**; and monitoring infants undergoing treatment. Hip ultrasound examinations are usually not performed on patients younger than 6 weeks of age because of the presence of physiologic laxity, unless indicated by an abnormal finding on physical examination.

Allowing infants to eat during the examination can increase their cooperation.

At the time of this publication, there are two CPT codes* for infant hips. The first is 76885, Ultrasound, infant hips, real-time with imaging documentation; dynamic (requiring physician or other qualified health care professional manipulation). The second code is 76886, Ultrasound, infant hips, real-time with imaging documentation; limited, static (not requiring physician or other qualified health care professional manipulation). Both codes cannot be billed on the same day.

Anatomy of the Infant Hip

The hip is a ball-and-socket joint in which the round femoral head is contained within the acetabulum. At birth, the proximal femur and most of the acetabulum are composed of cartilage, which is hypoechoic compared with soft tissue. The cuplike acetabulum is composed of both bone and cartilage and forms at the union of three pelvic bones: the ilium, ischium, and pubis. These structures are joined by the Y-shaped **triradiate cartilage**, which fuses by age 16. The labrum is a rim of soft cartilage that surrounds the acetabulum, adding stability by deepening the socket.

Ilium

The ilium is the most superior part of the pelvis, which, along with the ischium and pubis, forms the acetabulum. The ilium should be horizontal and appears echogenic with posterior shadowing.

Ischium

The ischium is the inferior and posterior portion of the acetabulum. The ischium appears as an echogenic structure deep to the femoral head that appears oval in the coronal plane and longer in the transverse plane.

Pubis

The pubis forms the anterior and inferior portion of the acetabulum. The left and right pubic bones join at the pubic symphysis. The pubis appears as an echogenic structure deep to the femoral head.

Triradiate Cartilage

The triradiate cartilage is a Y-shaped growth plate that connects the ilium, ischium, and pubis to form the acetabulum, or socket of the hip joint. It appears as a hyperechoic structure located between the ischium and pubis.

Labrum

The labrum is a ring of fibrocartilage that helps form and increase the depth of the acetabular hip socket. It is seen as an echogenic triangular structure inside the joint. The labrum is in contact with the femoral head and found lateral and distal to the anechoic hyaline cartilage roof inside the joint capsule.

Acetabulum

The acetabulum is the large cup-shaped cavity on the anterolateral part of the pelvis, which, along with the femoral head, forms the hip joint. It consists of the ilium, ischium, and pubis, which are separated by the triradiate cartilage. The acetabulum unossified components appear hypoechoic and the ossified components appear echogenic with posterior shadowing.

Femoral Head

The femoral head is the cartilaginous portion of the femur that, together with the acetabulum, forms the hip joint. It is a hypoechoic, unossified spherical portion of the femur and contains multiple echogenic speckles. It typically starts to ossify between 2 and 8 months of age.

Hip Maneuvers

Barlow Maneuver

The Barlow maneuver is designed to test and dislocate an unstable hip. The side being evaluated should have the knee flexed approximately 90 degrees, with the knee placed between the thumb and the rest of the fingers. The hip should then be adducted and the knee moved medially while providing pressure posteriorly (Fig. 18.2). The test is considered positive if the femoral head can be popped out of the socket. With a positive test a distinct clunk may be felt as the femoral heads pop out of joint.

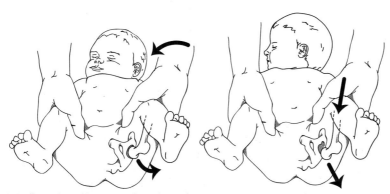

Fig. 18.2 Illustration of how to perform the Barlow maneuver. (From Henningsen C, Kuntz K, Youngs D. *Clinical Guide to Sonography,* 2nd ed. St. Louis, 2013, Mosby.)

Ortolani Maneuver

The **Ortolani Maneuver** is used to confirm the findings of the Barlow maneuver. It is performed immediately after the Barlow maneuver and is designed to identify a dislocated hip by manual reduction. The side being evaluated should have the knee flexed approximately 90 degrees, with the knee placed between the thumb and the rest of the fingers. The hip should then be abducted and the knee moved laterally while gently pulling anteriorly (Fig. 18.3). This maneuver typically reduces or relocates a dislocated hip and is considered positive when a clunk is heard.

Ultrasound of the Infant Hip

Patient Prep

There is no prep for this examination. Keep the baby as warm as possible during the examination of the hips. Feeding the baby during or immediately before the examination may help the baby be more cooperative. Coupling gel should be at body temperature. The diaper can be left on and the scan done with the tab on the side of the diaper opened for access to the hip.

Transducer

A high-frequency linear transducer of at least a 7.5–15 MHz should be used, which allows for adequate penetration and visualization of the soft tissues.

Patient Position

The scan can be done with the baby in the supine position and the baby's feet facing you. The baby can lie in a decubitus position with a pillow or other supporting structure at the baby's back.

Technical Tips

Evaluating infants younger than 4 weeks may create a false-positive result because of normal ligament elasticity. Evaluating infants older

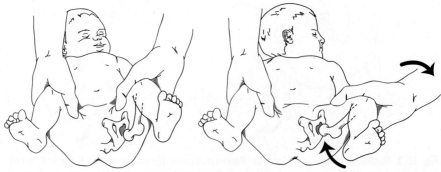

Fig. 18.3 Drawing of how to perform the Ortolani maneuver. (From Henningsen C, Kuntz K, Youngs D. *Clinical Guide to Sonography,* 2nd ed., St. Louis, 2013, Mosby.)

than 6 months may cause the examination to be limited because ossification of the femoral head reduces accuracy.

To evaluate the right hip, have the infant positioned with the head located toward the head of the bed. It may be easier if the transducer is held in the left hand, with the right hand stabilizing the leg.

To evaluate the left hip, hold the transducer with the right hand and stabilize the leg with the left hand. Another option would be to rotate the baby's position to scan each hip with the dominant hand instead of switching hands.

Both hips should be examined using two orthogonal planes, a coronal view in the standard plane at rest and a transverse view of the flexed hip with and without stress, which allows for an assessment of hip position, stability, and acetabular morphology, which is assessed at rest.

To properly measure the alpha and beta angles, the iliac bone echoes must be straight and parallel to the probe.

The stress maneuver, using the posterior push maneuver, is performed to evaluate for hip instability. Stress maneuvers are not performed when the patient is immobilized in a Pavlik harness or splint unless specifically requested.

When scanning the long axis of the femur in a coronal plane, make sure that the side being scanned is properly marked. There is no anatomic clue to differentiate between the right and left hip. When scanning in the transverse plane, the two sides will mirror each other.

Required Images

Scanning is performed from the lateral or posterolateral aspect of the hip. Coronal and transverse views are obtained in each position. For the sake of simplicity, the suggested annotations will say RT or LT. The actual side will be annotated on the image.

Hip • Coronal/Neutral or Flexed Evaluation

1. Also referred to as the standard plane. In this plane the evaluation is made with the leg in neutral position, which is 15 to 20 degrees, slightly flexed or in the flexed position, which is approximately 90 degrees flexed. The transducer should be rotated slightly posterior to display the ilium as a straight line. The femoral head position and coverage should be noted and documented. The acetabular alpha angle may be obtained in this view, which is normally 60 degrees or greater. Evaluation with stress in this plane is optional.

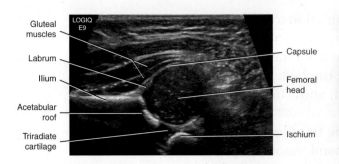

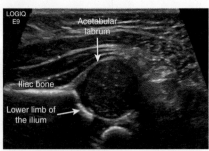

Suggested annotation: **LT CORONAL**

2. Measurement of the alpha and beta angles. A coronal image is needed with the ilium horizontal with a sharp ilium-roof angle and a centrally located, rounded femoral head seen. The ilium is the echogenic linear structure that ends at the femoral head. To measure the angles of the hip, three lines are drawn. The hip-measuring package on the unit will calculate the angles.

a. A horizontal line is drawn parallel along the echogenic line of the ilium.

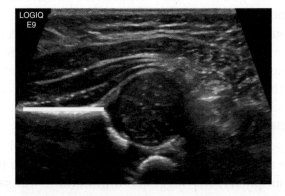

b. A line is drawn from the inferior edge of the osseous acetabulum to the most superior osseus rim.

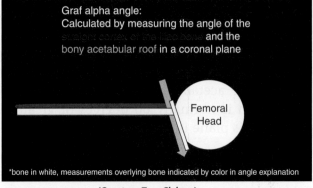

(Courtesy Tara Cielma.)

c. A line is drawn along the roof of the cartilaginous acetabulum from the lateral bony edge of the acetabulum to the labrum.

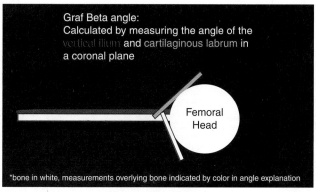

(Courtesy Tara Cielma.)

The intersection of line 1 and line 3 is called the alpha angle. The alpha angle is a measurement of the depth of the acetabulum and is the angle formed between the acetabular roof, line 3, and the ilium, line 1. The normal alpha angle is 60 degrees or greater. The intersection of line 1 and line 2 is called the beta angle. The beta angle is the angle formed between the ilium and the triangular labrum, line 2. It represents the acetabular cartilaginous roof modeling and is normally less than 77 degrees. Modeling is the process by which bone is altered in size and shape during its growth by resorption and formation of bone.

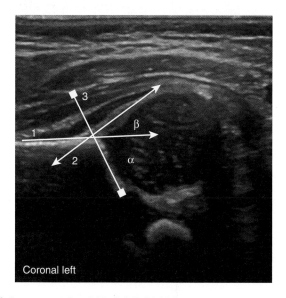

Suggested Annotation: **LT CORONAL**

3. Transverse/flex evaluation. With the leg flexed at 90 degrees, the hip should be evaluated in the transverse or axial plane, which places the transducer parallel to the femoral shaft. The femoral

head should be noted to rest on the ischium. The position of the femoral head should be evaluated at rest with passive abduction and adduction, which is also referred to as the Ortolani and Barlow maneuvers.

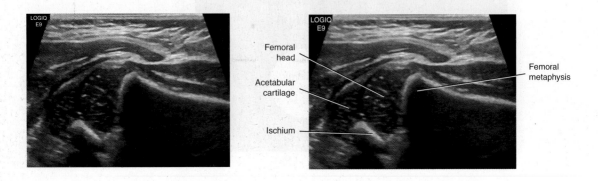

Suggested Annotation: **RT TRV** or **TRANS**

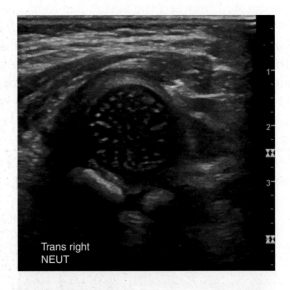

Suggested Annotation: **TRV** or **TRANS RT NEUT** or **NEUTRAL**

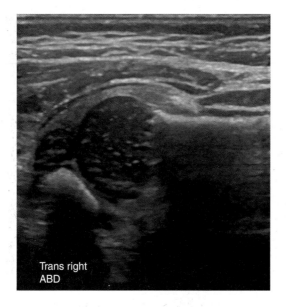

Suggested Annotation: **TRV or TRANS RT ABD or ABDUCTION**

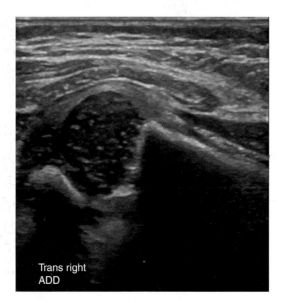

Suggested Annotation: **TRV or TRANS RT ADD or ADDUCTION**

4. Hip evaluation with stress. Evaluation with stress maneuvers can be difficult if the baby is fussy or moving the legs. Muscle activity may inhibit the movement of an unstable hip. Stress should not be performed while evaluating a patient in a Pavlik harness or splint device. Using the Barlow maneuver, the side being evaluated should have the knee flexed approximately 90 degrees, with the knee placed between the thumb and the rest of the fingers. The hip should then be adducted and the knee moved medially while providing pressure posteriorly. This maneuver forces the hip posterior and is best appreciated in real time. Subluxation or dislocation should be noted and documented. The normal views will be the same as the adduction views above. Any dislocation will be documented.

Musculoskeletal Scanning Protocol for Rotator Cuff, Carpal Tunnel, and Achilles Tendon

Ted Whitten

Keywords

Achilles tendon
Anisotropy
Aponeurosis
Biceps tendon
Bicipital groove
Bursae
Carpal tunnel
Crass position
Guyon's canal
Infraspinatus muscle/tendon
Kager's fat pad
Median nerve
Modified Crass position
Neutral position

Plantaris muscle
Retrocalcaneal bursa
Rotator cuff
Subacromial-subdeltoid bursa
Subcutaneous calcaneus bursa
Subscapularis muscle
Subscapularis tendon
Supraspinatus muscle
Supraspinatus tendon
Synovial sheath
Teres minor muscle
Teres minor tendon
Transverse ligament

Objectives

At the end of this chapter, you will be able to:

- Define the keywords.
- Describe the sonographic appearance of muscles, tendons, and ligaments and how to distinguish among them.
- Describe the transducer options for scanning the musculoskeletal system.
- Discuss and describe artifacts unique to musculoskeletal imaging.
- List the suggested patient position when scanning structures in the musculoskeletal system.
- Explain the order and exact locations to take representative images of the structures in the musculoskeletal system.

Overview

Musculoskeletal (MSK) ultrasound studies are performed in a variety of locations. These examinations can be performed in a radiology department, orthopedic department or office, physical therapy, anesthesia, rheumatology, sports medicine, pain management, emergency department and is used by podiatrists. MSK ultrasound studies are performed more commonly outside the United States because American radiologists prefer magnetic resonance imaging (MRI); however, MSK ultrasound is starting to gain some momentum in the United States especially outside of the Radiology department. MSK ultrasound has many advantages over MRI, especially as ultrasound can aid in the diagnosis of abnormalities that are seen only with movement of the joint, referred to as dynamic scanning, and ultrasound also has better spatial resolution. Ultrasound can also view joints from multiple planes and with the joint in different positions, unlike MRI, in which the joint is in one position for the entire scan, perform side-to-side comparisons and provide physiologic information. Ultrasound is also being used to guide joint injections and nerve blocks. Finally, it is easier to obtain an appointment quickly for an ultrasound examination, there are no claustrophobia or metal issues, and it is less expensive than MRI. Some insurance companies are now requiring an MSK ultrasound before an MRI is approved. The limitations of ultrasound are that the bony structures cannot be evaluated beyond the surface, pathologic conditions posterior to bones cannot be seen, the field of view is limited, and the skills of the sonographer and resolution quality of the ultrasound machine affect the results of the examination.

This chapter will be divided into the following three sections: MSK ultrasound of the shoulder, **carpal tunnel**, and Achille's tendon.

Ultrasound of the Shoulder

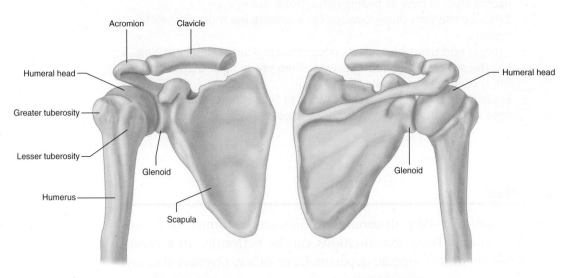

Anterior View   **Posterior View**

From Rumack CM, Levine D. *Diagnostic Ultrasound,* 5th ed. Philadelphia, 2018, Elsevier.

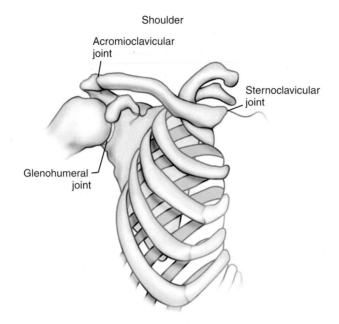

From Miller M, Thompson S. *DeLee, Drez and Miller's Orthopedic Sports Medicine,* Philadelphia, 2019, Elsevier.

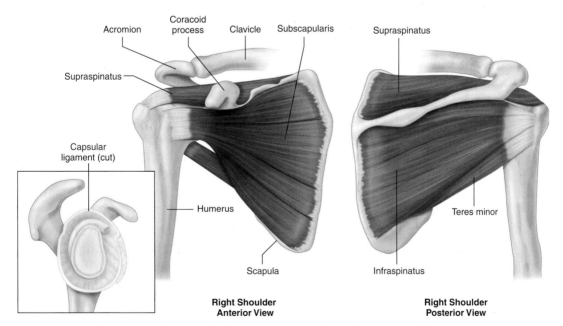

From Rumack CM, Levine D. *Diagnostic Ultrasound,* 5th ed. Philadelphia, 2018, Elsevier.

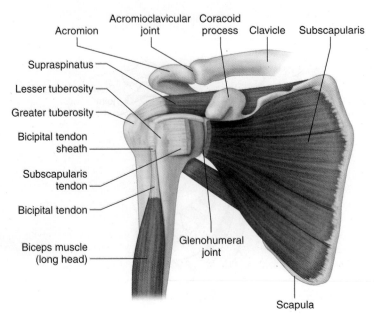

From Rumack CM, Levine D. *Diagnostic Ultrasound,* 5th ed. Philadelphia, 2018, Elsevier.

The most common indication for shoulder ultrasound is to evaluate for **rotator cuff** disease. Other reasons can include evaluating for tendinosis, joint effusion, masses, impingement, and bursitis. Ultrasound can be used in guiding needle aspiration and local injection therapy.

Anatomy

The shoulder is one of the most complex joints in the body, is formed where the humerus fits into the scapula, and is a ball-and-socket joint. The scapula is a large flat bone that has a prominent bony ridge on its posterior surface called the scapular spine. The other bony elements of shoulder anatomy include the acromion, which is a bony process off the scapula; the coracoid process, which is a small hook-like bony projection from the scapula that together with the acromion extends laterally over the shoulder; the clavicle, which meets the acromion in the acromioclavicular joint; and the labrum, which is cartilage that forms a cup in which the ball-like head of the humerus fits.

The primary tendons of the shoulder include the **biceps tendon** and the tendons of the rotator cuff. The rotator cuff comprises muscles and tendons that surround the shoulder, giving it support and stability and allowing a wide range of motion. The rotator cuff consists of four muscles and their corresponding tendons.

1. The **subscapularis muscle** is the largest muscle in the rotator cuff complex and fills the subscapular fossa. The subscapularis is a triangle muscle that originates from the medial two-thirds of the subscapular fossa, draping along the anterior surface of the scapula and inserting by way of the **subscapularis tendon** to the lesser

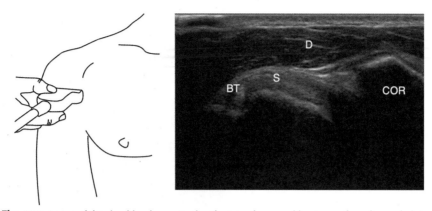

Fig. 19.1 Image of the shoulder demonstrating the transducer position to see the subscapularis tendon. *BT,* Bicep tendon; *COR,* coracoid process; *D,* deltoid muscle; *S,* subscapularis tendon.

tuberosity of the humeral head. The **transverse ligament** is a lateral extension of the subscapularis tendon that covers the anterior aspect of the bicep tendon, which is a landmark for locating rotator cuff anatomy (Fig. 19.1).

2. The **supraspinatus muscle** originates at the supraspinatus fossa and courses along the anterior and superior scapula, inserting by way of the **supraspinatus tendon** to the greater tuberosity. It is the most superior of the four rotator cuff muscles (Fig. 19.2).

3. The infraspinatus is a thick triangular muscle that originates in the infraspinous fossa and courses along the posterior scapular inferior to the supraspinatus, attaching by way of the **infraspinatus tendon** to the greater tuberosity. It is located at the back of the shoulder and occupies most of the dorsal surface of the scapula (Fig. 19.3).

4. The **teres minor muscle** is a cylinder-shaped muscle that originates on the lateral border or the scapula and courses inferior to the **infraspinatus muscle** along the posterior scapula, attaching by way of the **teres minor tendon** to the greater tuberosity (Fig. 19.4).

5. The tendon of the long head of the biceps originates on the superior margin of the supraglenoid tubercle of the scapula to pass through the **bicipital groove** of the humerus to insert on the radial tuberosity. The short head originates from the coracoid process of the scapula and also inserts on the radial tuberosity.

6. The rotator or cuff interval is a tetrahedron-shaped space between the anterior margin of the supraspinatus tendon and the superior edge of the subscapularis tendon and is bounded by the joint capsule anteriorly and the humeral head posteriorly. The rotator interval allows passage of the long head of biceps from the bicipital groove to insert on the glenoid labrum and supraglenoid tubercle (Fig. 19.5).

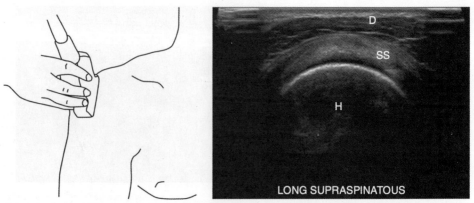

Fig. 19.2 Image of the shoulder demonstrating the transducer position to see the supraspinatus tendon. *D,* Deltoid muscle; *H,* humeral head; *SS,* supraspinatus tendon.

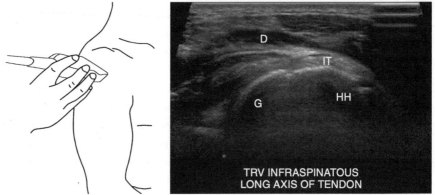

Fig. 19.3 Image of the shoulder demonstrating the transducer position to see the infraspinatus tendon. *D,* Deltoid muscle, *G,* glenoid; *HH,* humeral head; *IT,* infraspinatus tendon.

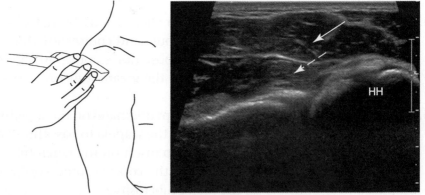

Fig. 19.4 Image of the shoulder demonstrating the transducer position to see the teres minor tendon. *Arrow,* Deltoid muscle; *dashed arrow,* teres minor tendon; *HH,* humeral head.

7. The shoulder contains several **bursae**, which are fluid-filled sacs that are found between skin, bone, tendons, and muscles. The fluid acts as a cushion to decrease friction between the different structures. The bursae in the shoulder include the subscapular,

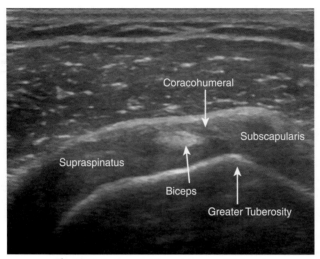

Fig. 19.5 An image of the rotator or cuff interval.

subacromial-subdeltoid bursa, subcoracoid, infraspinatus, and subcutaneous acromial bursae, with the subacromial delta bursa being the largest.

8. Also seen while imaging the rotator cuff is the deltoid muscle. It forms the rounded shape of the shoulder and is called the deltoid as it resembles the triangle shape of the Greek letter delta. It is attached by tendons to the clavicle, the acromion, and the spine of the scapula to insert on the deltoid tuberosity of the humerus. The deltoid is widest at the top of the shoulder and narrows as it travels down the arm. The fibers of the deltoid converge to insert on the deltoid tuberosity on the lateral shaft of the humerus. The deltoid works with the subscapularis to internally rotate the arm and when the arm is rotated medially, the deltoid assists with abduction of the arm. The deltoid is responsible for preventing dislocation of the humeral head while carrying a heavy load. The deltoid assists in other arm movements.

Physiology

The rotator cuff surrounds the shoulder joint, providing stability to the head of the humerus sitting in the glenoid fossa. The tendons provide the attachment for the muscles to the bones. The muscles and tendons creating the rotator cuff aid in movement of the shoulder and the arm.

1. The subscapularis muscle and tendon help with internal rotation and adduction of the arm and stabilize the anterior shoulder.
2. The supraspinatus muscle and tendon help with abduction of the arm.
3. The infraspinatus muscle and tendon help externally rotate the arm.
4. The teres minor muscle and tendon aid in external rotation of the arm with the infraspinatus.

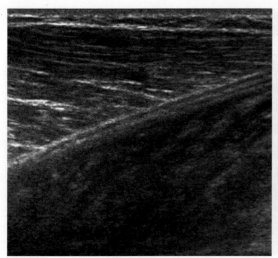

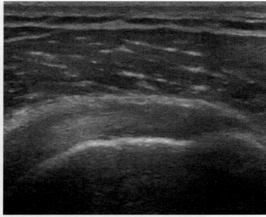

Fig. 19.7 The appearance of normal muscles in their short axis demonstrating the echogenic dot pattern.

Fig. 19.6 The appearance of normal muscles in their long axis demonstrating the feather appearance.

5. The bicep tendon is a noncontractile tendon that directs the humeral head with its motion, provides shoulder stability and support, and helps with flexion and supination of the forearm at the elbow.

Sonographic Appearance

The main function of the muscular system is movement, and the muscles are the only tissue in the body that have the ability to contract and thus move other parts of the body. Muscles are attached to bones by tendons. Muscles are hypoechoic with parallel echogenic lines running through them. They have a compartment-type feature caused by the connective tissue that surrounds the bundles of muscle fibers. Longitudinally, muscles appear fibrillar and have a pennate pattern, causing them to have a feather-like appearance (Fig. 19.6). Transversely, muscles appear as echogenic dots as a result of the perimysium separating the muscle fibers into small bundles (Fig. 19.7). The technique of rotating the transducer to confirm the change from speckled or dots to a striated appearance is helpful in distinguishing muscles from other structures. The **aponeurosis** is the tissue that binds muscle fibers together and aids in the connection to the bone. Sonographically it will appear as a bright reflecting linear structure. The borders of the muscle are easily defined because the epimysium surrounding the muscle is a highly reflective structure.

Tendons connect muscle to bone and have a characteristic sonographic appearance. The tendon is made up of parallel linear fibers that contain a high percentage of collagen and on sonography are seen as multiple echogenic parallel lines that act as specular reflectors. The tendon should be uniform in size and sonographic

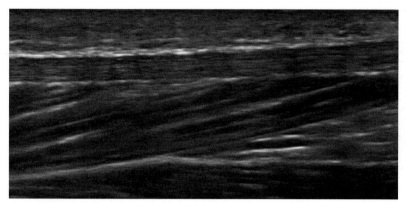

Fig. 19.8 An image of a normal tendon in long axis. Note the echogenic linear lines. A normal muscle is seen below the tendon.

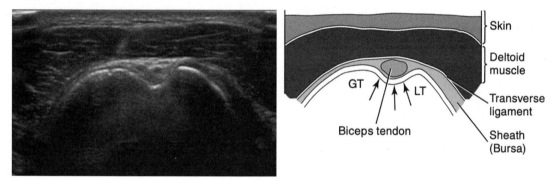

Fig. 19.9 A transverse image through the bicipital groove showing the speckled appearance of the bicep tendon. *GT,* greater tuberosity; *LT,* lesser tuberosity.

appearance (Fig. 19.8). On a transverse scan a tendon shows a bright speckled appearance (Fig. 19.9). Tendons appear mid-gray and have bright reflectors throughout that are hyperechoic to adjacent muscles. Some tendons, such as the bicep tendon, are surrounded by a **synovial sheath**, a membrane or bursa that contains a small amount of fluid or mucinous material, and aids in movement. The fluid will appear as a hypoechoic halo around the tendon (Fig. 19.10). Excess fluid may accumulate during some pathologic processes. There is low vascularity in a normal tendon. The tendon attaches to the bone by a narrow band of fibrocartilage and appears longitudinally as a triangular hypoechoic area in the distal tendon. Thickening of the insertion site can occur when there is injury. Normal tendons display an artifact called **anisotropy**, and this artifact is helpful when trying to locate normal tendons and also may be absent when evaluating an injured tendon. This artifact is dependent on the angle of incidence of the sound beam. When the sound beam is at an oblique angle, a critical angle occurs, and the tendon appears more hypoechoic (Fig. 19.11). When the beam is perpendicular to

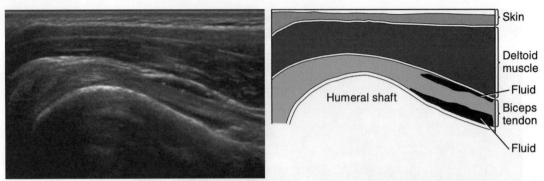

Fig. 19.10 An image demonstrating fluid in the sheath of the bicep tendon. This is an abnormal amount of fluid.

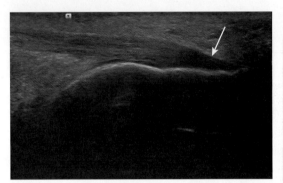

Fig. 19.11 The arrow is pointing to a hypoechoic area of the insertion of the Achilles tendon onto the calcaneus. Because of anisotropy, it appears as if the tendon is detached.

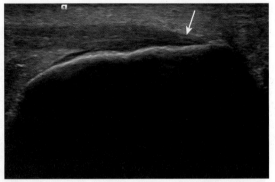

Fig. 19.12 Using a heel-toe maneuver the tendon is now perpendicular to the sound beam, showing that the tendon is normal and intact (arrow).

the imaged tendon, it creates a strong reflection that causes the tendon to be hyperechoic because the fibers are specular reflectors (Fig. 19.12).

Ligaments are thin structures that connect bone to bone and are best imaged by placing the transducer between the two bones. Ligaments appear as bandlike structures with a hyperechoic, striated appearance when imaged perpendicularly (Fig. 19.13) and will look hypoechoic because of anisotropy, like tendons. It may be difficult to see a ligament in a transverse plane because they blend in with the surrounding fat. Ligaments also may be difficult to see if the image is overgained or the time-gain compensation is set incorrectly.

The bursa is a fluid-filled structure and has echogenic borders that will deform with transducer pressure. They are easier to see on ultrasound when there is inflammation with fluid accumulation. If a bursa measures larger than 2 mm, it is considered enlarged and should be compared with the normal contralateral side.

Ultrasound can image the surface of the bone, and the normal bone is seen as a smooth hyperechoic surface with acoustic

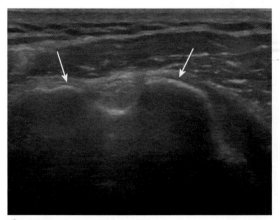

Fig. 19.13 The *arrows* are pointing to the normal transverse ligament.

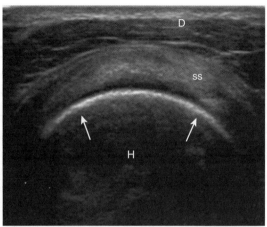

Fig. 19.14 The *arrows* are defining the arc of the head of the humerus. Bone should be bright white and smooth. *D,* Deltoid muscle; *H,* humeral head; *SS,* supraspinatus tendon.

shadowing (Fig. 19.14). Identifying the structures on the bone, such as the trochanter, will aid in evaluating attachment sites. Periosteal elevation or surface irregularity may be seen with trauma, infection, or tumor. Tears and inflammation can cause bone irregularity, and bone erosions can be seen with rheumatoid arthritis.

It is important to document any fluid collections and tears and to determine whether the tear is partial or full thickness. A complete full-thickness rupture will show separation of the two halves of the tendon with tendon retraction and fluid around the tendon. (Fig. 19.15).

Ultrasound of the Shoulder

Patient Prep

No prep is needed except the patient will need to take off clothes that will impede the scanning area. Men, if comfortable, can be shirtless, and women can keep their bra on, or the patient can be asked to wear a tank top style shirt or a type of shirt or top that does not cover the shoulder area. Gowns can be used to cover the patient for their privacy; however, the shoulder being scanned will not be in the sleeve of the gown.

Transducer

A linear array transducer is the transducer of choice because they have the highest frequencies and can image the most area under the transducer. A variety of frequencies may be used depending on the size of the patient's shoulder. Available frequencies should be as low as 5 MHz and up to a high of 18 MHz, with the appropriate frequency used for the best

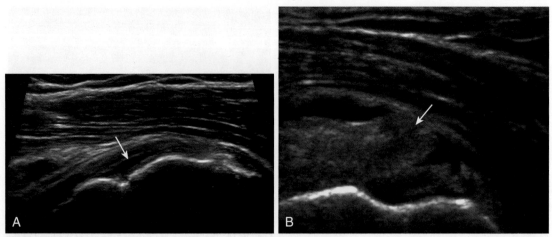

Fig. 19.15 A, The *arrow* is pointing to a partial tear in the bicep tendon. Note how the fluid is not superior to the tendon, which is compatible with a partial tear. **B,** The *arrow* is pointing to the ruptured end of the bicep tendon. Note the fluid above the tendon that is compatible with a full-thickness tear.

resolution on the area being evaluated. There are different transducer widths available, including what is called a "hockey stick" style transducer, and the width needed will be determined by the area being examined. Not every examination will need the transducer changed.

Breathing Technique

The patient will breathe normally during the examination.

Patient Position

The scan is performed with the patient in a sitting position, with the sonographer scanning either in front of or behind the patient. The patient should be on a stool, preferably without wheels, and, if possible, with some type of lower back support. Having the patient sit on a wheeled stool may cause the stool to move while scanning the patient. The patient can also sit on the edge of the stretcher if stable. The sonographer should sit on a stool with wheels to allow easy maneuvering.

It is important for the sonographer to scan in an ergonomic manner to reduce work-related injuries. When possible, the shoulder of the sonographer should be higher than the patient's shoulder, keeping the arm close to the body so as not to induce strain on the arm and shoulder. The editor always recommends holding the transducer at its end like a pencil or computer mouse because this gives the best control of the transducer, and the little finger can help stabilize the transducer and act as the sonographer's eyes while scanning. Holding the transducer like this allows finer motor control (think fulcrum) and takes the strain off the shoulder because the hand will be resting on the patient and not unsupported. Twisting of the sonographer's neck and body should also be avoided.

The arm is moved in different positions to optimize imaging of the various muscles and tendons. The arm positions are with the arm in neutral, external rotation, or in the **Crass position**, in which the dorsal aspect of the ipsilateral hand is placed behind the back, or the **modified Crass position**, in which the ipsilateral hand is placed in the back pocket and elbow extended posteriorly. With the hand in the "back trouser pocket" position, the supraspinatus and infraspinatus tendons can be clearly visualized because the extended and internally rotated position exposes the important distal end of the tendons from under the acromion. In the second part of the examination the patient's hand is placed on the ipsilateral thigh with the palm facing upward.

Technical Tips

The sonographer should develop a routine to follow to ensure the entire shoulder is scanned. Each step of the routine should identify the muscle or tendon of interest, scan the area in long- and short-axis planes, eliminate any artifacts, and document any pathologic condition.

Imaging of the shoulder can appear daunting at first. Like any aspect of ultrasound, it is important to learn the normal anatomy of the joint being scanned and to be able to tell the difference sonographically among muscles, tendons, and ligaments. If there is time during the day, scan yourself or a co-worker. Do not be embarrassed to scan with an anatomy book when first performing MSK examinations. Explain to the patient the complexity of the muscles and that the book is just a reference guide.

Understand the artifacts associated with MSK ultrasound. Because some tendons are curved, anisotropy may be present in that portion of the tendon that is not perpendicular to the soundbeam, therefore heel-to-toe rocking of the transducer is used to show the normal appearance of the tendon so that a tear or hematoma is not falsely diagnosed. Like with any aspect of ultrasound, pathologic findings should be documented in two planes.

Transducer orientation can get confusing while scanning. Check that orientation is correct when changing transducer positions.

The position of the arm will be important to properly evaluate the tendon. For example, it is important that the acromion is positioned so that the supraspinatus can be fully visualized.

Shoulder Required Images*

The tendons and muscles will not be in a true longitudinal or transverse plane but will usually be in an oblique plane. Like the pancreas, the long axis of some tendons will be with the transducer in a "transverse" appearance on the body and in a "longitudinal" position for the short axis. Because of this the anatomy is annotated long axis and short axis as opposed to long and transverse. The image should be marked RT for right and LT for left. Put the name of the muscle first so that you can backspace to change from long axis (LAX) to short axis (SAX).

1. *Biceps tendon short axis.* The patient should be sitting with the arm in a **neutral position** resting on the thigh with the hand facing upward. Begin with the transducer in a transverse orientation just inferior to the humeral head to demonstrate the biceps tendon within the bicipital groove of the humerus between the greater and lesser humeral tuberosities. The tendon appears as a mid-gray, ovoid structure with medium- to high-level echoes that are hyperechoic compared with the deltoid muscle. It may be normal to see a very small amount of anechoic fluid surrounding the tendon. The transverse ligament appears as a bright band sandwiched between the deltoid muscle anteriorly and biceps tendon posteriorly.

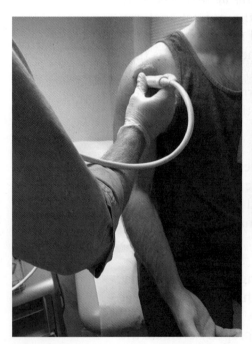

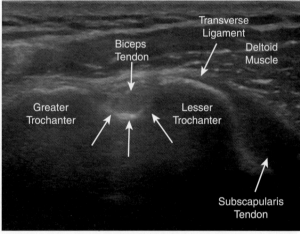

Suggested annotation: **BICEPS SAX.** The three arrows are outlining the bicipital groove.

---

*Images in this section courtesy Blake Randles.

2. *Biceps tendon long axis.* Rotate the transducer 90 degrees into the longitudinal plane to image the full length of the biceps tendon to demonstrate the tendon anterior to the humeral shaft and posterior to the deltoid muscle. Take note of the consistent architecture of the bicep tendon as any disruption is indicative of an abnormality.

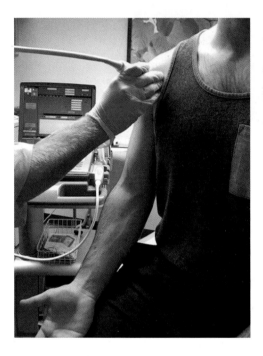

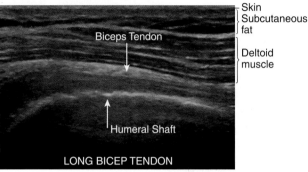

Suggested annotation: **BICEPS LAX or LONG**

3. *Subscapularis long axis.* The patient should begin with the arm in a neutral position.

Return the transducer to the transverse orientation and image the biceps tendon, then move the transducer slightly superior and medial toward the humeral head, to image the long axis of the subscapularis tendon. The long axis of the subscapularis tendon appears as a fibrillar band of medium-level echoes posterior to the deltoid muscle. The subscapularis is perpendicular to the long head of the biceps; therefore short axis and long axis are opposite to those of the biceps. Dynamic evaluation with the patient moving from internal to external rotation will help evaluate for biceps tendon subluxation, subcoracoid impingement, and to completely assess the subscapularis tendon.

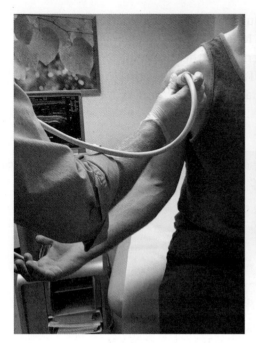

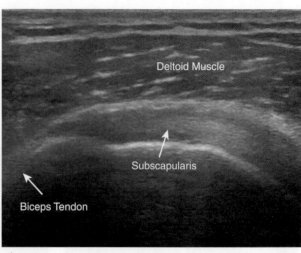

Suggested annotation: **SUBSCAP LAX**

4. *Subscapularis short axis.* With the patient still in the neutral position, rotate the transducer 90 degrees into the longitudinal plane. The subscapularis tendon will be seen in short axis just anterior to the humeral head.

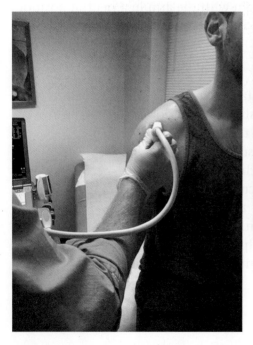

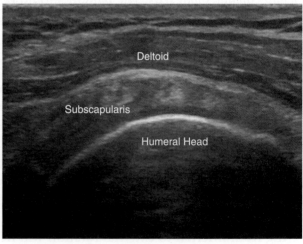

Suggested annotation: **SUBSCAP SAX**

5. *Supraspinatus long axis.* The patient should be placed into the Crass position, with the dorsal aspect of the ipsilateral hand placed behind the back, or the modified Crass position, with the ipsilateral hand in the back pocket and elbow extended posteriorly. Most references recommend using the modified Crass position because this pulls the supraspinatus tendon out from under the acromion for better visualization, offers a better view of the rotator interval, and is usually more comfortable for the patient. Orient the transducer approximately 45 degrees between the sagittal and transverse planes to obtain a longitudinal view. The medial edge of the transducer will be pointing in the direction of the patient's ear. In this oblique scanning orientation, move the transducer laterally, superiorly, and slightly posteriorly to fully evaluate the tendon. The long axis of the supraspinatus tendon can be evaluated just anterior to the echogenic line of the humeral head.

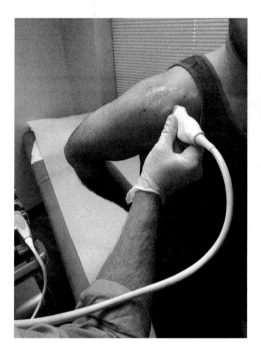 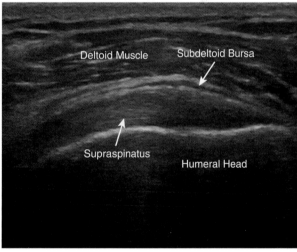

Suggested annotation: **SUPRASP LAX**

6. *Supraspinatus short axis.* Maintaining the Crass or modified Crass position, the supraspinatus tendon should be evaluated in a transverse plane by rotating the transducer 90 degrees from the previous position. Scan superiorly to inferiorly. The biceps tendon will be medial on the patient. The critical zone is an area approximately 8 to 15 mm from the insertion of the tendons onto the greater tuberosity and is about 1 cm lateral and posterior to the bicep tendon. The critical zone is an area of frequent tears, especially with the supraspinatus.

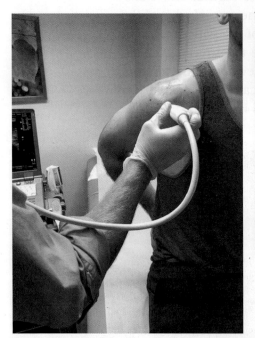
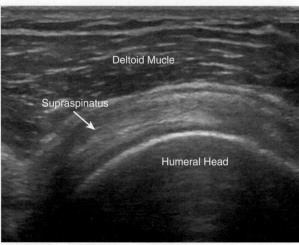

Suggested annotation: **SUPRASP SAX**

7. *Infraspinatus long axis.* Return the patient's arm to their lap, palm up, for the neutral position. Place the transducer just below the scapular spine, turn the transducer to an oblique axial plane to align with the infraspinatus tendon, and evaluate the insertion site on the greater tuberosity. Be careful not to confuse the insertion site with that of the teres minor. The transducer will seem to be in a transverse position for the long axis and in a longitudinal position for the short axis. Move the transducer posteriorly, medially, and laterally just inferior to the spine of the scapula to evaluate the entire tendon. The deltoid muscle is anterior to the echogenic-appearing infraspinatus tendon. The echogenic lines of the humeral head and scapula are posterior. Internal and external rotation or movement from neutral to hand reaching to opposite shoulder can be used for identification and evaluation. This position also can be used to evaluate the posterior labrum, the spino-glenoid notch, and the posterior glenohumeral joint.

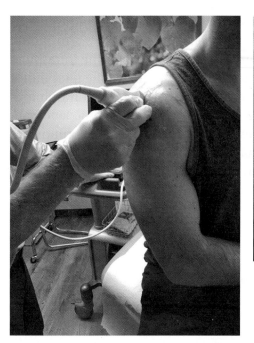
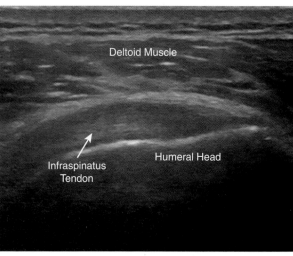

Suggested annotation: **INFRASP LAX**

8. *Infraspinatus short axis.* Turn the transducer 90 degrees to an oblique longitudinal orientation. The infraspinatus tendon is seen between the medially placed glenoid and the laterally placed humeral head. If the distal tendon is difficult to evaluate, have the patient grab the other shoulder because this will pull it anterior for better visualization.

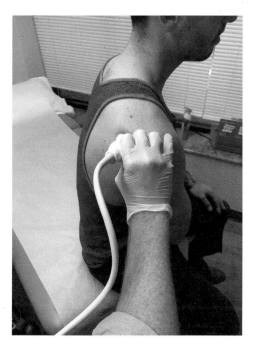
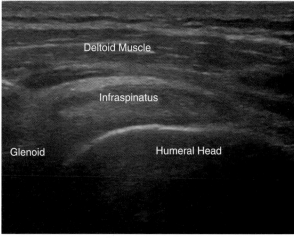

Suggested annotation: **INFRASP SAX**

9. *Teres minor.* The teres minor is seen while imaging the infraspinatus and will be inferior to the infraspinatus. The patient's arm should be in the neutral position. From the midportion of the infraspinatus muscle, glide the transducer caudally to image the teres minor muscle in its short axis. A bony ridge separates the infraspinatus from the teres minor and can be used as a sonographic landmark to differentiate between these two muscles. The teres minor has an appearance similar to that of the infraspinatus but should be approximately 50% smaller. Turn the transducer 90 degrees to image the trapezoidal shaped tendon in its long axis evaluating its insertion on the greater tuberosity. The humeral head will be lateral and the deltoid muscle anterior to the teres minor tendon.

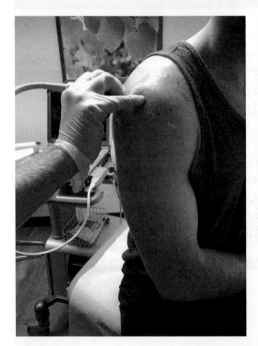
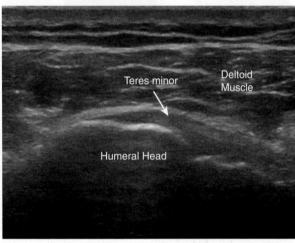

Suggested annotation: **TERES MINOR or TERES MIN or TM**

10. *Acromioclavicular (AC) joint.* With the arm dangling by the patient's side, place the transducer in a transverse plane at the apex of the shoulder over the acromion and distal clavicle to examine the AC joint for arthritis, infection, or trauma by sweeping the transducer anteriorly and posteriorly. The AC joint is the hypoechoic space between the clavicle and acromion, and the space should be less than 5 mm and not differ more than 2 to 3 mm between sides. Power Doppler can be used to evaluate for hyperemia. From this position move the transducer laterally and identify the supraspinatus and acromion. To evaluate for impingement, observe the motion of the supraspinatus under the acromion looking for snapping or catching. To document normalcy or abnormal motion, document with a video clip.

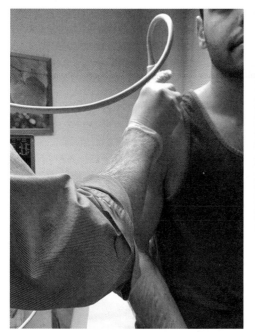
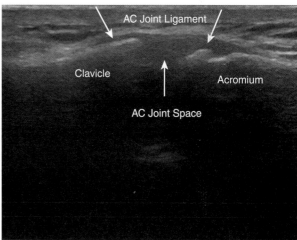

Suggested annotation: **AC JOINT**

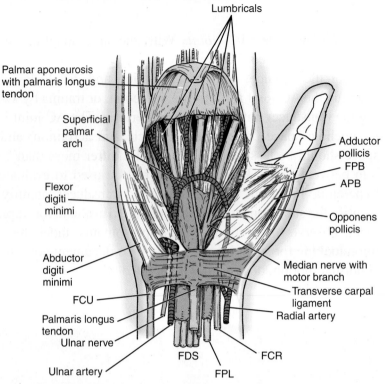

From Trumble TE, Rayan GM, Baratz ME, Budoff JE, Slutsky DJ. *Principles of Hand Surgery and Therapy*, 3rd ed. Philadelphia, 2017, Elsevier.

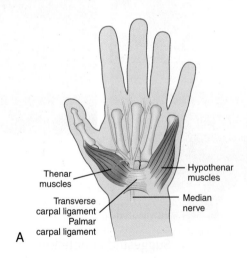

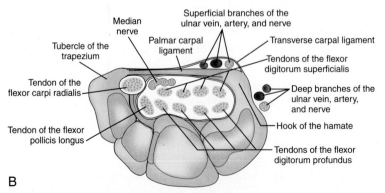

From Ferri F. *Ferri's Clinical Advisor 2020*. Philadelphia, 2020, Elsevier.

The carpal tunnel region is located along the mid-wrist proximal to the crease toward the forearm and distal to the wrist crease toward the fingers. The carpal tunnel houses bones, tendons, nerves, ligaments, muscles, and vessels, all providing the hand with the ability to function properly. Carpal tunnel syndrome (CTS), or **median nerve** compression, is one of the most common nerve entrapments and causes pain, numbness, weakness, and tingling in the hand and wrist that is felt by all the fingers except the little finger because it does not receive a branch of the median nerve. It is caused by the median nerve being compressed as it travels through the carpal tunnel. CTS is diagnosed by physical examination, electromyography (EMG) test, and nerve conductive velocity test (NCS), which is a painful test that helps confirm the diagnosis and can help determine the severity of CTS. Ultrasound can be used to diagnose CTS and is noninvasive and painless.

Anatomy

The carpal tunnel consists of a bundle of tendons coursing from the flexor muscles in the forearm through the wrist and into the hand. At the level of the mid-wrist, the superficial border to the tunnel is the transverse carpal tunnel ligament or flexor retinaculum. The tendons coursing through the tunnel are divided into two groups. The more posteriorly situated tendons originate from the flexor digitorum profundus muscle in the forearm and travel through the tunnel to the fingers as the flexor profundus tendons. The anteriorly placed tendons originate from the flexor digitorum superficialis muscle in the forearm and travel through the tunnel also to the fingers as the flexor superficialis tendons. The muscle and tendon aiding the thumb originate from the flexor pollicis longus muscle on the radial side of the forearm (Fig. 19.16). The tendons are all covered by a synovial sheath.

The carpal tunnel is a narrow passageway that protects the median nerve and is formed by the bones in the wrist and the flexor retinaculum on the palmar side through which pass the median nerve, flexor tendons, and tendon sheaths. The carpal tunnel is rigid and has very little ability to stretch. The ulnar nerve goes through **Guyon's canal**, which is formed by the hook of the hamate and pisiform bones.

Nerves are the conduits for impulses between the muscles and the central nervous system with muscle action controlled by the nerves. The nerve fibers are arranged into bundles called fasciculi and surrounded by dense insulating sheaths of myelin cells and connective tissue. The median nerve runs just anteriorly to the bundle of tendons and slightly toward the radial edge. The transverse carpal tunnel ligament or flexor retinaculum covers the tunnel transversely just anterior to the median nerve. The nerve is naturally elliptical and will flatten slightly as it courses distally into the hand.

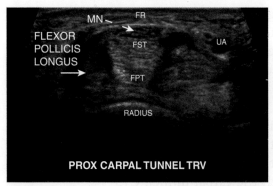

Fig. 19.16 The anatomy of the carpal tunnel showing the flexor pollicis longus muscle. *FPT,* flexor pollicis tendon; *FR,* flexor retinaculum; *FST,* flexor superficialis tendon; *MN,* median nerve; *UA,* ulnar artery.

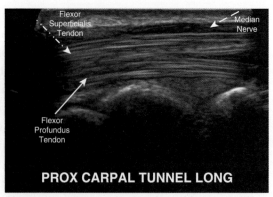

Fig. 19.17 A long axis of the tendons and median nerve in the proximal carpal tunnel.

The proximal carpal tunnel is located just before the crease in the wrist on the side of the forearm. Here, with the hand supinated, at the proximal region the pisiform stands as the bony landmark on the medial edge, scaphoid on the lateral edge, and lunate posteriorly. The profundus and superficialis tendons and median nerve are midline (Fig. 19.17). The flexor pollicis tendon courses laterally along the border of the scaphoid, and the ulnar nerve and artery course along the medial edge adjacent and slightly anterior to the pisiform border. The carpal tunnel anatomy is draped anteriorly by the flexor retinaculum.

The distal tunnel is located just past the crease in the wrist and is distinguished by the bony landmarks of the hamate medially, trapezium laterally, and capitate posteriorly. The profundus and superficialis tendons continue along the middle of the tunnel, with the flexor pollicis tendon far laterally along the border of the trapezium. The median nerve continues its course anteriorly and slightly laterally (Fig. 19.18). All of these structures continue to be draped anteriorly by the flexor retinaculum.

Physiology

The carpal tunnel houses the tendons that connect the muscles in the forearm to each of the digits in the hand. These tendons aid in movement of the fingers. Nerves coursing through the carpal tunnel, including the prominent median nerve, provide sensation and muscle function to the thumb, index finger, middle finger, and medial side of the ring finger. These structures are surrounded by a tunnel of bones that provide stability, not only for the structures inside the carpal tunnel but to the entire wrist and hand. The ulnar nerve goes to the little finger and to lateral side of the ring finger on both the palm and back side of the hand.

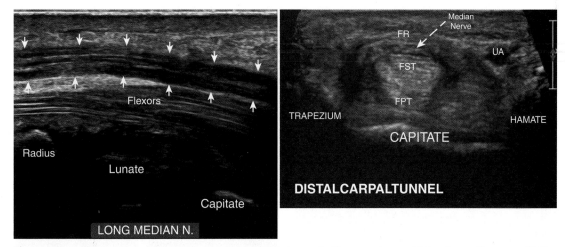

Fig. 19.18 A, The anatomy of the proximal carpal tunnel in long axis. The *arrows* are outlining the median nerve. **B,** The anatomy of the distal carpal tunnel in transverse. *FPT,* flexor pollicis tendon; *FR,* flexor retinaculum; *FST,* flexor superficialis tendon; *UA,* ulnar artery.

Sonographic Appearance

The tendons run midline through the carpal tunnel and will appear hypoechoic compared with adjacent structures and will move with flexion of the fingers. Sonographically, nerves look similar to tendons, but their nerve fibers are not as tightly packed and show less anisotropy (Fig. 19.19). The longitudinal image of a nerve shows parallel inner linear echoes similar to those of the tendon. The median nerve courses anterior to the tendons and will be hypoechoic relative to adjacent structures. On transverse views the median nerve will have a honeycomb-type appearance and the shape may be slightly elliptical with a thin hyperechoic ring seen around the periphery (Fig. 19.20).

Ultrasound of the Carpal Tunnel

Patient Prep

No patient prep is needed except that the patient should wear a short-sleeve or three-quarter sleeve shirt so that there is no shirtsleeve or cuff covering the wrist.

Transducer

A high linear array transducer with a frequency range of 10–18 MHz should be used. These studies are best performed with a small-width or footprint transducer. A hockey stick style transducer is good for these examinations.

Breathing Technique

The patient can breathe normally during the test.

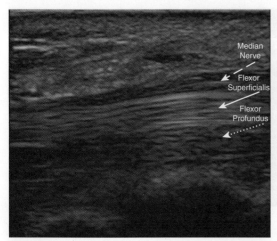

Fig. 19.19 A long axis of the normal median nerve and tendons of the wrist showing their sonographic appearance and relationship to each other and the surrounding anatomy.

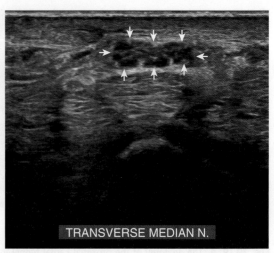

Fig. 19.20 A transverse image of the median nerve showing the hyperechoic border and the internal honeycomb appearance. The *arrows* are outlining the nerve.

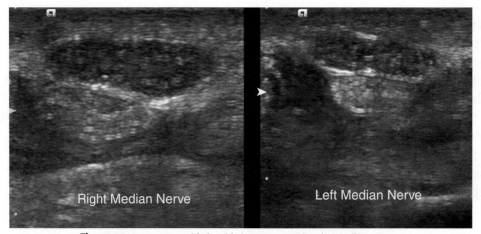

Fig. 19.21 A transverse side-by-side image comparing the median nerves.

Patient Position

The patient should be sitting with the arm at 90 degrees and the palm facing up in a resting position on a stable surface. A rolled towel placed under the wrist can add stability and aid with neutral positioning of the anatomy.

Technical Tips

The sonographer can be seated opposite the patient. Both wrists can be placed on the examination stretcher to easily allow side-to-side comparison (Fig. 19.21). A lot of gel, preferably thick, may be required because of the contours of the wrist and hand.

When measuring the median nerve, a cross-sectional area should be obtained, and according to the literature, the upper limits of normal ranges are between 9 and 12 mm². Another method of determining carpal tunnel syndrome is to measure the difference in median nerve area proximally at the pronator quadratus and distally at the carpal tunnel, with a diagnostic difference of 2 mm² or greater.

Carpal Tunnel Required Images

The image should be marked RT for right and LT for left. It is important that the side is properly labeled, as it is very difficult to tell the right from the left side on the images. Since the views are in traditional looking logitudinal and transverse planes, some sonographers may label the images as LONG and TRV as opposed to LAX and SAX.

Carpal Tunnel • Transverse Images

Start at the distal radius and ulna and scan through both rows of the carpal bones to the base of the palm.

1. Transverse image of the proximal carpal tunnel and median nerve.

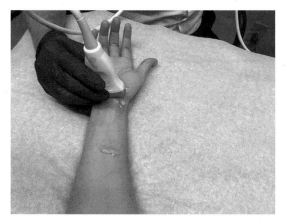 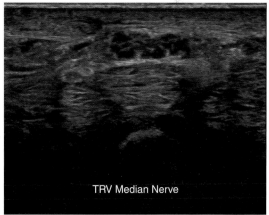

TRV Median Nerve

Suggested annotation: **TRV CARPAL TUNNEL or TRV MED NERVE**

2. Transverse image of the distal carpal tunnel and median nerve.

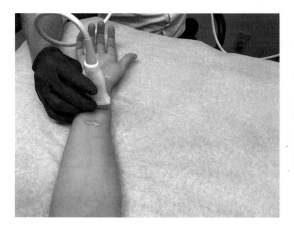 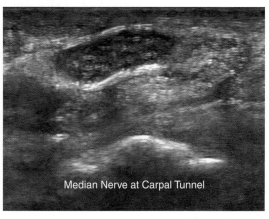

Median Nerve at Carpal Tunnel

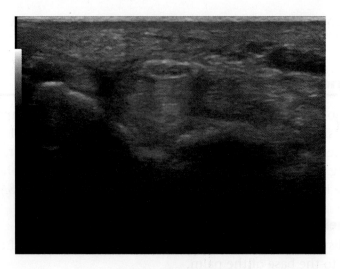

Suggested annotation: **TRV CARPAL TUNNEL or TRV MED NERVE**

3. Sagittal images of the median nerve from proximal to distal.

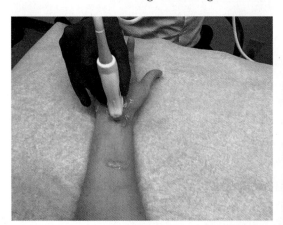

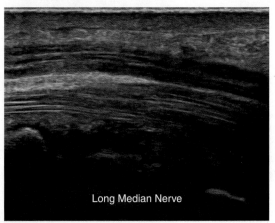

Long Median Nerve

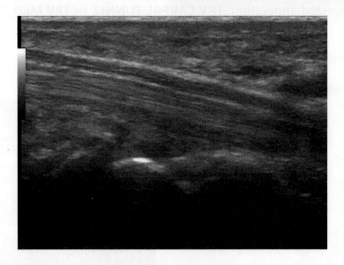

Suggested annotation: **SAG CARPAL TUNNEL or SAG MED NERVE**

Ultrasound of the Achilles Tendon

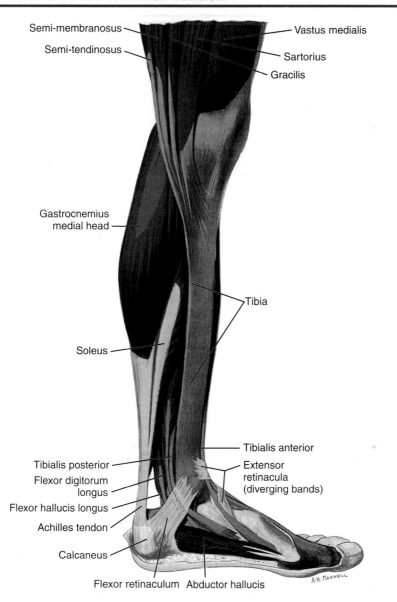

Semi-membranosus

Semi-tendinosus

Vastus medialis

Sartorius

Gracilis

Gastrocnemius
medial head

Tibia

Soleus

Tibialis anterior

Tibialis posterior

Extensor
retinacula
(diverging bands)

Flexor digitorum
longus

Flexor hallucis longus

Achilles tendon

Calcaneus

Flexor retinaculum Abductor hallucis

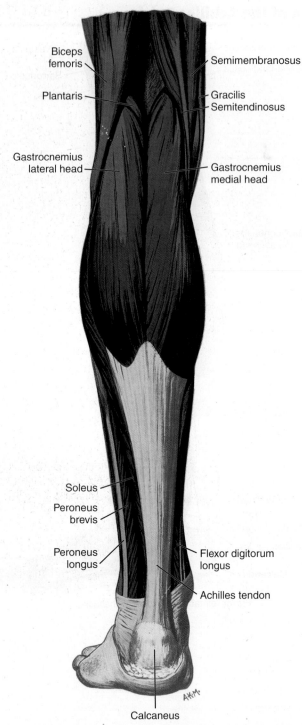

From Jacobson JA. *Fundamentals of Musculoskeletal Ultrasound,* ed 3. Philadelphia, 2018, Elsevier.

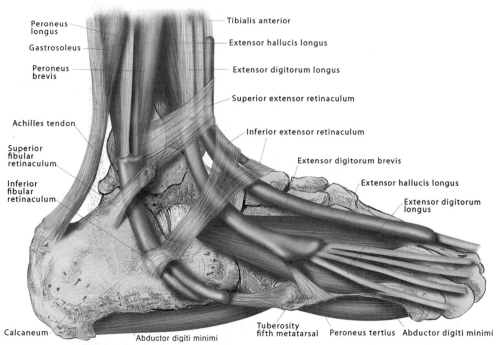

From Pope T, Bloem H, Beltran J, Morrison W, Wilson DJ. *Musculoskeletal Imaging,* 2nd ed. Philadelphia, 2015, Saunders.

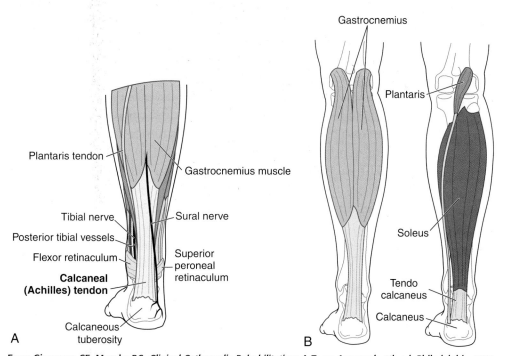

From Giangarra CE, Manske RC. *Clinical Orthopedic Rehabilitation: A Team Approach,* 4th ed. Philadelphia, 2018, Elsevier.

The **Achilles tendon** is the largest weight-bearing tendon of the body and is named after a figure in Greek mythology. Achilles was dipped in the waters of the river Styx as an infant, to make him invulnerable, except where he was held by his heel, resulting in a vulnerable spot. During the Trojan war, Paris shot Achilles in his heel with a poisoned arrow, resulting in Achilles' death. Injury to the Achilles tendon can make it difficult to walk without pain. Because there is a limited blood supply to the Achilles tendon, it has an increased risk for injury and a slow healing process. It is located at the back of the lower leg and is the thickest tendon in the human body; it is used to jump, walk, run, and stand on the balls of the feet. Excessive walking or exercise can cause tendonitis, especially in athletes, as can wearing poorly fitting shoes, sudden stops and changes in direction, not properly warming up, and wearing high heels. Abnormalities of the Achilles tendon include inflammation, rupture, and degeneration. Symptoms include pain or swelling around the tendon.

Anatomy

The Achilles tendon is about 6 to 10 inches long and connects the calf muscles to the calcaneus. The insertion of the Achilles tendon is positioned along the posterior calcaneus bone. The Achilles tendon continues to course along the posterior lower leg until it forms with the gastrocnemius and soleus calf muscles located in the mid to upper posterior lower leg. The Achilles tendon connects the lateral and medial gastrocnemius calf muscles and the soleus calf muscle to the calcaneus or heel bone. It does not have a tendon sheath, but rather a loose connective tissue surrounding it called the paratenon.

There are two bursae present, with one anterior and the other posterior to the tendon at the level of the calcaneus, that act as cushion pads. The **subcutaneous calcaneus bursa** sits along the posterior heel superficial to the tendon and is sometimes referred to as the retro-Achilles bursa and does not always contain fluid. The **retrocalcaneal bursa** is located between the posterior and superior aspect of the calcaneus bone and the Achilles. This bursa should normally contain fluid, which can make for easier identification.

Kager's fat pad is an area of fatty tissue located just posterior to the Achilles tendon that slides against the bursa and tendons to distribute the load of the body evenly through the tendon.

The posterior and superior edge of the calcaneus bone forms the inferior border, whereas the retrocalcaneal bursa will be located along the most inferior and posterior edge.

The plantaris muscle originates from the posterior aspect of the lateral femoral condyle. This very small, thin muscle then transitions into a very long and thin tendon that inserts into the medial aspect of the inferior Achilles tendon or may attach independently into the medial aspect of the calcaneus. Absence of this muscle is a normal variant. This muscle also may be intact in the presence of a full-thickness tear of the Achilles tendon.

Physiology

The Achilles tendon is the strongest tendon in the body and is able to receive a stress load about four times the body weight while walking and about eight times when running. The tendon aids in the movement of the foot downward and the ability to put weight and balance on the toes, which are necessary for walking and running motions. This tendon helps move the foot downward, push off when walking, and rise up on the toes.

Sonographic Appearance

In the longitudinal plane the Achilles tendon appears as a fibrillar pattern of thin echogenic lines having uniform thickness throughout the midsection. Distally at the muscle interface and proximally at the insertion, the tendon will become narrower. A thin echogenic border surrounds the tendon.

At the insertion point the echogenic border of the calcaneus bone will be seen posteriorly.

As the tendon continues superiorly up the leg and gets closer to the muscle interface, it will begin to appear less prominent and blend in with the surrounding muscular structure.

With dorsiflexion and plantar flexion of the foot the tendon will move in a sliding motion, which can be helpful for identification. At the midsection the tendon should measure between 4 to 6 mm in the anteroposterior dimension (Fig. 19.22). Transversely the tendon will appear elliptical and possibly slightly concave, with the same fibrillar pattern and thin echogenic rim (Fig. 19.23).

The retrocalcaneal bursa can be identified along the deep edge of the calcaneus bone by the small pocket of hypoechoic fluid

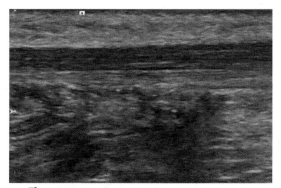

Fig. 19.22 The normal Achilles tendon in long axis.

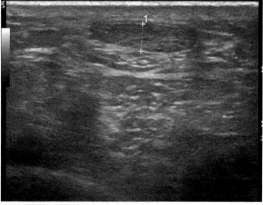

Fig. 19.23 A transverse image of the Achilles tendon with the anteroposterior dimension being measured.

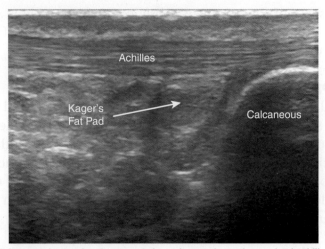

Fig. 19.24 A long-axis image showing Kager's fat pad, posterior to the proximal Achilles tendon and superior to the calcaneus.

surrounding it. Kager's fat pad adjacent to this bursa and just posterior to the Achilles tendon is more echogenic than the surrounding tissue and has an irregular shape on ultrasound (Fig. 19.24).

Ultrasound of the Achilles Tendon

Patient Prep
No patient prep is required. The patient, if not in shorts or a skirt, may need to remove his or her pants so that there is access to the back of the calf.

Transducer
A high-frequency linear array transducer with frequencies from 9–18 MHz should be used.

Breathing Technique
The patient can breathe normally.

Patient Position
The patient should be lying prone with the feet hanging off the end of the stretcher. The foot may be supported with a pillow or sheets for patient comfort. Patients who are unable to lie prone may be scanned while on the side with the leg of the injured Achilles tendon not on the stretcher so as to make transducer manipulation easier.

Technical Tips
The sonographer needs to pay special attention to the borders of Achilles tendon because they are prone to edge artifact, which may

mimic or hide pathologic conditions. Using an extra amount of thick gel may be helpful. As with any MSK ultrasound, it can be helpful to scan the patient while he or she is doing the motion that brings on pain or discomfort.

Achilles Tendon Required Images

The image should be marked RT for right and LT for left. It is important that the side is properly labeled, as it is very difficult to tell the right from the left side on the images.

Achilles Tendon • Longitudinal Images

1. Long-axis image of the Achilles tendon showing insertion onto the calcaneus. Begin scanning with the transducer placed along the posterior calcaneus bone. Make sure that there is not an anisotropic artifact that would falsely diagnosis a tendon rupture.

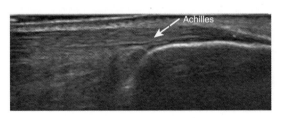
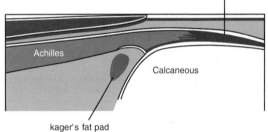

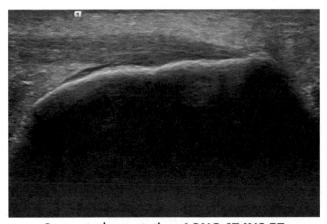

Suggested annotation: **LONG AT INS PT**

Some laboratories may use LAX for long axis.

2. Slowly move the transducer superiorly, following the tendon until it blends into the muscles at the distal end, approximately at the mid to upper calf. Sweep medially and laterally to evaluate the entire tendon.

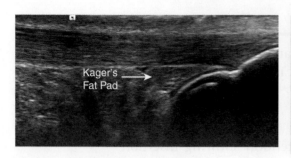
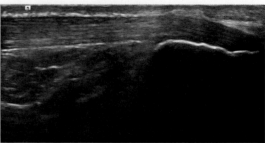

Suggested annotation: **LONG AT PROX**

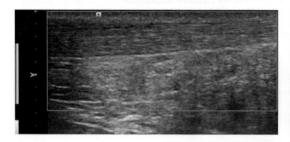
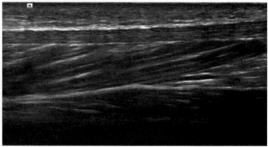

Suggested annotation: **LONG AT MID**

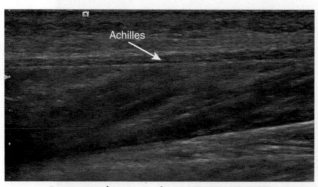

Suggested annotation: **LONG AT DST**

3. If available, a PANORAMIC VIEW of the entire length of Achilles tendon should be obtained.

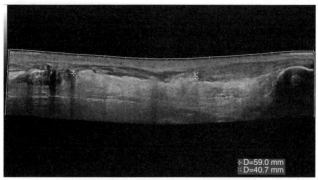

Suggested annotation: **LONG AT**

This example shows a complete tear about 4 cm above its insertion site. The length of the gap created by tendon retraction is measured.

Achilles Tendon • Transverse Images

1. Begin scanning with the transducer placed along the posterior calcaneus bone and identify the insertion point of the Achilles tendon. The width of the transducer will be wider than the tendon, creating an edge artifact along both medial and lateral borders of the tendon. Do not mistake the artifact for a tear.

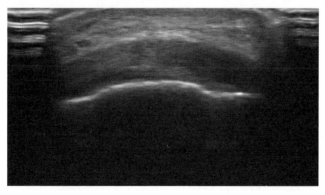

Suggested annotation: **TRV AT INS PT**

Some laboratories may use SAX for short axis.

2. Slowly move the transducer superiorly above the insertion site.

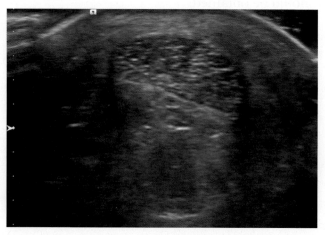

Suggested annotation: **TRV AT PROX**

3. Staying perpendicular to the tibia, follow the tendon until it blends into the muscles at the distal end approximately at the mid to upper calf. As the transducer moves up the calf, the soleal muscle can begin to be seen attaching to the deep part of the tendon; this should not be mistaken for a tendon tear or hematoma.

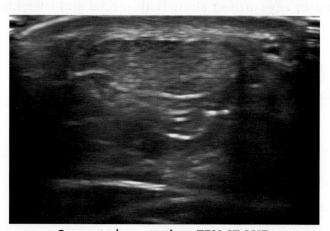

Suggested annotation: **TRV AT MID**

4. The tendon becomes thin distally. The *arrow* is pointing to the tendon.

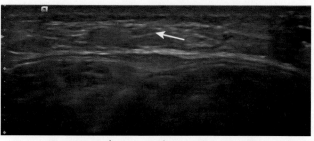

Suggested annotation: **TRV AT DST**

Achilles Tendon • Pathology Examples

1. A thick tendon from tendonitis is observed.

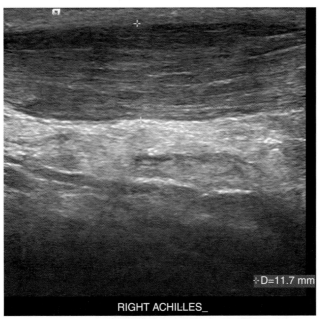

Suggested annotation: **PLANE AND LEVEL OF PATHOLOGY. THIS IMAGE IS LONG RT MID**

2. Power Doppler is helping to show the hyperemic flow. No flow will be seen with a normal tendon.

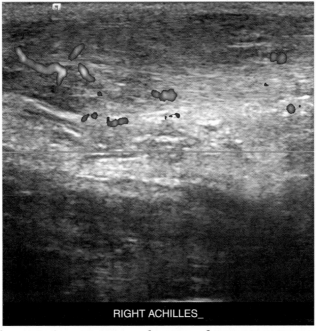

Suggested annotation: **PLANE and LEVEL of PATHOLOGY. THIS IMAGE is LONG RT MID**

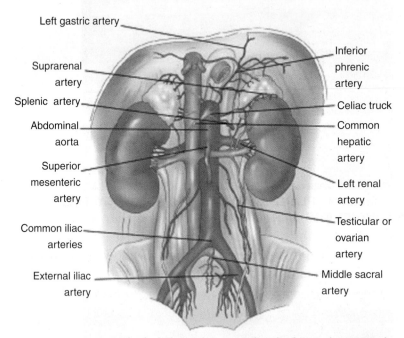

Left gastric artery

Suprarenal artery

Splenic artery

Abdominal aorta

Superior mesenteric artery

Common iliac arteries

External iliac artery

Inferior phrenic artery

Celiac truck

Common hepatic artery

Left renal artery

Testicular or ovarian artery

Middle sacral artery

From Hagen-Ansert SL. *Textbook of Diagnostic Sonography,* 8th ed. St. Louis, 2018, Mosby.

CHAPTER 20

Abdominal Doppler and Doppler Techniques

M. Robert DeJong

Keywords

Acceleration time
Angle correction control
Color Doppler
Color velocity scale
Doppler gain
Doppler shift
Hepatic vein
High-resistance waveform
Low-resistance waveform
Output power

Portal hypertension
Portal vein
Portal vein thrombosis
Power Doppler
Pulsatile waveform
Renal artery
Renal artery–to-aorta ratio
Renal artery stenosis
Renal vein
Resistive index

Objectives

At the end of this chapter, you will be able to:

- Define the keywords.
- Describe the anatomy of the abdominal vascular system.
- Differentiate low-resistance and high-resistance Doppler waveforms.
- Discuss how the color velocity scale affects the appearance of the color Doppler signal.
- List the additional views needed when a patient has portal hypertension.
- Describe the protocol for liver and renal Doppler examinations.

Overview

Doppler examinations of the abdomen are typically performed in the radiology or vascular department and, in some hospitals, the cardiology department. Sometimes specific examinations may be performed in a specific department with an agreement between the laboratories as to which laboratory will perform the examination, and in other places the laboratories may compete for the patient, with the ordering physician choosing the department where he or she prefers the examination be performed. Typically, if the test is requested by the vascular

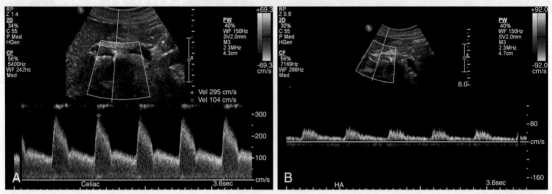

Fig. 20.1 A, An image of a stenosis at the origin of the celiac trunk. **B,** Image showing turbulent flow in the hepatic artery from the downstream stenosis of the celiac trunk.

surgery department, it will be performed in the vascular laboratory. Unfortunately for the radiology sonographer, he or she may discover the vascular disease but lose the patient to the vascular laboratory for follow-up or postoperative examinations because the vascular surgeon is usually the primary ordering physician. Unlike carotid or peripheral arterial examinations, a stenosis of the abdominal arteries is classified as greater than or less than 60% or 70%, or the percentage of stenosis that is on the chart with no other categories; for example, if there is a stenosis in the **renal artery**, it is either greater than or less than 60%.

In this chapter, Doppler examinations of the liver and kidneys will be highlighted. Mesenteric examinations for sudden abdominal pain with a concern for small bowel ischemia are best performed by computed tomography (CT) because small bowel ischemia is life threatening and may require emergency surgery. The diagnosis is made much quicker and with better accuracy with CT than with ultrasound. If atherosclerotic disease is suspected, ultrasound is a good screening examination, with color and spectral Doppler evaluating the origin of the celiac artery, superior mesenteric artery (SMA), and inferior mesenteric artery (IMA) (Fig. 20.1). Another examination that is not commonly ordered is to evaluate for median arcuate ligament syndrome (MALS), which is also known as celiac artery compression syndrome. MALS is an uncommon source of abdominal pain caused by the median arcuate ligament externally compressing the celiac artery and causing a hemodynamically significant stenosis during expiration. In these patients it is important to obtain the Doppler signal above the origin at the level where the median arcuate indents the wall of the celiac artery. In inspiration the color inside the artery will be a normal, uniform color. In expiration, the **color Doppler** will show an area of aliasing (Box 20.1) where the ligament is causing the stenosis. The Doppler sample volume will be placed in the area of aliasing, which will be above the origin of the celiac artery. Placing the sample volume at the origin is below the abnormality and

> **Box 20.1** Aliasing
>
> Aliasing occurs when the unit cannot process velocities quick enough, causing wrong colors to be assigned. Aliasing occurs with film, and for a good understanding, pay attention to the wheels on a car in a high-speed chase scene or the wheels on a stagecoach in a Western film. As the car starts to accelerate, the wheels are going in the proper direction. As speed increases, the wheels will momentarily stop and then appear to go backward! This is caused by the film unable to capture the position of the wheels quick enough.

a normal signal will be obtained, leading to a false-negative diagnosis. The diagnosis is made when there is an increased velocity of the waveform in expiration (Fig. 20.2, Color Plates 9 and 10). If the study is negative, there will not be a change in velocity between inspiration and expiration. If it is positive, the arcuate median ligament can be seen "punching" into the celiac artery on gray scale, and on color there will be a sudden appearance of color aliasing.

Abdominal Doppler

Doppler examinations of the abdomen can be very challenging technically because of the depth of the vessels, overlying bowel gas, respiratory motion causing the vessels to move, equipment settings, and sonographer experience. A Doppler examination also can be called a duplex examination, in which the image contains both gray-scale and color and/or spectral Doppler. On most ultrasound machines, duplex mode is an active gray-scale and color Doppler image or a frozen-gray-scale image, with or without color Doppler, and an active spectral Doppler waveform. Triplex is when gray-scale, color Doppler, and spectral Doppler are all in an active mode simultaneously. Triplex is very demanding on the machine and will result in decreased resolution in the image, with typically an aliased spectral Doppler signal. Doppler examinations can also refer to using a nonimaging continuous wave (CW) transducer for studies in which only the Doppler signal is obtained along with other nonimaging diagnostic equipment. Including Doppler in an examination can help make the diagnosis in a variety of ultrasound examinations by documenting the presence, direction, and velocity of flow; differentiating vascular structures from other tubular structures; demonstrating residual lumen; and helping with the investigation of vessels that are too small to be seen on the gray-scale image. Color Doppler can help with various aspects of the examination, including determining proper angle correction, showing where the highest velocity is located, and demonstrating perfusion of an organ.

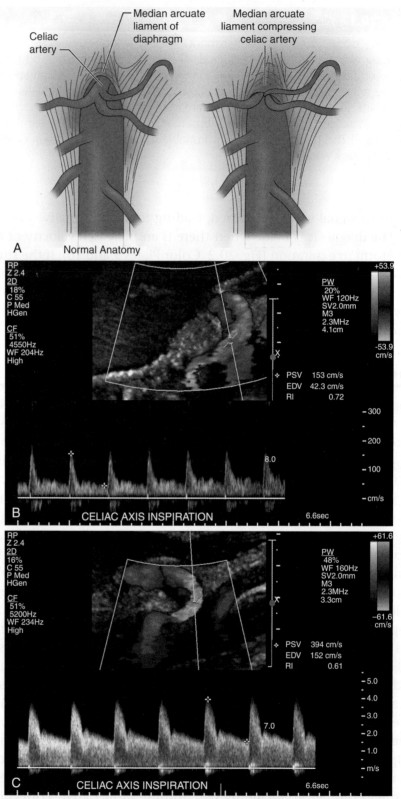

Fig. 20.2 **A,** A drawing of the mechanics behind median arcuate ligament syndrome. **B,** Spectral Doppler of the celiac at the level of the median arcuate during inspiration. **C,** Spectral Doppler of the celiac artery at the level of the median arcuate during expiration showing the increased velocities caused by the median ligament impinging on the outside of the artery causing a stenosis. See Color Plates 9 and 10. (*A,* from Sidawy AP, Perler BA. *Rutherford's Vascular Surgery and Endovascular Therapy,* 9th ed. Philadelphia, 2019, Elsevier.)

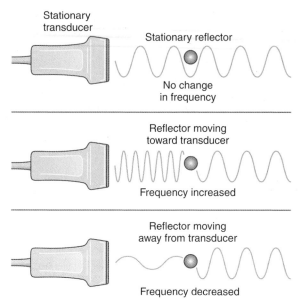

Fig. 20.3 A drawing demonstrating the Doppler effect. (From Soni NJ, Arntfield R, Kory P. *Point of Care Ultrasound,* 2nd ed. Philadelphia, 2020, Elsevier.)

To perform a Doppler examination, the sonographer should understand the following concepts, which will include the normal direction of blood flow in the vessel in relationship to the transducer and sound beam, the normal expected waveform for the vessel, the diagnostic criteria needed, any limitations of the procedure and how to optimize the ultrasound machine.

The **Doppler shift** is based on the angle between the emitted sound beam and the direction of the blood flow within the vessel and will determine whether the flow is toward the transducer or away from the transducer. When the blood is flowing toward the transducer, it will cause an increase in the returning echo frequencies. When the blood is flowing away from the transducer, it will cause a decrease in the returning echo frequencies (Fig. 20.3). To measure how fast the blood is flowing, the sonographer needs to determine this angle by using the **angle correction control**. Proper technique is to place the cursor line parallel to the walls of the vessel so that the measured angle is 60 degrees or less.

Diagnostic Criteria

In abdominal Doppler, the diagnosis may be determined from one or more of the following criteria:
1. Vessel patency: is the vessel allowing blood through (e.g., in renal vein thrombosis).
2. Flow direction: is the blood flowing in the proper direction (e.g., in portal hypertension).
3. Signal type: how much diastolic flow is seen in an arterial signal, and whether the flow is continuous or pulsatile in a venous signal (e.g., in the hepatic veins).

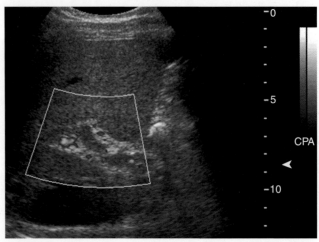

Fig. 20.4 Power Doppler image of the portal vein showing absence of flow. When a complete obstruction is seen, it is good practice to show the area with power Doppler because it is more sensitive to low flow.

4. Peak velocity measurement: how fast the blood is flowing in the vessel (e.g., in renal artery stenosis).
5. A ratio comparing the velocities of flow, such as comparing systole to diastole in the same vessel or the peak systolic velocity between two different vessels (e.g., in renal artery stenosis by calculating the **renal artery–to-aorta ratio**).
6. Resistance index (RI) is a comparison of systolic and diastolic flow that can help determine whether the signal is a high- or low-resistance signal (e.g., in renal disease).

Patency

Color, power, and spectral Doppler can verify vessel patency by showing that the lumen is patent and flow is easily demonstrated. It is important that the wall filters are at the lowest setting so that slow flow is not missed and a false diagnosis of thrombosis is made. The **color velocity scale** (CVS; pulse repetition frequency [PRF]) needs to be set properly for the vessel being investigated. If there is a partial thrombosis, color or **power Doppler** will outline the remaining lumen. Power Doppler is more sensitive and not as angle dependent as color Doppler; therefore, images using power Doppler are obtained to verify a complete obstruction in the vessel (Fig. 20.4) or a partial obstruction by outlining the residual lumen, including any "trickle" flow that might be present.

The color velocity scale is determined by the PRF. Some sonographers may say "Lower the PRF," which is the same as lowering the CVS. Since the numbers are now displayed as cm/sec and not in Hertz, as in earlier ultrasound machines, the term PRF has been replaced by color velocity scale.

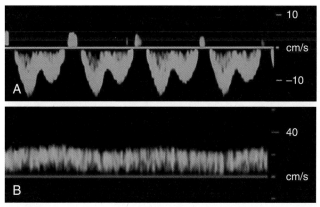

Fig. 20.5 A, An example of normal venous pulsatile flow. **B,** An example of normal venous continuous flow.

Flow Direction

Spectral or color Doppler can be used to assess the direction of blood flow in the vessel. If the unit has directional power Doppler, that also can be used. Determining flow direction is very important in the **portal vein**, splenic vein, and abdominal shunts. It is important to understand the normal direction of blood flow in relation to the transducer and sound beam. When determining flow direction, the CVS should be set so that there is little to no aliasing. Flow direction also should be documented, with a spectral Doppler signal. It is best to display flow in its true direction and not use the spectral invert control, to help avoid potential confusion and misdiagnosis. It is permissible to use spectral invert in certain examinations in which flow reversal is highly unlikely, such as in carotid and renal artery examinations, displaying the arterial flow above the baseline.

Spectral Doppler Waveform Analysis

Besides understanding the normal flow direction, it is also important to know the characteristic waveform for the vessel being investigated. For arteries in the abdomen, the normal characteristic patterns are described as a high-resistance or a low-resistance signal, and for veins either continuous flow or pulsatile flow (Fig. 20.5). These normal patterns may be altered in the presence of disease; for example, the normal pulsatile **hepatic vein** waveform becomes a continuous waveform in a cirrhotic liver (Fig. 20.6). **High-resistance waveforms** are associated with high resistance distally; that is, during diastole the capillaries are closed. The high-resistance signal will have little to no flow in diastole or even possibly reversed diastolic flow. Examples of high-resistance waveforms are the distal aorta, the external carotid artery, and the preprandial SMA (Fig. 20.7). **Low-resistance waveforms** will have forward flow in diastole and are associated with low resistance distally; that is, during diastole the capillaries remain open. Examples of low-resistance signals are the renal arteries, postprandial SMA, and the internal carotid artery (Fig. 20.8).

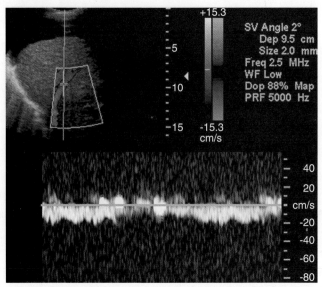

Fig. 20.6 The hepatic vein should be a pulsatile signal because of its close proximity to the heart. This signal shows a continuous waveform, which can be expected in patients with cirrhosis, as seen in this image. Ascites is also seen on this image.

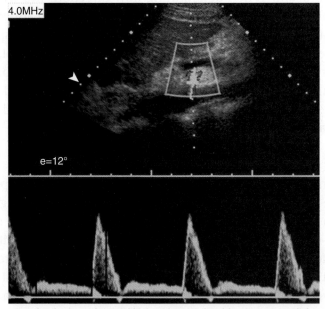

Fig. 20.7 An example of a normal arterial high-resistance signal from a preprandial superior mesenteric artery.

Peak Velocity Measurements

Peak velocity measurements are used to determine the velocity of blood flow in an artery or vein. The velocity is then compared with a chart to determine the percentage of stenosis or if the flow is a normal velocity. When measuring peak velocity, angle correction must be used properly. Color Doppler can help with determining the sample volume placement and aid with determining the angle. Proper angle correction

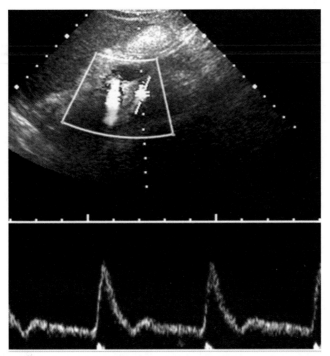

Fig. 20.8 An example of a normal arterial low-resistance signal from a postprandial superior mesenteric artery, which is the normal expected response.

must be less than 60 degrees, with the cursor parallel to the vessel walls. Some examinations may not need a peak velocity to make a diagnosis.

Resistive Index

The RI is a comparison of systolic and end diastolic flow and is determined by the following formula:

$$(\text{Peak systole} - \text{End diastole}) / \text{Peak systole}$$

The end of diastole is measured right before the next systolic upstroke, not where diastolic flow ends. The sonographer should ensure that noise, venous flow, or a mirror image artifact is not measured as end diastolic flow, because this will give a false number that will affect the diagnosis (Fig. 20.9, Color Plates 11 and 12). Evaluating the color Doppler image for a few cycles will give you an idea of the RI. If arterial flow completely disappears during diastole, creating a flashing appearance on the screen, the RI is 1, because there is no flow at the end of diastole (Fig. 20.10, Color Plates 13 and 14). If the arterial flow nearly disappears on the screen, the RI will be greater than 0.8 (Fig. 20.11, Color Plates 15 and 16). If there is good arterial flow during diastole, the RI will be less than 0.7 (Fig. 20.12). The calculation package on the ultrasound unit automatically calculates the RI by the sonographer placing a cursor at peak systole and a cursor at end diastole. If an RI is needed and was not measured on the unit, it can be calculated by hand. RI measurements are angle independent, and therefore angle correction is not used.

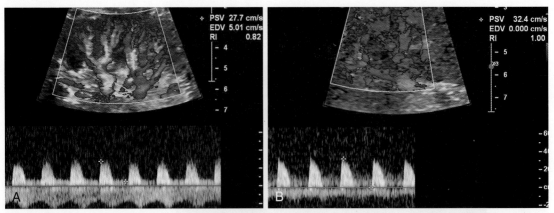

Fig. 20.9 A, An example of the resistive index (RI) measuring noise in the spectrum as end diastolic flow. **B,** An example of the RI measuring end diastolic flow correctly. The sonographer should evaluate the diastolic signal because the brightness is the same as that of the vein, with the arterial signal being brighter. See Color Plates 11 and 12.

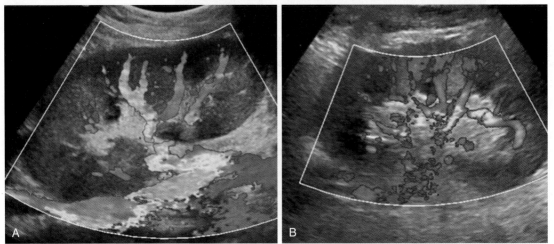

Fig. 20.10 A, A Doppler image of the kidney in systole. **B,** A Doppler image of the same kidney in diastole showing only diastolic flow. The resistive index for this kidney would be 1.0. See Color Plates 13 and 14.

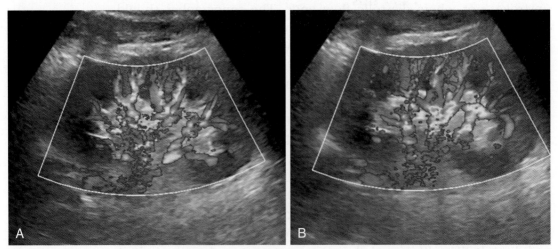

Fig. 20.11 A, A Doppler image of the kidney in systole. **B,** A Doppler image of the same kidney in diastole showing minimal systolic flow remaining. The resistive index for this kidney would be greater than 0.8. See Color Plates 15 and 16.

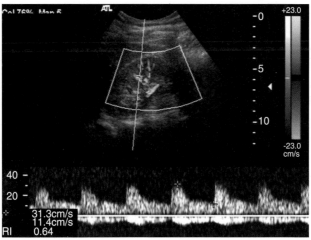

Fig. 20.12 An example of a normal resistive index in a kidney in which diastolic flow is well seen.

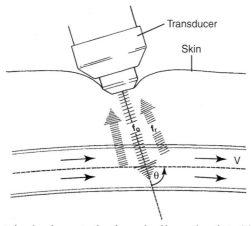

Fig. 20.13 A drawing demonstrating the angle of insonation, theta (θ). V, velocity.

Doppler Techniques and Tips

Acquiring the Doppler aspect of the examination may require different scanning techniques than are used in gray-scale imaging. A good Doppler signal will not always accompany an aesthetically appealing two-dimensional (2D) image. For gray-scale imaging, perpendicular angles are used, while scanning angles of less than 60 degrees to blood flow are required to obtain the best Doppler signal. For normal imaging the higher frequencies in the bandwidth are used, and when Doppler is activated, the lower frequencies are used. On some units you will notice degradation of the gray-scale image when obtaining the spectral Doppler waveform. Modern equipment has helped to maintain a high-resolution image when color Doppler is activated.

Doppler Angle

To obtain the best Doppler signal, it is necessary to optimize the sound beam–to-vessel angle (Fig. 20.13). Remember that the cosine between the sound beam and blood flow influences the velocity scale and therefore the measurements. To optimize this angle, it may be necessary to change the position of the patient and/or transducer. In vessels parallel to the skin, such as the aorta, flow will be perpendicular to the sound beam. Therefore, creating a good Doppler angle requires the sonographer to use what is called a "heel-toe" maneuver. This is done by angling the transducer superiorly or inferiorly, causing the vessel to go from a parallel course across the screen to an oblique course, thus creating a 45- to 60-degree angle with the sound beam. This technique is for vector/sector and curved linear array transducers because a linear array transducer can "steer" the sound beam into an angle away from perpendicular. When it is hard to get below 60 degrees, one trick is to place the angle correction at 60 degrees and angle the transducer until the walls are parallel to the cursor (Fig. 20.14). When performing the heel-toe maneuver, the edge of the transducer may no longer be in contact with the skin, creating a loss of image on the side where the transducer is not touching the skin.

Signal-to-Noise Ratio

Optimizing the signal-to-noise ratio helps to display the Doppler signal and the color Doppler image with little or no background noise. This is accomplished by using the correct transducer frequency to counteract the effects of attenuation, using the proper gain setting for all aspects of the image—color, spectral, and 2D—by placing the focal zone at or right below the area of interest or by increasing the **output power**. A clue that the output power needs to be increased is when there is a lot of background noise in the spectral or color Doppler aspect of the image, as this indicates the spectral or color gain is at a high setting in order to see the signal. Doppler signals do not have the same signal intensity as the gray-scale echoes and are much weaker. Increasing the output power will increase the intensity of the sound beam, thus increasing the intensity or strength of the returning Doppler signals, giving them the boost that they need to make it back to the transducer. When increasing the output power, the intensity of the gray-scale echoes will be increased and the overall 2D gain should be decreased (Fig. 20.15). Increasing the output power should not increase the risk to the patient as long as the proper preset is used.

To set the color gain properly, turn up the color gain until the background fills with color speckles, then decrease the color gain until the speckles disappear (Fig. 20.16, Color Plates 17 and 18). The color gain is now at a proper setting. If the 2D gain is too high or there is a lot of artifact in the lumen of the vessel, the machine may not be able to overwrite the gray-scale echo with a color echo. If this happens, adjust the overall image gain, clean up the vessel with the time-gain compensation (TGC), or adjust the gray-scale/image contrast control by making the gray-scale image more contrasty, thus eliminating

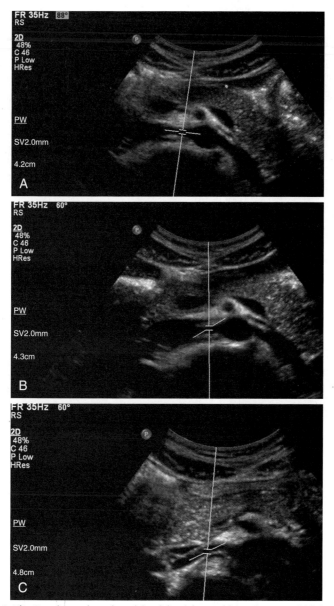

Fig. 20.14 A, The Doppler angle at the origin of the right renal is 70 degrees, which is an unacceptable Doppler angle. **B,** The angle correction is placed at 60 degrees to help determine how to heel-toe the transducer. Because the cursor is not parallel to the vessel walls, it cannot be used to obtain the waveform. **C,** The transducer is angled so that the artery is now parallel to the cursor and a waveform can now be obtained.

low-level gray-scale echoes. Some units have what is called a priority control that will allow the sonographer to determine whether to display the grayscale or color echo. This control can be used on a frozen image. The **Doppler gain** is similarly adjusted by turning up the gain until speckles are seen in the background and then turning the Doppler gain down until they disappear (Fig. 20.17). Sometimes, to see a full spectrum from an especially weak signal, it may be necessary

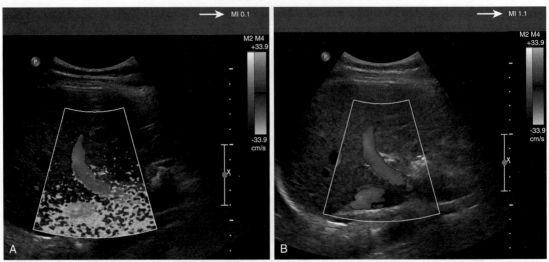

Fig. 20.15 A, The output power, *MI,* is very low, making both the gray-scale and Doppler echoes faint. To see flow inside the portal vein the color gain has to be increased to the point that there is color noise in the image. **B,** The same liver as in **A** with the MI increased to 1.1; both the gray-scale echoes and color Doppler are well seen.

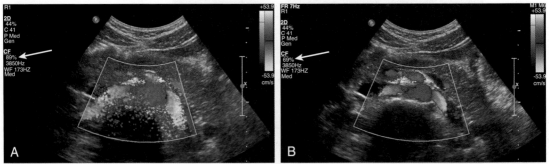

Fig. 20.16 A, The color signal is overgained at 89% *(arrow),* causing background color noise. **B,** The color gain is decreased to 69% *(arrow),* and the noise is gone. See Color Plates 17 and 18.

to display a "noisy" spectrum. Remember that small vessels, such as the hepatic or interlobar arteries, will not have a systolic window.

Color Velocity Scale

Vessel fill-in is determined by using the proper CVS setting, which also may be termed PRF. The CVS concentrates and displays the color Doppler signal based on the number above and below the color scale bar. I like to think of the CVS as a combination of a filter and color gain. With high numbers the unit is concentrating on velocities around that number and may not display color Doppler echoes above or below certain velocities. If this control is set too high, the machine is looking for fast velocities and color may not be displayed in a vessel with slower flow, thus leading to an incorrect diagnosis of vessel thrombosis or occlusion. When this control is set with low numbers, the unit is looking for slow velocities, and color aliasing will occur because the velocities are too fast for the machine to process, making the determination

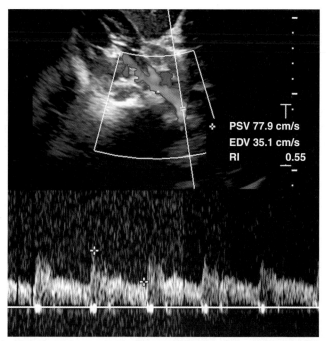

Fig. 20.17 The beginning of the trace has background noise, and as the trace scrolls across the screen, the Doppler gain is decreased until the noise disappears. What do you notice about the image? The sample volume is placed in the bend, making it difficult to determine angle correction that was possibly not applied or a zero degree angle was used, as the angle correction cursor is not seen. By moving the sample volume either lower to the straight section or moving it up above the angle, the angle correction could be properly used.

of flow direction difficult (Fig. 20.18, Color Plates 19, 20, and 21). Slow-flow settings of less than 6–7 cm/s should be used when looking for "trickle" flow or in very slow-flow states. On some units, when the CVS is at the lowest setting, the unit is looking to process very slow velocities and may not display normal flow, which again may falsely cause an impression of a thrombosis or occlusion. When looking for slow flow, evaluate the image with each increment of the CVS control until either color is seen inside the vessel or the lowest setting is obtained. If color is still not seen, then a thrombosis or occlusion can be suspected. If no flow is seen the output power and color gain should be increased until flow is seen. If flow is still not seen, because of its increased sensitivity for slow flow, power Doppler should be used to determine if any flow is present. A compromise with aliasing may be required to have proper vessel fill-in.

A starting point for the CVS is between 10 and 20 cm/s for venous flow and between 20 and 30 cm/s for arterial flow. These values are a starting point and need to be adjusted according to the patient and the patient's flow states. For example, with a young healthy patient these numbers will be increased, and with a patient in congestive heart failure these numbers will need to be decreased.

Frame Rate

Color Doppler places a great demand on the processing power of the machine, resulting in a sacrifice in frame rate. The frame rate is determined in part by the depth of the image setting and the width of the color box. The frame rate can be improved by using the smallest image scale size possible. This will also help maximize your spectral Doppler scale by improving the PRF. For example, when evaluating the hepatic veins, it is not necessary to see 4–5 cm beyond the diaphragm because this is empty space. By decreasing the image depth from a 20-cm scale size to a 16-cm scale size, the PRF will be increased, rewarding the sonographer with a faster frame rate as well as increasing the spectral Doppler velocity scale before aliasing will occur. Minimizing the width of the color sample box will help improve color sensitivity and increase the frame rate. The width of

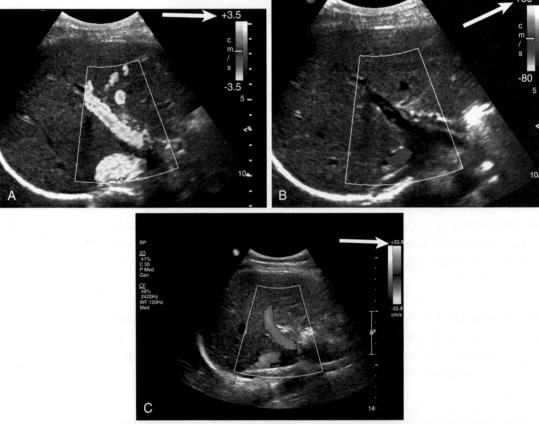

Fig. 20.18 A, The color velocity scale is too low at 3.5 cm/s *(arrow)*, causing aliasing that makes determining flow direction impossible. **B,** With the color velocity scale (CVS) at 80 cm/s *(arrow)*, no flow is seen inside the portal vein, giving the illusion of portal vein thrombosis. Flow is seen in the hepatic artery because the flow is faster. **C,** The CVS is set properly at 33.9 cm/s *(arrow)*, and vessel fill-in is seen and flow direction can be determined. These examples show how crucial the CVS setting is and how it can affect the flow seen inside a vessel. It is important to double check this setting when there appears to be no flow in the vessel. See Color Plates 19, 20, and 21.

the box will determine the number of color lines used in the image. The greater the number of color lines, the more processing is needed, and there will be a reduction in frame rate. The height of the box will not affect the frame rate because the number of color lines will be the same.

Doppler Tips

On small vessels, such as the hepatic artery, enlarge the area with preferably a write zoom or a read zoom. A write zoom will have the sonographer define the area to be enlarged, which will preserve resolution and can be performed only on an active image (Fig. 20.19). Each of the ultrasound manufacturers has their own name for the write zoom control. A read zone enlarges the area and can be performed on a frozen image. As the image is enlarged, it will start to get blurry because it enlarges only what has already been received (Fig. 20.20). Again, each manufacturer may have a different name for this control, although zoom is a common name. Zoom features will make these small vessels easier to see. Use the enlarged image for sample volume placement to obtain the Doppler spectral waveform.

If the Doppler spectrum is weak or noisy, freeze the 2D image. This will improve the appearance of the spectrum by allowing the machine to concentrate on obtaining the spectral Doppler waveform. If an artery has a high velocity and the peak is not crisp, increase the Doppler wall

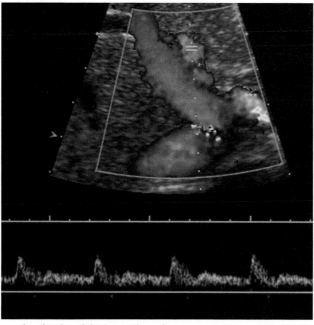

Fig. 20.19 Increasing the size of the image through a zoom control can help identify and place the sample volume on small vessels such as the hepatic artery.

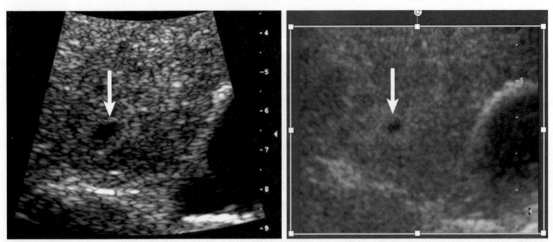

Fig. 20.20 **A,** Using a write zoom the resolution of the image is maintained and even may be increased. *Arrow,* Cyst. **B,** The same cyst *(arrow)* in the liver using a read zoom. Note how the borders are blurry and thickened, making the size of the cyst appear smaller in size.

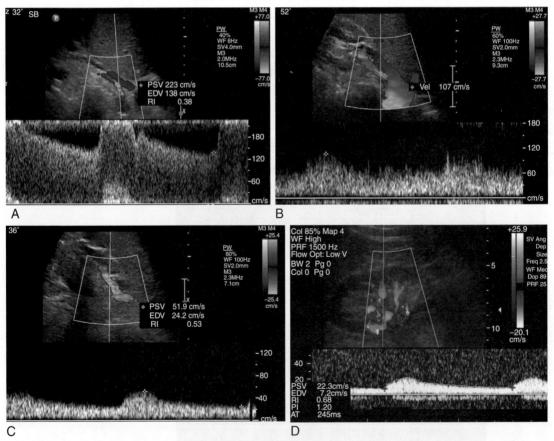

Fig. 20.21 **A,** An example of a high-grade stenosis at the origin of the right renal artery. The peak systolic velocity is aliasing, and the peak of the seen signal is measured, which is acceptable. **B,** The Doppler signal past the area of stenosis showing turbulent flow causing a ragged appearance to the waveform. **C,** The signal from the distal artery showing classic rounding of the signal, the tardus-parvus signal. **D,** The intrarenal signal also showing a tardus-parvus signal with an acceleration time of 245 ms, an increase of over the normal less than 70 ms. See Color Plates 22 and 23.

filter. This allows the machine to concentrate on the higher velocities and will improve visualization of the peak of the Doppler waveform.

Because patients will need to hold their breath during the actual examination, do not tire them out while setting the controls (image scale size, color maps, baseline shift, filters, Doppler scale, CVS, and 2D, color, and Doppler gains). Set all of these parameters with the patient breathing normally. If patients have difficulty holding their breath, only a small amount of signal (one or two beats) may be obtained. However, one or two beats can be just as diagnostic as a full screen of five or more beats. Only one beat and the next systolic upstroke are needed to determine flow presence, type, and direction and measure peak systole and end diastole and the RI.

When documenting a stenosis, it is important to "walk" the sample volume before the stenosis, through the stenosis, and past the stenosis, looking for the highest velocity. These images will be added to the protocol. Doppler is audible, and you may hear the high-pitched stenosis before you see it. Once the highest velocity is documented, continue moving downstream and document any poststenotic turbulence that is present (Fig. 20.21, Color Plates 22 and 23). Further downstream the arterial signal may display a tardus-parvus waveform.

Doppler Study of the Kidneys

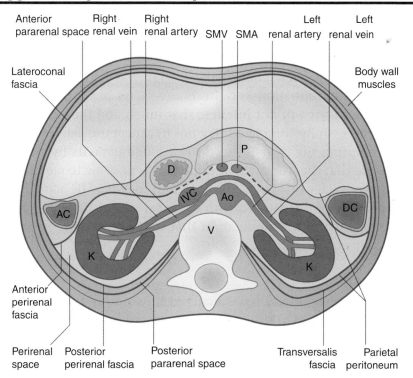

AC, ascending colon; *AO,* aorta; *D,* duodenum; *DC,* descending colon; *IVC,* inferior vena cava; *K,* kidney; *P,* pancreas; *V,* vertebral body. (From Allan PL, Baxter GM, Weston MJ. *Clinical Ultrasound,* 3rd ed. Edinburgh, 2011, Churchill Livingstone.)

Refer to Chapter 9 to review the anatomy, physiology, sonographic appearance, and protocol for imaging the kidney. In some laboratories the only gray-scale images obtained will be a long-axis view of each kidney with length measurements, whereas other laboratories may require a full renal sonogram depending on the date of the last renal examination. Renal Doppler studies are performed on the arteries to evaluate unexplained or uncontrolled hypertension caused by renal artery stenosis and on the veins to evaluate for clot or tumor thrombus. A renal arterial study would evaluate the entire length of the artery from the aorta to the renal hilum and the intrarenal arteries and include a **renal vein** waveform at the hilum. Renal vein studies would include evaluating the entire length of the renal vein from renal hilum to the IVC and a renal arterial signal at the hilum. Remember that inflow and outflow must be documented to be able to charge for a complete study.

Patient Prep

The purpose of patient prep is to help reduce bowel gas. Most laboratories ask the patient to not have anything to eat or drink (NPO) after midnight except medications with water. Diabetic patients should be scheduled as the first patient of the morning. If the patient will be scanned in the late morning or afternoon, advise the patient to avoid gas-producing foods, such as beans, peas, cabbage, onions, broccoli, cauliflower, foods with sorbitol or fructose, apples, or pears; not to drink carbonated beverages or beer; not to suck on hard candies; and not to smoke or chew gum. If the patient has had food or drink, attempt the examination because many views are from a coronal approach and gas will not interfere that much and the examination may be successfully completed. Try not to cancel the patient without first attempting the study. Also do not judge patients by their size and decide that the study will be limited. It is possible to see the renal vessels very nicely on "large" patients, and they may be actually easy to scan. Some of the patients with the most gas are patients who are very thin, so that an examination that may appear easy is actually technically challenging.

Transducer

The sonographer should have a curved linear array transducer that includes frequencies in the 3–5 MHz range and a phased/vector array transducer with frequencies in the 1–3 MHz range. For large patients, do not use the lower-frequency transducer without first trying to use the curved linear array transducer. Curved linear array transducers are better and more comfortable to the patient when pushing gas out of the way. The phased/vector array transducers are best when images need to be obtained between the ribs. The author typically used a combination of both transducers on some patients. For pediatric and newborn patients, use a sector/vector array with frequencies in the 5–8 MHz range and/or a tightly curved array, such as the transducer used for neonatal brain sonograms, with frequencies in the same range.

Breathing Technique

Having the patient take in a deep breath and hold it is not always the best way to image the renal vessels. When scanning intercostal, the patient may need to stop breathing on expiration. Sometimes having patients breath normally or having them take in and hold small breaths is acceptable. Some patients may be able to stop breathing on command when the vessel is in the image. Remember to let patients breath normally as controls are optimized so as not to tire them out.

Patient Position

Many different positions will be used when performing imaging of the renal arteries. Typically, the patient starts out supine, turned in right and left posterior obliques, right and left lateral decubitus positions, and sometime even prone. Sometimes both the patient and the sonographer get a workout! Renal veins are not as challenging, and the examination usually can be performed with the patient supine and using other positions as needed.

Technical Tips

Use the renal preset for performing any renal Doppler examination. The machine will optimize controls, including some "controls" inside the machine to which the sonographer does not have access. The Doppler settings needed for the kidney are different from those needed for the other abdominal organs. Not using the renal preset may make the examination difficult for the color Doppler aspect (Fig. 20.22). As for any aspect of ultrasound examination, when you see it, grab it! You can always make it better, but you will never get it again! This may mean that the right and left images may be intermingled and not in a right/left sequence.

The right renal artery may need to be scanned in multiple positions. Start with the patient supine and obtain the aorta waveform. Scan the IVC in a longitudinal plane and look for a small circle underneath it. This is the right renal artery. This image is also good to determine whether there are multiple renal arteries, because there will be

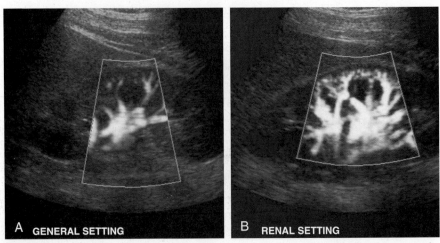

Fig. 20.22 A, A power Doppler image of the kidney using the general preset. Notice the poor perfusion that is seen. **B,** The same patient using the renal preset and showing good renal perfusion. All other controls were the same.

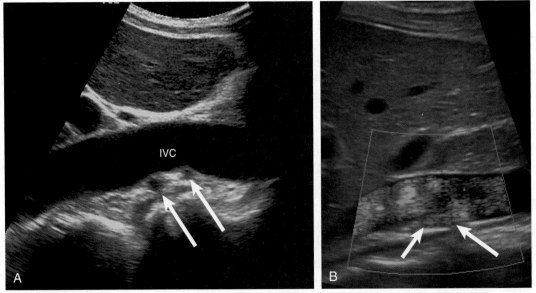

Fig. 20.23 A, A longitudinal image with the *arrows* pointing to duplicate right renal arteries seen under the inferior vena cava *(IVC)*. **B,** A longitudinal image of the IVC with power Doppler image. The *arrows* are pointing to the duplicated renal arteries.

two or more circles posterior to the IVC (Fig. 20.23). While keeping the right renal artery in site, turn the transducer counterclockwise to try to view the artery in its long axis. The origin of the right renal artery usually presents itself with an angle greater than 60 degrees, making it difficult to obtain a Doppler signal. Sliding the transducer laterally while angling the sample volume to the origin of the artery may help create an angle less than 60 degrees. This is the heel-toe maneuver. The origin often can be imaged very nicely by scanning coronally and lining up the IVC, aorta, and liver in the same view.

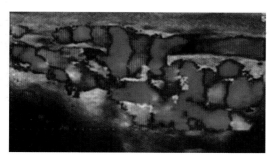

Color Plate 1 Color Doppler image of the increased flow seen with a Valsalva maneuver in a patient with a varicocele. (See Fig. 15.30B.)

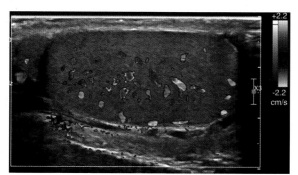

Color Plate 2 Color Doppler image demonstrating flow in the normal right testicle. (See Fig. 15.32A)

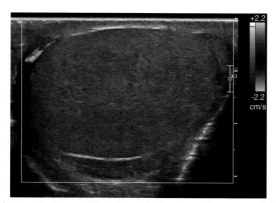

Color Plate 3 Color Doppler image of the left testicle showing no flow, compatible with testicular torsion. Some peritesticular flow is seen, and the sonographer should not confuse that with intratesticular flow. The color velocity scale is at a low setting of 2.2 cm/s, which is the same setting as the patient's right testicle seen in Color Plate 2. (See Fig. 15.32B)

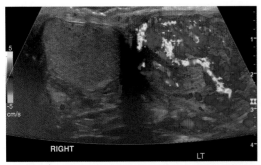

Color Plate 4 Side-by-side image of both testicles showing the increased flow in the left testicle, compatible with orchitis. (See Fig. 15.33A.)

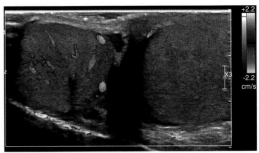

Color Plate 5 Side-by-side image of both testicles showing absence of flow in the left testicle, compatible with torsion. (See Fig. 15.33B.)

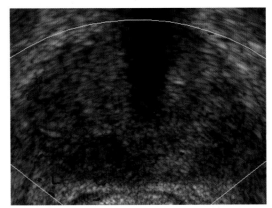

Color Plate 6 Color Doppler image of the prostate showing the increased flow of a prostate cancer. (See Fig. 15.69.)

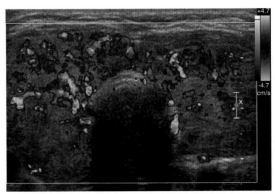

Color Plate 7 Image of the increased color Doppler seen in a patient with Hashimoto's disease. (See Fig. 16.15C.)

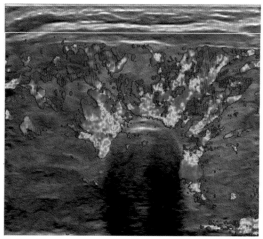

Color Plate 8 Image of the markedly increased color Doppler, thyroid inferno, seen in a patient with Grave's disease. (See Fig. 16.16B.)

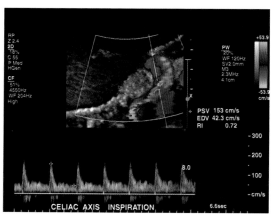

Color Plate 9 Image of the celiac trunk at the level of the median arcuate during inspiration. (See Fig. 20.2A.)

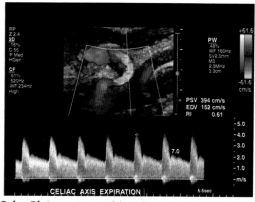

Color Plate 10 Image of the celiac trunk at the level of the median arcuate during expiration showing increased velocities in the same patient as in Color Plate 9. (See Fig. 20.2B.)

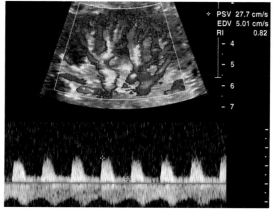

Color Plate 11 An example of incorrectly measuring the resistive index by mistaking an artifact for end diastolic flow. (See Fig. 20.9A.)

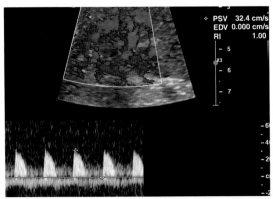

Color Plate 12 Same patient as in Color Plate 11 with the proper end diastolic measurement at the baseline. (See Fig. 20.9B.)

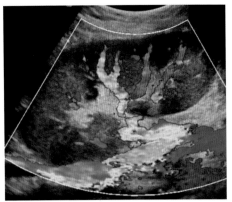

Color Plate 13 Using color Doppler to help determine the resistive index. This image is during peak systole. (See Fig. 20.10A.)

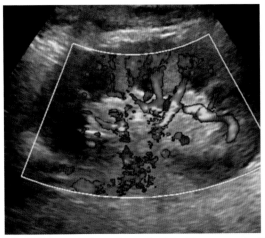

Color Plate 14 Same patient as in Color Plate 13 now in diastole. Note that there is no red, which would represent systolic flow. The resulting RI will be 1.0. (See Fig. 20.10B.)

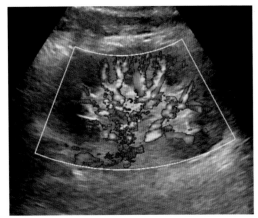

Color Plate 15 Another example of a patient with a high resistive index. This image is during peak systole. (See Fig. 20.11A.)

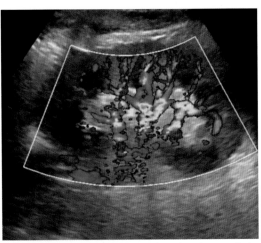

Color Plate 16 Same patient as in Color Plate 15 during diastole showing the decrease in systolic flow that almost disappears but is still present at end diastole, compatible with an resistive index greater than 0.8. (See Fig. 20.11B.)

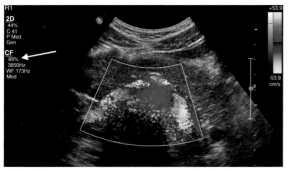

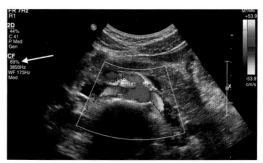

Color Plate 17 Note all the color noise on the image compatible with too much gain, which is set at 89%. (See Fig. 20.16A.)

Color Plate 18 Same patient as in Color Plate 17 with the gain properly set at 69%. (See Fig. 20.16B.)

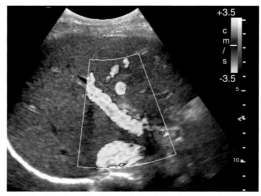

Color Plate 19 Image of the portal vein showing aliasing as the color velocity scale is too low at 3.5 cm/s. (See Fig. 20.18A.)

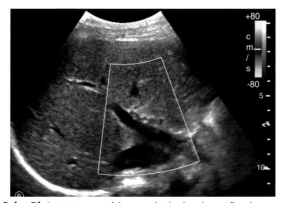

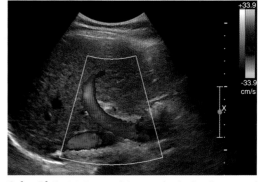

Color Plate 20 Image of the portal vein showing no flow because the color velocity scale is too high at 80 cm/s. (See Fig. 20.18B.)

Color Plate 21 Image of the portal vein showing normal flow with the color velocity scale at the proper setting of 33 cm/s. (See Fig. 20.18C.)

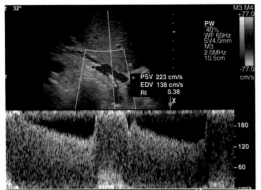

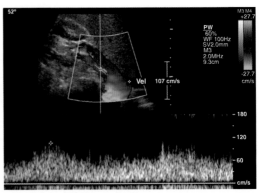

Color Plate 22 Image of the right renal artery with the sample volume near the origin in the area of aliasing, which represents the area of high flow. Because obtaining a full signal was not technically possible, the top of the seen signal is measured, which is 223 cm/s. This value is greater than 200 cm/s, which is compatible with a greater than 60% stenosis. Because of the depth of the renal arteries, it is common for the signal to alias when there is a stenosis. The diagnostic criterion is a single value to determine a greater than 60% stenosis; thus, the true peak is not needed. (See Fig. 20.21A.)

Color Plate 23 Same patient as in Color Plate 22 showing poststenotic turbulence and the return to a homogeneous color in the artery. (See Fig. 20.21B.)

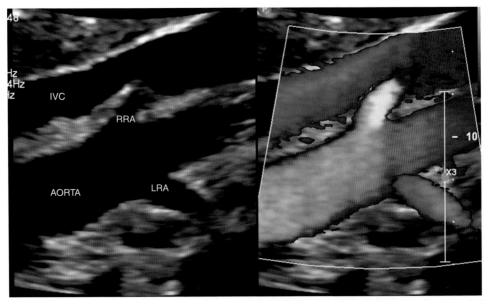

Color Plate 24 Gray-scale and color Doppler images of the origins of the renal arteries obtained from the coronal plane, the "banana peel" view. *IVC,* Inferior vena cava; *LRA,* left renal artery; *RRA,* right renal artery. (See Fig. 20.24.)

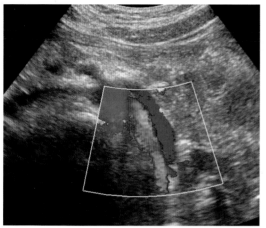

Color Plate 25 Color Doppler image of the left renal artery from the aorta to the left kidney with the patient in the supine position. Note the uniformity of color suggesting a normal artery. (See Fig. 20.28.)

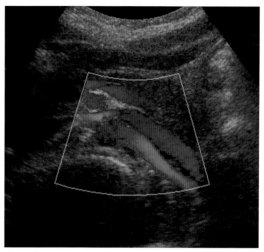

Color Plate 26 Color Doppler image of the left renal vein from the left kidney to the inferior vena cava showing patency. The area of *black* is due to the flow being perpendicular to the sound beam. (See Fig. 20.29.)

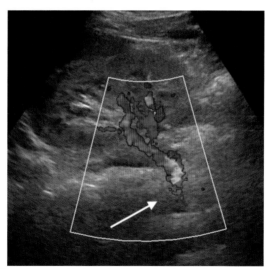

Color Plate 27 Image of the left renal artery, with the patient in the right lateral decubitus position, showing the entire length of the artery. The aliasing at the origin is due to a stenosis. The *arrow* is pointing to the aorta, which does not demonstrate flow because of being perpendicular to the sound beam. (See Fig. 20.30.)

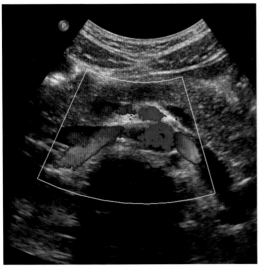

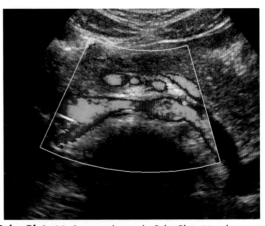

Color Plate 28 The origin of the right renal artery does not fill in with color because it is perpendicular to the sound beam. There is a good Doppler angle on the left side, and the origin of the left renal artery is nicely seen. (See Figure 20.31A.)

Color Plate 29 Same patient as in Color Plate 28, using power Doppler to show the patency of the origin of the right renal artery. Power Doppler is able to show perpendicular flow. (See Fig. 20.31B.)

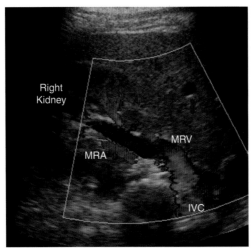

Color Plate 30 The right renal vein seen from the right kidney to the inferior vena cava *(IVC)*. *MRA,* Main renal artery; *MRV,* main renal vein. (See Fig. 20.35.)

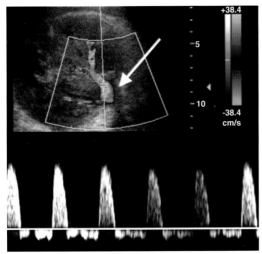

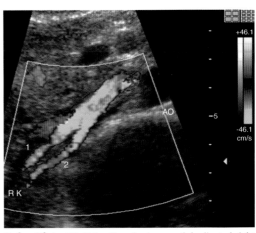

Color Plate 31 A biphasic arterial signal associated with renal vein thrombosis *(arrow)*. (See Fig. 20.37.)

Color Plate 32 Color Doppler image of duplicated right renal arteries. These are two separate arteries arising side by side from the aorta. *RK*, Right kidney; *AO*, aorta. (See Fig. 20.38.)

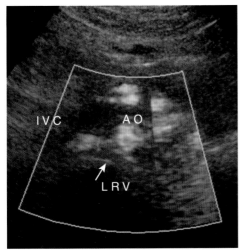

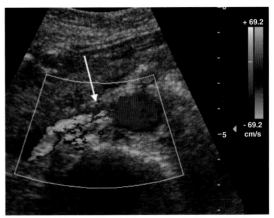

Color Plate 34 Color Doppler showing the reduced lumen and aliasing of a stenosis at the origin of the right renal artery *(arrow)*. (See Fig. 20.41.)

Color Plate 33 Power Doppler image showing a retroaortic left renal vein. It was difficult to show flow through the vein with color Doppler because it is perpendicular to the sound beam. *AO,* Aorta; *IVC,* inferior vena cava; *LRV,* left renal vein. (See Fig. 20.39.)

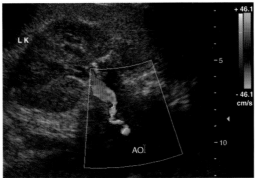

Color Plate 35 A patient with fibromuscular dysplasia in the left renal artery. Note the mid-vessel area of aliasing. Patient is in the right lateral decubitus position. *AO,* Aorta; *LK,* left kidney. (See Fig. 20.43.)

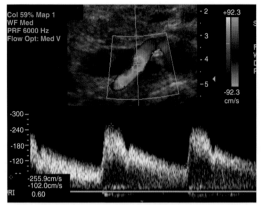

Color Plate 36 Spectral Doppler image with elevated velocities from the right renal artery in a patient with fibromuscular dysplasia. (See Fig. 20.44A.)

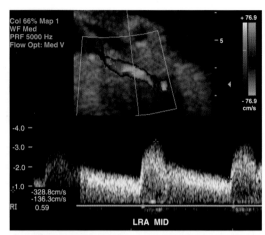

Color Plate 37 Same patient as in Color Plate 36 showing high velocities from the left renal artery from a patient with bilateral fibromuscular dysplasia. (See Fig. 20.44B.)

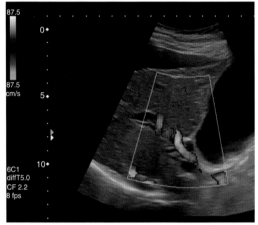

Color Plate 38 The hepatic artery is seen with tortuous flow. The patient has cirrhosis and ascites. No flow is seen in the portal vein. All of the findings are suggestive of portal vein thrombosis. Evaluating the color velocity scale shows that the values are very high at 87.5 cm/s, which might be the reason that there is no flow seen in the portal vein. (See Fig. 20.60A.)

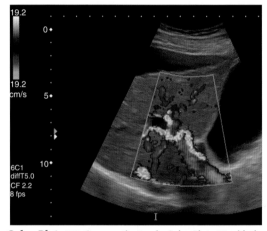

Color Plate 39 Same patient as in Color Plate 38 with the color velocity scale lowered to 19.2 cm/s, a more normal value for venous flow. The hepatic artery is now aliasing. (See Fig. 20.60B.)

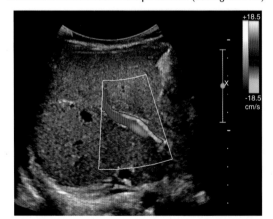

Color Plate 40 Normal color Doppler image of the slower portal vein flow, *darker orange,* and the faster flow of the hepatic artery, which is a *brighter orange.* The colors on the color bar closer to the middle, darker shades are the slower flows, and the colors on the end, brighter shades are the faster flows. (See Fig. 20.60C.)

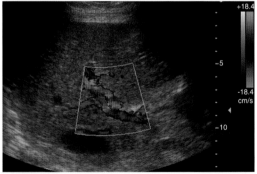

Color Plate 41 Image of portal hypertension with the portal vein in *blue,* going away from the liver and transducer, and the hepatic artery in *red,* going into the liver and toward the transducer. The color bar has red on top. (See Fig. 20.62A.)

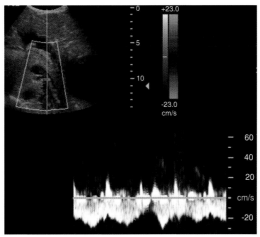

Color Plate 42 Color and spectral Doppler showing reversed flow in the splenic vein. Blue is on the bottom of the color bar and the splenic vein is in *blue* going away from the transducer back toward the spleen. (See Fig. 20.64.)

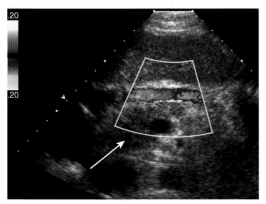

Color Plate 43 This is a collateral that the author mistook for a splenic vein with reversed flow until the radiologist pointed out that it was above the pancreas. The *arrow* is pointing to the head of the pancreas. The lesson is to carefully evaluate the entire image and not just where your eyes are focused. (See Fig. 20.66A.)

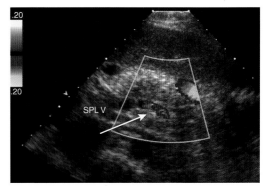

Color Plate 44 Same patient as in Color Plate 43, with the real splenic vein *(SPL V)*, which is small with retrograde flow. The *blue* above the pancreas is the collateral. (See Fig. 20.66B.)

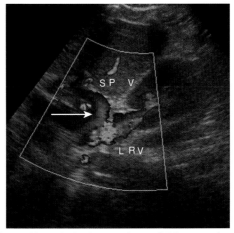

Color Plate 45 The body is amazing, and here the body created a conduit between the splenic vein *(SP V)* and left renal vein *(LRV)* so that the portal blood could return to the systemic circulation. The *arrow* is pointing to the created splenorenal shunt. (See Fig. 20.68A.)

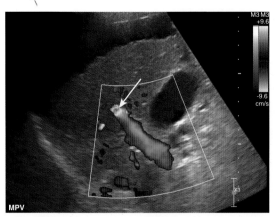

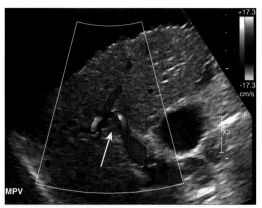

Color Plate 46 An image of the portal vein that the sonographer thought was normal until the radiologist asked why there is aliasing at the end of the vein *(arrow).* The lesson is to pay close attention to the details. In this image the portal vein should be a uniform color, and the aliasing was a sign that something was not right and needed to be explained. (See Fig. 20.73A.)

Color Plate 47 Same patient as in Color Plate 46 with the color velocity scale increased from 9.6 to 17.3 cm/s. At the higher scale setting the clot is now seen that was "hidden" by the color signal *(arrow).* (See Fig. 20.73C.)

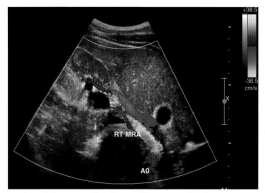

Color Plate 48 Normal color Doppler of the normal right renal artery and vein. *Ao,* Aorta; *RT MRA,* main renal artery. (See Chapter 20, unnumbered figure 15, p. 47.)

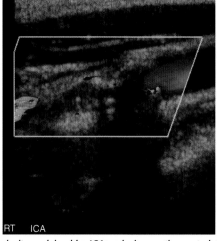

Color Plate 49 An abnormal high velocity explained by ICA occlusion on the contralateral side. The aliasing flow on the left side of the image is from the jugular vein as the CVS is at a very low setting. (See Fig. 21.1)

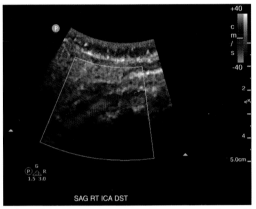

Color Plate 50 Color image of the distal internal carotid artery using an abdominal curved area transducer. (See Fig. 21.16B.)

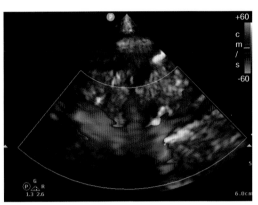

Color Plate 51 Using a low-frequency phased array transducer to document the origins of the common carotid artery *(CCA)* and subclavian artery off of the aortic arch. (See Fig. 21.17E.)

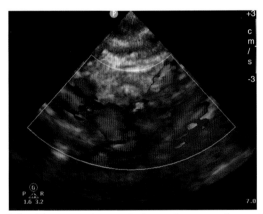

Color Plate 52 Color Doppler image shows a small area of color aliasing at the left common carotid artery origin, indicating the area of the stenosis. (See Fig. 21.22C.)

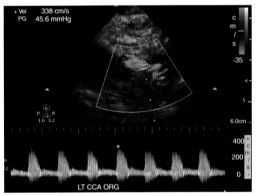

Color Plate 53 Color Doppler image showing an area of aliasing where an elevated velocity and turbulent waveforms were seen, confirming significant disease of the origin of the common carotid artery CCA. (See Fig. 21.22D.)

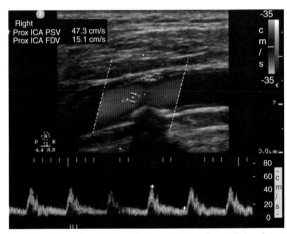

Color Plate 54 An example of a stenosis less than 50% with the color Doppler outlining the residual lumen. (See Fig. 21.26A.)

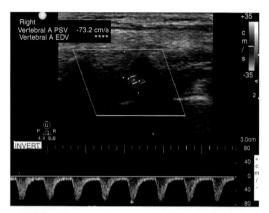

Color Plate 55 The vertebral artery is *blue* away from the transducer and head and compatible with reversed flow. (See Fig. 21.28B.)

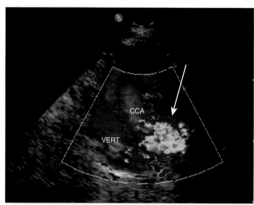

Color Plate 56 An image showing a color bruit *(arrow)* of the distal innominate artery that is associated with a stenosis. The color bruit is caused by the vibration of the tissue in response to the stenosis. *CCA,* Common carotid artery. (See Fig. 21.28C.)

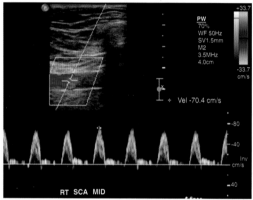

Color Plate 57 The subclavian artery is *red,* which is away from the transducer in this image. The subclavian vessels will go in the opposite direction as they originate from the center of the chest and run laterally. This is why the color bar is inverted to keep the artery red in this normal subclavian artery. With this same angle on the left side, the normal flow would be blue. *RT SCA MID*, Right subclavian artery mid vessel. (See Fig. 21.28E.)

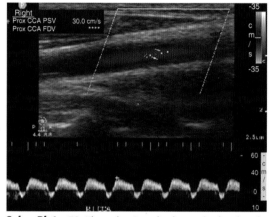

Color Plate 58 The color Doppler image is showing the reduced lumen in this common carotid artery. An abnormal carotid waveform is seen resulting from an occlusion of the innominate artery. *RT CCA*, Right common carotid artery. (See Fig. 21.28F.)

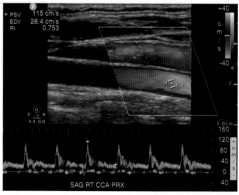

Color Plate 59 Normal color Doppler image of the common carotic artery and jugular vein. Note that the color does not completely fill in the jugular vein because of the higher color velocity scale needed for the artery. *SAG RT CCA PROX*, Sagittal right common carotid artery proximal. (See Chapter 21, unnumbered figure 2 in protocol section).

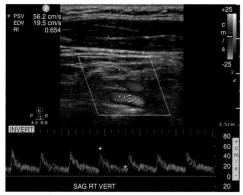

Color Plate 60 Image of the normal vertebral artery and the vertebral vein superior to the artery. Note in this image that they are about the same diameter. (See Chapter 21, unnumbered figure 14 in protocol section).

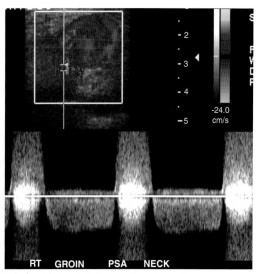

Color Plate 61 Color Doppler of a pseudoaneurysm (PSA) showing the yin-yang sign. Blue in on the top of the color bar. The blood enters the PSA, *blue,* and flows clockwise to exit the PSA, *red.* (See Fig. 22.8.)

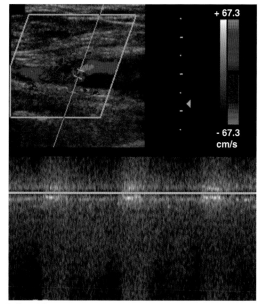

Color Plate 62 The sample volume is in the area of aliasing, which is the location of the connection between the artery and the vein. Note the color bruit in the area. The diastolic flow is almost aliasing, giving the illusion that the Doppler tracing is all noise. However, a high-pitched signal is heard with distinct systolic and diastolic components. This demonstrates the importance of listening to the audible Doppler signal. (See Fig. 22.11.)

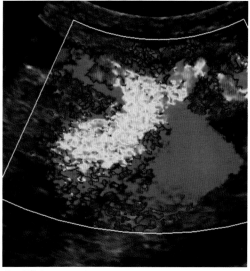

Color Plate 63 An example of a color Doppler image showing the color bruit of the surrounding tissue in a patient with an arteriovenous fistula. (See Fig. 22.12.)

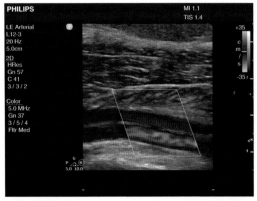

Color Plate 64 There is no flow seen against the walls in the vein, giving the illusion of a nonobstructive thrombus. This is caused by the color velocity scale being optimized for the artery. In this type of situation, it might be good to take a color Doppler image at the same level with the color scale optimized for the vein to show that the vein does completely fill in. (See Fig. 22.36.)

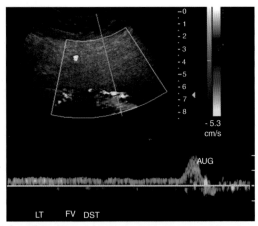

Color Plate 65 Using a lower-frequency curved linear array to optimally see the distal femoral vein. The superficial femoral artery is the area of aliasing above the vein caused by the low color velocity scale. The artery was normal. (See Fig. 22.37.)

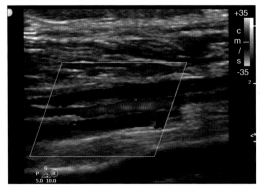

Color Plate 66 Color Doppler image of the two posterior tibial veins on either side of the posterior tibial artery. (See Fig. 22.43C.)

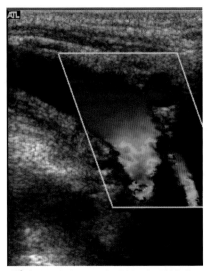

Color Plate 67 Color Doppler image in which the color is masking the clot underneath. (See Fig. 22.47A.)

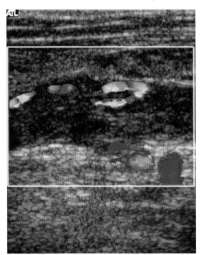

Color Plate 68 Color Doppler image of an acute deep vein thrombosis showing recanalized flow. (See Fig. 22.48B.)

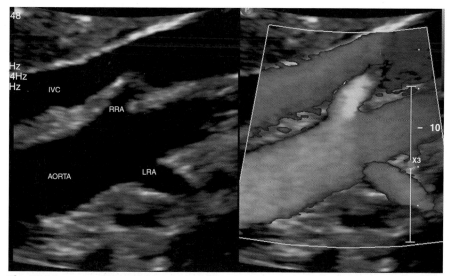

Fig. 20.24 A gray-scale and color Doppler image of the origins of the renal arteries form a coronal plane. This is the "banana peel" view. Ever notice how we equate findings with food in medicine? See Color Plate 24. *IVC,* Inferior vena cava; *LRA,* left renal artery; *RRA,* right renal artery.

This usually shows both origins at the same time, with Doppler angles less than 5 degrees. This is typically called the "banana peel" view because the aorta looks like a peeled banana with the arteries mimicking the peel (Fig. 20.24, Color Plate 24). Start with the patient supine and find the right kidney. Start to angle medially until the IVC is seen, and keep angling until the aorta comes into view. If unsuccessful with the patient in the supine position, roll the patient into a 30- to 45-degree left posterior oblique (LPO) position and repeat the previously described steps. If still unsuccessful, roll the patient into a 60-degree LPO position. This view takes some practice to be able to routinely obtain. Try to imagine the liver, IVC, and aorta aligned and how much to turn the patient to make that happen and where to place the transducer. With both origins nicely visualized, obtain Doppler signals from each one and the aorta if you could not see the aorta from the supine position (Fig. 20.25). This is also a good position to look for duplicated renal arteries (Fig. 20.26). Do not just obtain the right renal artery and come back later to obtain the origin of the left renal artery (Fig. 20.27). This increases scanning time, and there is no guarantee that you will be able to find it again, or you may struggle to duplicate the image. Evaluate the rest of the right renal artery with the patient in an LPO position using the kidney as an acoustic window. The transducer can be held in a longitudinal or transverse plane. Line up the renal hilum with the aorta using color Doppler to find the artery and vein. The entire right renal artery usually can be seen with this view. Note the color of the artery. If it is uniform, the artery

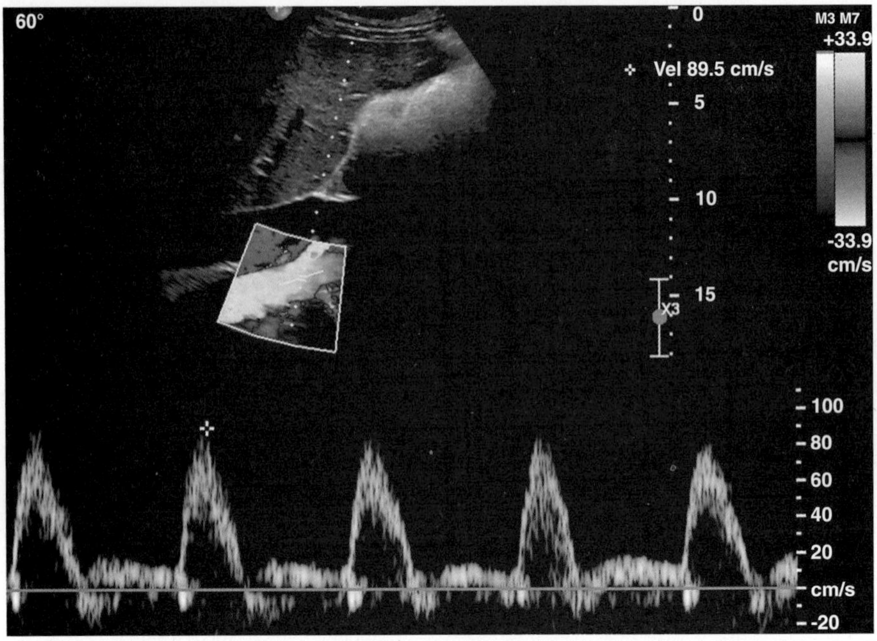

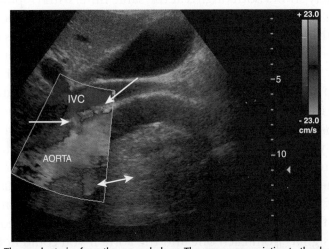

Fig. 20.25 A Doppler waveform from the aorta from the coronal plane. This is a good alternative if getting a waveform from the supine approach is difficult.

Fig. 20.26 The renal arteries from the coronal plane. The *arrows* are pointing to the duplicated right renal arteries and the *double-headed arrow* to the left renal artery. *IVC,* Inferior vena cava.

will be normal. If aliasing is seen, there is probably a stenosis, and this is where good Doppler waveforms should be obtained and velocities measured. Some patients may need to be in a steeper oblique or even in a left lateral decubitus position for the artery to be seen.

The left renal artery is shorter than the right and is about 3–4 cm in length. In some patients the left renal artery may be seen with the patient supine from the aorta to the hilum (Fig. 20.28, Color Plate 25). The artery usually appears with a good Doppler angle at the origin. With some patients, using slight transducer pressure applied over

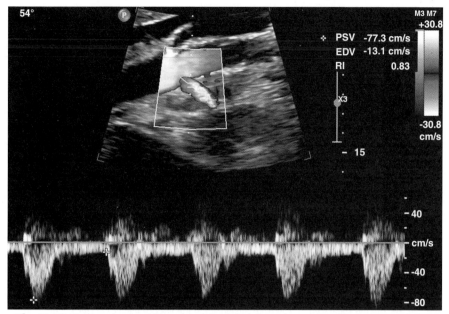

Fig. 20.27 The Doppler signal from the origin of the left renal artery from the banana peel view.

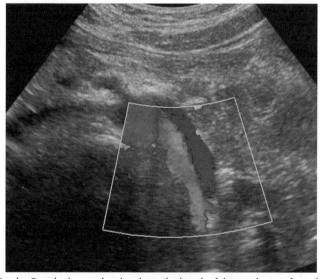

Fig. 20.28 A color Doppler image showing the entire length of the renal artery from the aorta to the kidney. The renal vein is seen superior to the artery. See Color Plate 25.

the aorta with a curved linear array will show the artery. The left renal vein can be used to locate the artery and serve as an acoustic window (Fig. 20.29, Color Plate 26). If there is too much gas, turn the patient into a right lateral decubitus, left side up, position and line up the kidney and the aorta in the same plane. With color Doppler the artery and vein can be located (Fig. 20.30, Color Plate 27). If the Doppler angle is zero, angle correction will not be used. The aorta may be devoid of color because flow will be perpendicular to the

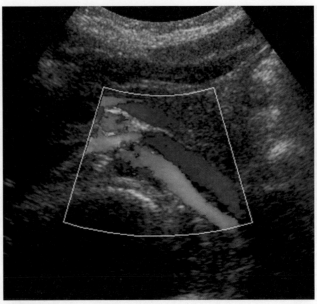

Fig. 20.29 The left renal vein is seen from the kidney to the inferior vena cava *(IVC)* anterior to the left renal artery and is being used as an acoustic window. See Color Plate 26.

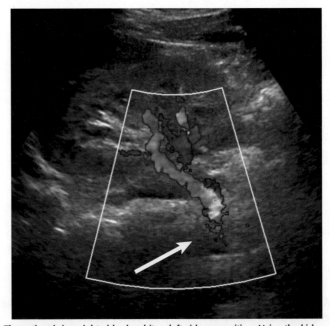

Fig. 20.30 The patient is in a right-side-decubitus, left-side-up position. Using the kidney as an acoustic window, the entire length of the artery is seen. The *arrow* is pointing to the aorta, where flow is not seen because it is perpendicular to the sound beam. See Color Plate 27.

sound beam. The origin of the left renal artery can be seen if it has not been imaged earlier in the examination. Again, look for uniformity in color or areas of aliasing.

Both renal arteries should be evaluated from the aorta to the renal hilum using angles less than 60 degrees. In some patients the origin of the renal arteries may be seen in a supine position, but it may be difficult to obtain an angle of 60 degrees or less for the waveform. The patency of the origin of the arteries can be demonstrated with color Doppler or power Doppler, because it is less angle dependent, if the origin is too perpendicular and will not fill in with color (Fig. 20.31, Color Plates 28 and 29). As with any type of Doppler examination, the Doppler angle should never be greater than 60 degrees and the angle correction cursor parallel to the walls of the renal artery (Fig. 20.32). At the hilum the main renal artery will bifurcate into the segmental arteries. In some patients the renal artery may start bifurcating before the hilum. The diagnosis of **renal artery stenosis** is made by measuring the peak systolic velocity and obtaining a ratio of renal artery–to–aortic velocity (RAR) using the peak velocities in each vessel. This is called a direct evaluation as the renal arteries themselves are being investigated. The Doppler criteria commonly referenced are a peak systolic measurement of greater than 180 to 200 cm/s and a renal artery–to-aorta ratio greater than 3 or 3.5. These numbers will correspond to a 60% diameter reduction of the renal artery. Because of the depth of the renal artery, it is not always possible to see the peak velocity. Remember that aliasing occurs at half the PRF, the Nyquist limit, which is influenced by the image depth. Because any number more than 200 cm/s is compatible with a greater than 60% stenosis, the true peak value is not needed and the top of the seen waveform measured and recorded is acceptable and diagnostic.

Evaluating the segmental or interlobar arteries is called an indirect evaluation. The sweep speed should be increased to stretch out the signal for more accurate measuring of the **acceleration time** (AT) and index (AI). If using automatic Doppler measuring, check that the AT is measured correctly, because some automatic traces measure to peak systole, which may not be the same as first systolic peak. This will give a false reading of prolonged acceleration time. When this occurs, do a second measurement tracing the start of systole to the first systolic peak and hit end (Fig. 20.33). This will measure the AT correctly. A prolonged AT will usually have a tardus-parvus type of waveform, indicating an upstream stenosis. A normal AT should be less than 0.07 second or 70 ms. Some machines will display the value in seconds (s), whereas others may use milliseconds (ms). Because of the delayed upstroke, a value greater than 70 ms is compatible with a stenosis greater than 60%. The AT can be used to look for differences between the segmental or interlobar arteries obtained from the upper, mid, and lower poles. If one segment is abnormal this might indicate the presence of a stenotic accessory or segmental artery. If a difference is noted between the kidneys, this may be an indication that the one with the prolonged time has a stenosis (Fig. 20.34). Normal intrarenal signals should have a sharp systolic upstroke with a normal acceleration index > 300 cm/s^2. On technically challenging examinations, for portable examinations, and when scanning patients on a ventilator, the intrarenal signals may be used as an indirect method to raise the suspicion of a hemodynamically significant

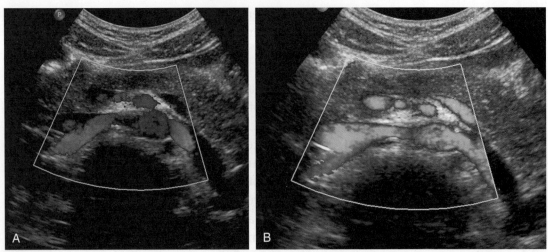

Fig. 20.31 A, A Doppler image of the renal arteries with the patient in the supine position. Note that there is no flow seen at the origin of the right renal artery because of angle issues. **B,** Using power Doppler, flow is seen in the origin and proximal segment because power Doppler is not as angle dependent. See Color Plates 28 and 29.

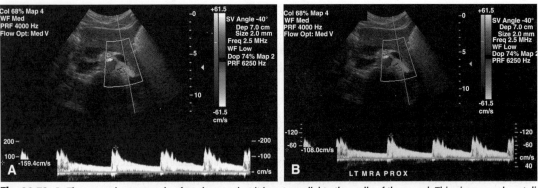

Fig. 20.32 A, The cursor is at an angle of 60 degrees, but it is not parallel to the walls of the vessel. This gives a peak systolic measurement of 159.5 cm/s. **B,** The cursor is now properly positioned parallel to the vessel walls, giving an angle of 40 degrees and a correct velocity measurement of 108 cm/s, which is 50 cm/s less than when the cursor was improperly placed.

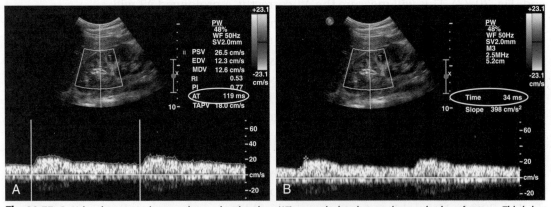

Fig. 20.33 A, Using the automatic trace, the acceleration time (AT) was calculated at an abnormal value of 119 ms. This is because the machine used peak systole as opposed to the early systolic peak. There was no evidence of arterial disease to explain the prolonged value, which was caused by technical issues. **B,** Same kidney using a manual trace. The cursor is placed at the start of systole, the second cursor at the early systolic peak, and the measurement ended. The machine is now only calculating the AT and the slope. This gives a normal value of 34 ms. Lesson learned: Always check measurements when obtained by an automatic method because sometimes they can be incorrect, causing confusion as to why there is an abnormal value suggestive of disease.

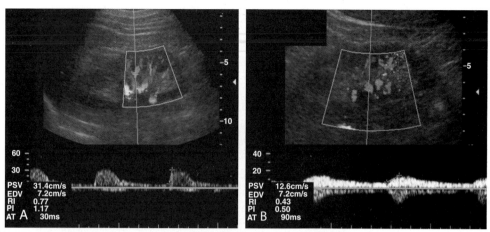

Fig. 20.34 A, The waveform from a normal interlobar artery from the right kidney showing a sharp upstroke and a normal acceleration time (AT) of 30 ms. **B,** The waveform from the left kidney showing an abnormal interlobar artery affected by renal artery stenosis. The signal is rounded and diminished in size with an AT of 90 ms.

stenosis. If there is still a concern for a renal artery stenosis with normal indirect findings, the patient may need to be scanned again when they are able to hold their breath and move into different positions.

Renal veins have larger diameters and are usually easier to see (Fig. 20.35, Color Plate 30). The average diameter of the vein is 9–12 mm compared to 5–6 mm for the arteries. The right renal vein is shorter than the left renal vein, which has to go over the aorta on its way to the IVC. If the right renal vein cannot be seen with the patient supine, try imaging with the patient in an LPO position. The left renal vein may need to be imaged in two positions if the entire vein cannot be seen with the patient supine. With the patient in the supine position, obtain the image of the left renal vein as it goes between the aorta and the SMA as it empties into the IVC (Fig. 20.36). If the origin and proximal portion cannot be evaluated, turn the patient into a right posterior oblique or a right lateral decubitus position. The renal veins appear as a low-velocity, continuous signal. When renal vein thrombosis is present, the kidney may enlarge and be echogenic, with loss of corticomedullary definition. The vein will be filled with low-level echoes, and the renal artery may show to-and-fro flow because the arterial blood cannot leave through the vein and will return back to the aorta because of the increased pressure in the kidney, which is greater than in the aorta in diastole (Fig. 20.37, Color Plate 31). If a renal mass is present and there appears to be renal vein thrombosis, evaluate the vein with color Doppler. If flow is seen inside the vein, a Doppler signal must be obtained to see if it represents arterial or venous flow. If arterial flow is seen, this is compatible with extension of the renal cell carcinoma into the vein and is called tumor thrombus. If thrombus is seen in the renal vein, the IVC must be evaluated for extension of the clot or tumor. If an IVC clot is discovered, the renal veins must be evaluated for extension of the clot. Because the renal veins empty through the side walls of the IVC, it is very easy for thrombus to spread from the IVC into the renal vein and vice versa.

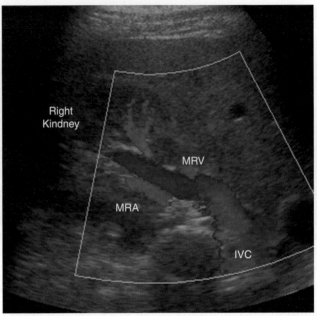

Fig. 20.35 A color Doppler image showing the entire right renal vein from the kidney to the inferior vena cava *(IVC)*. Note that it is bigger in diameter than the artery. See Color Plate 30. *MRA,* main renal artery; *MRV,* main renal vein.

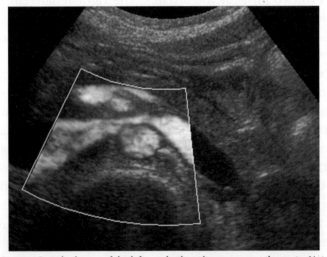

Fig. 20.36 A power Doppler image of the left renal vein as it crosses over the aorta. Note how the left renal vein is seen separately from the right renal artery, showing the better spatial resolution of power Doppler. With color Doppler the two vessels tend to blend together as one big vessel. Because they are both flowing in the same direction, they will be the same color.

The sonographer needs to observe for vascular anomalies, and the renal system is no exception. As discussed earlier in the chapter a patient may have multiple renal arteries. If multiple renal arteries are discovered, each artery needs to be completely evaluated for any evidence of a stenosis (Fig. 20.38, Color Plate 32). Besides multiple renal arteries, another anomaly is the retroaortic left renal vein, in which

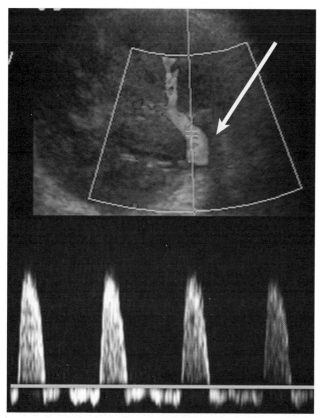

Fig. 20.37 The *arrow* is pointing to the thrombosed right renal vein. The arterial signal is biphasic, which can be seen with renal vein thrombosis. See Color Plate 31.

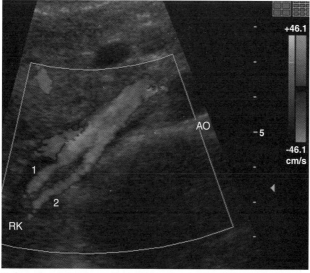

Fig. 20.38 A Doppler image from a supine position showing two right renal arteries. See Color Plate 32. *AO,* Aorta.

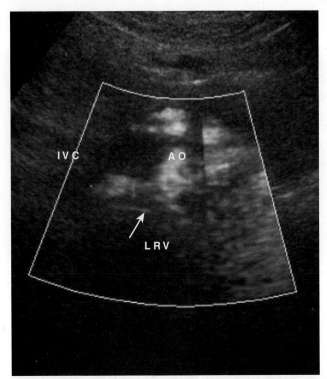

Fig. 20.39 The *arrow* is pointing to a left retroaortic renal vein. Power Doppler was helpful in seeing the vessel because of the increased spatial resolution that separated it from the aorta and the fact that it is not as angle dependent. Care should be taken to look posterior to the aorta when a vein is not seen crossing between the aorta and superior mesenteric artery so as not to assume that there is a renal vein thrombosis. Even though variants are rare, the sonographer needs to think about them while scanning. See Color Plate 33. *IVC,* Inferior vena cava; *LRV,* left renal vein;

the vein goes under the aorta as opposed to above the aorta (Fig. 20.39, Color Plate 33). This can occur in about 3% of the population.

Renal artery stenosis can be caused by atherosclerotic disease or fibromuscular dysplasia (FMD). It is important for the sonographer to recognize the sonographic differences between atherosclerotic disease and FMD. Renal artery stenosis caused by atherosclerotic disease typically affects the origin and proximal portions of an artery. On the gray-scale image, the plaque can be seen at the origin (Fig. 20.40). With color Doppler the narrowing of the lumen is appreciated and color aliasing is seen (Fig. 20.41, Color Plate 34). The Doppler findings of a stenosis are seen in Fig. 20.21.

FMD is a nonatherosclerotic arterial disease that primarily affects young women. It is a disease of the walls of the artery that occurs in the mid and distal portions of the artery, causing small stenoses with areas of post dilatation or small aneurysms. FMD can be found in any artery, but it is primarily found in the renal and internal carotid arteries. It can be found in both renal arteries in up to 60% of patients and in both the renal and internal carotid arteries in about 15% of patients. On angiography the characteristic pattern is called a "string of beads" because of the alternating areas of stenoses and dilation.

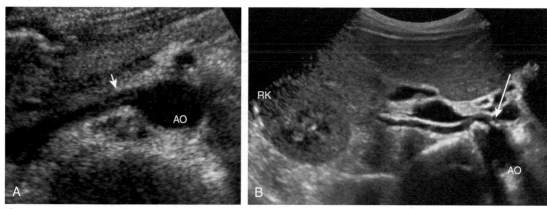

Fig. 20.40 A, The *arrow* is pointing to a thrombus seen with gray scale inside the right renal artery. *AO,* Aorta. **B,** Another example of the importance of gray scale because it shows calcifications *(arrow)* at the orifice of the renal artery that may be originating from inside the aorta *(AO)*. *RK,* Right kidney.

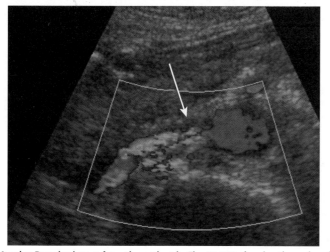

Fig. 20.41 A color Doppler image from the patient in Fig. 20.40A showing the reduced lumen *(arrow)*. See Color Plate 34.

On gray scale, the artery will appear normal because the areas of stenosis are too small to be appreciated (Fig. 20.42). On ultrasound, FMD is suspected when there is aliasing of the color signal in the mid to distal artery (Fig. 20.43, Color Plate 35). A Doppler waveform in this area will show elevated velocities (Fig. 20.44, Color Plates 36 and 37).

Do not be afraid to do renal artery examinations and do not get a defeatist attitude when you have a difficult study. Remember that an image does not have to be textbook perfect, but it does need to be diagnostic. Use the kidney as the acoustic window to see the artery. Learn the controls on the machine so you can use that control when needed. Use different patient positions as discussed, as well as various transducer positions. Once you have a good view of the artery, hold still and walk down or up the artery. You may need different positions to see the entire artery. The right kidney can be scanned with the patient in supine, oblique, or decubitus position. The left kidney can be scanned with the patient in the supine or decubitus position. Oblique views may work as well. Doppler waveforms signals can be obtained with the patient prone (Fig. 20.45). As you are moving the sample volume through the artery, listen for those high velocities. Use color Doppler to find areas of high velocity and to help with angle correction. It can be easy to forget about angle correction as you sample the artery. It is appropriate to move the sample volume as you search for high velocities; however, when you are ready to take the image, angle correction needs to be checked. It is best to do

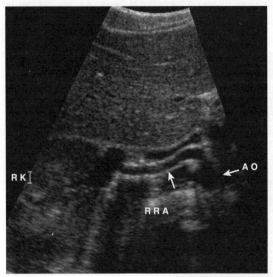

Fig. 20.42 The right renal artery (RRA) of a patient with fibromuscular dysplasia. Note how the artery looks normal with gray scale. *AO,* Aorta; *RK,* right kidney.

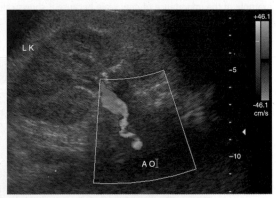

Fig. 20.43 A color Doppler image of the left renal artery showing mid-vessel aliasing. See Color Plate 35. *AO,* Aorta; *LK,* left kidney.

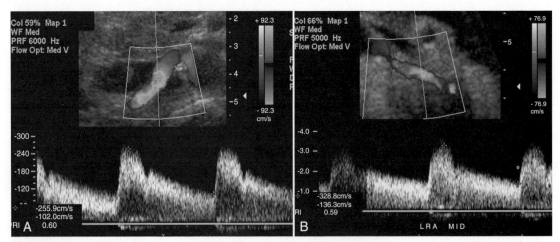

Fig. 20.44 A, The Doppler signal from mid-artery showing an elevated flow of 255 cm/s compatible with fibromuscular dysplasia (FMD). **B,** A Doppler signal from the left midrenal artery with a velocity of 328.8 cm/s, again compatible with FMD. This patient had bilateral FMD of the renal arteries. See Color Plates 36 and 37.

angle correction while scanning and not adjust on a frozen image, because it can be easy to subconsciously angle the transducer when trying to obtain the best signal. If that happens, the angle used for color Doppler may not match the angle used for spectral Doppler.

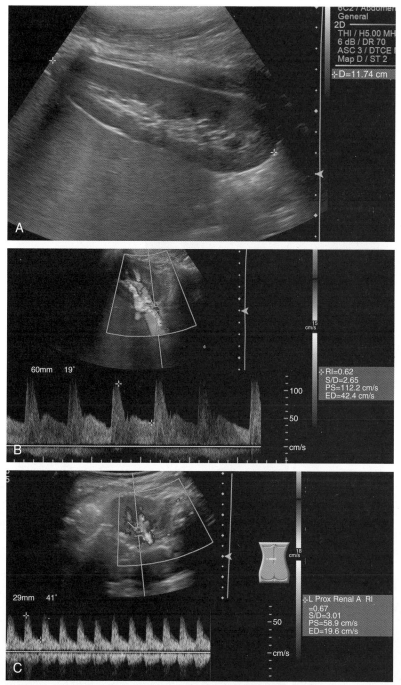

Fig. 20.45 A, An image of the left kidney from a prone position. The spleen is seen posterior to the patient. Of note, it is rare to see the spleen. **B,** Obtaining a waveform from the proximal renal artery with the patient in the prone position. **C,** Obtaining a waveform from an interlobar artery with the patient in the prone position. As can be seen, good images and Doppler waveforms can be obtained from a prone position.

If having trouble, turn off the color and scan with real-time 2D and spectral Doppler. Make sure you evaluate the kidneys for any pathologic conditions. If the patient is scheduled for examination to rule out hypertension and you discover that the patient has adult polycystic kidney disease, you have the answer to the hypertension, and evaluation of the renal artery may not be necessary. Always confirm with the interpreting or ordering physician first. Renal artery studies can be challenging at first, but as you perform more of these studies, your skills will improve and you may discover that you like the challenge they provide. If you have time, practice the banana peel view on routine renal studies. Mastering this view is a skill and very helpful for evaluating the renal artery origins.

If asked to evaluate the renal veins for a thrombus, the diagnosis is made using color or power Doppler to show vessel patency, no flow, or partial flow (Fig. 20.46). The kidney on the affected side will

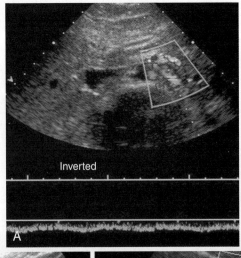

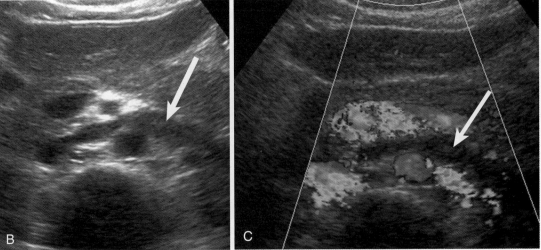

Fig. 20.46 A, A waveform from the left renal vein showing a normal waveform. The waveform has been inverted so that the flow is under the baseline. This is not necessary and not usually done. The author always preferred not to invert the baseline except for carotid and renal arteries. **B,** A gray-scale image in which the *arrow* is pointing to a thrombus in the left renal vein. **C,** A color Doppler image showing absence of flow in the left renal artery *(arrow).*

enlarge and become echogenic. If there is a clot, the IVC needs to be evaluated for extension of the clot. Spectral Doppler of the vein really adds no benefit to the examination, but some laboratories will want a sample taken from the normal or thrombosed vein. As stated earlier, the Doppler signal from the artery will typically show biphasic flow because of the increased pressure from the outlet obstruction.

Kidney Required Images

Kidney • Longitudinal Images

1. Long axis image with the longest length measured.

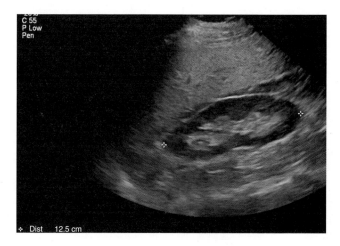

Suggested annotation: **RT KID**

2. This may be optional in some laboratories. Perfusion image of the kidney with color or power Doppler.

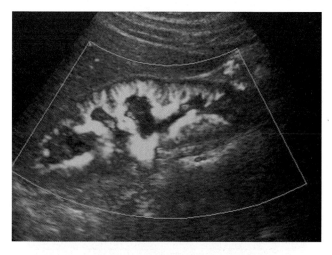

Suggested annotation: **RT KID**

Kidney • Doppler Images

> **NOTE:** All measurements must be angle corrected with peak velocity and end diastole measured. Some labs may only measure end diastole in the intrarenal arteries. The following images are from a variety of patients to provide the reader example images from different patients.

1. Doppler signal of the aorta just distal to the SMA in the region of the origin of the renal arteries. May be with or without color Doppler with the peak velocity measured.

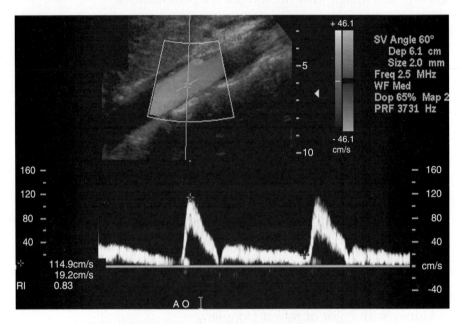

Suggested annotation: **AORTA or AO**

2. Transverse image of the aorta at the level of the origin of the renal arteries. In some patients the view of this area may be obstructed by gas, and the sonographer would go to the coronal banana peel view.

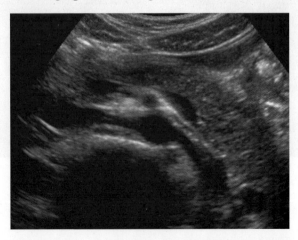

Suggested annotation: **TRV AO ORIGIN MRAS**

3. Color Doppler image of the aorta at the level of the origin of the renal arteries.

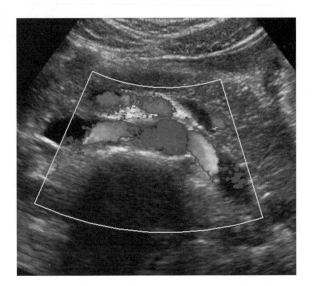

Suggested annotation: **TRV AO ORIGIN MRAS**

4. If the left renal artery can be seen, a color Doppler image of the length of the renal artery or of the part that seen.

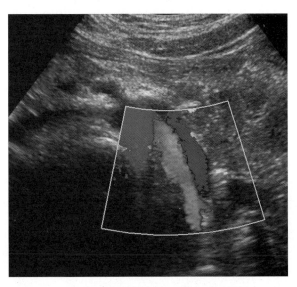

Suggested annotation: **LRA**

5. If the left renal artery can be seen, a Doppler waveform of the origin and/or proximal portion with systolic and diastolic velocities measured.

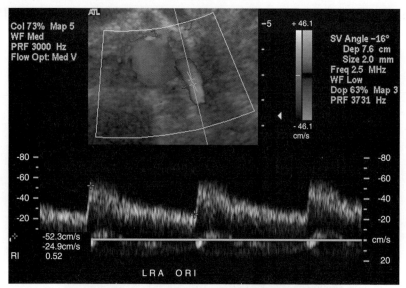

Suggested annotation: **LRA ORI or ORI/PROX**

In some patients the mid to distal segments will be obscured by bowel gas. If the entire length of the left renal artery is well seen, obtain Doppler waveforms from the mid and distal artery. You can continue with the left kidney to obtain the intrarenal signals, but this usually involves the patient being in a right lateral decubitus position. While the patient is supine, obtain Doppler signals from the right renal artery. My routine was to obtain what can be seen with the patient in the supine position of the renal arteries and then go to the banana peel view.

6. In some patients it may be difficult to obtain a good angle for the origin of the right renal artery. If the proximal portion is seen, obtain a waveform or go to the banana peel view.

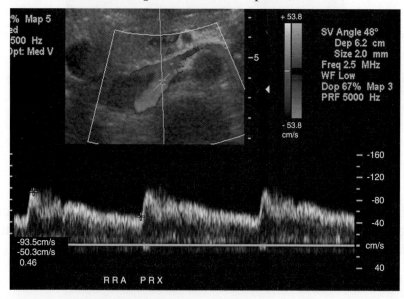

Suggested annotation: **RRA ORI or PROX depending on where the waveform was obtained**

If obtaining the origin was successful, obtain the proximal segment or obtain the waveforms from the right renal artery from the oblique position. I would usually not obtain Doppler signals from the right side with the patient in the supine position.

7. Determine the best position for the patient and the transducer to obtain the renal arteries in the coronal plane, the banana peel view. Once found, take a gray-scale image of the aorta and the origins of the renal arteries. In some patients the left renal artery *(LRA)* can be tricky to line up. Do not waste a lot of time frustrating yourself or the patient if the right renal artery *(RRA)* is seen, especially if the left renal artery was seen and documented from the supine position. The origin of the left renal artery is also well seen when the patient is in the right lateral decubitus position.

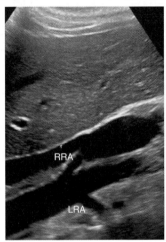

Suggested annotation: **ORIGIN MRAS; some sonographers may annotate on the screen RT MRA, LT MRA; some sonographers may also annotate as CORONAL MRAS**

8. Color Doppler of the origin of the renal arteries. *LRA,* Left renal artery; *RRA,* right renal artery.

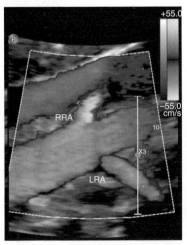

Suggested annotation: **ORIGIN MRAS**

9. If the left renal artery is seen, obtain a Doppler waveform of the origin measuring peak systole and end diastole. The angle may vary but will always be less than 60 degrees, and in some patients it may even be zero and angle correction is not used.

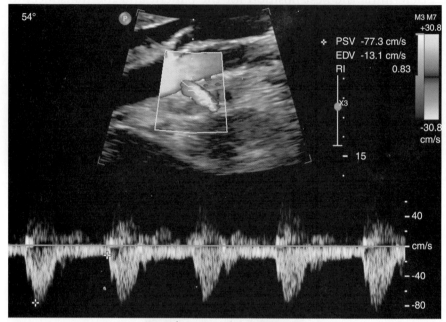

Suggested annotation: **ORIGIN LRA**

10. Color Doppler and waveform of the origin of the right renal artery with measurements.

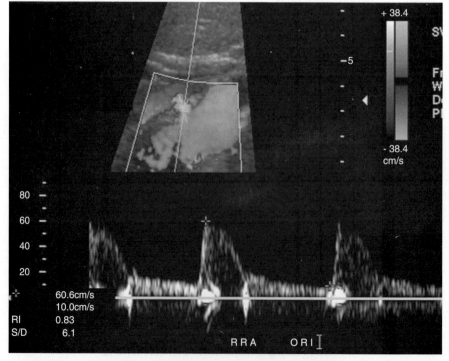

Suggested annotation: **ORIGIN RRA**

11. Color Doppler image of the length of the entire renal artery. *RT MRA*, main renal artery.

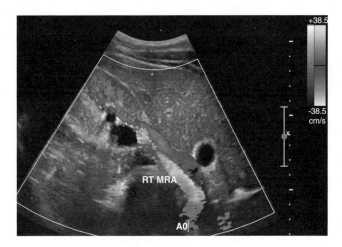

Suggested annotation: **RRA**

At this point the sonographer can Doppler from distal to proximal or proximal to distal. The author preferred distal to proximal.

12. Doppler waveform of the distal segment of the right renal artery with peak systole and end diastolic velocities measured.

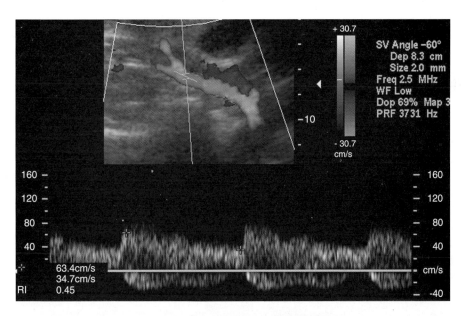

Suggested annotation: **RRA DIST**

13. Doppler waveform of the mid segment of the right renal artery with measurements.

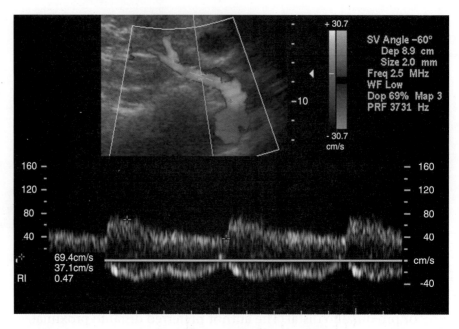

Suggested annotation: **RRA MID**

14. Doppler waveform of the proximal segment of the right renal artery with measurements.

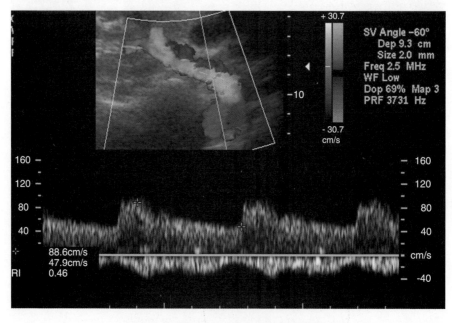

Suggested annotation: **RRA PROX**

15. Doppler waveform of the origin of the right renal artery with measurements if not already obtained from other views.

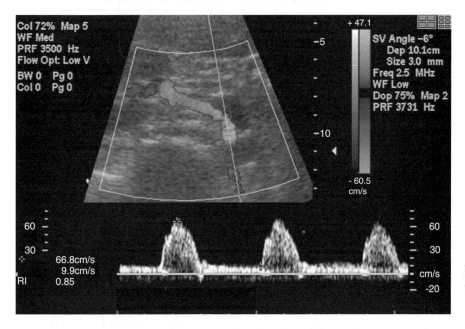

Suggested annotation: **RRA ORI**

16. Angle-corrected waveform from the segmental or interlobar artery from the upper pole of the kidney with peak systole, end diastole, RI, and AT measured. Some laboratories may also include the AI. You can start anywhere in the kidney; just make sure that all three poles are evaluated.

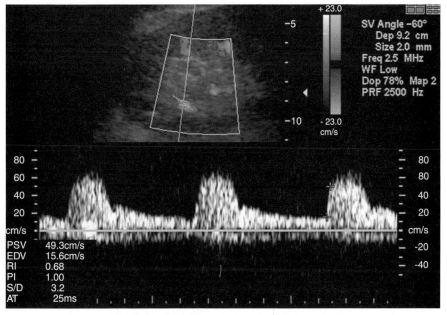

Suggested annotation: **RT SEG/ILA UP**

17. Angle-corrected waveform from the segmental or interlobar artery from the mid-pole of the kidney with peak systole, end diastole, RI, and AT measured. Some laboratories may also include the AI.

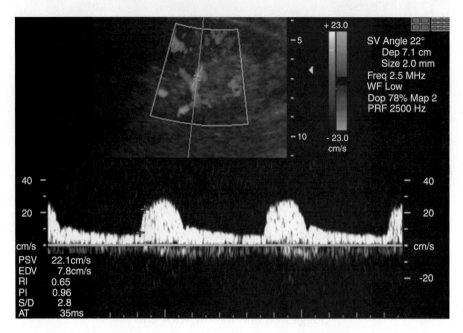

Suggested annotation: **RT SEG/ILA MID**

18. Angle-corrected waveform from the segmental or interlobar artery from the lower pole of the kidney with peak systole, end diastole, RI, and AT measured. Some laboratories may also include the AI.

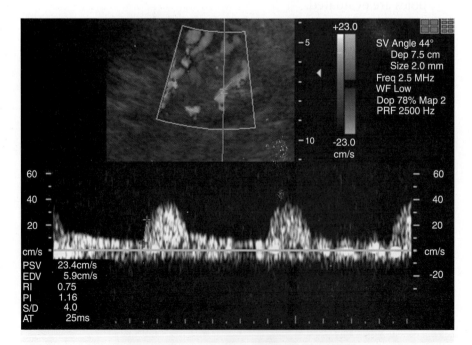

Suggested annotation: **RT SEG/ILA LOW**

19. Doppler waveform from the renal vein at the hilum.

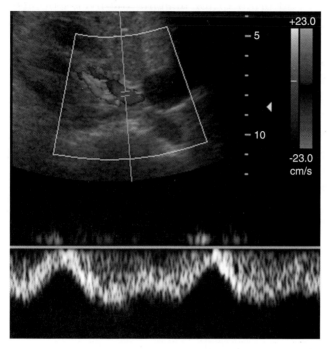

Suggested annotation: **RRV**

20. Repeat for the left kidney. Images that were obtained with the patient in the supine or coronal position do not need to be repeated, although some sonographers may repeat them to have a consistent flow of signals obtained from the same position at the same time. Turn the patient into the right lateral decubitus position and line up the left kidney and the aorta.

Liver Required Doppler Images

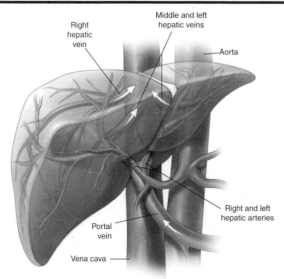

Hilscher MB, Kamath PS. The liver in circulatory disturbances. *Clin Liver Dis* 2019;23(2): 209–220.

Refer to Chapter 6 to review the anatomy, physiology, sonographic appearance, and protocol for imaging the liver. Doppler studies of the liver are performed when portal hypertension or thrombosis is suspected and when hepatic vein thrombosis is suspected. Except in liver transplants, the hepatic artery is rarely the concern for causing liver problems. In a liver Doppler examination, the main portal vein, the right and left branch of the portal vein, the main hepatic artery, and the right, middle, and left hepatic veins are evaluated with gray-scale, color, and spectral Doppler. If the patient has a liver transplant, then the right and left hepatic arteries need to be evaluated as well.

Patient Prep

The patient is typically NPO after midnight for two reasons: first, because typically the biliary system is evaluated; and second, portal vein velocities are based on the preprandial state of the portal vein. Portal vein velocities will increase after the patient has had something to eat or drink. If the biliary system does not need to be properly evaluated and the velocity in the portal vein is not required, the study may be performed on a patient who was not NPO.

Transducer

A curved linear array that includes frequencies in the 3–5 MHz range or a phased/vector array transducer with frequencies in the 1–3 MHz range for patients with a fatty liver and larger patients, although the patient should be first imaged with the curved linear array and switched to a lower frequency only if needed. A phased/vector array transducer may be needed for intercostal views. For pediatric and newborn patients use a sector/vector array with frequencies in the 5–10 MHz range or a tightly curved array, such as the transducer used for neonatal brain sonograms, with frequencies in the same range or a curved linear array with frequencies in the 5–9 MHz range.

Breathing Technique

The patient will need to suspend breathing at times during the examination. Depending on the vessel being evaluated, the patient may need to take in a deep breath and hold it, take in a small to medium breath and hold it, suspend respiration when instructed, hold the breath on expiration, or breathe normally.

Patient Position

Typically, the scan is done with the patient in the supine position and turned into an LPO position to better evaluate the vessels as needed. If the gallbladder needs to be examined, left lateral decubitus views will be needed.

Technical Tips

To evaluate the hepatic vasculature, the sonographer should be knowledgeable about the different variations in the vessels, especially the hepatic arteries. A replaced right hepatic artery occurs when it originates from the SMA (Fig. 20.47).

The three main hepatic veins are the right, middle, and left hepatic veins. The most common normal variant is a right inferior or accessory hepatic vein, which is separate from the right hepatic vein and drains the right posterior lobe (Fig. 20.48). The right hepatic vein is the largest of the three veins. In a common variant the left and middle hepatic veins join to form a single vein before entering the IVC. The hepatic veins have a pulsatile flow pattern because of their close proximity to the right atrium. Their pattern is influenced by pressure changes in the right atrium. The normal pattern of the hepatic vein is described as pulsatile, multiphasic, or even triphasic. The Doppler spectral pattern shows an above and below baseline flow pattern. The flow above the baseline is caused by the right atrial contraction, which sends blood back into the liver. During ventricular systole, blood will be below the baseline as it flows into the right atrium. The majority of the signal will be below the baseline, emptying into the IVC (Fig. 20.49). This

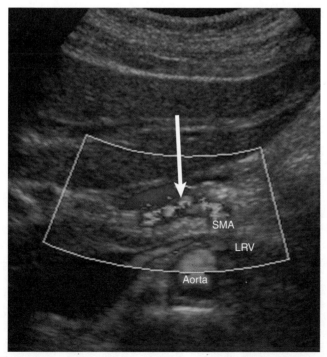

Fig. 20.47 The *arrow* is pointing to a replaced right hepatic artery that is originating from the superior mesenteric artery *(SMA)*. If there was also the normal right hepatic artery coming off of the main hepatic artery, this would be called an accessory right hepatic artery. *LRV,* Left renal vein.

pattern can become exaggerated in right-sided heart failure (Fig. 20.50) or monophasic as a result of increased intrahepatic pressure as seen with patients who have cirrhosis (Fig. 20.51). The hepatic veins can be seen in a transverse subxiphoid or subcostal view. The veins should be seen with color or power Doppler to drain into the IVC, because it is possible to have thrombosis just at this level. The right hepatic vein may be seen with color Doppler, but it may be hard to obtain a Doppler signal because of its perpendicular

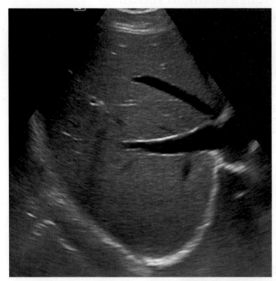

Fig. 20.48 An example of an accessory right hepatic vein. Note the bright walls caused by a specular refection.

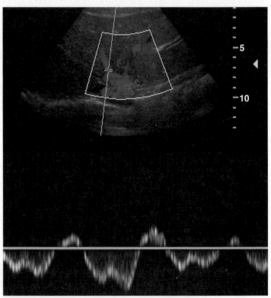

Fig. 20.49 An example of a normal hepatic vein waveform showing the pulsatile waveform caused by the close proximity to the heart.

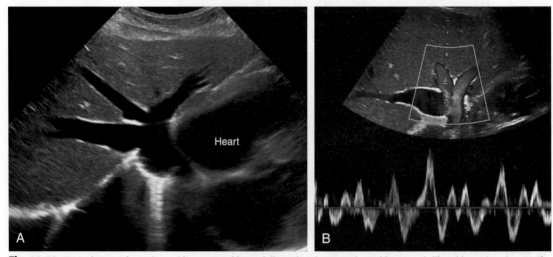

Fig. 20.50 A, An image of a patient with congested heart failure showing an enlarged heart and dilated hepatic veins. **B,** The Doppler waveform from the middle hepatic vein from a patient with right-sided heart failure. The waveform almost looks upside down from a normal waveform. Note the exaggerated flows back into the liver.

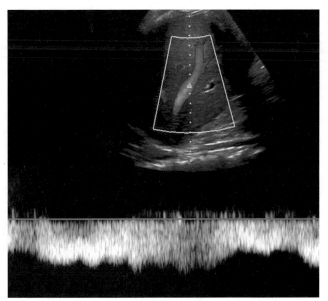

Fig. 20.51 An example of a "portalized" hepatic vein, so called because the flow resembles that found in the portal vein. These patients have increased hepatic pressure that keeps the blood flowing into the heart. This waveform is usually seen in patients with cirrhosis.

course. In these patients, move the transducer laterally to obtain a better angle or move to an intercostal approach to improve the Doppler angle. Thrombosis of the hepatic veins, Budd-Chiari syndrome, can be diagnosed with color and power Doppler by observing the lack of hepatic veins or the inability to visualize the hepatic veins draining into the IVC (Fig. 20.52). Enlargement of the caudate lobe may be seen in patients with hepatic vein thrombosis; hepatic blood flow will drain into the caudate lobe, causing volume overload because the caudate lobe drains directly into the IVC via the caudate veins, which are rarely seen by ultrasound. An enlarged caudate lobe is an indirect sign of hepatic vein thrombosis (Fig. 20.53). In some patients one or more of the hepatic veins may be affected. These patients may also develop portal vein hypertension.

The portal vein is formed by the confluence of the splenic and superior mesenteric veins. On entering the liver at the hilum, the main portal vein divides into right and left branches (Fig. 20.54). The portal vein should have a low-velocity signal that is almost continuous with slight variations in respiration (Fig. 20.55). Because the flow of the portal vein is an "uphill" flow toward the hilum of the liver and the transducer, flow will be displayed in a positive deflection above the baseline. Normal portal flow is termed hepatopetal, sometimes written as hepatopedal, and reversed portal flow is termed hepatofugal flow. Hepatopetal is considered the proper term, as *hepato* refers to the liver and *petal* comes from the Latin *petere*, which

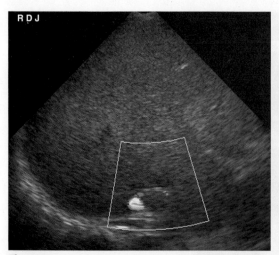

Fig. 20.52 Transverse image in the area of the hepatic veins. Flow is seen in the inferior vena cava, but there is no evidence of the hepatic veins.

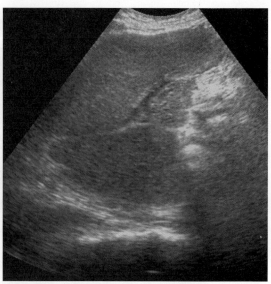

Fig. 20.53 A patient with an enlarged caudate lobe, which is seen in patients with hepatic vein thrombosis, (Budd-Chiari syndrome). The caudate lobe enlarges as a result of volume overload as the liver sends its blood to the caudate lobe that empties directly into the inferior vena cava by the caudate veins.

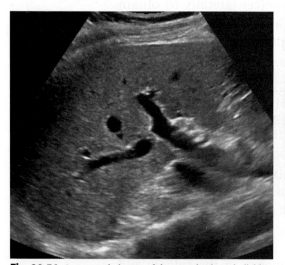

Fig. 20.54 A gray-scale image of the portal vein as it divides into its right and left branches.

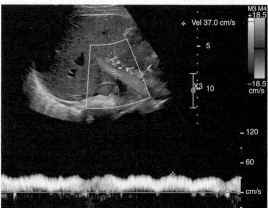

Fig. 20.55 A normal waveform from the portal vein.

means traveling toward; together they translate as traveling toward the liver. A good rule of thumb is that both the hepatic artery and the portal vein will flow in the same direction (Fig. 20.56). The right portal vein as it courses into the right lobe will flow away from the transducer and therefore will be below the baseline (Fig. 20.57). It is important to evaluate the portal vein with color or power Doppler to show complete vessel fill-in (Fig. 20.58). An intercostal approach may be needed to evaluate the portal vein in a longitudinal view and an intercostal and subcostal approach for transverse views.

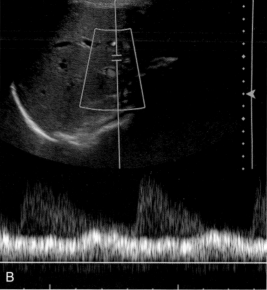

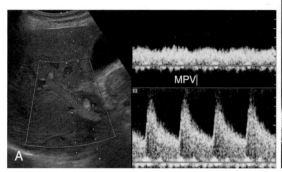

Fig. 20.56 A, An ultrasound unit that has the ability to obtain two Doppler tracings at the same time. This image shows normal hepatopetal portal vein and hepatic artery flow. **B,** The flows in the portal vein and hepatic artery need to be documented to show that both are flowing in the same direction. By positioning the sample volume just right, a Doppler signal from both can be seen on one tracing. *MPV,* main portal vein.

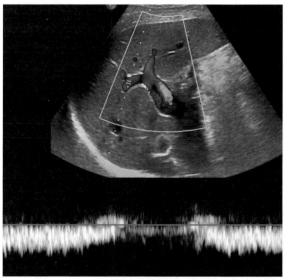

Fig. 20.57 The normal flow direction for the right portal vein is away from the transducer because it sends blood to the right posterior lobe. If a patient had portal hypertension, blood would be flowing toward the transducer.

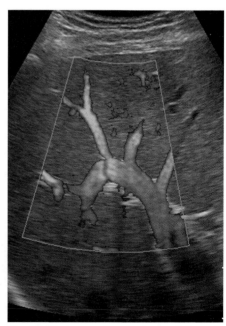

Fig. 20.58 A power Doppler image of the main portal vein and branches.

The sonographer needs to be able to differentiate between the hepatic veins and the portal veins. This is easily done in one of two ways. Remember that the portal triad is enclosed by Glisson's capsule, which is highly reflective on ultrasound. This means that no matter how small the portal vein is, it will have bright walls. Hepatic veins are not covered by any highly reflective covering and appear to blend in with the parenchyma (Fig. 20.59). Do not be fooled by "echogenic" walls of the main hepatic vein, usually the right, because this brightness represents a specular reflection, and the left and main veins will not have bright walls because they are not perpendicular to the sound beam. The second way is to obtain a Doppler waveform, as portal veins will have a continuous waveform and the hepatic veins a pulsatile one. The normal patterns may be altered with certain disease processes, making the two waveforms appear similar in appearance. In these instances, the bright walls of the portal vein will help differentiate between the two.

The sonographer should pay attention to the CVS when evaluating the portal vein and the hepatic artery. The CVS will be at a higher number to see the hepatic artery without aliasing. This may give the impression of a thrombus in the portal vein if flow is not seen. Decreasing the CVS to optimize portal vein flow may cause the hepatic artery to alias. Each vessel may need to be worked up independently for the best optimization of each vessel (Fig. 20.60, Color Plates 38 and 39). In most patients one CVS setting may work for both vessels (Fig. 20.60, Color Plate 40). This can be the challenge in the liver of optimizing for one vessel at the sacrifice of the other. Before assuming that there is an issue with a vessel, check the CVS setting. Usually the portal flow is the problem. When no or poor flow is seen in the portal vein, it is important to reduce the CVS.

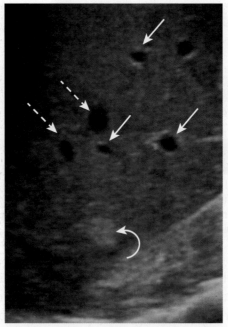

Fig. 20.59 The *solid arrows* are pointing to the echogenic portal veins. The *dashed arrows* are pointing to the "wall-less" hepatic veins. Note that no matter how small the portal branch is, it has an echogenic wall, and that even the larger hepatic veins do not have echogenic walls. The *curved arrow* is pointing to an hemangioma.

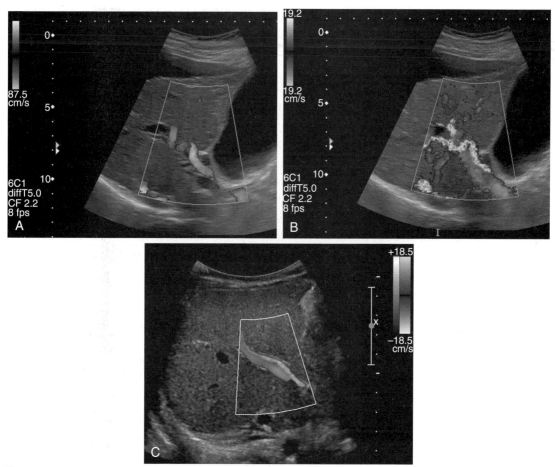

Fig. 20.60 A, The color velocity scale (CVS) is at 87.5 cm/s, removing the aliasing from the hepatic artery but is not showing the flow in the portal vein. Because the patient has cirrhosis and ascites, this technical setting could be misleading for portal vein thrombosis. **B,** By reducing the CVS to 19.2 cm/sec, flow is now seen in the portal vein. **C,** A color Doppler image showing normal flow in both the portal vein and the hepatic artery. See Color Plates 38, 39, and 40.

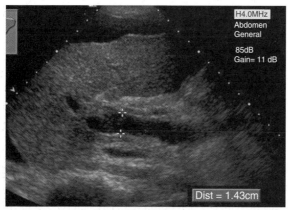

Fig. 20.61 An image measuring the diameter of the portal vein, which is over 13 cm, compatible with portal hypertension.

Portal hypertension is caused by an increase in resistance to flow in the hepatocytes, as can be seen in patients with cirrhosis. Sonographically, an enlarged portal vein measuring greater than 13 mm may be seen with hepatopetal flow in the early stages (Fig. 20.61). The portal vein diameter should be measured just above the IVC where the hepatic artery crosses the portal vein with the patient in quiet respiration. Eventually the flow will become hepatofugal, with the hepatic artery and portal vein flowing in opposite directions. The hepatic arterial flow will enter the cell and be forced to take the path of least resistance, which is to exit the damaged cell through the portal vein. It is important that the CVS be set appropriately so that the portal flow direction can be determined, which will be away from the liver with portal hypertension (Fig. 20.62, Color Plate 41). This may cause aliasing in the hepatic artery, and an image optimized for the artery should be obtained. Spectral Doppler waveforms should be obtained from each vessel. In some patients the sample volume may be positioned to obtain both signals simultaneously (Fig. 20.63). The baseline should never be inverted when evaluating the portal vein because this can lead to a misdiagnosis. It is much easier to see that the flow is below the baseline as opposed to trying to locate the word "invert" or the + and – symbols on the scale.

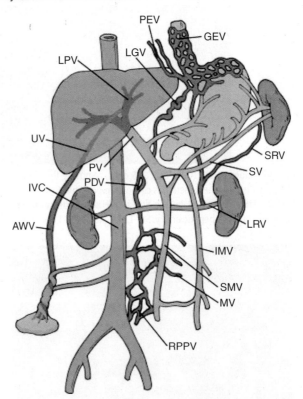

Drawing illustrates the collateral vessels in portal hypertension: *AWV,* abdominal wall vein; *GEV,* gastroesophageal vein; *IMV,* inferior mesenteric vein; *IVC,* inferior vena cava; *LGV,* left gastric vein; *LPV,* left portal vein; *LRV,* left renal vein; *MV,* mesenteric vein; *PDV,* pancreaticoduodenal vein; *PEV,* paraesophageal vein; *PV,* portal vein; *RPPV,* retroperitoneal-paravertebral vein; *SMV,* superior mesenteric vein; SRV, splenorenal vein; *SV,* splenic vein; *UV,* umbilical vein. (From Gore RM, Levine MS. *Textbook of Gastrointestinal Radiology,* 4th ed. Philadelphia, 2015, Saunders.)

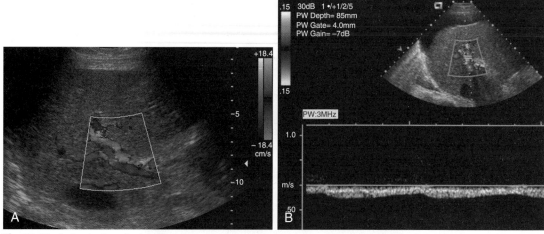

Fig. 20.62 A, A color Doppler image of the portal vein and hepatic artery. The portal vein is a dark color from the bottom half of the color bar. This is compatible with portal hypertension. **B,** A Doppler waveform from the portal vein showing flow beneath the baseline consistent with portal hypertension. See Color Plate 41.

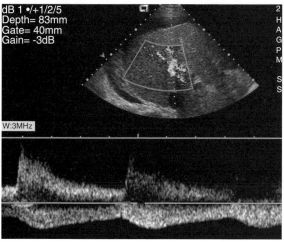

Fig. 20.63 An image with the Doppler sample volume positioned to show that the flow is in opposite directions with the hepatic artery above the baseline and the portal vein flow below the baseline.

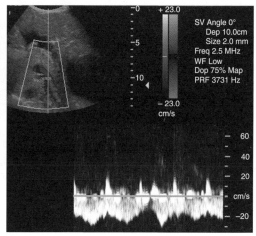

Fig. 20.64 A Doppler waveform from the splenic vein showing flow back toward the spleen. See Color Plate 42.

With the portal blood unable to get into the systemic circulation to get back to the heart, the body will try to find a way to get the blood where it needs to go. This will cause the formation of varices and collaterals, and the sonographer will see vessels where there should be no vessels. The splenic vein should be evaluated for possible reversed flow, because the portal blood will flow back toward the spleen, which may cause splenic varices and splenomegaly. The best way to evaluate the splenic vein is to evaluate the segment from the splenic hilum to midline because that portion will always be flowing toward the transducer in a normal patient (Fig. 20.64, Color Plate 42). With red on the top part of the color bar, normal flow will be red and reversed flow will be blue. The abdomen should be evaluated for

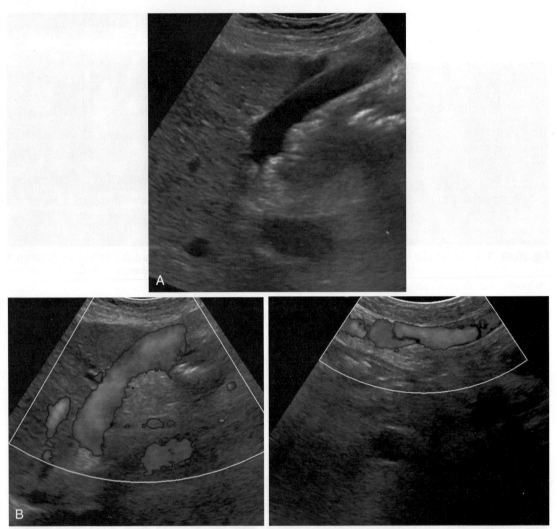

Fig. 20.65 A, A gray-scale image of a reconstituted umbilical vein as it heads to the surface. **B,** Doppler image of the reconstituted umbilical vein. **C,** Doppler image of the reconstituted umbilical vein underneath the skin as it heads toward the umbilical area.

other problems caused by portal hypertension, such as a recanalized umbilical vein, collateral vessels, varices, and ascites. A recanalized umbilical vein arises from the left portal vein and courses toward the abdominal wall as it travels to the umbilicus (Fig. 20.65), where it causes the superficial epigastric veins to dilate, called the caput medusa. It is important not to mistake a collateral for a normal vein (Fig. 20.66, Color Plates 43 and 44), because the body makes new vessels to try to find a way back into the systemic system. Varices may be seen around the esophageal junction or the splenic hilum (Fig. 20.67). These esophageal varices can burst, causing gastrointestinal bleeding. In some patients a collateral may be seen that connects the splenic vein with the left renal vein, creating a splenorenal shunt that will allow the portal blood to get into the systemic system via the renal vein. A Doppler signal in the renal vein will show turbulent flow (Fig. 20.68, Color Plate 45). The extent of ascites should be

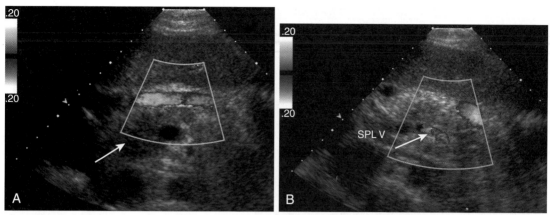

Fig. 20.66 A, An image of a collateral vein superior to the pancreas that was initially thought to be the splenic vein until it was noticed that the vessel was above the pancreas. The *arrow* is pointing to the head of the pancreas. **B,** The same patient with the *arrow* pointing to a small splenic vein that is flowing back toward the spleen. See Color Plates 43 and 44. *SPL V,* Splenic vein.

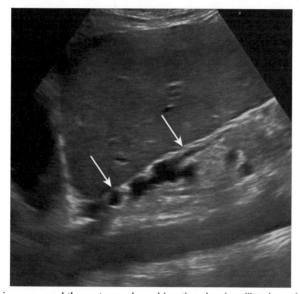

Fig. 20.67 An image around the gastroesophageal junction showing dilated esophageal veins *(arrows)* compatible with esophageal varices.

documented (Fig. 20.69). Portal hypertension causes a lot of issues as the portal blood tries to find a way to return to the systemic circulation. The standard protocol will need to be expanded to evaluate the abdomen to look for any of these complications among others that were not discussed, caused by portal hypertension.

Portal vein thrombosis can occur in patients with portal hypertension, hypercoagulable states, or intestinal inflammation, such as appendicitis and diverticulitis. Ultrasound will demonstrate either an enlarged or normal vein that is filled with low-level echoes and a lack of flow by spectral, color, or power Doppler (Fig. 20.70). The hepatic artery will enlarge and become tortuous, sometimes called the corkscrew sign, because of it bringing in more blood to compensate for the lost portal blood. It may be so enlarged that it may have the

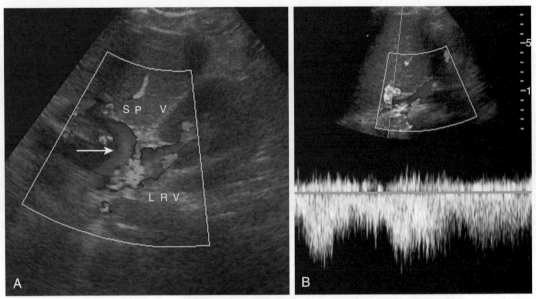

Fig. 20.68 A, The *arrow* is pointing to a splenorenal shunt that is joining the splenic vein *(SP V)* and the left renal vein *(LRV).* **B,** A Doppler signal from the left renal vein showing turbulent flow where the splenic flow is emptying into the left renal vein. See Color Plate 45.

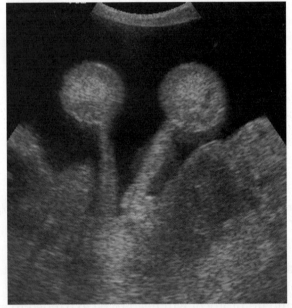

Fig. 20.69 Some alien eyes seen in ascites. Sonographers have good imaginations and can see fun things in some images!

appearance of a portal vein. A spectral Doppler signal from the vessel is needed to verify that this is an enlarged hepatic artery, especially when only one vessel can be seen (Fig. 20.71). Portal vein thrombosis does not usually cause complications like portal hypertension does, and therefore the protocol does not need to be expanded.

In some patients with congestive heart failure the flow in the portal vein may become pulsatile (Fig. 20.72) like the hepatic veins.

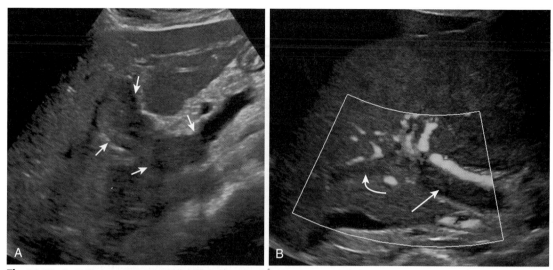

Fig. 20.70 A, A dilated portal vein filled with echoes, outlined by the *arrows,* compatible with portal vein thrombosis. **B,** The *arrow* is pointing to a thrombosed main portal vein that is extending into the right portal vein, indicated by the *curved arrow.* An enlarged hepatic artery is seen anterior to the vein.

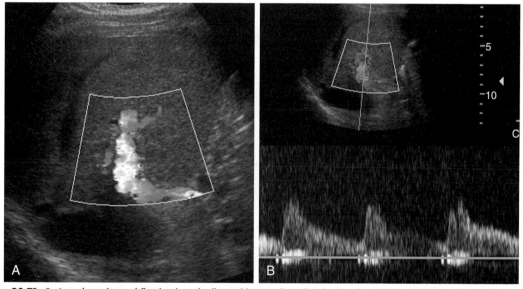

Fig. 20.71 A, An enlarged vessel flowing into the liver with some branches having the appearance of a portal vein; however, only one vessel is seen, and a Doppler signal needs to be obtained to identify the vessel. Never assume what a vessel is without obtaining a Doppler signal. **B,** The Doppler waveform from the same patient documenting that this vessel is an enlarged hepatic artery resulting from portal vein thrombosis.

As you scan, evaluate the whole image and see if there is a clue that you are missing. It can be easy to overlook pathologic conditions as you concentrate on other pathologic conditions. Color Doppler can give a lot of information, and if you are not looking at the detail, you will overlook the disease. Often a small area of aliasing may be overlooked and even ignored. In a renal transplant a small area of fast flow, brighter color, or aliasing can indicate an arteriovenous fistula after biopsy. Finding an area of fast flow in a vein can be unusual; however, it can happen as a result of a small nonobstructive clot (Fig. 20.73, Color Plates 46 and

47). Changes in color, changes in waveforms, and changes in flow direction from normal need to be explained. Being a sonographer can be like being Sherlock Holmes as we look for those subtle clues to solve the mystery of what might be wrong with our patient. The game is afoot!

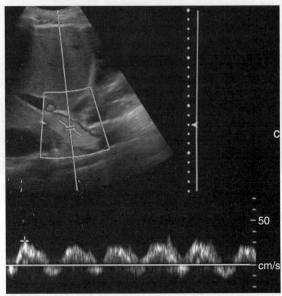

Fig. 20.72 An example of pulsatile flow in the portal vein in a patient with right-sided heart failure.

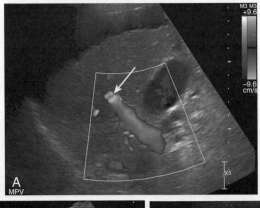

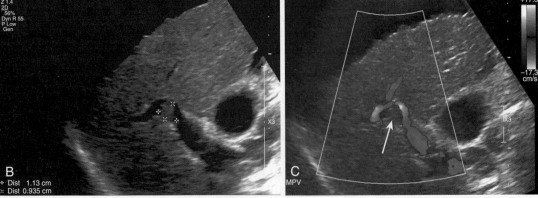

Fig. 20.73 A, The *arrow* is pointing to an area of aliasing at the end of the portal vein. **B,** Gray-scale image of the portal vein showing a thrombosis in the portal vein that was covered by color Doppler. **C,** Same patient with the color Doppler scale increased so that the thrombus is now seen *(arrow)*. See Color Plates 46 and 47.

Liver Required Images

Liver • Longitudinal and Transverse Images

1. A liver sonogram should be performed as outlined in Chapter 6 to evaluate for liver pathologic conditions. In some laboratories the study concentrates on the liver and the liver vasculature, and the gallbladder and biliary system are not formally evaluated.

Liver • Doppler Images

1. Image of the main portal vein in gray scale.

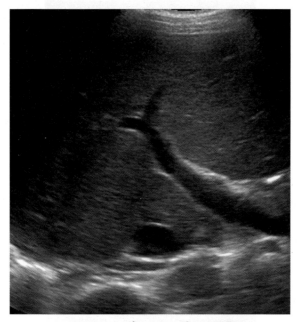

Suggested annotation: **MPV**

2. Color Doppler image of the main portal vein evaluating fill-in and flow direction.

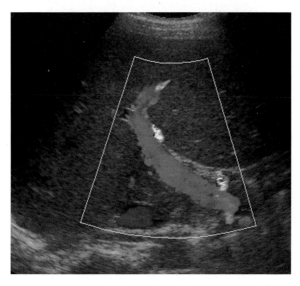

Suggested annotation: **MPV**

3. Doppler waveform of the main portal vein. If the velocity of flow is needed, angle correction should be used.

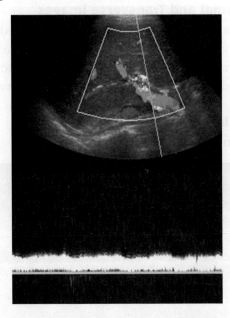

Suggested annotation: **MPV**

4. Doppler waveform of the main hepatic artery.

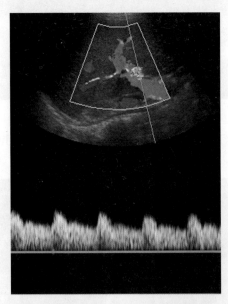

Suggested annotation: **MHA**

5. Doppler waveform of the right portal vein.

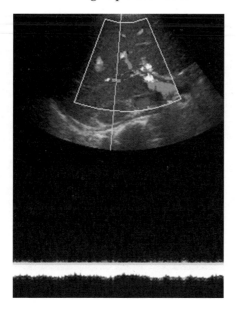

Suggested annotation: **RPV**

6. Doppler waveform of the left portal vein.

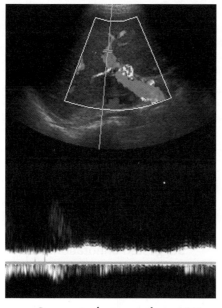

Suggested annotation: **LPV**

7. Gray-scale image of the hepatic veins.

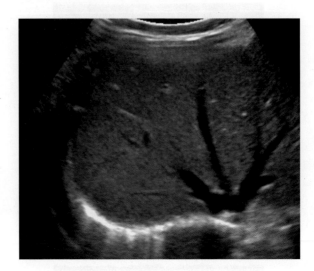

Suggested annotation: **HVS**

8. Color Doppler image of the hepatic veins.

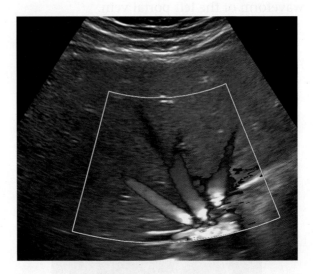

Suggested annotation: **HVS**

The Doppler waveforms of the hepatic veins can be obtained in any order.

9. Doppler waveform of the right hepatic vein.

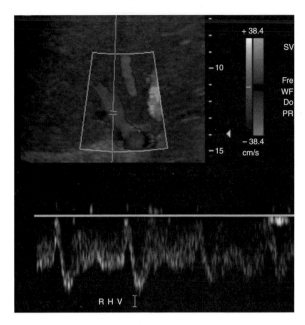

Suggested annotation: **RHV**

10. Doppler waveform of the middle hepatic vein.

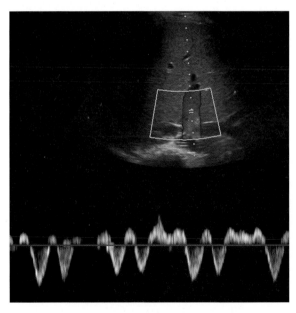

Suggested annotation: **MHV**

11. Doppler waveform of the left hepatic vein.

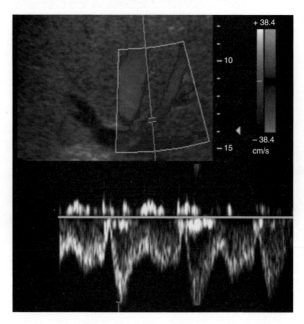

Suggested annotation: **LHV**

12. Gray-scale image of the IVC as it passes through the liver, intra-hepatic portion.

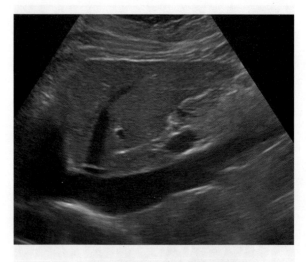

Suggested annotation: **IVC**

13. Doppler signal from the intrahepatic portion of the IVC.

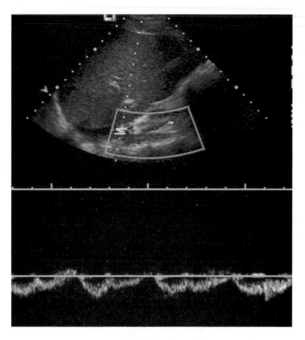

Suggested annotation: **IVC**

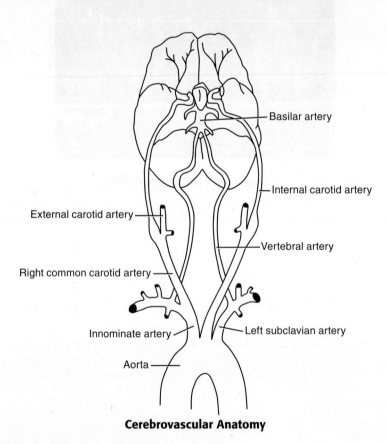

Cerebrovascular Anatomy

CHAPTER 21

Cerebrovascular Duplex Scanning Protocol

Aubrey J. Rybyinski

Keywords

Anterior cerebral circulation
Basilar artery
Carotid bifurcation
Common carotid artery (CCA)
External carotid artery (ECA)
High-resistance vascular beds
Internal carotid artery (ICA)
Innominate artery

Low-resistance vascular beds
Posterior cerebral circulation
Spectral window
Subclavian artery
Vertebral artery

Objectives

At the end of this chapter, you will be able to:

- Define the keywords.
- Discuss the normal anatomy of the extracranial cerebrovascular system and indicate common anatomic variations.
- Discuss the signature waveform patterns associated with vessels supplying low- and high-resistance vascular beds.
- Explain issues relating to choice of transducer type.
- Detail appropriate patient and sonographer positioning for sonographic evaluation of the extracranial cerebrovascular arteries with emphasis on correct application of ergonomics.
- Describe the duplex scanning survey of the extracranial cerebrovascular system and detail the locations to take representative images that are required to ensure an accurate interpretation.

Overview

Carotid Doppler examinations evaluate blood flow to the brain. These studies are performed in a vascular laboratory, in the radiology department, and in some hospitals the cardiac department. Vascular surgeons may also perform carotid examinations in their private office. If carotid surgery is needed, typically the vascular laboratory performs any follow-up examinations.

The carotid arteries are the major blood vessels in the neck that deliver blood and oxygen to the brain. Carotid artery disease is the progressive blockage of these vessels as a result of the buildup of plaque, which is composed of cholesterol, calcium, and fibrous tissue, that deprives the brain of oxygen. More than 700,000 strokes occur each year, and carotid artery disease is one of the most preventable causes.

Carotid artery examinations are performed to evaluate the presence of a hemodynamically significant stenosis. Although the percentage of stenosis is largely based on the peak systolic and end diastolic velocities, the diagnosis of a hemodynamically significant stenosis is best determined by looking at all the components of the examination by evaluating the gray-scale images, color Doppler images, and the Doppler waveform. The gray scale will demonstrate any plaque, the color Doppler the residual lumen, and the spectral Doppler waveform the velocity of the blood. All three aspects of the examination should point to the same conclusion, and if not, the outlier must be explained. For example, a high velocity is obtained in the **internal carotid artery** (ICA) compatible with a high-grade stenosis but there is no evidence of a plaque on gray scale, nor is there any vessel narrowing seen with color Doppler. The high velocity must be explained because it is not agreeing with the gray scale or the color Doppler information. When examining the contralateral side, an occlusion of the ICA is discovered and compensatory flow explains the high velocity found (Fig. 21.1).

Common indications to perform extracranial duplex examinations include, but are not limited to, evaluating a carotid cervical bruit, known stenosis follow-up; symptoms of cerebrovascular accident; symptoms of transient ischemic attack; postintervention follow-up from endarterectomy, stent, or bypass placement; pulsatile neck mass; syncopal episodes; and subclavian steal syndrome. Good knowledge of anatomy and pathophysiology is essential to perform a thorough and diagnostic examination.

Anatomy

As with any sonographic examination, the sonographer should have a thorough knowledge of anatomy, physiology, and pathophysiology of the extracranial arterial system. The **common carotid artery** (CCA) lies medial to the internal jugular vein, lateral to the thyroid gland, and posteromedial to the sternocleidomastoid muscle (Fig. 21.2). The right CCA originates from the innominate or brachiocephalic artery, and the left CCA originates directly from the aortic arch. On each side at the superior border of the thyroid cartilage, around C2-C3, the CCA bifurcates into an anteromedial **external carotid artery** (ECA) and a posterolateral ICA. The level and anatomic configuration of the bifurcation can be variable. The ICA usually has a larger diameter than the ECA, although this is variable. The ECA may lie posterior and lateral or posterior and medial to the ICA and can be differentiated

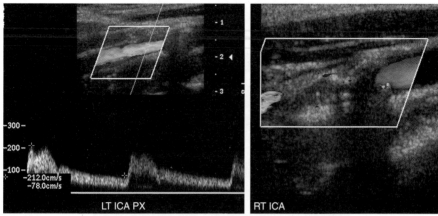

Fig. 21.1 The left internal carotid artery (ICA) has a velocity of 212 cm/s, which is compatible with a 50% to 69% stenosis. The color Doppler shows that the lumen is widely patent. The right ICA image shows that it is occluded. The left ICA has increased velocities because there is an increase of flow through the left ICA as it helps to bring blood to the right side of the brain, called compensatory flow. (see Color Plate 49).

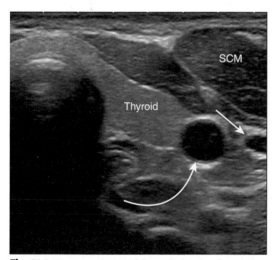

Fig. 21.2 Transverse image of the neck showing the relationship of the common carotid artery (CCA) to other structures in the neck. The curved *arrow* is pointing to the CCA and the *straight arrow* to the internal jugular vein. *SCM,* Sternocleidomastoid muscle.

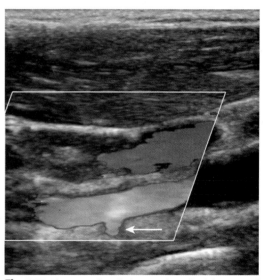

Fig. 21.3 The *arrow* is pointing to a branch of the external carotid artery.

from the ICA by the presence of branches within the neck (Fig. 21.3), as the ICA does not have extracranial branches.

The common, internal, and external carotid arteries form the **anterior cerebral circulation**. The **vertebral artery** originates from the **subclavian artery** and courses superiorly and posteriorly, entering the transverse processes of the vertebrae at C6 and exiting between C1 and C2 (Fig. 21.4). The left vertebral artery is often greater in diameter than the right. The vertebral arteries join to form the **basilar artery**, and together these vessels make up the **posterior cerebral circulation**.

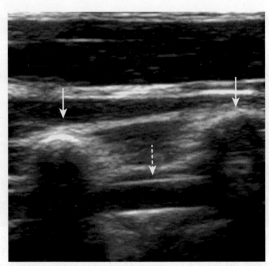

Fig. 21.4 Longitudinal image of the mid-neck showing the vertebral artery. The *dotted arrow* is pointing to the vertebral artery, and the *solid lines* to the shadows caused by the transverse processes of the spine.

Physiology

The CCA provides blood flow to both low- and high-resistance vascular beds. Approximately 70–80% of the blood flow from the CCA enters the ICA to supply blood flow to the low-resistance vascular tissues of the brain and eye. The remaining 20–30% of the blood flow volume enters the ECA to supply the high-resistance muscular tissues of the face and scalp. The Doppler spectral waveform from the CCA is influenced by both the ICA and ECA flow, resulting in a low-resistance waveform, although with less diastolic flow than the ICA.

The Doppler waveform pattern of the ICA is characterized by constant forward diastolic flow (Fig. 21.5). The Doppler waveform pattern of the ECA is characterized by low or absent diastolic flow (Fig. 21.6). The vertebral artery provides blood flow to the low-resistance vascular bed of the posterior cerebral hemispheres. Thus, its Doppler waveform pattern is characterized by a constant forward flow in diastole.

Low-resistance vascular beds consist of tissues that require blood flow throughout the cardiac cycle because they have high metabolic demands and oxygen usage. In addition to the internal carotid and vertebral arteries, examples of low-resistance waveforms include the renal and hepatic arteries. In contrast, **high-resistance vascular beds** are formed of tissues that normally have a low metabolic demand in the resting state and thus exhibit low diastolic flow. In addition to the ECA, examples of high-resistance waveforms include the common femoral artery and the superior mesenteric artery in a patient who is fasting.

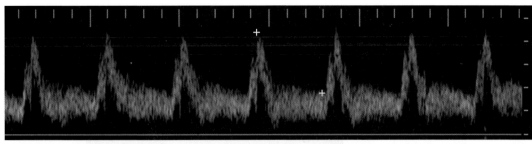

Fig. 21.5 An example of a low-resistance waveform from the internal carotid artery. Note that the diastolic flow is about one third of the next systolic peak.

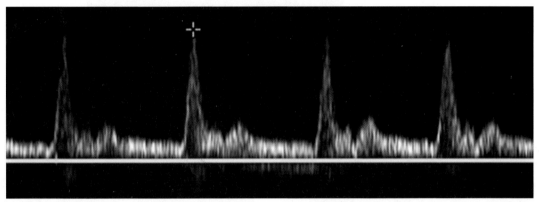

Fig. 21.6 An example of a high-resistance waveform from the external carotid artery. Note that the diastolic flow approaches the baseline.

Sonographic Appearance

The lumen in a normal vessel should be completely echo free. Arterial walls have three layers, the inner intima, the middle media, and the outer adventitia. With ultrasound the layers are seen as an echogenic line from the lumen-intima interface, a hypoechoic area that corresponds to the media, and another echogenic line from the media-adventitia interface (Fig. 21.7). The three layers produce two echogenic parallel lines that are best seen when imaging the artery perpendicularly, causing them to be echogenic, as they are specular reflectors. With a normal artery the intimal reflection should be straight, thin, and parallel to the adventitial line.

The CCA should be a straight tube that widens at the distal aspect of the artery to become the carotid bulb (Fig. 21.8). The carotid bulb can be seen before the bifurcation of the ICA and ECA, in the proximal ICA or in the proximal ECA (Fig. 21.9). The ICA is typically larger and posterolateral to the ECA, although there are variations, so this is not an accurate method to distinguish between the two arteries. The ICA will dive deep toward the back of the neck, whereas the ECA proceeds to go anteriorly toward the face. The Doppler signal from the ICA will have more diastolic flow than the ECA. The ECA should have a good response to a temporal tap maneuver demonstrating

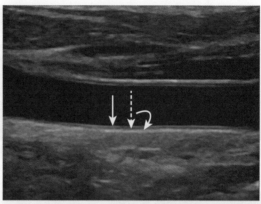

Fig. 21.7 The layers of the carotid wall. The *solid arrow* is pointing to the inner echogenic intima. The *dotted area* to the hypoechoic media layer, and the *curved arrow* to the outer adventitia later.

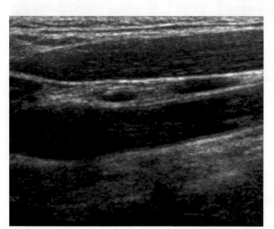

Fig. 21.8 An image of the common carotid artery and where it widens to become the bulb.

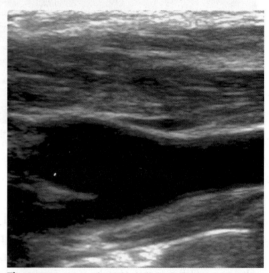

Fig. 21.9 An example of the bulb in the internal carotid artery.

oscillations in diastolic flow (Fig. 21.10). However, the best way to distinguish between the two is by finding a branch off of the ECA (Fig. 21.11).

NOTE: To properly perform a temporal tap, first feel for the pulsations of the superficial temporal artery. You need to feel the pulsation. Once located, tap the artery using two fingers. Your fingers should leave the skin. If you tap by pressing and releasing the artery and keep in contact with the skin, this can move the skin under your fingers and can cause dampened or false oscillations from skin motion, which could also affect the ICA making identification of the ECA difficult or falsely labeling the ICA as the ECA. Also, do not wiggle your fingers while you are pressing on the artery as this can also cause skin motion and misleading results.

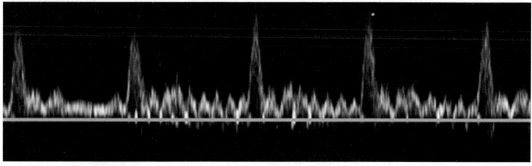

Fig. 21.10 The external carotid artery waveform is disturbed from the temporal tap maneuver.

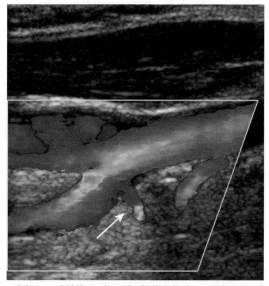

Fig. 21.11 An image of the carotid bifurcation. The bulb is in the anterior vessel, which is the internal carotid artery. The *arrow* is pointing to a branch in the posterior vessel, confirming that it is the external carotid artery.

All three arteries should display a sharp systolic upstroke with a narrow spectral envelope called a **spectral window**. The waveforms and velocities in these arteries should be symmetric between both sides. The CCA bifurcates and will supply blood to both the ICA and the ECA. Its waveform reflects the two vessels that it feeds, with a waveform showing continuous forward flow in diastole, but less than the diastolic flow seen in the ICA (Fig. 21.12). The normal ICA waveform has continuous forward flow in diastole, with a thicker spectral envelope (Fig. 21.13). The normal ECA waveform has a thinner spectral envelope with little diastolic flow and typically has an early diastolic or dicrotic notch, which is caused by the closure of the aortic valves (Fig. 21.14). The amount of diastolic flow that is seen in the ECA will vary among patients.

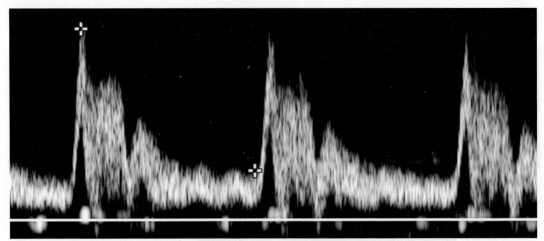

Fig. 21.12 An example of a normal common carotid artery waveform. Note that it has the dicrotic notch of the external carotid artery and the diastolic flow of the internal carotid artery.

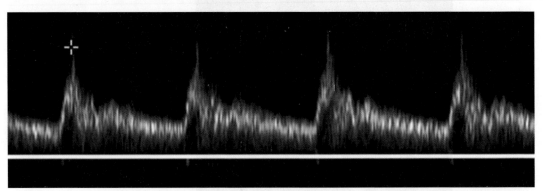

Fig. 21.13 An example of a normal waveform from the internal carotid artery with good forward flow in diastole.

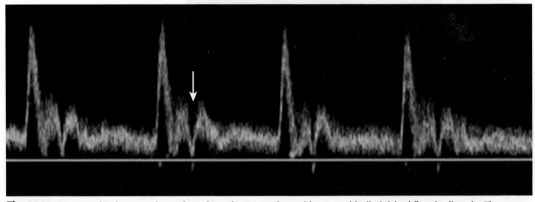

Fig. 21.14 An example of a normal waveform from the external carotid artery with diminished flow in diastole. The *arrow* is pointing to the dicrotic notch.

A clean spectral window is seen when there is smooth, laminar flow of the red blood cells using a small sample volume size in the middle of the vessel. The spectral window will be filled with echoes if the sample volume is too large, in the case of vessel tortuosity, and with a stenosis and is called spectral broadening. Spectral broadening of the waveform

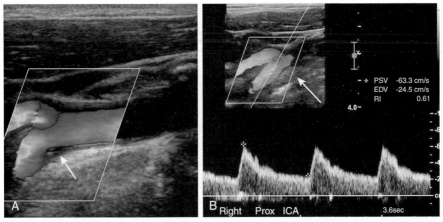

Fig. 21.15 A, Color Doppler image showing a decreased lumen from a plaque *(arrow)*. **B,** Doppler waveform showing spectral broadening caused by the plaque.

indicates the presence of a large range of flow velocities and can be an indication of turbulence caused by a plaque or thrombus (Fig. 21.15).

Patient Prep

There is no patient prep for a carotid duplex examination. If the patient has a neck brace or bandages on the neck, the nurse taking care of the patient will need to remove them if permitted. If they cannot be removed, the sonographer should see what access to the neck is available and obtain images and Doppler signals from those areas. Usually the main area of concern is the distal CCA and proximal ICA, so every effort should be made to scan those areas.

Transducers

A linear array transducer with a frequency of at least 7.5 MHz should be used, scanning with the transducer that offers the best resolution with adequate penetration. If the vessels lie deep within the neck, a transducer with a lower frequency should be used that will allow better penetration. In some patients, using the curved linear array or a sector transducer will improve visualization of the distal ICA (Fig. 21.16). Additionally, a 2–4 MHz curved linear or sector transducer is also useful for imaging the innominate and proximal left CCA.

Patient Position

Patients are scanned in a supine position with the chin slightly elevated, with the pillow under the patient's shoulder and the neck slightly extended. This will allow better access to the bifurcation under the mandible if the patient has a high bifurcation. Avoid hyperextension of the neck because this can make the skin taut,

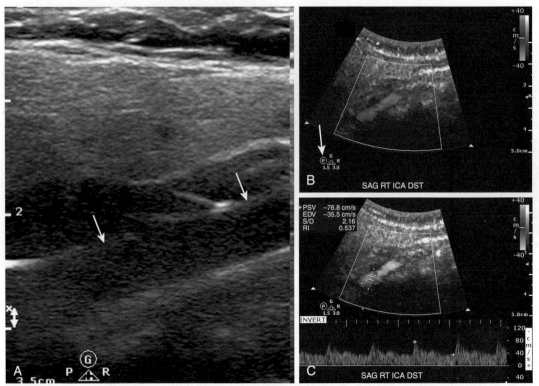

Fig. 21.16 A, The *arrows* are pointing to the distal internal carotid artery (ICA), which is difficult to see because of its depth and the frequency of the transducer being used. **B,** Same patient with better visualization of the distal ICA using a lower frequency curved linear array transducer. (see Color Plate 50). **C,** The Doppler waveform from the distal ICA. The spectral broadening is due to the lower frequency and the wider sample volume.

making it difficult to maintain transducer contact with the skin. Once situated, the patient should turn his or her head slightly away from you to scan the right carotid and toward you to scan the left carotid.

There are two methods of scanning the carotids, and you should use the position that you find the most ergonomic. The first way is the preferred position used by most vascular sonographers that work in a vascular laboratory. In this position the patient's feet are by the console and you sit at the head of the examination table with the patient's head directly in front of you. In this position, scanning the right carotid is easy because you should be able to rest your elbow on the corner of the table or the end of the pillow. This allows for a good ergonomic position for your arm and shoulder. When scanning the left carotid, you will have to turn your hand toward the patient's neck and it can be difficult to find a comfortable position for your arm and shoulder. You could also scan the left side with your left hand and reach over with your right hand to manipulate the controls.

The second way is the "radiology" method, in which you stand beside the examination table like when scanning the thyroid. In this position the left carotid is easy to scan and you will need to turn your hand and shoulder in toward the neck for the right side, trying to scan as ergonomically as possible.

Technical Tips

It is important to use all of the tools in the sonographer's toolbox. Patients with a short and/or thick neck may present a challenge to adequately image the carotid arteries using a linear array transducer. Some companies make linear array transducers in different widths. Trying to use a high-frequency transducer used for thyroid scanning will make the examination difficult because the transducer face is wider and the frequencies are too high for adequate penetration. Switching to a curved linear array transduder, especially if there is a higher frequency available, can help with completing the study. The curved linear array transducer is particularly helpful in evaluating the distal-most segment of the ICA. Additionally, using either the curved linear array or sector transducer may help with visualization of the innominate or right subclavian artery origin (Fig. 21.17). By using multiple scan planes, the sonographer should be able to image and evaluate the CCA, the **carotid bifurcation**, and the external and internal carotid and vertebral arteries for any disease that is present. Pay attention to the Doppler waveform because it can tell you about proximal and distal flow. Loss of diastolic flow in the CCA is a sign of a distal occlusion. If the ICA is patent, it too will have no diastolic flow and the occlusion is intracranial.

Vertebral Arteries

Finding the vertebral arteries can be challenging in some patients. In 75% of the population the two vertebral arteries are asymmetric in size, with usually the left vertebral artery being the larger artery. In 15% of the population one artery, typically the left, is atretic or hypoplastic. One technical reason that the vertebral artery may not be seen is because it is off the screen. It is important to note that the vertebral artery courses fairly deep in the neck as it travels through the vertebral bodies of the cervical spine. If using the CCA as a landmark to find the vertebral artery, remember to increase your depth; otherwise it may not be seen (Fig. 21.18). Once the depth is increased, the artery should be visible. Another technical issue is that the color velocity scale is set too high and will need to be lowered for the slower vertebral flow. The sonographer should look for a vessel going between the vertebra. Use caution calling a vessel the artery until you have obtained a Doppler signal, because the vertebral vein can be prominent in some people (Fig. 21.19). Use power Doppler to help find the vertebral artery, as it is

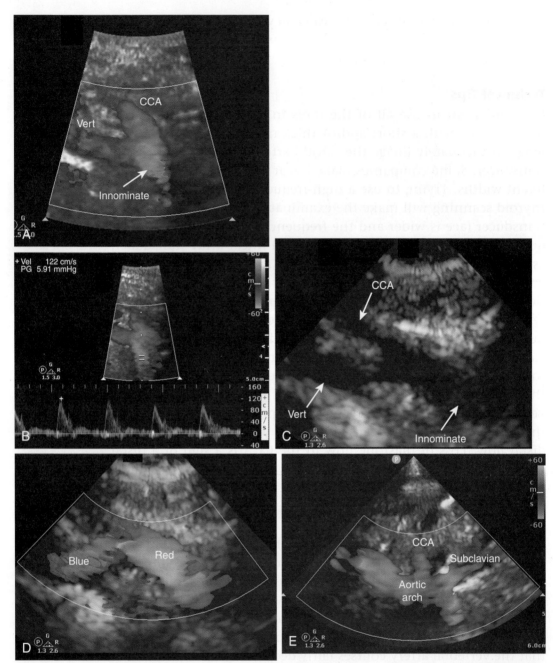

Fig. 21.17 A, Using a curved abdominal probe to evaluate the innominate artery and the origins of the common carotid artery *(CCA)* and vertebral artery *(Vert)*. **B,** Waveform from the innominate artery. **C,** Same patient now using a lower frequency sector transducer to evaluate the innominate artery. Note how the lower frequency affects image quality. **D,** Color Doppler image of the distal innominate artery using a lower-frequency sector transducer. The image may not be pretty but it is diagnostic, and that is what matters. **E,** Color Doppler image of the aortic arch and the origins of the CCA and subclavian artery using a lower-frequency sector. (see Color Plate 51).

more sensitive to flow and is not as angle dependent (Fig. 21.20). If unable to visualize the vertebral artery, slide the transducer down to the clavicle and the subclavian area and attempt to find the vertebral artery origin and follow it to the mid-neck (Fig. 21.21).

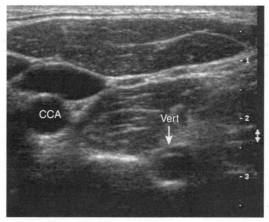

Fig. 21.18 Transverse image of the neck. The *arrow* is pointing to the vertebral artery *(Vert),* which is deeper than the common carotid artery *(CCA).*

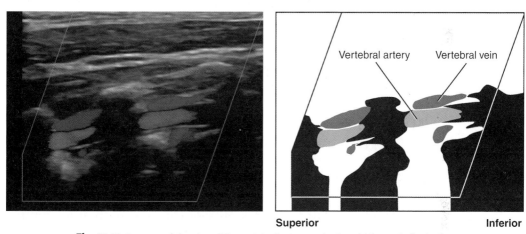

Fig. 21.19 Image and drawing of the vertebral artery and vein, which are similar in size.

Angle Correction

To use 60 degrees or not to use 60 degrees? That is the question. To accurately measure the velocity in a blood vessel, the sonographer must input the missing piece of information to complete the Doppler equation, which is the angle between the sound beam and the flowing blood. Sixty degrees was chosen because in the early days of carotid Doppler, there was no duplex and a nonimaging handheld continuous wave (CW) Doppler transducer was used. Although not perfect, it was decided that the sonographer could judge and maintain a 60-degree angle while obtaining the Doppler signals. When duplex came onto the scene, so did angle correction capabilities. It was decided to mimic the 60-degree angle that was used with CW Doppler to be able to use the existing charts. Somehow the carotid Doppler world became stuck with 60 degrees and passed it down from generation to generation. In a perfect world the ideal angle

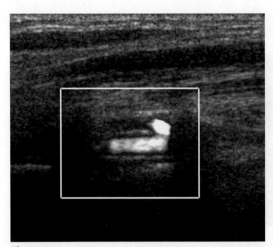

Fig. 21.20 Doppler image of the vertebral artery. Note how the Doppler angle is at 90 degrees and there is still good color fill-in. One benefit of power Doppler is that it is less angle dependent.

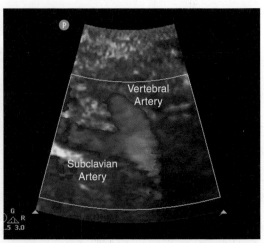

Fig. 21.21 Image of the origin of the right vertebral artery from the subclavian artery.

would be 0, because the cosine of this angle is 1, and would give the greatest possible frequency shift. But because a 0-degree angle is not possible, the ultrasound community decided that angles from 30 to 60 degrees are acceptable to use for measuring carotid arterial flow with Doppler.

Miscellaneous Tips

Ultrasound can be highly accurate in skilled hands and with sonographers who can think outside the box to obtain a complete and diagnostic study. This will save the patient from unnecessary additional imaging such as a computed tomography (CT) scan that uses radiation and nephrotoxic contrast media. Imaging of the aortic arch is not routinely part of the cerebrovascular protocol, but it is important to know how to visualize it if this can aid in the diagnosis of disease. Indications to evaluate the arch would be asymmetric CCA spectral Doppler waveforms or a significant difference in the calculated peak systolic velocities because they should be similar (Fig. 21.22). A good rule of thumb when evaluating bilateral vessels is that when one side is affected, blame the vessel, and if both sides are affected, blame the heart. It is important to note that the heart plays an important role in hemodynamics and will affect the Doppler waveform. The Doppler waveforms on patients with aortic insufficiency can vary depending on the degree of insufficiency, from a bisferiens waveform, which has two peaks, to diastolic flow reversal (Fig. 21.23). Patients with aortic valve stenosis will have tardus-parvus carotid waveforms, which are small, rounded waveforms.

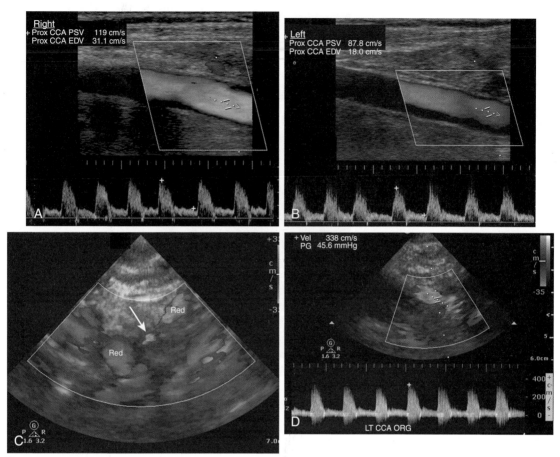

Fig. 21.22 A, Mid–common carotid artery (CCA) showing a waveform with mild changes from turbulence. **B,** Proximal CCA demonstrating spectral broadening from poststenotic turbulence. **C,** The abnormal looking signals in the proximal and mid-CCA prompted the sonographer to evaluate the origin of the CCA. The image shows color aliasing *(arrow)* of the left CCA origin. (see Color Plate 52). **D,** Elevated velocity and turbulent waveforms confirming significant disease of the origin of the CCA. (see Color Plate 53).

Often sonographers assess the carotid artery with an anterior approach, but the mandible will get in the way. By sliding the transducer to a posterolateral approach, you can use the jugular vein as an acoustic window to not only better visualize but also appreciate a longer segment of the ICA. Power Doppler imaging may be used in a similar manner as a complement to the color Doppler images. The addition of power Doppler may be useful to confirm areas of possible vessel occlusion or low flow states. A complete occlusion should have an image using power Doppler to show that there is no trickle flow.

Quick Survey

It is a good idea to do a quick gray-scale survey in the transverse plane to locate the position of the ICA and ECA and look for any plaque. Place the transducer in a transverse plane and slide the transducer from the proximal CCA to the proximal ICA. Discovering the

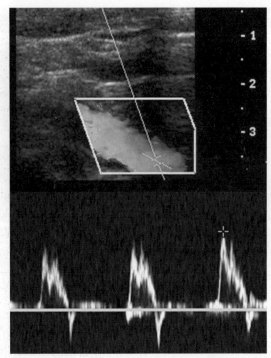

Fig. 21.23 The abnormal looking waveform from a CCA that is otherwise normal, resulting from aortic insufficiency.

relationship of the position of the ICA to the ECA can help obtain the correct angle and approach to get the "tuning fork" view if it is possible to obtain (Fig. 21.24)

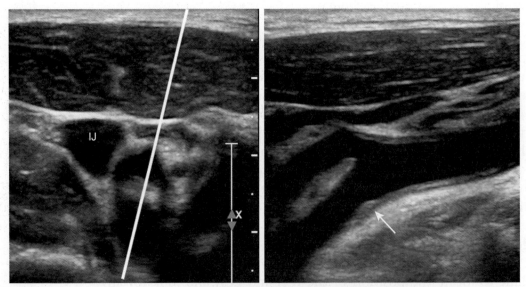

Fig. 21.24 A, Transverse image at the bifurcation. The *line* shows the angle needed to get a "tuning fork" image of both origins at the same time. **B,** The resulting tuning fork view. The *arrow* is pointing to a small plaque in the proximal ICA. *IJ,* Internal jugular (vein).

Color Doppler

Color Doppler also needs angles that are less than 60 degrees for proper fill-in of the vessel. This may require the sonographer to adjust the steering angle to maintain an angle less than 60 degrees to blood flow. The color box may be angled toward the patient's feet for the CCA but will then need to be angled toward the patient's head to evaluate the ICA and ECA. The color Doppler controls should be adjusted as needed to assess the quality of flow and identify regions of aliasing or absent flow. The velocity of flow will increase between the CCA and ICA, so it may be necessary to increase the color velocity scale for ICA flow so as not to have any aliasing.

Angle Correction

Carotid duplex examinations are not a "one size fits all" type of examination. The study involves imaging vessels at different depths and with different velocities; therefore, the gray scale and Doppler controls must be continuously evaluated and adjusted as needed. The Doppler angle of insonation should always be 60 degrees or less, with the angle correction cursor placed parallel to the vessel walls. The American Institute of Ultrasound in Medicine (AIUM) recommends keeping the angle between 45 and 60 degrees as much as possible, understanding that the angle used is governed by the patient's anatomy and may be lower than 45 degrees but should never be above 70 degrees because there is increased risk for inaccurate measurements. The angle correction needs to be continually fine-tuned as you move the cursor through the vessel. When there is a stenosis with an eccentric jet, some resources recommend angling to the jet using color Doppler as your guide, whereas others recommend keeping the cursor parallel to the vessel walls. It is important that all sonographers use the same angle correction technique in a lab. Follow the current recommendation of ultrasound's governing and accrediting bodies or the decision made by the department. In angle correction with a tortuous vessel, try not to place the sample volume in the curve because hemodynamics may cause a falsely elevated velocity. Try to place the sample volume in the straightest portion if possible.

Wall Filters

A low Doppler and color Doppler wall filter should be used throughout the examination. If set too high, low flows may not be seen, leading to a potential misdiagnosis. Even in the absence of a visible pathologic condition, it is important to carefully image the carotid bifurcation because this area is more prone to atherosclerosis resulting from shear forces imposed on the arterial wall by the moving

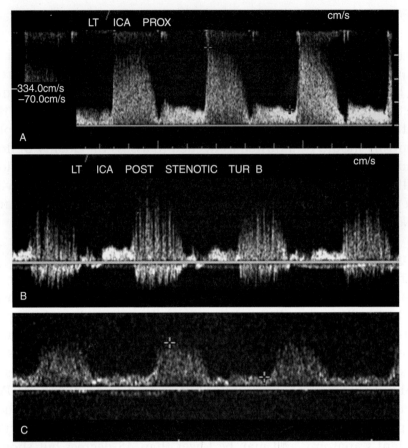

Fig. 21.25 A, Doppler image showing the high velocity from a greater than 80% internal carotid artery (ICA) stenosis. **B,** An image of poststenotic turbulence, which supports a greater than 80% stenosis. **C,** A Doppler signal from the mid ICA showing a tardus-parvus waveform resulting from the greater than 80% stenosis.

blood and the geometry of the region. Stenotic lesions often remain asymptomatic until they produce a pressure-flow gradient by reducing the diameter of the carotid lumen by more than 60%. Lesser lesions may be detected only with careful, thorough scanning in the transverse and longitudinal planes.

Documenting a Stenosis

If a stenosis is found, the sonographer should obtain a waveform before the stenosis, slowly moving the cursor through the area of stenosis to locate the highest velocity, to past the stenosis. Some sonographers call this "walking through the stenosis." If there is any poststenotic turbulence, it should be documented and a signal obtained when flow returns to a normal-appearing waveform, although the signal may be a tardus-parvus type of signal, which is a small, rounded appearing waveform (Fig. 21.25).

Table 21.1 Current Diagnostic Criteria				
Primary Parameters			**Additional Parameters**	
Degree of Stenosis	**ICA PSV (cm/s)**	**Plaque Estimate (%)**	**ICA/CCA PSV Ratio**	**ICA EDV (cm/s)**
Normal	<125	None	<2.0	<40
<50%	<125	<50	<2.0	<40
50%–69%	125–230	≥50	2.0–4.0	40–100
>70% but less than near occlusion	>230	≥50	>4.0	>100
>80% but less than near occlusion	>230	≥50	>4.0	>140
Near occlusion	High, low, or undetectable	Visible	Variable	Variable
Total occlusion	Undetectable	Visible, no detectable lumen	N/A	N/A

CCA, Common carotid artery; EDV, end-diastolic volume; ICA, internal carotid artery; PSV, peak systolic velocity.
Modified from Grant EG, Benson CB, Moneta GL, et al. Carotid artery stenosis: Gray-scale and Doppler US diagnosis–Society of Radiologists in Ultrasound Consensus Conference. Radiology. 2003;229:340–346.

Diagnostic Criteria

Current validated diagnostic criteria to determine the percentage of stenosis in the ICA uses the highest angle-corrected peak systolic velocity (PSV) obtained in the proximal ICA with the presence of plaque. Additional parameters that are used include the end-diastolic velocity (EDV) and ICA/CCA ratio, which is the highest angle-corrected velocity in the ICA over the systolic velocity of the CCA from 2 to 4 cm proximal to the carotid flow divider, which is where the ICA and ECA branch off of the CCA.

The Society of Radiologists in Ultrasound (SRU) consensus chart is presented in Table 21.1 and lists the diagnostic criteria used to grade ICA disease. A consensus panel brings together experts from different medical specialties to discuss a medical issue or problem. This consensus panel was sponsored by the SRU; it did not comprise solely radiologists, but also included other experts who diagnose and treat carotid disease. It is recommended that the reader use the following link (https://www.sru.org/Education-Content/US-Consensus-Statements)

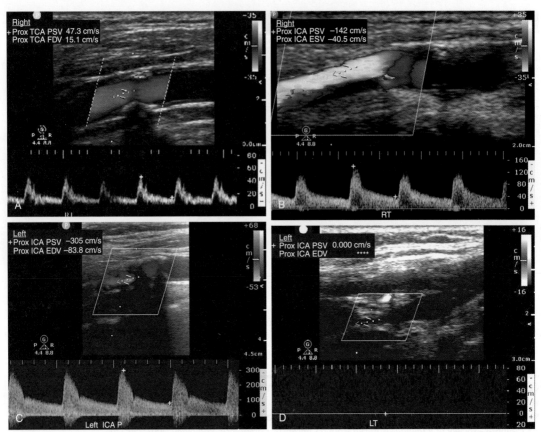

Fig. 21.26 A, An example of a less than 50% stenosis. An acoustic shadow can be seen posterior to the calcified plaque. (see color Plate 54). **B,** A Doppler waveform from a 50% to 69% stenosis. **C,** A high-velocity signal with spectral broadening as it leaves a calcified plaque compatible with a 70% to 99% stenosis. **D,** A lack of color inside the internal carotid artery (ICA) and inability to elicit a Doppler signal, which is compatible with an occluded ICA.

and read The SRU Carotid Consensus article. It is important to be aware that other published criteria are available, and a laboratory should use criteria that are the most accurate for their patient population. It is a best practice for sonographers to familiarize themselves with the diagnostic criteria used by the department. Accreditation demands that the same chart be used by the entire staff, including the interpreting physicians, and the same angle correction techniques be used by all staff.

Commonly used categories to grade the percent stenosis are less than 50%, 50% to 69%, 70% to 99%, near occlusion, and total occlusion (Fig. 21.26). Carotid examinations are not about just plugging an ICA velocity measurement into a chart. The sonographer should pay attention to the velocities seen within the CCA. Younger, healthy patients have more compliant arteries, and the measured velocity in the ICA may fall into a significant disease category; however, there is no plaque inside the artery to account for the high velocity. For these patients the ICA/CCA ratio is helpful; it will be normal because the velocity in the CCA also will be high. In patients with poor cardiac output the velocity in the ICA may never reach a high-grade stenosis level despite the amount of plaque seen and the small residual lumen. In these patients the ICA/CCA ratio will be abnormal, indicating the degree of stenosis. This is why understanding basic hemodynamics is important for sonographers so they can adjust an examination to include images that will help with the diagnosis.

For something to be considered stenotic there needs to be three components present, which include plaque causing narrowing of the lumen, elevated systolic velocity, and poststenotic turbulence (see Fig. 21.25). When plaque is present, the vessel is sampled proximally, within the area of the plaque, and distal to the plaque to evaluate for high velocities and the presence of poststenotic disturbed flow. Any plaque should be measured in the transverse and sagittal planes, and some laboratories perform a percentage of area stenosis that involves using the area measurement tool and outlining the ICA and the residual lumen, which is best performed using power Doppler. The images of the plaque should be able to define its acoustic properties of homogeneous or heterogeneous, and its surface characteristics of smooth or irregular. If there is calcified plaque, it may be difficult to obtain a signal underneath it because of the high attenuation rate from the plaque. Not all calcified plaques cause a mid- to high-grade stenosis, and it may just be a calcification in the arterial wall. With an understanding of hemodynamics, the sonographer can evaluate the color flow before the area of calcification and after the area. If the color after the plaque does not demonstrate any aliasing and is approximately the same color as before the plaque, then any stenosis is probably a low percentage. However, if the exiting color is aliasing or a brighter color, which indicates a faster flow, a significant stenosis may be present. Sometimes using a lower-frequency curved linear array transducer may be able to obtain a Doppler signal under the area of the plaque.

Some laboratories use the term "bulb" to describe the bulbous area of the carotid artery. The confusion with requiring a dedicated bulb velocity is that its location is variable because it can be part of the distal CCA or extending into the ECA or ICA; it can be solely in the proximal ICA, at the level of bifurcation only, or the individual may not have a bulbous segment at all. Accreditation does not require a spectral Doppler signal from the bulb for these reasons. It is important to know the bulb is an anatomic feature of the

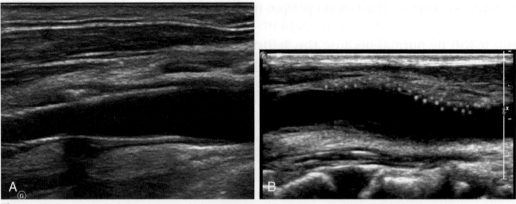

Fig. 21.27 A, Longitudinal gray-scale image demonstrating a carotid stent. Note the bright walls of the stent in comparison to the nonstented artery. **B,** Image of a carotid endarterectomy site showing the suture line, which is represented by the *bright white dots.*

carotid bifurcation region, not a specific location. Using correct, unambiguous terminology is very important in our examinations and reports.

If plaque or turbulent flow is visualized in the subclavian artery, or **innominate artery**, bilateral brachial pressures may be obtained to evaluate for a discrepancy of 20 mm Hg or greater between the two arms. This is not performed in most radiology departments and is more frequently performed in the vascular laboratory.

If the examination indication is a follow-up after an intervention such as endarterectomy or stent, representative images of the intervention site should be documented. These images include proximal, within, and distal to the intervention site. Stent evaluation should include velocities of the vessel before the stent, proximal stent, mid-stent, and distal stent and the vessel after the stent (Fig. 21.27).

The severity of ICA stenosis is commonly divided into the clinically relevant categories of greater than 70% or greater than 80% diameter reduction. The primary differentiation of the two categories is based on the EDV. The criteria from the SRU panel is to use an EDV greater than 100 cm/s to distinguish more than a 70% stenosis, whereas the criteria from University of Washington uses an EDV greater than 140 cm/s to signify a stenosis above 80%. It is up to the laboratory to decide which criteria they think best serves their patient population.

Although the primary reason for a cerebrovascular duplex is to evaluate for ICA disease, an abnormal Doppler signal from either the CCA or vertebral artery may suggest a stenosis of the innominate or subclavian arteries and should be investigated. A biphasic or reversed flow direction in the vertebral artery suggests a subclavian steal syndrome. The term *subclavian steal* describes retrograde blood flow in the vertebral artery associated with proximal ipsilateral subclavian artery stenosis or occlusion, just past the origin of the vertebral artery. The reversed flow in the vertebral artery acts as a collateral to supply blood to the arm (Fig. 21.28). Figs. 21.29 to 21.31 are bonus images to enjoy.

Carotid Required Images

Sonographers sometimes have a preferred way to perform a study, or it may be dictated by the reading physicians. In this example of a protocol the longitudinal and transverse images are taken side by side in a split screen. If you scan with this method, it is important to evaluate the entire CCA with transverse imaging and not just at the representative sites.

Another method is to take the gray-scale image of the vessel, with the next image being the color Doppler and spectral Doppler together. This would have the sonographer obtaining the long-axis views from the proximal, mid, and distal CCA and bifurcation, followed by the transverse images of the proximal, mid, and distal CCA and one of the bulb, with and without color, and then one of the origins of the ICA and ECA, with and without color. Next would be documentation of either the ICA or ECA, including the bifurcation, followed by color Doppler and spectral Doppler images. For the ECA just two images are obtained, one gray scale and the other the color, and spectral Doppler waveform. For the ICA this sequence needs to be repeated for the proximal, mid, and distal segments. It is best to integrate the color and Doppler images with the gray-scale images because it is inefficient to obtain all the gray-scale images and then go back and obtain all the color and spectral Doppler images. If obtaining the ICA was challenging, you would not want to lose that place and have to find it again because that is frustrating for both you and the patient and unnecessarily prolongs room use and examination time.

At the time of publication, the AIUM/SPR/SRU extracranial guidelines recommend a spectral Doppler signal of the proximal and mid–distal CCA 2 to 3 cm below the bifurcation and of the proximal and distal ICA, while the Intersocietal Accreditation Commission Vascular Testing (IAC-VT) standards recommend a proximal and mid–distal CCA and proximal and as distally as possible in the ICA. It is always appropriate to do more than the standards, and some laboratories may still obtain a mid-CCA and ICA Doppler waveforms.

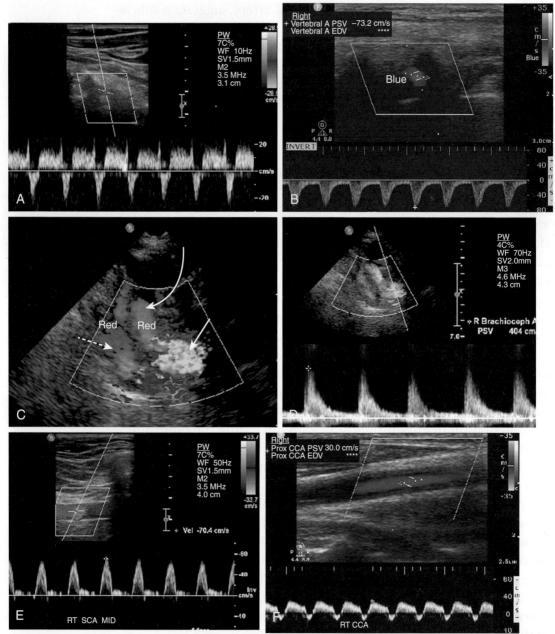

Fig. 21.28 A, Bidirectional vertebral artery waveform demonstrating a mid-systolic flow reversal, which is sometimes referred to as the bunny sign. This waveform is associated with a presteal. With these waveforms, in some laboratories the sonographer may have the patient raise their arm for 30 to 45 seconds or until it starts to ache and then reevlauate the waveform, which should now be completely retrograde. Any waveforms of the distal subclavian and brachial arteries will show monophasic signals in a subclavian steal. (see Color Plate 55). **B,** Complete flow reversal, retrograde flow, in the vertebral artery consistent with an occluded or very high stenosis of the subclavian artery. **C,** An abnormal-looking common carotid artery (CCA) signal prompted the sonographer to evaluate the origin of the CCA. An image showing a color bruit of the distal innominate artery, which is associated with a stenosis. The color bruit is caused by the vibration of the tissue in response to the stenosis. The *arrow* is pointing to the color bruit, the *curved arrow* to the CCA, and the *dotted arrow* to the vertebral artery. (see Color Plate 56). **D,** The Doppler waveform of the distal innominate artery showing an elevated velocity. Note that a sector probe was used to better evaluate the artery because of its depth. **E,** Delayed systolic upstroke is seen in the mid-subclavian artery. The patient had brachial pressures obtained that were found to be asymmetric, calculated as 90 mm Hg on the right and 140 mm Hg on the left artery. (see Color Plate 57). **F,** An abnormal carotid waveform in the right CCA. This patient has total occlusion of the innominate artery. The right carotid system is receiving blood from the retrograde ipsilateral vertebral artery. The bidirectional flow pattern is from blood demand alternating between the carotid system and the right arm arterial system. (see Color Plate 58).

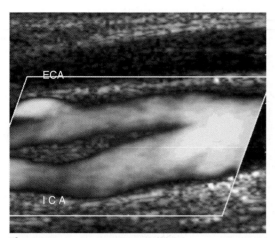

Fig. 21.29 Power Doppler image of the external carotid artery *(ECA)* and internal carotid artery *(ICA)* from origin to mid-artery.

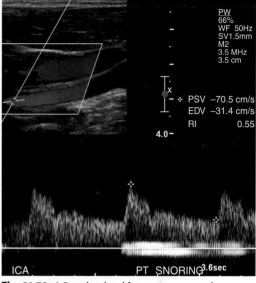

Fig. 21.30 A Doppler signal from someone snoring.

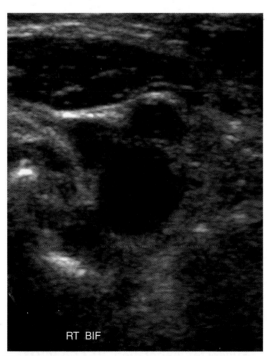

Fig. 21.31 Hidden Mickeys are everywhere. The jugular vein is his right ear, the external carotid artery his left ear, and the bulb/internal carotid artery is Mickey's head. A hidden Mickey also can be found in the porta hepatis.

Carotid • Longitudinal Images

1. Longitudinal and transverse image of proximal CCA.

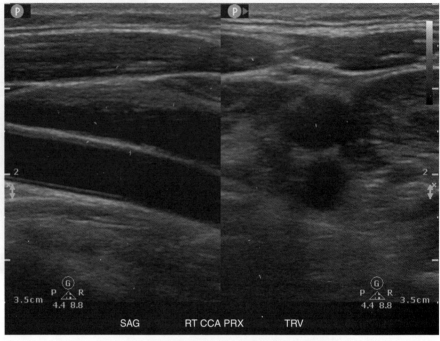

Suggested Annotation: **RT CCA PROX**

> **NOTE:** You can start on either side. The right side is just being used for the example protocol.

2. Color and spectral Doppler of proximal CCA with angled corrected peak systole and end diastole measured. (see Color Plate 59).

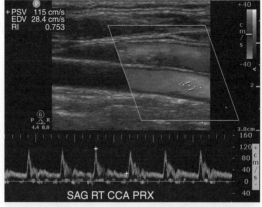

Suggested Annotation: **RT CCA PROX**

3.   Longitudinal and transverse image of mid–distal CCA.

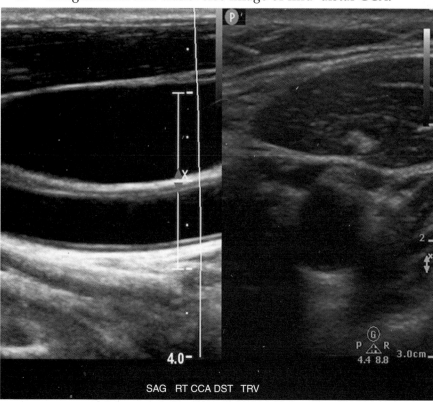

Suggested Annotation: **RT CCA DST or MID/DST**

4.   Color and spectral Doppler of mid–distal CCA with angled
corrected peak systole and end diastole measured.

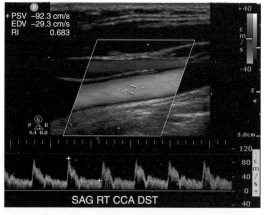

Suggested Annotation: **RT CCA DST or MID/DST**

5.   Longitudinal and transverse image of the bifurcation.

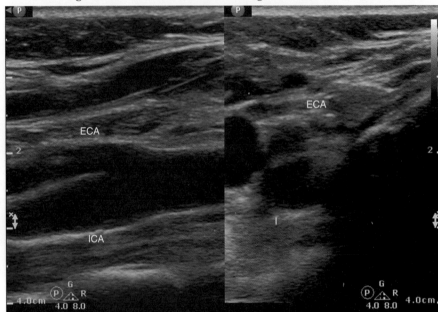

Suggested Annotation: **RT BIFUR**

6.   Longitudinal and transverse images of the origin of the external carotid artery *(ECA)*.

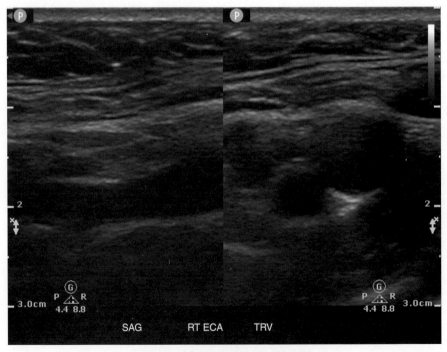

Suggested Annotation: **RT ECA**

7. Color and spectral Doppler of the origin of the ECA with angled corrected peak systole and end diastole measured.

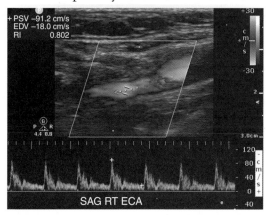

Suggested Annotation: **RT ECA or RT ECA PROX or RT ECA ORI**

8. Longitudinal and transverse image of the origin of the ICA.

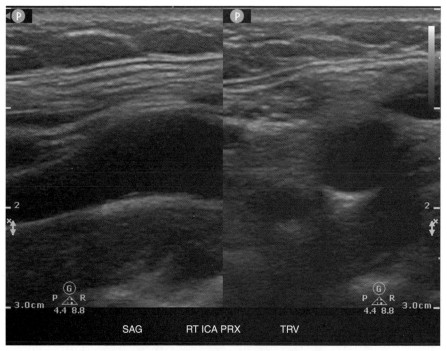

Suggested Annotation: **RT ICA PROX or RT ICA ORI**

9. Color and spectral Doppler of the proximal/origin of the ICA with angled corrected peak systole and end diastole measured.

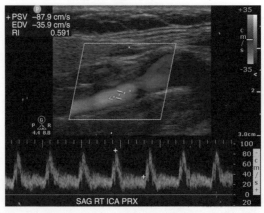

Suggested Annotation: **RT ICA PROX or RT ICA ORI**

10. Longitudinal and transverse image of mid–distal ICA (AIUM protocol).

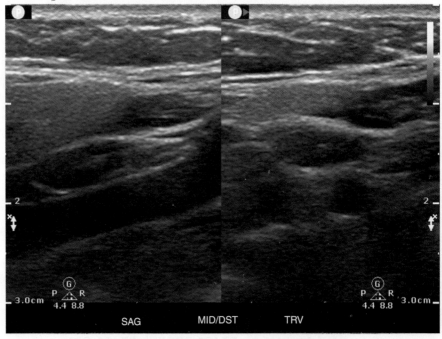

Suggested Annotation: **RT ICA MID/DST**

11. Color and spectral Doppler of mid–distal ICA with angled corrected peak systole and end diastole measured. (AIUM protocol).

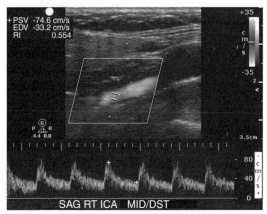

Suggested Annotation: **RT ICA MID/DST**

12. Longitudinal and transverse images of distal ICA (IAC-VT standard).

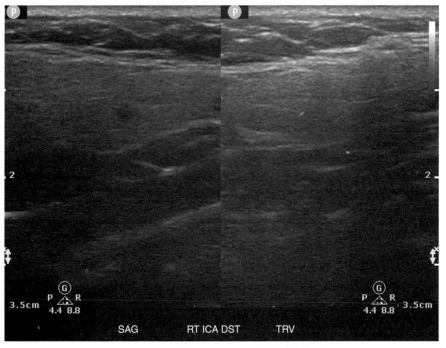

Suggested Annotation: **RT ICA DST**

13. Color and spectral Doppler of distal ICA with angled corrected peak systole and end diastole measured. (IAC-VT standard).

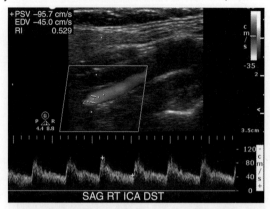

Suggested Annotation: **RT ICA DST**

14. Color and spectral Doppler of the vertebral artery, usually proximal–mid neck. (see Color Plate 60).

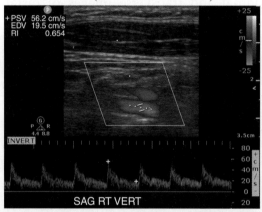

Suggested Annotation: **RT VERT**

15. Repeat for left side.

16. Long axis of right subclavian artery. (This is required in some laboratories, although not by AIUM or IAC vascular.)

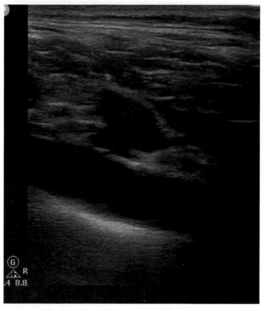

Suggested Annotation: **RT SCA or RT SUBCLAV**

17. Color and spectral Doppler of right subclavian artery with angled corrected peak systole measured.

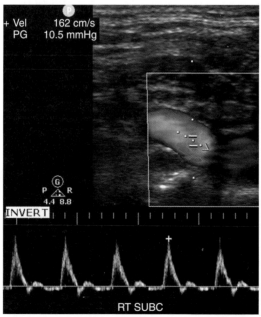

Suggested Annotation: **RT SCA or RT SUBCLAV**

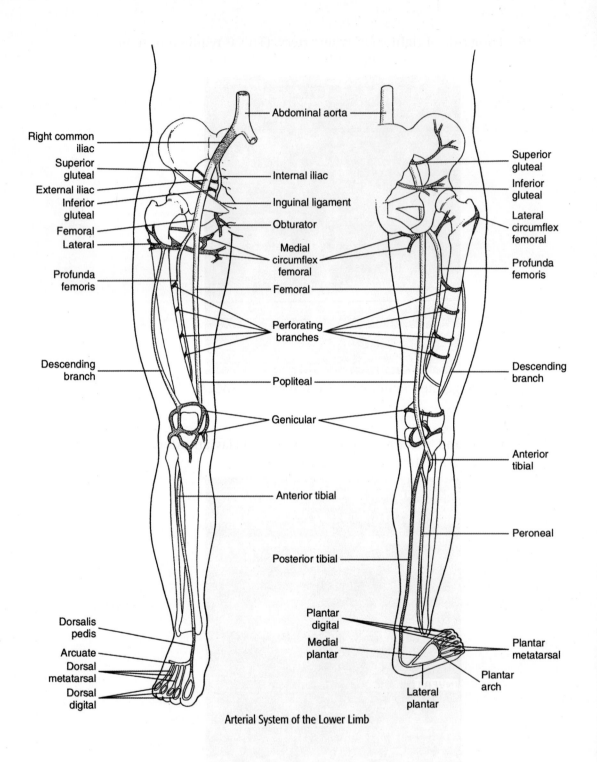

Arterial System of the Lower Limb

Right common iliac

Superior gluteal

External iliac

Inferior gluteal

Femoral

Lateral

Profunda femoris

Descending branch

Dorsalis pedis

Arcuate

Dorsal metatarsal

Dorsal digital

Abdominal aorta

Internal iliac

Inguinal ligament

Obturator

Medial circumflex femoral

Femoral

Perforating branches

Popliteal

Genicular

Anterior tibial

Posterior tibial

Plantar digital

Medial plantar

Lateral plantar

Superior gluteal

Inferior gluteal

Lateral circumflex femoral

Profunda femoris

Descending branch

Anterior tibial

Peroneal

Plantar metatarsal

Plantar arch

CHAPTER 22

Peripheral Arterial and Venous Duplex Scanning Protocols

Aubrey J. Rybyinski

Keywords

Augmentation	Medial malleolus
Coapt	Pulsatile flow
Compressibility	Respiratory phasicity
Continuous flow	Spontaneous flow
High vascular resistance	Triphasic
Lateral malleolus	Valves
Low vascular resistance	Valvular competence

Objectives

At the end of this chapter, you will be able to:

- Describe the normal anatomy of the lower extremity arterial system and indicate common anatomic variations.
- Discuss the blood flow patterns associated with arteries supplying the high resistance vascular bed of the lower leg muscles.
- Explain how to choose the proper transducer frequency and type.
- Detail appropriate patient and sonographer positioning for sonographic evaluation of the lower extremity arteries and veins with emphasis on correct application of ergonomic principles.
- Describe the normal anatomy of the lower extremity deep, superficial, and perforator venous systems and indicate common anatomic variations.
- Discuss normal and abnormal venous blood flow patterns.

Overview

This chapter will be divided into two parts, lower extremity arterial and lower extremity venous duplex studies. Although they are two distinctly different systems, there are common generalized indications to perform either one. If you think the incorrect examination was ordered, it is appropriate to reach out to the ordering physician to ensure that the patient receives the correct examination. Ultrasound plays a vital role in the diagnosis and management of vascular disease in patients. The results will help determine the best treatment for the patient. The goal of any sonographer or vascular technologist should be to provide a detailed, diagnostic examination to avoid patients being referred for additional imaging examinations that can be invasive or use radiation. In addition, examinations calling for nephrotoxic contrast agents can be expensive.

Peripheral Arterial Overview

Peripheral arterial duplex examinations are typically performed in a vascular laboratory because nonimaging studies are usually performed at the same visit. They may be performed in the radiology department for specific reasons, for example, to rule out arterial occlusion when a patient presents in the emergency department with a sudden cold foot. In some hospitals the cardiology department may also perform these examinations.

Peripheral arterial disease (PAD) is very common, affecting more than 3 million people a year. Over time the lower extremity arteries can become narrowed, and when the demand for blood cannot be met, the result is calf pain known as claudication. Ultrasound is an excellent diagnostic tool that accurately reports the extent of arterial insufficiency or occlusive disease while localizing and quantifying stenoses with a noninvasive approach. Some of the reasons to perform an arterial study include evaluating for exertional leg pain, claudication, rest pain, ulcer, and evaluation after endarterectomy, angioplasty, stent placement, or bypass graft placement. Ultrasound is very helpful in the ability to differentiate true claudication, which is caused by vascular disease, from pseudoclaudication, which is usually caused by neurologic issues. Claudication is usually defined by how many blocks a patient can walk before developing calf pain that is relieved with rest. For example, patients with three-block claudication can walk three blocks before calf pain causes them to stop walking and rest. Usually, after 30 to 45 seconds of resting the pain subsides and they can walk another three blocks before they must stop and rest again.

The arterial duplex examination will evaluate the leg from the femoral artery down to the ankle to provide diagnostic information that can be used to determine the best type of treatment for the patient. Depending on the patient symptoms or if abnormal findings are discovered during the examination, it may be expanded to cover the aorta, common iliac arteries, and external iliac arteries.

The ankle-brachial index, usually referred to as ABI, plays an important role in the evaluation of PAD. Duplex is an anatomic evaluation, whereas the ABI provides physiologic information. The examinations are complementary to each other and provide important pieces of the patient management puzzle.

Anatomy

The thoracic aorta becomes the abdominal aorta at the aorta hiatus of the diaphragm and lies to the left of the midline, coursing through the retroperitoneum until it bifurcates into the iliac arteries around the level of the umbilicus. The common iliac artery runs inferior and laterally for about 4 cm and then bifurcates into the external and internal arteries. The internal iliac artery, also known as the hypogastric artery, courses medially to supply blood to the pelvis and pelvic organs, and the external iliac artery courses toward the leg, where it becomes the common femoral artery (CFA), just proximal to the inguinal ligament. The CFA lies lateral to the common femoral vein (CFV) and bifurcates into the superficial femoral artery (SFA) and the deep femoral artery, which was previously called the profunda femoral artery (Fig. 22.1). The deep femoral artery lies lateral and posterior to the SFA and gives rise to branches that supply blood to the region of the femoral head and the deep thigh muscles. In a small percentage of patients, the deep femoral artery will originate medially from the CFA. The SFA lies anterior to the femoral vein and courses along the anteromedial aspect of the thigh. It courses deep as it enters the adductor canal in the distal thigh, where it becomes the popliteal artery. The popliteal artery lies within the popliteal fossa and lies anterior and medial to the popliteal vein. It branches into the anterior tibial artery and the tibioperoneal trunk (Fig. 22.2). The anterior tibial artery passes superficial to the interosseous membrane and courses anteriorly along the membrane. Distally, the anterior tibial artery courses along the anterior aspect of the

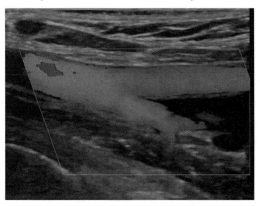
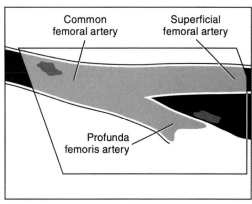

Superior   Inferior

Fig. 22.1 Color Doppler image and drawing of the common femoral artery bifurcating into the superficial femoral artery and profunda femoris (deep femoral) artery.

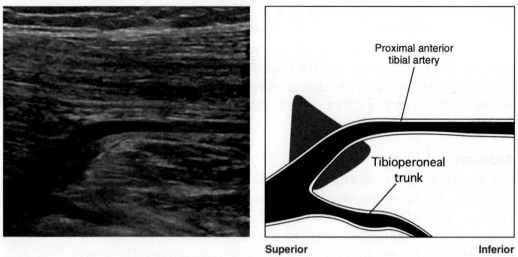

Fig. 22.2 Gray-scale ultrasound image of the popliteal artery bifurcating into the anterior tibial artery and the tibioperoneal trunk.

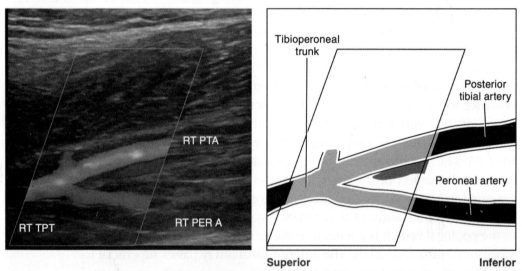

Fig. 22.3 Color Doppler image and drawing of the tibioperoneal trunk artery bifurcating into the posterior tibial artery and the peroneal artery.

tibia and becomes the dorsalis pedis artery after crossing the ankle joint. The tibioperoneal trunk gives rise to the posterior tibial and peroneal arteries that supply the calf muscles (Fig. 22.3). The posterior tibial artery originates between the tibia and the fibula and courses along the medial aspect of the calf to a midpoint between the **medial malleolus** and the heel (Fig. 22.4). The peroneal artery originates from the tibioperoneal trunk and courses obliquely along the medial aspect of the fibula. The peroneal artery lies deep to the posterior tibial artery and in close apposition to the fibula.

Physiology

The lower extremity arteries supply blood to the muscles of the thigh and calf. Normal resting muscle has a low demand for blood and

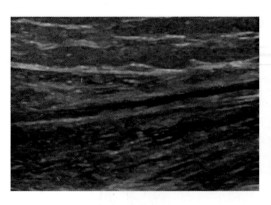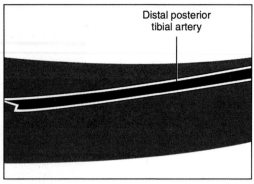

Distal posterior
tibial artery

Superior   Inferior

Fig. 22.4 Gray-scale ultrasound image of the posterior tibial artery.

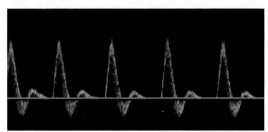

Fig. 22.5 Spectral Doppler waveform of a normal triphasic signal.

displays a high-resistance Doppler waveform (Fig. 22.5). In contrast, exercising the muscles requires a significant increase in flow volume to oxygenate the muscles and carry away exercise-related toxins, causing a low-resistance Doppler waveform.

Sonographic Appearance

The normal vessel lumen should be echo-free with echogenic arterial walls caused by the acoustic properties of collagen fibers found within the intima and media of the arterial wall. Arteries will have more echogenic walls than veins (Fig. 22.6). Using multiple scan planes, the sonographer should be able to image the vessel bifurcations, which are usually in an oblique plane.

Arterial Duplex

Patient Prep

There is no patient prep for a lower arterial examination. If the aorta and iliac arteries are evaluated, some departments may have the patient on nothing by mouth (NPO) after midnight except for clear liquids and medications in the morning to reduce bowel gas to help visualize the aorta. When the patient needs to be NPO, the tests should be scheduled in the morning. Because patients with diabetes

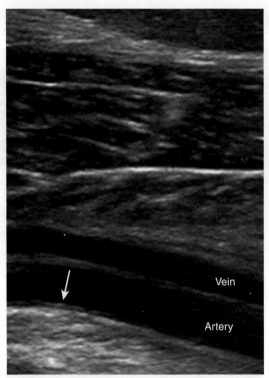

Fig. 22.6 Gray-scale image comparing a vein and an artery. The *arrow* is pointing to the echogenic wall of the artery.

are at risk for PAD, they should be the first patient in the morning or they should be given a modified prep. Some departments do not have the patient be NPO and will schedule patients throughout the day.

Transducers

A 5–7.5 MHz linear array transducer is used for the thigh and calf and is usually sufficient for the majority of patients. A 2–4 MHz curved linear array transducer is used for the abdominal aorta and iliac arteries. It also may be used to image the thigh vessels in patients with large thighs. In some patients using the curved linear array transducer will improve visualization of the distal SFA as it courses through the adductor canal. It is of utmost importance to fully evaluate this area because it is prone to atherosclerosis. A sonographer should always try to use the highest-frequency transducer that offers adequate depth penetration with clean far fields.

Breathing Technique

The patient can breathe normally during the examination. Suspended respiration may be needed for the imaging aorta.

Patient Position

The examination is performed with the patient in the supine position with the leg rotated outward and the knee slightly flexed in a

Table 22.1 Ankle-Brachial Index	
>1.3	Arterial calcification
1.0–1.3	Normal
0.9–1.0	Mild arterial compromise with only mild symptoms
0.5–0.9	Mild to moderate ischemia with mild to moderate claudication
0.3–0.5	Moderate to severe ischemia with severe claudication or rest pain
<0.3	Severe ischemia with rest pain or gangrene

frog-leg position. This allows good access to the medial portion of the thigh and the popliteal fossa. Make sure that appropriate ergonomic positioning techniques are followed and that your arm is supported and not at a right angle to your body. The examination table should be raised to a height that is comfortable for you and the monitor and keyboard are at the appropriate height and position.

Ankle-Brachial Index

The severity of blood flow compromise in the lower extremities may be assessed by using the ABI (Table 22.1). The ABI is a nonimaging examination and does not provide anatomic detail. Blood pressure is measured in both brachial arteries and in the dorsalis pedis and posterior tibial arteries of both lower legs. Any patient with newly diagnosed PAD should have an ABI performed as a baseline. For reimbursement, in addition to pressure measurements, waveforms must be obtained from both tibial arteries using continuous-wave Doppler or from the ankle using pulse volume recording.

The equation for calculating the ankle-brachial index is:

Higher of the two tibial pressures/Highest brachial pressure

Beginning with the patient in a supine position, obtain bilateral brachial systolic blood pressures using an appropriately sized blood pressure cuff (the width of the cuff bladder should exceed 20% of the limb diameter) and a continuous-wave Doppler transducer. Inflate the cuff until the Doppler signal disappears and slowly release pressure until a Doppler signal returns. This is the systolic pressure. Save the waveform as an image on the ultrasound unit or the physiologic testing machine. Record the blood pressure reading in the appropriate place, typically a worksheet, if not recorded on the unit. In a similar manner, obtain bilateral ankle systolic pressure measurements from the dorsalis pedis and posterior tibial arteries by placing an appropriately sized blood pressure cuff above the ankle. Record the ankle pressures in the same manner as the brachial pressures and calculate the

ABI for both legs by dividing the highest ankle pressure for each leg by the highest brachial pressure. The highest brachial pressure reading is used, regardless of arm, for calculating the ABI for both ankles.

Artifactually elevated tibial artery pressures may be found in patients with stiff, calcified vessels. When the ABI is uninterpretable or unreliable, the systolic pressures may be measured in the great toe because the digital arteries infrequently calcify. The blood pressure may be obtained by using a photoplethysmography (PPG) sensor. Diabetic patients may also need a blood pressure obtained on their great toe. This is achieved with a PPG sensor and a smaller blood pressure cuff, usually 2.5 cm. The toe brachial index is calculated by dividing the great toe pressure by the highest brachial pressure. The blood pressure in the great toe is usually 70% of the brachial pressure. Therefore a normal toe-brachial index exceeds 0.7. An unreliable ABI measurement would be one that is calculated in the "normal" range, but the continuous wave Doppler waveforms are clearly abnormal.

Puncture Complications

Patients who have had femoral punctures for catheterization or other reasons are at risk for developing a postprocedural complication. Hematoma, pseudoaneurysm (PSA), and arteriovenous fistula (AVF) are the three main complications and are easily distinguished from one another with ultrasound. Patients will be referred if a pulsatile mass is discovered in the groin or the patient reports pain at or near the puncture site. A hematoma may push the artery deeper in the thigh, necessitating use of a curved linear array transducer (Fig. 22.7). Noticing a color bruit can help locate the area of the hematoma. A PSA will show

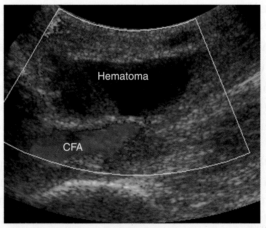

Fig. 22.7 An image of a patient status post cardiac catheterization that developed a painful swollen groin. Using a lower-frequency curved linear array transducer, a complex mass that was primarily cystic was seen that was compatible with a hematoma that was pushing the common femoral artery (*CFA*) posteriorly.

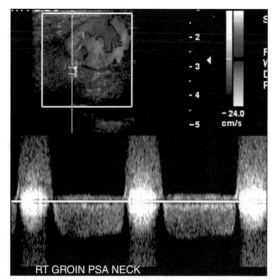

Fig. 22.8 A patient with a pseudoaneurysm (PSA) displaying the classic to-and-fro flow from the neck of the PSA and the swirling color Yin-Yang sign in the PSA sac. (see Color Plate 61).

a vessel coming off the artery going to a sac-like structure. The vessel, called the neck, will display to-and-fro flow as the blood enters and leaves the sac. The sac will display the Yin-Yang sign as the blood enters the sac during systole and swirls around to leave the sac in diastole (Fig. 22.8). This causes half of the sac to be red and the other half blue. A color bruit may be seen around the neck and the sac. It is important not to call a prominent arterial branch seen coming off of the CFA a PSA because this vessel will have a **high vascular resistance** and seem to disappear into the muscle. An AVF is a connection that is formed between the artery and the vein. This is easy to diagnose with just two Doppler waveforms. Before the connection, blood will be flowing into the low-pressure vein causing the arterial signal to have diastolic flow (Fig. 22.9). After the connection the blood is flowing to the high-pressure leg and will revert back to a triphasic or a high-resistance signal (Fig. 22.10). A color bruit will usually point to where the connection is located. Increasing the color velocity scale can help eliminate the bruit and show the fast velocity of the AVF (Fig. 22.11). The Doppler waveform in the vein will be pulsatile, and it is important not to mistake it for an artery. Obtaining a Doppler signal at the mid-femoral vein should show a normal Doppler signal. Scanning slowly in a transverse plane with color Doppler from the mid SFA to the CFA can help locate the color bruit and the area to be investigated (Fig. 22.12).

Doppler Waveforms

Doppler waveform terminology continues to be a controversial issue in the field of vascular ultrasound in the absence of standardization.

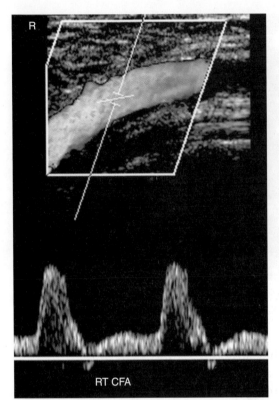

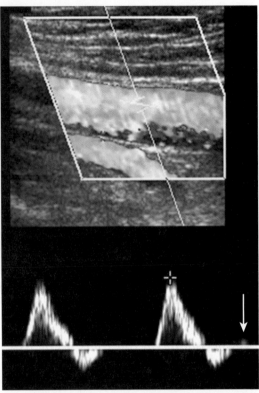

Fig. 22.9 A Doppler waveform from the common femoral artery (CFA) above the connection between the artery and the vein. The CFA should be a high-resistance, triphasic signal but instead shows forward flow in diastole.

Fig. 22.10 A Doppler waveform from the common femoral artery below the connection between the artery and the vein from the same patient as in Fig. 22.9 showing a normal triphasic signal. The *arrow* is pointing to the third component that is just above the inherent Doppler wall filter.

Using appropriate terminology will communicate the severity of the disease and may have an impact on diagnosis and treatment. It is important to keep in mind that terminology describes a waveform and does not diagnose a condition or the cause for the abnormal waveform. This section should be used for reference, and it is important to use the terminology determined by the department and interpreting physicians. The ultrasound community is trying to develop a standardization to describe the various Doppler waveforms, and the sonographer should stay aware of current recommendations.

Triphasic waveforms also can be referred to as a multiphasic waveform and has a rapid upstroke and deceleration in systole, early diastolic flow reversal, and a late diastolic forward flow component. The reverse flow component is caused by vasoconstriction in the arteriolar capillary bed of the normal resting lower extremity (Fig. 22.13).

Biphasic waveforms can be found in normal arteries and arteries with lesions that are not yet reducing flow (<50%–60% stenosis). This waveform has a rapid systolic upstroke and

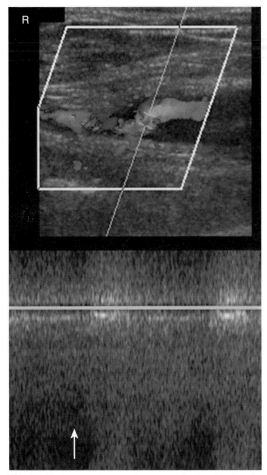

Fig. 22.11 Same patient as Fig. 22.9 and 22.10 showing the high-velocity, low-resistance, turbulent waveform from the connection between the artery and the vein. The *arrow* is pointing to end diastole. The findings are compatible with an arteriovenous fistula. (see Color Plate 62).

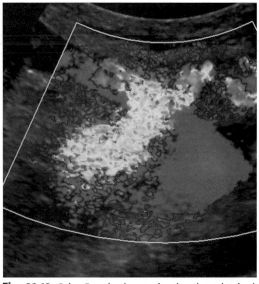

Fig. 22.12 Color Doppler image showing the color bruit of the surrounding tissue in a patient with an arteriovenous fistula. (see Color Plate 63).

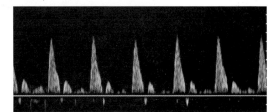

Fig. 22.13 An example of a triphasic waveform.

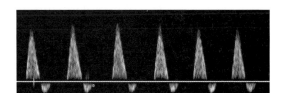

Fig. 22.14 An example of a biphasic waveform.

deceleration from systole to a brief period of early diastolic flow reversal. There is the possibility that the forward flow component is small and is filtered out by the inherent wall filter of the machine. A biphasic signal can be considered abnormal if there is a clear transition from a **triphasic** signal along the artery. This waveform also may be seen in geriatric patients or patients with arterial wall calcification or loss of vessel wall elasticity and compliance (Fig. 22.14).

Monophasic waveforms do not cross the zero-velocity baseline. These waveforms have a rapid systolic upstroke and deceleration in systole, with no diastolic flow (Fig. 22.15).

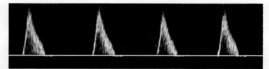

Fig. 22.15 An example of a monophasic waveform. Note the lack of diastolic flow.

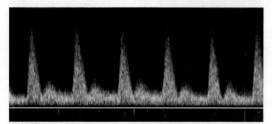

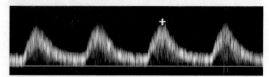

Fig. 22.17 An example of a monophasic and continuous waveform also showing a more rounded and diminished waveform, called the tardus-parvus sign, from a patient with a proximal hemodynamically significant waveform.

Fig. 22.16 An example of a monophasic and continuous waveform. This patient had recently been stressed on a treadmill.

Table 22.2 Lower Extremity Arterial Normal Velocities	
Common femoral artery	80–100 cm/s
Popliteal artery	60–80 cm/s
Tibial arteries	40–60 cm/s

Monophasic and continuous waveforms have a systolic peak followed by diastolic forward flow and can be seen in patients with vascular disease and after arterial stress exercise testing (Fig. 22.16). Waveforms with blunting of the systolic portion of the signal with continuous diastolic flow are seen distal to a flow-limiting lesion (Fig. 22.17).

Lower Extremity Arterial Velocities

The peak systolic velocity range for each artery is given as a guide only (Table 22.2). Most often, a ratio of the prestenotic velocity to the stenotic velocity is used to determine the hemodynamic significance of a lesion. A velocity ratio greater than 2.0 suggests at least a 50% diameter-reducing stenosis, whereas a ratio greater than 4.0 suggests at least a 75% stenosis.

Examples of Arterial Disease

A biphasic waveform will be found in 1% to 49% of cases of stenosis (Table 22.3). Plaque is visualized in the artery, but it does not appear to occupy more than 50% of the vessel and the velocity is not elevated. As the stenosis approaches 49%, the amount of spectral broadening will increase (Fig. 22.18).

Table 22.3 Lower Extremity Arterial Duplex Diagnostic Criteria

% Stenosis	Waveform	Spectral Broadening	Velocity/Ratio	Distal Waveform
Normal	Triphasic or biphasic	None	None	Normal
1%–19%	Triphasic or biphasic	Minimal	<30% increase in PSV compared with proximal segment	Normal
20%–49%	Triphasic or biphasic	Pansystolic	30%–100% increase in PSV compared with proximal segment	Normal
50%–74%	Biphasic or mono-phasic	Pansystolic possible turbulence	>100% increase in PSV compared with proximal segment; 2:1 ratio	Monophasic distally
75%–99%	Biphasic or mono-phasic	Pansystolic possible turbulence	Four fold increase in PSV compared with proximal segment; 4:1 ratio	Monophasic distally
Occluded	No flow	None	None	Collaterals are mono-phasic with reduced PSV

PSV, Peak systolic velocity.

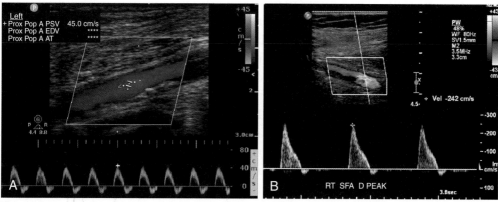

Fig. 22.18 A, Plaque is visualized in the artery but does not appear to occupy more than 50% of the vessel, the velocity is not elevated, and a clear systolic window is present. **B,** A patient with a moderate, 20–49% stenosis with a biphasic waveform with pansystolic spectral broadening.

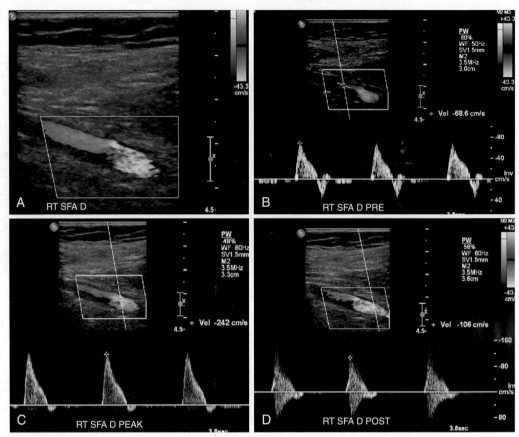

Fig. 22.19 A, Color Doppler image of a patient from the distal superficial femoral artery with a 50% to 74% stenosis demonstrating narrowing of the lumen and aliasing. **B,** Spectral Doppler waveform before the stenosis with a velocity of 68.6 cm/s. The signal has a triphasic appearance with marked spectral broadening. **C,** Peak spectral Doppler waveform velocity of 242 cm/s. There is an increase from 69 to 242 cm/s for a ratio of 3.5 consistent with a 50% to 74% stenosis. **D,** Spectral Doppler waveform after the stenosis has a velocity of 106 cm/s. The signal has marked spectral broadening with poststenotic turbulence and below-baseline flow, and is now a monophasic signal.

A biphasic or monophasic waveform will be seen in patients with a 50% to 74% stenosis. The pre, peak, and post velocities will demonstrate a velocity increase and a ratio greater than 2. Color Doppler images will demonstrate narrowing of the artery (Fig. 22.19).

A biphasic or monophasic waveform will be seen in patients with a 75% to 99% stenosis. The pre, peak, and post velocities will demonstrate a velocity increase and a ratio greater than 4. The post velocity will usually have a turbulent waveform. Color Doppler images will demonstrate narrowing of the artery (Fig. 22.20).

Monophasic waveforms are abnormal, and when they are visualized in the CFA, the examination should extend into the aorta and iliac arteries to find the area of disease. If only one side is abnormal, it will be from iliac disease. If both sides are abnormal, it will be from aortoiliac disease (Fig. 22.21).

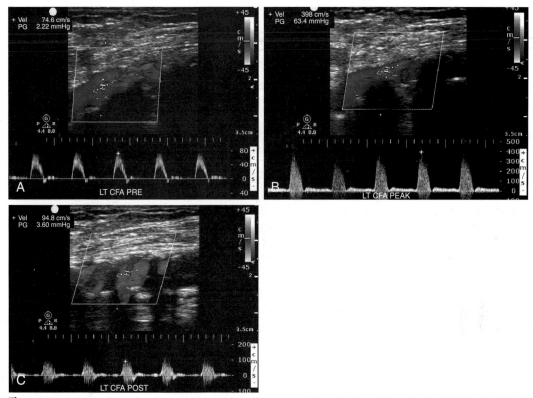

Fig. 22.20 A, Spectral Doppler prestenosis signal from the common femoral artery with a velocity of 74.6 cm/s. **B,** Peak velocity of 398 cm/s with a ratio of 5.3 compatible with a 75% to 99% stenosis. Color Doppler demonstrates the decreased arterial lumen. **C,** Poststenotic turbulent monophasic signal with some diastolic flow and a velocity of 94.8 cm/s.

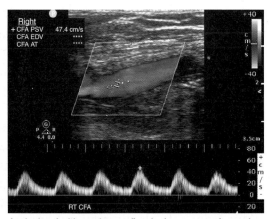

Fig. 22.21 A monophasic signal with continuous flow in the common femoral artery (CFA), prompting an investigation into the iliac artery and discovery of a high-grade stenosis. The contralateral CFA was normal, so the aorta was not imaged.

Spectral broadening is when the clear systolic window begins to fill in with echoes. In the leg this is usually caused by disease, because plaque, even a small plaque, will disrupt normal laminar flow. Spectral broadening is seen in small arteries in which the diameter of the artery is

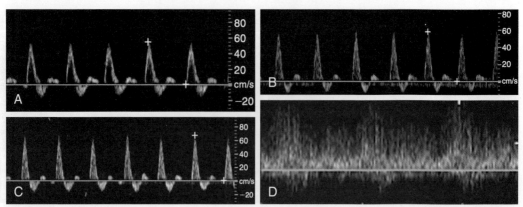

Fig. 22.22 A, A normal triphasic signal with a clear systolic window from the common femoral artery, where the sample volume is small and in center stream flow. **B,** Minimal spectral broadening is seen in this signal from the posterior tibial artery. The artery is too small, and the sample volume encompasses the whole artery. Venous flow is seen below the baseline. **C,** Pansystolic spectral broadening is demonstrated in this signal from the posterior tibial artery that is being caused by the signal being overgained. **D,** An example of a poststenotic waveform right past a high-grade stenosis where the artery has widened back to normal diameter.

not that much wider than the sample volume; therefore, center stream flow is not possible to sample and, instead, the entire artery's velocity profile is sampled. If the Doppler gain is too high, it can add noise to the spectral window and mimic spectral broadening (Fig. 22.22).

Technical Tips

Ultrasound can be highly accurate in skilled hands, and thinking outside of the box can help obtain a complete, diagnostic study. It is worth pointing out that angiography and CT scans provide only anatomic information, not physiologic information, and interpretation can vary among the interpreting physicians. Patients with PAD may also have renal disease and are unable to receive contrast for fear of damaging their kidneys.

Critical thinking should guide the examiner while evaluating the lower extremity arteries, as they focus on image optimization. Adjusting the controls is not just performed once at the beginning of the examination but rather is done throughout the examination. It might seem visually appealing to adjust the image contrast or the overall gain so that the vessel appears completely anechoic, but low-intensity reflections from soft plaque may not appear on the image and will be missed.

It is important to choose the correct frequency for imaging because transducers allow several frequencies to be chosen by using either the frequency adjustment control or PEN/RES/GEN control, which is PEN for penetration, GEN for general, and RES for resolution. Choosing PEN activates the lower frequencies of the transducer, GEN the middle frequencies, and RES the higher frequencies. The frequencies may need to be changed during the course of the examination. For example, higher frequencies, RES or GEN, may be used for the CFA and proximal SFA, but as the artery dives deeper into the leg, lower frequencies, or PEN, are needed.

Patients with large thighs may be a challenge to adequately image the arteries using a linear array transducer. The curved "abdominal" probe is particularly helpful with these patients and for evaluating the distal SFA in other patients. The distal SFA and popliteal artery also could be evaluated using a posterior approach, either by finding the popliteal artery and working cephalad to the posterior thigh or by positioning the patient prone with the feet slightly elevated on a pillow or rolled towel or dangling off the end of the scanning stretcher to allow access to the popliteal fossa.

It is very important to keep in mind the physical principles of Doppler and to keep all Doppler angles less than 60 degrees. With color Doppler, the pulse lines are parallel to the sides of the color box. To maintain proper angles with the artery, it is often necessary to change the steering angle as the course of the artery changes. Adjust the color Doppler controls as necessary to assess the quality of flow and identify regions of disordered, turbulent, or absent flow. For the spectral Doppler waveform, adjust the Doppler angle of insonation to be 60 degrees or less with the cursor parallel to the vessel walls. A low spectral and color Doppler wall filter should be used throughout the examination. If the wall filter is too high, it will not display low flows, which could lead to a false diagnosis of occlusion or make a biphasic signal appear to be monophasic. Power Doppler imaging may be used to complement color Doppler because it is more sensitive to flow and not as angle dependent. The use of power Doppler is helpful to confirm areas of possible vessel occlusion or low-flow states. The frame rate is determined by depth of the image, number of focal zones, and lines per frame. Depth and frame rate are inversely related; when using color Doppler imaging, increasing depth will cause the frame rate to decrease. While scanning in the transverse plane, keep the sector width of the color box as small as possible because, like depth, increasing sector width will decrease the frame rate. The height of the color box does not affect frame rate.

Finally, finding the optimal acoustic window will help improve visualization. Plaque can attenuate the sound beam, and a color Doppler image and spectral Doppler waveform under the plaque will not be possible. When plaque is encountered, slide the transducer into a position in which the sound beam does not go through the plaque, for example, by using a more posterior approach. The proximal aorta can be better visualized by placing the transducer near the level of the sternum and having the patient take a breath in and hold it, which moves the liver inferiorly, which then becomes an acoustic window. The examination of the iliac arteries may be facilitated by having the patient lie in a lateral decubitus position and placing the transducer medial to the anterior iliac spine and parallel to the iliac wing.

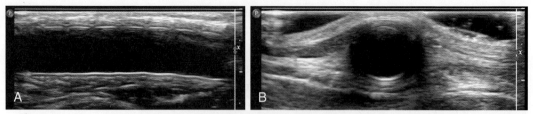

Fig. 22.23 A, Longitudinal image of a polytetrafluoroethylene (PTFE) bypass graft. Note the *double line sign* that is characteristic of this material. **B,** Transverse image of the PTFE bypass graft.

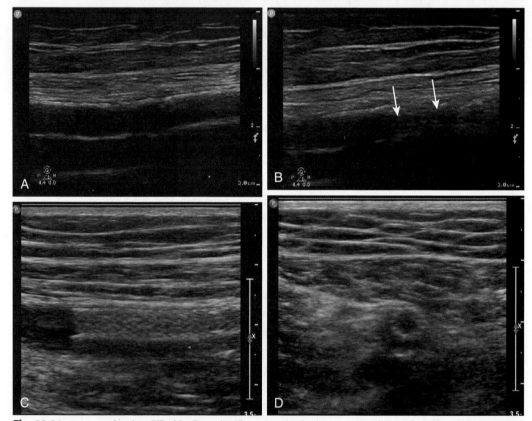

Fig. 22.24 A, Image showing difficultly discerning the stent edge in the presence of arterial calcifications. **B,** Rocking the transducer side to side reveals a subtle mesh appearance of the stent (arrows). **C,** Example of a peripheral stent in the long axis. **D,** Example of a peripheral stent in the transverse plane.

Arterial stents can be difficult to distinguish from calcified vessels (Fig. 22.23). Because stents need to be thoroughly evaluated, it is important to be able to distinguish their location. When evaluating the artery, rock the transducer side to side to see the mesh appearance of the stent. This also can be performed in the transverse plane to confirm location (Fig. 22.24).

Lower Arterial Evaluation Required Images

The aortic and iliac arteries are not routinely evaluated as part of the lower extremity arterial examination. The sonographic examination would be extended into the iliac arteries and the aorta if the Doppler spectral waveforms from the CFA demonstrated delayed systolic upstroke consistent with proximal flow-limiting disease, or if the patient's presenting symptoms indicated the likelihood of an aortoiliac lesion.

1. Longitudinal image of the CFA.

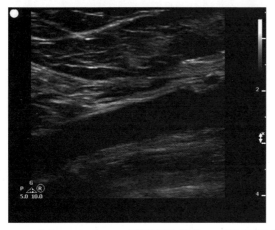

Suggested Annotations: **SAG RT CFA or SAG LT CFA**

NOTE: The images in this section will be labeled RT for ease and consistency.

2. Color Doppler image and Doppler spectral waveform with color from the CFA with peak systolic velocity measured.

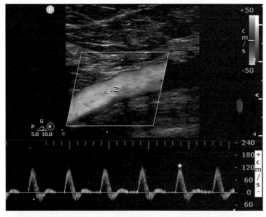

Suggested Annotations: **SAG RT CFA**

3. Longitudinal image of the proximal deep femoral artery.

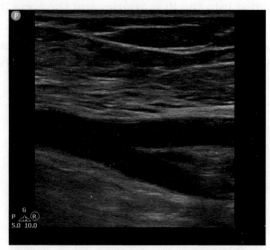

Suggested Annotations: **SAG RT PFA**

NOTE: It is acceptable to have one gray-scale image for the PFA and PROX SFA with a suggested annotation of SAG RT CFA BIF or SAG RT BIF.

4. Color Doppler image and Doppler spectral waveform from the proximal deep femoral artery with peak systolic velocity measured.

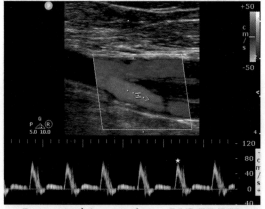

Suggested Annotations: **SAG RT PFA**

5. Longitudinal image of the proximal SFA.

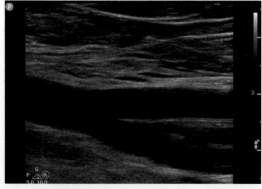

Suggested Annotations: **SAG RT SFA PROX**

6. Doppler spectral waveform from the proximal SFA with peak systolic velocity measured.

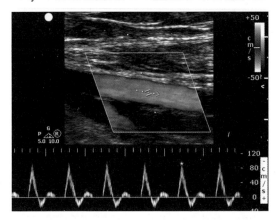

Suggested Annotations: **SAG RT SFA PROX**

7. Color Doppler image and Doppler spectral waveform from the mid-SFA with peak systolic velocity measured. If there is not any plaque present, some labs may incorporate the color Doppler image with the spectral Doppler waveform and not have a separate gray-scale image of the artery.

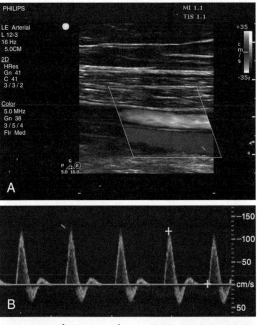

Suggested Annotations: **SAG RT SFA MID**

8. Color Doppler image and Doppler spectral waveform from the distal SFA with peak systolic velocity measured.

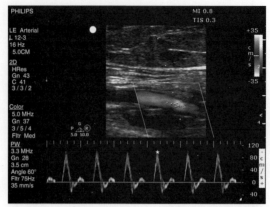

Suggested Annotations: **SAG RT SFA DST**

9. Longitudinal image of the popliteal artery.

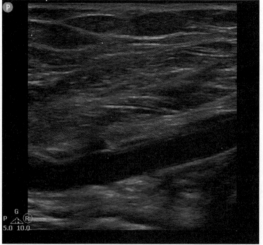

Suggested Annotations: **SAG RT POP**

10. Color Doppler image and Doppler spectral waveform from the popliteal artery with peak systolic velocity measured.

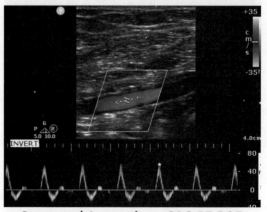

Suggested Annotations: **SAG RT POP**

11.   Longitudinal image of the proximal anterior tibial artery and tibioperoneal trunk.

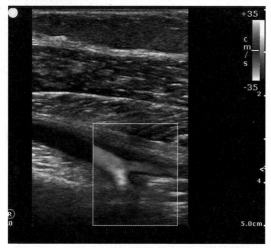

Suggested Annotations: **SAG RT POP BIF or RT ATA/TPT**

12.   Color Doppler image and Doppler spectral waveform from the proximal anterior tibial artery with peak systolic velocity measured.

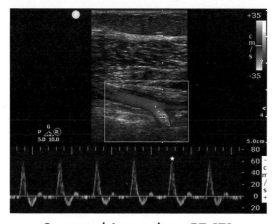

Suggested Annotations: **RT ATA**

13. Color Doppler image and Doppler spectral waveform from the tibioperoneal trunk with peak systolic velocity measured.

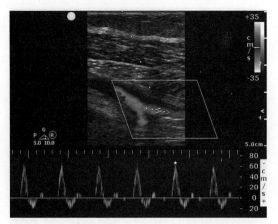

Suggested Annotations: **RT TPT**

14. Doppler spectral waveform from the posterior tibial artery with peak systolic velocity measured.

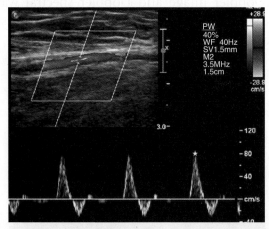

Suggested Annotations: **RT PTA with location such as PROX or MID**

Some departments may require Doppler signals from the proximal, mid, and distal portions.

    The mid to distal part of the artery may be too small to see without color or power Doppler.

Note: Both the American Institute of Ultrasound in Medicine (AIUM)/American College of Radiology (ACR) and the Intersocietal Accreditation Commission Vascular Testing (IAC-VT) require imaging and waveforms only from the tibial artery. The department may require the peroneal and anterior tibial arteries to be evaluated and documented.

Venous Duplex of the Lower Extremity

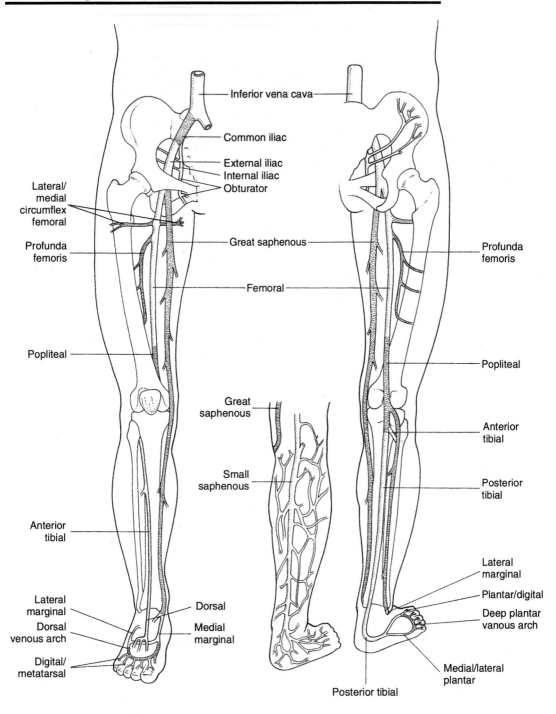

Deep vein thrombosis (DVT) and pulmonary embolism (PE) are a major public health concern because of the number of deaths and the associated health system costs. Venous thromboembolism (VTE) is when a blood clot forms in a vein, a DVT, and part of it breaks off, travels in the bloodstream, and ends up in the lungs, causing

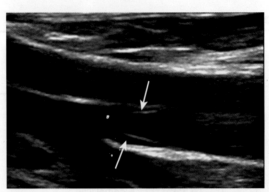

Fig. 22.25 Image demonstrating valve leaflets *(arrows)* in the vein.

a PE. Venous duplex examinations are one of the most frequently performed ultrasound examinations in a hospital and can be performed in the radiology department or the vascular laboratory. In some hospitals, the departments may compete for the same patient or the referring service may have a department that they prefer to perform their patient's examinations. Some emergency departments may perform a full or an abbreviated protocol, and some cardiology departments may also perform venous duplex examinations.

Examinations of the lower extremity venous system are performed to evaluate for the presence of a thrombus. Indications to perform a venous duplex study include but are not limited to swelling, pain, tenderness, palpable cord, and follow-up of a known DVT. The diagnosis of a DVT is important to help prevent the patient from having a PE, which can be fatal.

The diagnosis of DVT in the lower extremity is made when the walls of the vein cannot touch with compression maneuvers because of the intervening thrombus. When the vein collapses and the walls can touch completely with probe pressure, the diagnosis of a thrombus-free vein at that location can be made.

The Centers for Disease Control and Prevention (CDC) estimates that there are as many as 900,000 people in the United States affected with a DVT and that 60,000 to 100,000 people will die of a VTE, which is more than the total number of people who lose their lives each year to acquired immunodeficiency syndrome (AIDS), breast cancer, and motor vehicle accidents combined. One problem with patients with a DVT is that they may be asymptomatic or that the leg with a DVT is asymptomatic and the symptomatic leg does not have a DVT.

The lower extremity veins contain **valves** that keep the blood moving in one direction, toward the heart (Fig. 22.25). When these valves malfunction, blood pools in the legs and can cause symptoms that include pain, swelling, visible varicose veins, venous stasis ulcers, or a "heaviness" feeling in the leg. Venous Doppler can evaluate the leg for leaking valves, called venous insufficiency. These examinations are very challenging and are typically performed by experienced sonographers and will not be discussed in this chapter. Besides being performed in a hospital, venous insufficiency examinations are also performed in vein clinics.

Anatomy

Thorough knowledge of venous anatomy and its variations is important to perform a high-quality diagnostic examination. It is important to use the correct vein names because they have changed in recent years. The superficial femoral vein is now called the femoral vein because the word *superficial* created confusion with either the great saphenous vein, which is a superficial vein, or the word *superficial* caused some physicians to treat the femoral vein as a superficial vein and not treat it as a deep vein when DVT was present. Other name changes are the profunda femoris, which is now called the deep femoral vein; the greater saphenous vein, which is now called the great saphenous vein; and the lesser saphenous vein, which is now called the small saphenous vein.

The external iliac vein, as it crosses the inguinal ligament, becomes the CFV, which lies medial to the CFA. The CFV receives blood from the great saphenous vein and will bifurcate into the femoral vein and the deep femoral vein. The femoral vein lies posterior to the SFA and follows a medial course along the inner curve of the thigh. The femoral vein is duplicated in approximately 20% to 30% of the population, and when a duplicated vein is found, each vein must be evaluated separately. The deep femoral vein is found posterior to the femoral vein, where they join to form the CFV, which runs deeper in the thigh. The deep femoral vein is hard to evaluate after the bifurcation, and usually only the proximal portion is evaluated. At the adductor canal the femoral vein becomes the popliteal vein, which lies posterior and lateral to the popliteal artery. The popliteal vein is formed by the anterior tibial vein and the tibioperoneal trunk joining together.

The veins of the calf include the anterior tibial, posterior tibial, and peroneal veins and are seen as pairs on both sides of the same-named artery. In some patients there will be more than two veins with the same named artery. The paired anterior tibial veins originate as the dorsalis pedis veins and course on top of the interosseous membrane, lateral to the tibia. The anterior tibial veins and artery are found above the echogenic interosseous membrane between the tibia and the fibula. Just below the knee the veins join together to become the common anterior tibial trunk, which penetrates the proximal end of the membrane to join with the tibioperoneal trunk and insert into the popliteal vein. The anterior tibial veins do not communicate directly with the soleal sinus veins in the calf, unlike the posterior tibial and peroneal veins, and do not commonly develop venous thrombosis. Imaging of the anterior tibial veins is not a requirement of either the IAC-VT or AIUM protocol. The posterior tibial veins are formed by the plantar veins of the foot and they lie behind the tibia. They accompany the posterior tibial artery posterior to the medial malleolus and course superiorly along the medial calf to form the common tibial trunk in the lower popliteal space. The peroneal veins course along the lateral aspect of the calf in a posteromedial aspect to the fibula. The paired veins converge to form the common peroneal trunk and join the posterior tibial trunk to form the tibioperoneal trunk, which then drains into the popliteal vein. The posterior tibial and peroneal veins are typically visualized together in the same image.

The great saphenous vein is the longest vein in the body and lies within the subcutaneous tissues of the leg. The great saphenous vein originates on the dorsum of the foot, passes anteriorly to the medial malleolus, courses medial to and then posterior to the medial aspect of the tibia, around the medial aspect of the knee, and then continues in the medial aspect of the thigh to drain into the femoral vein at the saphenofemoral junction just below the inguinal ligament. There are venous valves along the length of the great saphenous vein. The small saphenous vein also runs subcutaneously, originating from the lateral aspect of the dorsal veins of the foot to course inferior and posterior to the lateral malleolus, then along the posterior aspect of the calf, usually at midline, to drain into the popliteal vein usually at or above the knee joint at about the same level as the gastrocnemius vein. The small saphenous and the gastrocnemius veins may join together and form a common trunk. The small saphenous vein has variations in where it joins the deep venous system and may bypass the popliteal vein and join with either the femoral vein or great saphenous vein, where it is called the Giacomini vein.

There are two groups of veins in the calf muscles: the gastrocnemius and the soleus veins. The soleal veins or soleal sinus veins are found in the deep soleus muscles of the calf and drain into the posterior tibial and peroneal veins. Clots can form in the soleal sinus veins when the calf muscles are not active and can become a common source for popliteal vein DVT. This is why it is important to squeeze your calf muscles when sitting for an extended period, such as on a long air flight or drive. The gastrocnemius veins are located in the more superficial gastrocnemius muscles and drain into the popliteal vein at the level of the small saphenous vein. A gastrocnemius vein will branch from the popliteal vein as a single trunk and then quickly bifurcate into two veins accompanied by an artery. A way to

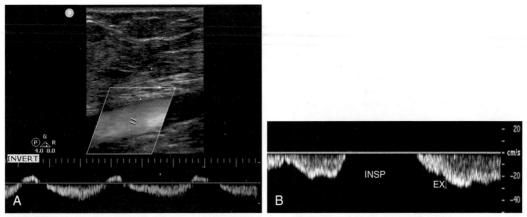

Fig. 22.26 A, Spectral Doppler waveform demonstrating normal respiratory phasicity. **B,** Doppler waveform with inspiration marked on the image causing cessation of flow as a result of increased intraabdominal pressure and with flow returning in expiration as the pressure decreases.

differentiate a gastrocnemius vein from a posterior tibial vein is to follow the vein to see if it goes all the way to the foot. If it does, it is a posterior tibial vein because the gastrocnemius veins stay within the gastrocnemius muscle.

With the exception of the soleal veins, valves are located in all of the lower extremity veins to move the blood in one direction and prevent retrograde venous flow. The number of valves is greatest in the tibial veins of the calf.

Sonographic Appearance

The normal vein should have thin walls with an echo-free lumen. If slow flow is present, low-level swirling echoes may be seen inside the vein. It is important to not confuse these low-level echoes with a thrombus. Venous valves can be seen opening and closing, especially in the larger veins. They should appear as thin echogenic structures.

Angle correction is not used during a venous duplex examination because the peak velocity is not being measured. What is important is the characteristics of the waveform. The spectral Doppler signal is evaluated for **spontaneous flow** with respiratory variations. **Augmentation** and Valsalva maneuvers can add additional information about the vein. Spontaneous flow is continuous and present without using any augmentation maneuvers. **Respiratory phasicity** causes the Doppler flow patterns to vary in amplitude because of changes in intraabdominal and intrathoracic pressures associated with respiration. Flow decreases during inspiration as a result of the increased intraabdominal pressure and increases with expiration because the intraabdominal pressure decreases (Fig. 22.26). **Continuous flow** with no noticeable respiratory variation suggests a proximal obstruction (Fig. 22.27). Augmentation should demonstrate a sharp upstroke from the rapid increase in venous velocity

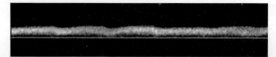

Fig. 22.27 Venous waveform with dampened respiratory variations.

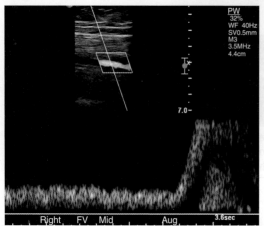

Fig. 22.28 Doppler waveform from mid femoral vein with a normal augmentation. Note the quick and sharp upstroke and aliasing of the Doppler waveform. These Doppler characteristics are showing that the "tube" is open from the calf, where the augmentation pressure was applied, to mid femoral vein.

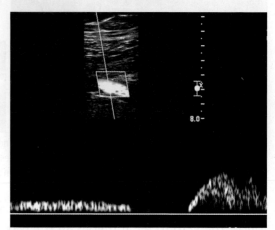

Fig. 22.29 Note the difference in the augmentation of this signal. There is no sharp or quick upstroke, nor is there aliasing. This signal was obtained from the distal femoral vein. These findings could be caused by a poor squeeze, a swollen calf where it was difficult to apply the needed pressure, or possibly a nonobstructive thrombus in the popliteal vein.

with distal limb compression by squeezing the calf (Fig. 22.28). This finding indicates the absence of a vein thrombosis between the transducer and the point of compression. The absence or a lower increase in velocity with a rounded shape, much like the tardus-parvus signal in an artery, suggests that there is possible partial obstruction between the transducer and point of compression (Fig. 22.29).

The following are additional maneuvers that are not performed in all laboratories. By using proximal compression, by pressing down on the abdomen at the level of the umbilicus or by having the patient perform a Valsalva maneuver, **valvular competence** can be evaluated. This maneuver causes the blood flow in the vein under the transducer to stop if the valves are competent (Fig. 22.30). If the valves are leaking, there will be retrograde flow seen while pressing on the abdomen or having the patient perform a Valsalva maneuver, which will return to proper flow direction once the maneuver is stopped (Fig. 22.31). A minimal amount of retrograde flow may be noted if a quick, hard compression is performed because this does not allow enough time for the valve leaflets to close adequately (Fig. 22.32). Venous flow variations should occur with the respiratory cycles and not with each heartbeat. Venous **pulsatile flow** suggests congestive heart failure or tricuspid insufficiency (Fig. 22.33).

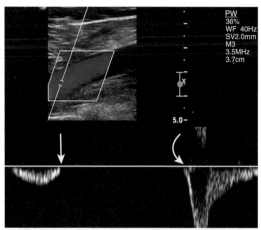

Fig. 22.30 A normal response to a proximal augmentation, which is performed by pressing on the abdomen at the level of the umbilicus. An alternative method is to have the patient perform a Valsalva maneuver. This is a normal response that indicates that there is no valvular regurgitation at the level of the sample volume. The *arrow* is pointing to when pressure was applied that caused flow to stop. The *curved arrow* points to when pressure was stopped and flow returned.

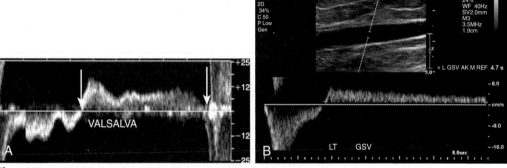

Fig. 22.31   A, A patient with valvular incompetence. When the patient bears down, the flow reverses, going back down the leg, and when the patient stops, the flow resumes with a rush back to forward flow. The *arrows* mark the beginning and end of the Valsalva maneuver. **B,** Doppler spectral waveform from the great saphenous vein demonstrating prolonged valvular incompetence (retrograde flow, reflux) occurring after the augmentation maneuver, consistent with severe superficial insufficiency.

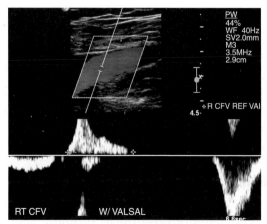

Fig. 22.32 An example of a quick reflux at the start of Valsalva. Note the quick upstroke and that the reflux does not extend throughout the entire Valsalva maneuver.

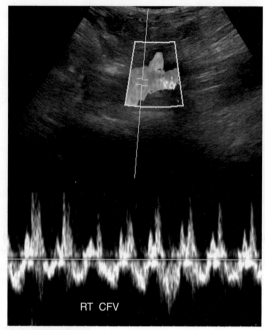

Fig. 22.33 An example of a pulsatile venous waveform on a patient with severe tricuspid regurgitation.

Venous Duplex of the Lower Extremity

Patient Prep

The patient will need to undress from the waist down except for their underwear. Socks should come off so that the veins in the ankle can be evaluated. Tuck a pillowcase or hand towel in the leg of the underwear to protect it from the gel. Men wearing boxers may have to remove them. All patients should be covered with a sheet folded to expose the skin on the side being examined. Patients with leg braces or removable casts will need them removed. If the patient is not sure if they can be removed, then the patient's physician will need to be contacted for permission.

Transducer

A 5-10 MHz linear array transducer is used to image the veins. A 1–5 MHz curved linear array transducer is used for imaging the pelvic and abdominal veins, the iliac veins, and the distal FV, as needed, and for large or swollen legs to obtain greater depth of penetration (Fig. 22.34). As with any aspect of diagnostic ultrasound, the highest frequency should be used that allows good penetration with little to no noise in the image.

Patient Position

Patients are evaluated supine with the examination table placed in the reversed Trendelenburg position to promote venous pooling in

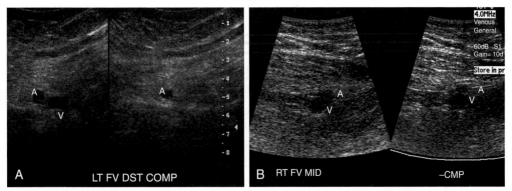

Fig. 22.34 A, An image of a normal compression on the distal femoral vein using a curved linear array transducer on a patient with a large leg. To bring out the veins and eliminate the noise inside them the contrast control was adjusted to make the image more black and white. This eliminates the low-level echoes and needs to be used with understanding and caution. **B,** An image of an abnormal compression on the mid femoral vein using a curved linear array transducer on a patient with a large leg. Because of the use of the contrast control the echoes inside the vein are not seen, and it is only through the compression maneuver that the clot is seen, illustrating the need to use this control with caution and understanding. *A,* Artery; *V,* vein.

the legs, when possible. To access the medial aspect of the leg the patient can externally rotate the leg out. For patient comfort, place a pillow under the knee. For the popliteal vein the leg may need to be rotated more or have the patient rotate on their side until the thigh is on or almost on the table.

Technical Tips

Compressions are performed in the transverse plane starting above where the great saphenous vein empties into the CFV. Enough pressure is used to compress the vein so that the vein walls touch, or **coapt**. Continue compressing the vein at 1–2 cm intervals down the leg to the tibioperoneal trunk, so as not to skip over a small thrombus. In some departments the compression views are documented with small ciné clips. Compressions should be performed with gray-scale imaging unless it is very difficult to see the vein, and then color Doppler may be used. If the leg is large and difficult to compress, place your hand under the leg below the transducer and push up while pushing down with the transducer. Once the walls of the vein touch, free up a hand to hit freeze and then ciné back to obtain the image of the compression. This technique is also good to use to compress the distal femoral vein in the adductor canal. In some patients with edematous or swollen legs it may be difficult to obtain good compression without also causing the artery to compress. With edematous legs the transducer will temporarily leave an indentation in the leg until the fluid fills it back up. A tip for large legs, including edematous ones, is to press lightly with the transducer to get the veins nearer to the transducer but not enough to make them start to collapse, as this may sharpen up the vein by bringing it closer to the transducer; freeze the image and then perform the compression aspect, freeze the image, and then document the image. With the extra pressure being used, be aware of your joints to reduce a musculoskeletal injury. If a clot is found in a vein, compressions should proceed with care so as not to knock off a piece and cause a PE.

Finding a thrombus in a duplicated vein can be difficult, especially if the entire vein is filled with a thrombus. Carefully evaluating the vein while compressing may enhance visualizing the thrombosed vein or identifying one of the connections.

For noisy legs try adjusting the contrast or compression control of the gray-scale image to increase the contrast, making sure it does not eliminate low-level echoes from a clot. Increasing the contrast may help "clean up" the vessels. Fresh acute thrombus may be anechoic, and it is the lack of compression that alerts the sonographer that a clot is present. Sometimes increasing the overall gain may help bring out echoes in the vein.

Color Doppler is used on longitudinal images of the vein to evaluate patency, demonstrate partially occlusive thrombus, and help locate vessels, especially those that are deep. Augmentation with color Doppler will aid in locating veins in technically challenging situations. Augmentation maneuvers are performed by squeezing the calf to cause the blood to flow rapidly up the leg. Augmentation maneuvers should not be performed when there is free-floating or partially occlusive thrombus, because dislodgement and potential embolization may occur.

All Doppler spectral waveforms should be obtained from the longitudinal view of the vein with an angle of less than 60 degrees. Augmentation maneuvers may be used to help demonstrate vein patency and improve visualization of blood flow in patients with slow flow. Do not squeeze the calf hard but rather apply a gentle continuous squeeze, so as not to cause a rapid upstroke but rather an even amplitude. The spectral sweep speed should be properly adjusted to show venous flow below the baseline before augmentation or Valsalva maneuver and to show flow reversal above the baseline and the return of flow to below the baseline.

Optimization of the image is not a one-time adjustment at the beginning of the examination, but rather it is done multiple times during the examination. It might seem appealing to adjust the overall gain so low that the vessels appear completely anechoic, but low-intensity signals such as thrombus can be missed (Fig. 22.35). The venous preset should be used and the color velocity scale adjusted to a setting that allows color filling the lumen from wall to wall (Fig. 22.36).

Patients with large thighs may present a challenge to adequately image the veins using the linear array transducer. The curved abdominal probe is particularly helpful in evaluating the distal FV and may be necessary in evaluating the veins throughout the leg in obese

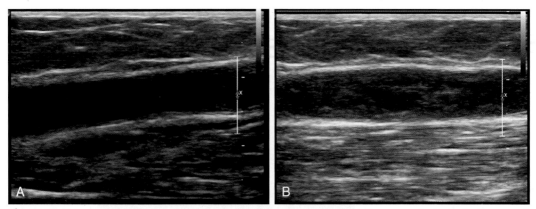

Fig. 22.35 A, Image of vein with gain settings too low so that it appears normal. **B,** The same patient as in **A** with appropriate gain settings demonstrating intraluminal echoes consistent with thrombus.

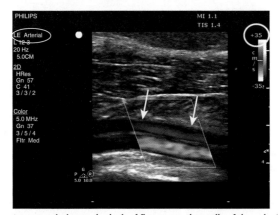

Fig. 22.36 The *arrows* are pointing to the lack of flow up to the walls of the vein. The *oval* points out that the wrong preset was used and is set on arterial and not venous, causing the color velocity scale, indicated by the *circle,* to be too high for the vein and eliminating the slower flow against the walls. This gives the illusion of a nonobstructive thrombus. (see Color Plate 64).

patients (Fig. 22.37). The distal femoral and popliteal vein could also be evaluated using a posterior approach, either by finding the popliteal vein and moving superiorly to the posterior thigh or by positioning the patient prone with the feet slightly elevated on a pillow or rolled towel to allow access to the popliteal fossa.

If the vascular laboratory or the department is accredited by IAC-VT or the ACR, a requirement for a unilateral examination is that spectral Doppler waveforms from both CFVs or both external iliac veins, if the department's protocol includes evaluating the external iliac veins, be obtained. It is a best practice to start the examination with the contralateral limb and then move to the symptomatic limb. This enables the examiner to see any variations between the CFVs and whether the iliac veins should be evaluated, as well as the inferior vena cava. If the iliac veins are evaluated and there is a difference in waveforms, the common iliac veins should be evaluated and the distal IVC (Fig. 22.38).

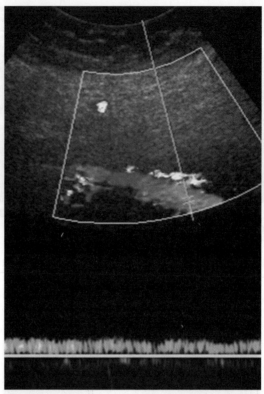

Fig. 22.37 Using a curved linear array transducer to obtain a Doppler signal from the distal femoral vein. (see Color Plate 65).

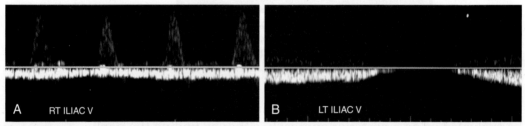

Fig. 22.38 A, A Doppler signal from the right iliac vein demonstrating loss of respiratiry variations. **B,** The same patient as in **A** showing normal respiratory variations in the left iliac vein. This caused the sonographer to evaluate the left common iliac vein, which was positive for thrombus.

Calf veins may be easier to find distally and trace to their confluence. A low spectral and color Doppler velocity scale should be used for examination of the calf veins. Careful optimization should be performed so as to not make the veins appear abnormal. Sometimes it can be difficult to stay on the calf vein and obtain a waveform. In this situation, scanning without color can help obtain the Doppler waveform because this allows the two-dimensional (2D) image to be active while the signal is obtained (Fig. 22.39). In the calf veins, absence of spontaneous flow can be a normal finding.

For patients with pain and tenderness in the calf, it is helpful to examine the calf muscle in the region of pain. Thrombus can originate

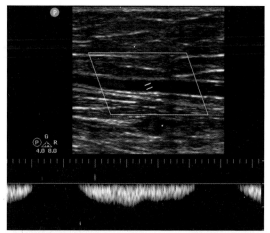

Fig. 22.39 The color map was removed to see the vein better for good sample volume placement.

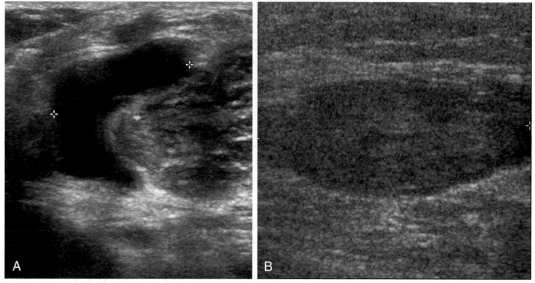

Fig. 22.40 A, An example of a patient with a Baker's cyst found incidentally while performing a dep vein thrombosis (DVT) examination. Finding and documenting incidental pathologic conditions will tell the physician the cause of the leg pain or swelling, especially when there is no evidence of a DVT. **B,** An image of an enlarged lymph node in the groin of the patient. Note its oval shape and the faint hyperechoic echoes in the center compatible with an enlarged lymph node resulting from an infectious process. Groin nodes can be tender, and it might be painful trying to compress the common femoral vein, especially if the nodes are under the transducer.

in the soleal veins in the calf and cause pain or discomfort. Look for large, swollen soleal veins filled with thrombus. The soleal veins normally drain into the posterior tibial and peroneal veins.

Not all leg pain is vascular in origin, and the sonographer should be on the lookout for any pathologic condition, such as enlarged lymph nodes, fluid collections, or muscle pathologic findings (Fig. 22.40). While performing the venous study, the sonographer should pay attention to the arterial system because unsuspected arterial disease could be the cause of the pain (Fig. 22.41).

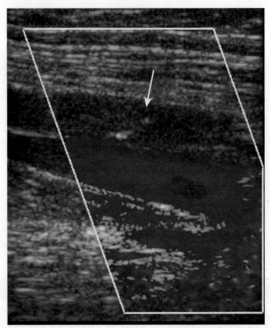

Fig. 22.41 The patient was referred for a venous duplex for leg pain. While performing the study the sonographer noticed that the common femoral artery (CFA) was occluded. The *arrow* is pointing to the occluded CFA.

Scanning Tips and Tricks

Begin scanning in a transverse scanning plane with the patient lying supine with the lower limb rotated outward and the knee slightly flexed in a frog-leg position to gain access to the common femoral and popliteal veins. Start the examination above the inguinal canal and locate the CFV and CFA. Assess compressibility of the vein by applying slow, firm pressure over the vein and confirm that the vein walls coapt (Fig. 22.42). The walls of the CFA should not deform with adequate compression of the vein. Continue to scan and compress inferiorly to the level of the saphenous-femoral junction and then to the CFV bifurcation. Follow the course of the femoral vein along the medial aspect of the thigh. Document **compressibility** of the femoral vein in the proximal, mid, and distal thigh continuing through Hunter's canal to the popliteal vein. Place the transducer in the popliteal fossa, document compression, and continue to scan through to the anterior tibial and tibial-peroneal trunk. Finish the compressions by scanning the posterior tibial and peroneal veins down to the ankle. The peroneal and posterior tibial veins and their accompanying arteries lie inferior to the interosseous membrane with the peroneal veins being deeper than the posterior tibial veins (Fig. 22.43). Compressing the calf veins usually makes the veins appear as if they are winking. Accreditation does not dictate the number of images needed to document compressions of the calf veins, and the department will

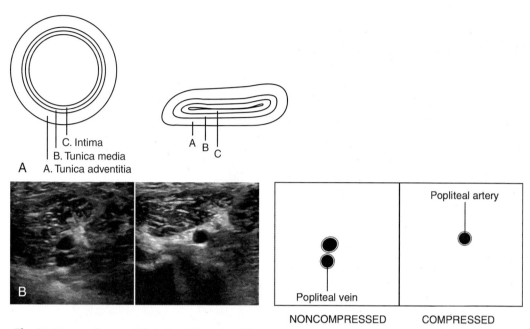

C. Intima
B. Tunica media
A. Tunica adventitia

A   B   C

NONCOMPRESSED   COMPRESSED

Fig. 22.42 A, A diagram of the veins of the wall and how the walls touch when there is no clot present.**B,** Image and diagram of a normal compression of the popliteal vein.

decide how many and at what levels. If required to evaluate the gastrocnemius veins, start at the popliteal vein and follow it inferiorly to the gastrocnemius veins. The examiner should follow them into the upper calf and assess compressibility of the veins (Fig. 22.44). Per accreditation, the following levels must be documented: CFV, saphenofemoral junction, deep femoral vein with or without the proximal femoral vein, proximal femoral vein, mid femoral vein, distal femoral vein, popliteal vein, posterior tibial veins, and peroneal veins. These levels are the minimum levels, and the department can expand on the areas of compression.

The next part of the examination is the color Doppler and Doppler spectral waveforms. The IAC-VT requires at a minimum a spectral Doppler waveform demonstrating spontaneous venous flow, phasicity, and/or flow augmentation from the right and left CFVs and the popliteal vein. The department may obtain additional waveforms from other levels. Remember, for unilateral examinations, spectral Doppler waveforms must be documented from the right and left CFVs or external iliac veins. The AIUM guidelines are a little different and require color and spectral Doppler waveforms from the long axis at each of the following levels: right and left common femoral or external iliac vein and popliteal vein on the symptomatic side or on both sides if the examination is bilateral. Bilateral CFV or external iliac vein waveforms are needed to determine whether there is any disease in the common iliac veins or the IVC. A unilateral loss of

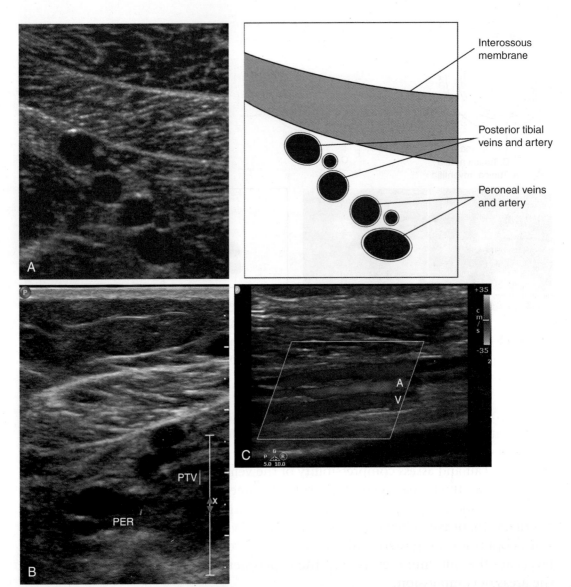

Fig. 22.43 A, Image and diagram of the posterior tibial veins and artery and peroneal veins and artery posterior to the interossus membrane just past the popliteal fossa. **B,** Image of the posterior tibial vein *(PTV)* and peroneal veins *(PER)* and their accompanying arteries lying inferior to the interosseous membrane in the calf. **C,** Color Doppler image of the two posterior tibial veins on either side of the posterior tibial artery. (see Color Plate 66). *A,* Artery; *V,* vein.

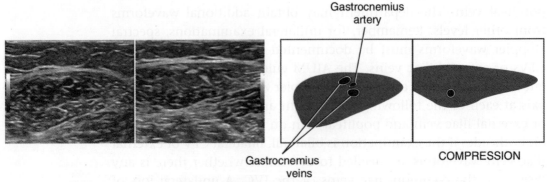

Fig. 22.44 Image and diagram of the gastrocnemius veins and artery with and without pressure.

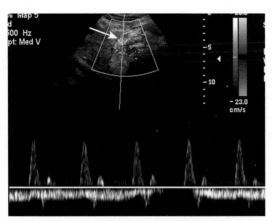

Fig. 22.45 An image of the external iliac vein and artery. The *arrow* is pointing to the more anterior artery. As seen here, it is possible to get a Doppler signal from both the artery and vein because the sample volume is three-dimensional and is obtaining signals "in back of" and "in front of the screen." Because venous flow is nicely seen, this is an acceptable image. To isolate the venous flow, adjust the placement of the sample volume to a more distal aspect of the vein.

phasicity of the CFV or external iliac vein Doppler waveforms can indicate proximal or occlusive thrombus or extrinsic compression. Bilateral flattening of the CFV and external iliac vein Doppler waveforms can indicate IVC compression by tumor or occlusive thrombus. Note that neither organization requires a Doppler waveform from the femoral vein, deep femoral vein, great or small saphenous vein, or calf veins.

The external iliac veins may be required in some departments because isolated iliac vein thrombus has been reported. A 1–5 MHz curved linear transducer will be needed because the veins are deep and the transducer fits well into the depression of the iliac crest. The faster-velocity iliac arteries are typically easy to see where they go over the iliac crest, and the external iliac veins are directly posterior to the artery. If the vein is not seen, the color velocity scale should be decreased until venous flow is seen, possibly causing color aliasing of the artery, which is acceptable as we are evaluating the vein. The vessels run in an oblique course toward the common iliac vein and IVC, so angle the transducer toward the umbilicus (Fig. 22.45).

Examples of Venous Disease

The diagnosis of a DVT is made when the vein walls do not touch and echogenic material is seen inside the vein. Both should be seen to confirm a diagnosis of DVT (Fig. 22.46). However, in an acute thrombosis the thrombus may be anechoic and difficult to visualize. In these cases, turn up the 2D gain to see if echoes can be elicited, evaluate the area with color or preferably power Doppler to see if there is any detectable flow inside the vein, or perform a distal augmentation to see if that ilicits flow. If color or power Doppler do show vessel patency,

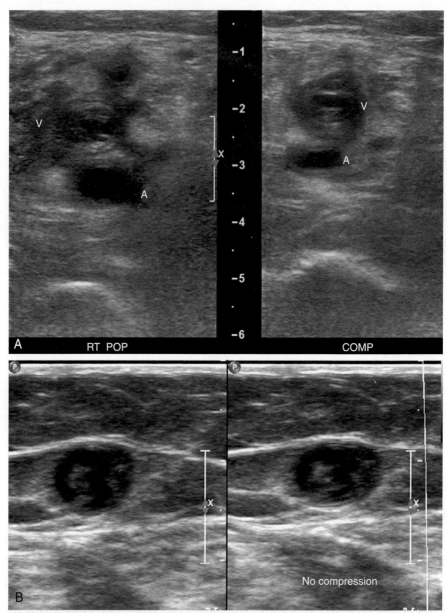

Fig. 22.46 A, Image of a thrombus seen in the popliteal vein. Note that with compression the vein becomes better defined. **B,** Split-screen transverse images of noncompressed and compressed thrombus-filled great saphenous vein showing lack of compressibility. Notice how the vein becomes oval with compression. *A,* Artery; *V,* vein.

the sonographer should try to discover the cause of noncompressibility, which might include poor patient positioning or a proximal obstruction. Another maneuver is to compress until the artery starts to collapse, making sure to warn the patient before increasing pressure because this may be uncomfortable for them. If the artery compresses and the vein does not, that is suspicious for a thrombus. Care should be taken in using color Doppler alone to evaluate the venous lumen because it can overwrite a nonocclusive clot (Fig. 22.47)

Imaging Criteria for Normal vs Abnormal Examination

Normal Examination

Compressibility: The vein walls coapt completely with moderate probe compression, and there is no evidence of intraluminal echoes.

Flow pattern: The Doppler spectral waveform demonstrates spontaneous flow with respiratory phasicity in all venous segments.

Abnormal Examination

Compressibility: The vein walls do not touch or are partially compressible, and there is evidence of intraluminal echoes.

Flow pattern: The Doppler spectral waveform is absent in a complete occlusion and is continuous, nonphasic flow with a nonobstructing thrombus. The Doppler signal in the vein distal to the clot is continuous.

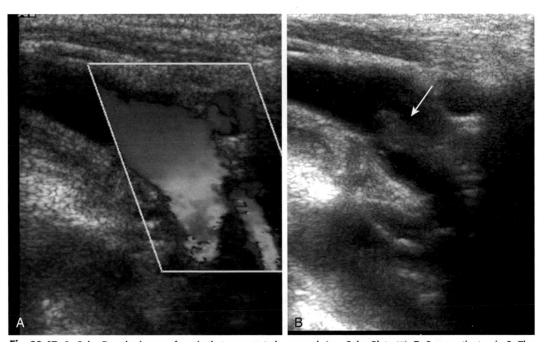

Fig. 22.47 A, Color Doppler image of a vein that appears to be normal. (see Color Plate 67). **B,** Same patient as in **A.** The *arrow* is pointing to a free-floating clot that was masked by the color Doppler.

Acute vs Chronic DVT

Acute thrombus usually expands the vessel, causing the diameter of the vein to be larger than the artery. The thrombus is generally anechoic to slightly hypoechoic in echogenicity. The vein may

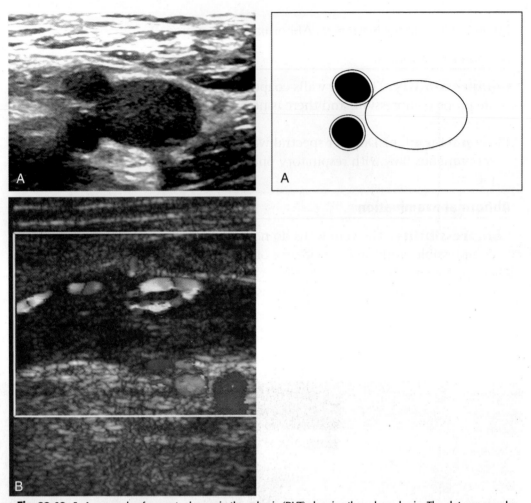

Fig. 22.48 A, An example of an acute deep vein thrombosis (DVT) showing the enlarged vein. The clot was seen by increasing the overall gain to bring out the low-level echoes. **B,** A color Doppler image of an acute DVT with recanalized flow seen. (see Color Plate 68).

show a very slight compression when doing the compression view. Recanalization is when venous flow starts to return to a previous occluded vein. The color velocity scale should be decreased or power Doppler used to try and see if there is any flow. Ensure that the color wall scale is at the minimal setting and adjust the color gain control to a proper setting (Fig. 22.48).

Generally, as a thrombus becomes more chronic, it increases in echogenicity and retracts in size. Thus, chronic or residual DVT becomes more eccentric and focal in location, resulting in a decrease in diameter of the vein (Fig. 22.49)

Sonographic Characteristics of an Acute vs a Chronic Deep Vein Thrombosis

Characteristics of Acute Deep Vein Thrombosis

1. Hypoechoic or anechoic thrombus
2. Poorly attached or "floating" thrombus
3. Spongy-texture thrombus
4. Compressible or deformable thrombus
5. Dilated or expanded vein

Characteristics of Chronic Deep Vein Thrombosis

1. Brightly echogenic thrombus
2. Well-attached thrombus
3. Rigid texture of thrombus
4. Contracted vein
5. Large collaterals
6. Thickened vein walls

Lower Extremity Venous Duplex Required Images

The suggested annotations are using RT for simplicity.

1. Split-screen images of noncompressed and compressed CFV. *A,* Artery; *V,* vein.

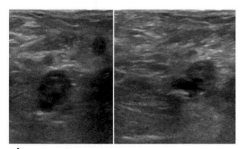

A

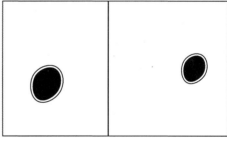

NONCOMPRESSED   COMPRESSED

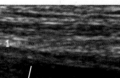

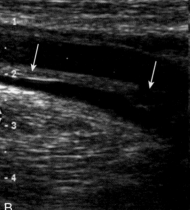

B

Fig. 22.49 A, Image of a patient with a chronic deep vein thrombosis (DVT) demonstrating a heterogenous thrombus. **B,** An image of a patient with a chronic DVT. The *arrows* are pointing to the thin caliber of the vein and the thickened walls.

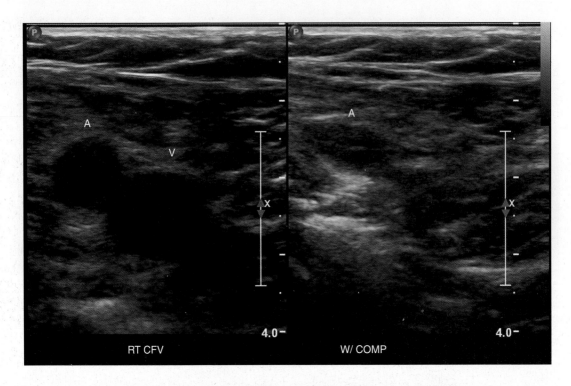

Suggested Annotations: **RT CFV and COMP or W/COMP**

Some departments annotate the arteries and veins, others only annotate when the vein does not compress, and some departments do not annotate at all. Another variation is to annotate NO COMP when the vein does not compress. Use the annotation method that the department uses.

2. Split-screen axial images of noncompressed and compressed saphenofemoral junction. *A*, Artery; *V*, vein.

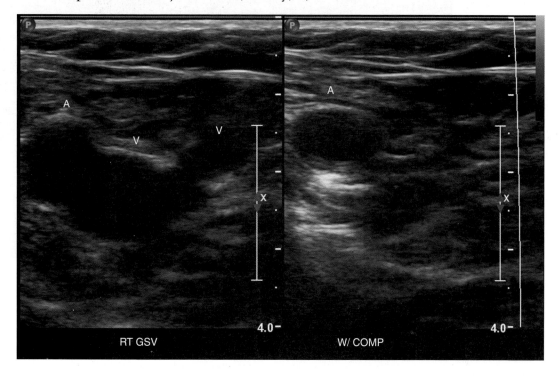

Suggested Annotations: **RT GSV, SFJ, or CFV/GSV and COMP or W/COMP**

3. Split-screen axial images of noncompressed and compressed deep femoral vein *(DFV)*. *A*, Artery; *FV*, femoral vein.

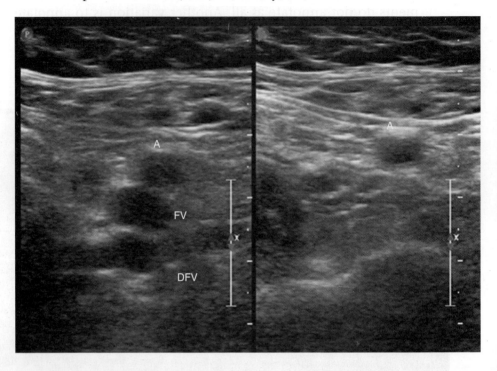

Suggested Annotations: **RT PROX DFV and COMP or W/COMP; if proximal femoral vein is seen, annotation could be RT PROX FV/DFV**

4. Split-screen axial images of noncompressed and compressed proximal femoral vein. *A*, Artery; *V*, vein.

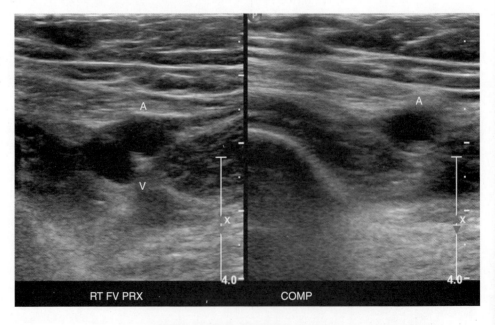

Suggested Annotations: **RT FV PRX or PROX and COMP or W/COMP**

NOTE: Type FV first so that you only have to backspace and type the location.

5. Split-screen axial images of noncompressed and compressed mid femoral vein.

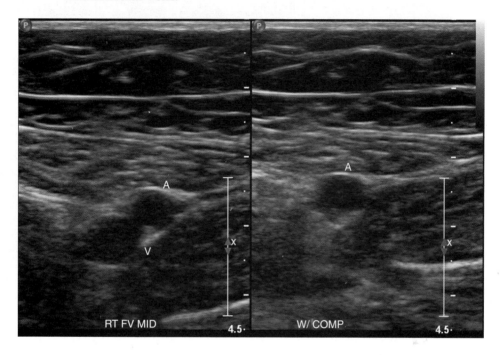

Suggested Annotations: **RT FV MID and COMP or W/COMP**

6. Split-screen axial images of noncompressed and compressed distal femoral vein.

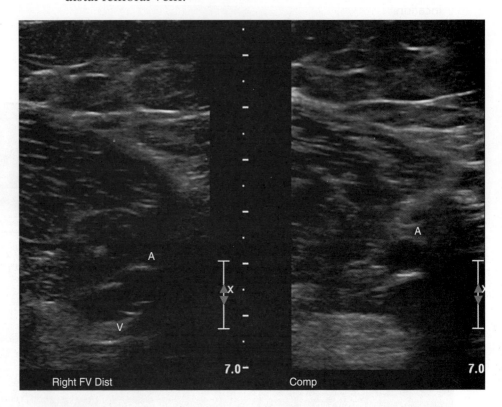

Suggested Annotations: **RT FV DST or DIST and COMP or W/COMP**

7. Split-screen axial images of noncompressed and compressed popliteal vein. *A,* Artery; *V,* vein.

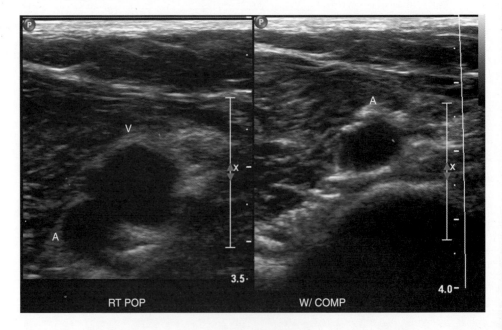

Suggested Annotations: **RT POP and COMP or W/COMP**

8. Split-screen axial images of noncompressed and compressed posterior tibial and peroneal vein. *A,* Artery; *V,* vein.

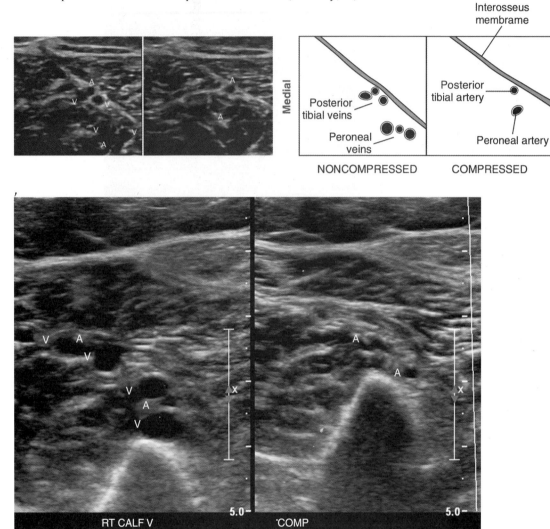

Suggested Annotations: **RT PTV/PER and COMP or W/COMP**

9. Longitudinal right CFV, with or without color, spectral Doppler waveform, with or without augmentation. NOTE: Although the images are demonstrating augmentation maneuvers, they are no longer required. However, some labs are still performing them.

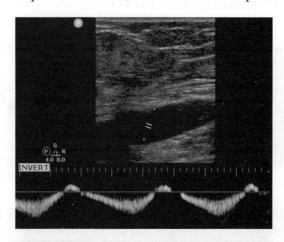

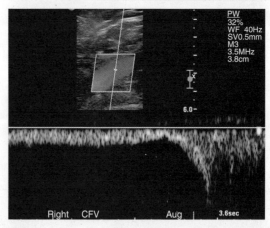

Suggested Annotations: **RT CFV; if augmentation is performed, most departments annotate AUG at the point that the calf was squeezed.**

10. Longitudinal left CFV, with or without color, and spectral Doppler waveform, with or without augmentation.

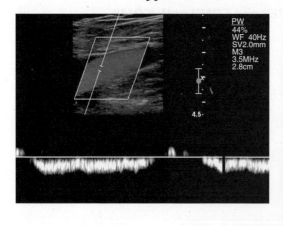 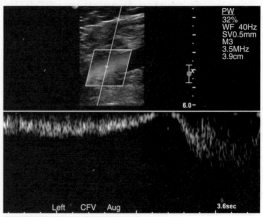

Suggested Annotations: **LT CFV; if augmentation is performed, most departments annotate AUG at the point that the calf was squeezed.**

11. Longitudinal popliteal vein, with or without color, and spectral Doppler waveform, with or without augmentation.

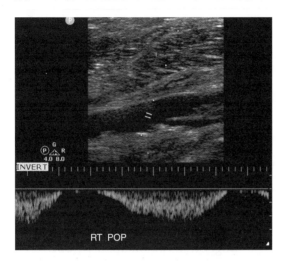

Suggested Annotations: **RT POP; if augmentation is performed, most departments annotate AUG at the point that the calf was squeezed.**

The following are examples of images that used to be required and that some laboratories may still perform today.

1. Image of the great saphenous vein with anteroposterior measurement and compression. This image is the classic "Egyptian eye" appearance of the great saphenous vein.

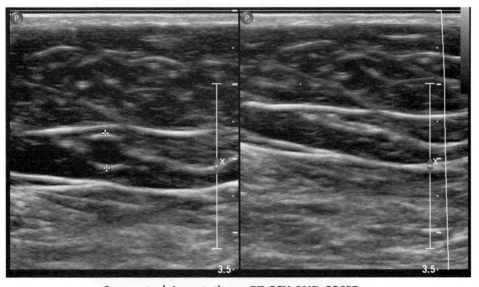

Suggested Annotations: **RT GSV AND COMP**

2. Spectral Doppler of the great saphenous vein before the saphenofemoral junction.

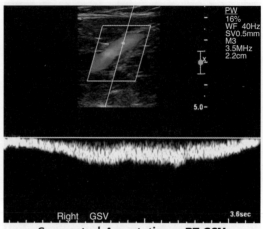

Suggested Annotations: **RT GSV**

3. Spectral Doppler of proximal, mid, and distal femoral vein.

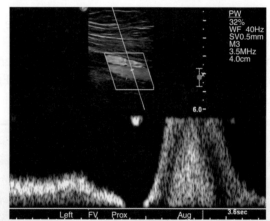

Suggested Annotations: **RT FV (PROX, MID, DIST)**

4. Spectral Doppler of deep femoral vein *(DFV)*. *FV,* Femoral vein; *PFA,* profunda femoral artery; *SFA,* superficial femoral artery.

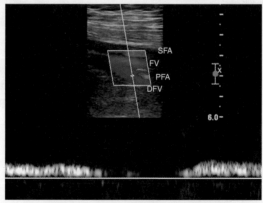

Suggested Annotations: **RT DFV**

Infection Prevention

Hospital-acquired infections (HAIs) are infections that a patient develops while in the hospital. HAIs add a financial burden to the health care system, costing billions of dollars. According to the Centers for Disease Control and Prevention (CDC), about 1 in 31 hospital patients has at least one HAI, affecting an estimated 687,000 patients annually. Approximately 72,000 patients die of an HAI each year.[1] HAIs are a serious problem in health care and are a worldwide problem.

Recently evidence has shown that the ultrasound department has been the source of patients' infections. As a sonographer it is important to do our part in reducing the number of HAIs. Why? Besides affecting the health of the patients, many payers, including Medicare, consider HAIs to be preventable. Therefore, they will not reimburse the facility for the cost to care for the patient due to the HAI. This means the hospital itself will have to assume the costs of the care for the patient, resulting in increased expenses to the hospital. Paying this additional money has to come from somewhere, and that can mean decreased annual raises, increased cost for benefits, and inability to purchase new units.

Most pathogens such as vancomycin-resistant enterococci (VRE), methicillin-resistant *Staphylococcus aureus* (MRSA), and *Clostridium difficile* (C. diff), will last weeks on surfaces. As sonographers we need to protect our patients, but just as important is protecting ourselves and our family. Properly washing our hands before and after each patient, before we eat, and after using the restroom is essential to help reduce the number of HAIs. Most of these pathogens can be found on our hands, and the pathogens can enter our body through our mouths, thereby infecting us. Because we are infected does not mean that we will develop the disease, but we will be a carrier who can infect others.

The sonographer must ensure that the ultrasound unit and transducers are properly disinfected. The manufacturer's website will have a section devoted to cleaning and disinfecting the unit and transducers. It is important to only use the products that the manufacturer has deemed safe to use on their equipment. Not all transducers on a unit may be able to be cleaned with the same disinfectant product; therefore, a product that can be used on all transducers is preferred, so that the wrong product is not accidentally used on a transducer. Using the wrong product can void any warranties.

How the transducer was used will determine what type of disinfection is required and is based on Spaulding's classification. A transducer that touches mucous membranes, was used in a procedure, or that touches body fluids (even though a cover was used) must undergo high-level disinfection (HLD). All other transducers can be treated with low-level disinfection (LLD). In regard to HLD options, it has been shown that there are pathogens on the handles of both endovaginal (EV) and transrectal (TR) transducers; therefore, using a device that can undergo HLD on the handle is preferred. Studies have shown the number of pathogens left on transducers after LLD therefore, if possible, HLD should be performed on all transducers.

HLD of all transducers is easier to perform if the transducers can be disinfected in the scanning room. Use of 35% hydrogen peroxide for HLD is popular in health care. There are devices that can spray an HLD in a room that had been occupied by an infected patient, making it safe for the next patient. There are products in ultrasound that use insonated 35% hydrogen peroxide, for example the Trophon, allowing for in-room HLD of the transducer. In addition, there are newer technologies using ultraviolet radiation, such as Antigermix S1. Current research has shown that not all HLD methods kill human papillomaviruses (HPVs), which have been found on EV transducers after HLD. [2] If the department performs a lot of EV examinations, a method that kills the HPV virus should be used so as not to infect patients. Refer to the American Institute of Ultrasound in Medicine (AIUM) official statement: Guidelines for Cleaning and Preparing External and Internal-Use Ultrasound Transducers Between Patients, Safe Handling, and Use of Ultrasound Coupling Gel.

There are other aspects of infection prevention, such as transducer storage and use of gel, that the sonographer needs to understand. It is beyond the scope of this book to go into the detail needed to truly learn about disinfection and the ultrasound department, and the reader is urged to talk to the infection preventionists in the hospital, read more about the subject, attend lectures, or listen to webinars on infection prevention. The ultrasound community is helping sonographers and sonologists to learn about the importance of infection prevention and ultrasound.

References

1. Magill, S. S., O'Leary, E., Janelle, S. J., Thompson, D. L., Dumyati, G., Nadle, J., et al. (2018). Emerging Infections Program Hospital Prevalence Survey Team. Changes in prevalence of health care-associated infections in U.S. hospitals. *New England Journal of Medicine*, *379*(18), 1732–1744. https://doi.org/10.1056/NEJMoa1801550.

2. Meyers J, Ryndock E, Conway MJ, Meyers C, Robison R. Susceptibility of high-risk human papillomavirus type 16 to clinical disinfectants. *J. Antimicrob Chemother.* 2014;69:1546–1550.

Top 10 Tips for the Sonographer

1. All pathologic areas need to be documented in at least two planes. A mass may not have been seen in a sagittal plane but suddenly is seen in a transverse plane. In this scenario the sonographer needs to bring out the mass in a sagittal or coronal plane. Failure to see the mass in two planes raises the suspicion that the area is being artifactually created.

2. Measurements are very important, because an abnormal measurement can suggest a pathologic condition. In follow-up examinations they are important to determine any changes in size, especially with patients undergoing therapy. Poor measurement techniques can cause a lot of confusion on future examinations or when comparing between imaging modalities. Never fudge your measurements to protect another sonographer. That is not good patient care.

3. Not every image will be worthy of hanging in The Louvre, but they should be diagnostic. It is better to have a diagnostic image that is not "pretty" than a nondiagnostic "pretty" image.

4. Speaking of images that are not pretty, take the image if it demonstrates what you need to show. An old ultrasound proverb is, *You can always get it better, but you can never get it again.* Maybe an image you have taken is not the greatest-looking fetal spine image, so you decide to unfreeze and try to get a better one. However, the fetus is bored and decides to move, making spine images impossible to get, and of course the fetus stays in that position the rest of the examination. The pancreas are another good example: as you try to get a better image, gas can move in the way and the pancreas disappear for good.

5. Before documenting or "taking" an image, take a second to look at the image for quality. Sonographers are required to use their critical-thinking skills. When we scan, we should be subconsciously evaluating the image to see if we can improve or tweak the image. Good sonographers realize that with the technical aspects of the examination, "one size does not fit all," and continually think about if or how the image can be improved. They know which control is needed to help improve the image. Be open to learning how all of those controls affect the image. Try

693

to learn one or two controls a day and see how they can change the appearance of the image. Do this by turning the control to its lowest setting and then start increasing until the maximum setting is achieved, noticing the effects on the image with every adjustment. You cannot "hurt" the patient by adjusting controls, but you can "hurt" the patient by not doing so, meaning you might not see or demonstrate an abnormality by not optimizing the image. Learn your machine and how all the controls affect the image, including the Doppler controls, so you know which control to adjust as needed. It is not as overwhelming as it seems.

6. Always admit it if you miss something. It happens to all of us at times as we put the blinders on and only see what we are working up. However, the radiologist/sonologist is used to looking at the whole picture and sometimes may see an area of concern. Do not try to cover it up and say it was gas or an artifact. Instead, admit that you did not see it and offer to go back and work up that area again. If you try to pass it off as nothing and the radiologist wants to scan that area and finds a pathologic area, you just lost trust with the radiologist, who may now have concerns with your work and your integrity. There is a sacred bond of trust between the sonographer and the sonologist, and it can take time to repair it once it is broken. Remember that the sonologist is relying on the sonographer to be his or her eyes to obtain a diagnostic examination.

7. Never be afraid to try new examinations. With so much information and so many tutorials on the internet, it can be easy to find the information that you need to perform the examination. Be an autodidact and be proud to be one. (*Auto-* means "self," and *didact* comes from the Greek word for "teach," so an autodidact is a person who is self-taught—a cool word to describe yourself to friends and family!) If you are working on a new examination with a physician, combining their knowledge of anatomy, physiology, and pathology with your knowledge of ultrasound and image optimization can create beautiful images. What a great feeling and confidence booster.

8. Keep a positive attitude. The only thing that can cause you to have a bad or poor attitude is yourself. Do not let situations control your attitude. The 5 o'clock Friday add-on DVT study does not want to be there any more than you do. It is not like the patient planned it. Do not take out your frustrations on the patient. You have chosen a profession that is subject to life's unexpected situations. Be understanding and respectful of your co-workers. Things happen in life, and instead of talking about

others behind their back to other co-workers, see if they want to talk about the situation and ask if you can do anything to help them. The other person's problem might be as simple as an issue with taking a child to a new school and trying to figure out new traffic patterns. Team members who get along and support one another create a happy work environment.

9. Take care of your body. There is a lot of information available about scanning ergonomically. There are many, many sonographers out there who wished they had "listened" to their body. When you start to routinely feel aches or pain as you scan, do not think the pain will go away. It probably will only get worse over time. Discuss your pain with your primary care physician. Try to get a physical therapy appointment to learn exercises to help protect and strengthen your joints. To protect yourself, in case you require surgery, report your pain to your supervisor or manager and try to go to occupational health clinic. It is against the law for your supervisor to retaliate if you seek help from Workman's Compensation or Occupational Health clinic. It is important to start documenting your pain so that if it gets worse and you need surgery, you will be covered under workers' compensation. However, there are pros and cons to claiming your injury under workers' compensation. Have someone in workers' compensation explain the process. Make sure that you understand the Family and Medical Leave Act (FMLA), short-term disability (STD), and long-term disability (LTD) insurance that you have. One misconception is that you receive pay through FMLA. FMLA is for job security and does not pay the employee. Shoulder surgeries can require months to heal before you can return to work, especially if there are complications. You want to protect yourself financially. Usually the employer will pay for STD and the employee pays LTD insurance. It might be that the employee has to pay both premiums. For the small monthly premium cost, you will have the peace of mind of continuing to receive a paycheck, although it may be reduced. If you are going to have any type of surgery, talk to someone, usually in the human resources department, about how the process works and what needs to be done if you need to transition from STD to LTD so as to not interrupt receiving pay.

10. Make sonography a profession, not a 9-to-5 job. Join national societies such as the Society of Diagnostic Medical Sonography (SDMS). Attend local and national meetings. This allows you to network and make new friends, learn new technologies and techniques to stay current, earn Continuing Medical Education (CME) credits, and have a good time. If you do not know about

a pathologic condition your patient had, go home and search for and learn about it on the internet. Read selected articles in ultrasound journals. Keep abreast of changes in the profession, such as state licensure. Consider writing case studies or journal articles. Give lectures. Start at a staff meeting or to students. Once you feel confident with the lecture, talk to your local society about giving it at a meeting. Submit to the annual SDMS conference, adhering to deadlines for submission. Some societies, even local ones, give an honorarium, usually per lecture. Look into getting involved with your local society or the SDMS. Consider applying to the SDMS to be on a committee. If you are a member, you would receive an e-mail calling for nominations. Decide on a career path. Do you want to be in management, in education, or work for an ultrasound company? Look at the positive and negative aspects of each career path and start your journey. Do you need a higher degree? What type of courses should you take? See if your employer helps pay for any of your higher education. Finally, get registered in each aspect of sonography in which you practice. This shows your commitment to your career and looks great on a resume. Some employment requirements may call for the applicant to be registered in certain specialties. It is a gift and privilege to be able to help people with their health care. Your special skills and dedication affect the care of that patient. Be proud.

Documentation of an Ultrasound Examination

The following are proposed guidelines based on the guidelines that can be found on the American Institute of Ultrasound in Medicine (AIUM) website under Resources and Practice Parameters.

Accurate and complete documentation is essential, and there must be good communication among all the members of the diagnostic ultrasound team for high-quality patient care. All communication should be performed in a manner that respects patient confidentiality and complies with current Health Insurance Portability and Accountability Act (HIPAA) regulations. Images from the ultrasound examination should be recorded and stored in a retrievable format.

Proper documentation is essential for patient care and to protect the facility in legal situations. There should be a permanent record of the ultrasound examination and its interpretation. Images of the organ(s) and/or areas of concern, both normal and abnormal, should be documented and stored. Variations from normal size should be accompanied with measurements. The ultrasound examination must be stored and kept for as long as stated by the guidelines of national and state standards.

As per the AIUM Practice Parameter for Documentation of an Ultrasound Examination found under Practice Parameters of the Resource tab on the AIUM website, http://www.aium.org, ultrasound examinations should be recorded in a manner that will allow subsequent review for adequacy and for diagnostic purposes. Although for some examinations still images may be all that is needed, archiving of video or ciné loops may be required for some examinations as stated in the Practice Parameters found on the AIUM website.

Whether still-frame images, ciné images, or both are captured, the archived images should contain the following:

- Patient's name and other identifying information
- Facility's identifying information
- Date and time of the ultrasound examination
- Output display standard of the thermal index (TI) and mechanical index (MI)
- Label of the anatomic location and laterality, when appropriate
- Image orientation when appropriate
- Some type of identification as to who performed the study, such as initials or a numerical code

A good practice is to follow the ALARA (*as low as* reasonably *a*chievable) principle when adjusting controls that affect the acoustic output or power. However, sacrificing image quality to keep a low output power does not help the patient get a diagnosis; they may then require additional imaging that uses radiation and/or nephrotoxic contrast agents. The U.S. Food and Drug Administration (FDA) has limited the output power of diagnostic ultrasound units to keep patients safe. These limits change according to the preset used, with the obstetrics presets having the lowest acoustical output. Although the acoustic output allows good gray-scale imaging, it may not be strong enough for the Doppler aspects of the examination, especially in the abdomen. Increasing the output power is acceptable, especially if it improves the image quality and Doppler sensitivity. If there is a lot of noise artifact in the image or Doppler signal, consider increasing the output power.

Guidelines for Performance of the Abdominal and Retroperitoneal Ultrasound Examination

The following are proposed guidelines based on the guidelines that can be found on the AIUM website under Resources and Practice Parameters.

These guidelines have been developed to provide assistance for sonographers performing ultrasound studies of the abdomen and retroperitoneum. The guidelines describe the examination to be performed for each abdominal organ or region in the abdomen and retroperitoneum. Organs for which documentation is needed for a complete abdominal or retroperitoneal examination are found in their respective chapters. A limited examination would include one or more of these areas, but not all of them.

Ultrasound has its limitations and cannot allow visualization of all pathologic conditions. It is the hope that following guidelines found on the AIUM website will maximize the probability of finding pathologic conditions that occur in the abdomen and retroperitoneum. In some patients, additional and/or specialized examinations, such as a biopsy or other imaging modality, may be necessary to determine a diagnosis.

Equipment

Abdominal and retroperitoneal ultrasound studies should be performed using a phased array transducer, a curved linear array transducer, or a combination of both. The transducer should be the highest frequency that allows proper penetration. The frequencies used for an abdominal or retroperitoneal ultrasound study are between 2.0 and 9.0 MHz.

Liver

An ultrasound examination of the liver should include images obtained from longitudinal and/or sagittal views, transverse views, and other views, such as coronal, as needed. Images should provide a good representation of the liver, documenting both normal and abnormal tissue of all three lobes: the right, left, and caudate. Images comparing the echogenicity of the liver to the right kidney and images of the aorta and the inferior vena cava (IVC), in the region of the liver should be documented. The regions of the ligamentum teres in the left lobe and of the dome of the liver in the right lobe, along with the right hemidiaphragm and right pleural space should be imaged and documented. The length of the liver should be measured. The liver surface can be imaged with a high-frequency linear array transducer to evaluate for surface nodularity in patients at risk for cirrhosis. Patients with nonalcoholic fatty liver disease (NAFLD), alcoholic liver disease, cirrhosis, hepatitis, and other indications should have a liver elastography examination to assess for liver fibrosis. This can be performed in conjunction with an ordered liver sonogram, with the appropriate order placed, or the patient can return for just the liver elastography study.

Images of the right and left lobes should include the hepatic veins and the main, right, and left branches of the portal vein. A Doppler signal showing flow direction in the portal vein should be considered in all studies. The common bile duct and the intrahepatic bile ducts should be evaluated for dilatation.

Gallbladder and Biliary Tract

A gallbladder ultrasound study should be performed on an adequately distended gallbladder and include multiple long-axis and transverse views with the patient in the supine position. When needed, a measurement of the length of the gallbladder should be obtained. The thickness of the wall of the gallbladder should be measured. Left lateral decubitus, right side up, of the gallbladder in multiple long-axis and transverse views should be done to evaluate for mobility of structures seen inside the gallbladder and to look for stones that were not seen in the supine position. Erect views are performed when the patient cannot roll on the side or to further clarify pathologic areas seen. Tenderness over the gallbladder with transducer compression, sonographic Murphy's sign, should be assessed in patients with right upper quadrant or abdominal pain.

The intrahepatic ducts are evaluated by obtaining multiple views of the liver. The extrahepatic ducts are evaluated in supine and left lateral decubitus positions with semi-erect positions as needed. Color Doppler can be used to differentiate hepatic arteries and portal veins from bile ducts. The intrahepatic and extrahepatic bile ducts should be evaluated for dilatation, wall thickening, intraluminal findings, and other abnormalities. The bile duct in the porta hepatis should be measured and documented. When possible, the distal common bile duct in the pancreatic head should be evaluated and measured.

Pancreas

The pancreatic head, uncinate process, body, and tail of the pancreas should be identified in transverse and sagittal views. When visible, the pancreatic duct can be measured. To help better visualize the pancreas, the patient can be given water or other fluid to distend the stomach, and changes in patient positioning, such as upright and oblique positions, may afford better visualization of the pancreas.

The following should be assessed with a sonographic examination of the pancreas:
1. Parenchymal abnormalities, such as masses, cysts, and calcifications.
2. The pancreatic duct should be evaluated for dilatation and, if possible, the cause.
3. The distal common bile duct in the region of the head of the pancreas, if visualized, should be measured.
4. The peripancreatic region should be evaluated for adenopathy and fluid.

Spleen

Multiple views of the spleen in long-axis and transverse planes should be obtained. The length of the spleen should be measured, especially if splenomegaly is a concern. If splenic volume is needed, the width and anteroposterior (AP) measurements should be added. The echogenicity of the upper pole of the left kidney should be compared with that of the spleen, and an attempt should be made to demonstrate the left pleural space.

Kidneys

Longitudinal views of each kidney should be obtained demonstrating the cortex and renal pelvis through the medial, mid, and lateral aspects of each kidney. The length of the kidney should be measured, and the renal cortex thickness assessed. Transverse views of both the left and right kidney at the upper pole, midpole at the renal hilum, and lower pole. The echogenicity of the kidney should be compared with the adjacent liver and spleen. When appropriate, images of the bladder should be obtained. The patient should be scanned in the best position to provide diagnostic images of the kidneys. Patient scanning positions can include supine, prone, oblique, decubitus, or any combination of these positions. Color Doppler can be helpful to assess for regions of flow void and decreased flow to the capsule, verifying a tubular structure in the hilum as a blood vessel, and identifying the twinkling artifact in detecting renal stones.

Aorta

The aorta is imaged in long-axis and transverse planes from the diaphragm to the bifurcation, including images of the common iliac arteries. The AP diameter should be measured in a sagittal plane at proximal, mid, and distal areas. If an abdominal aortic aneurysm is discovered, a transverse image at the level of the renal arteries needs to be obtained.

Inferior Vena Cava

The IVC should be imaged in long-axis and transverse planes from the diaphragm to the bifurcation, including the common iliac veins. Color Doppler is needed to evaluate the patency of an IVC filter. If thrombus is found in the IVC, the renal veins need to be evaluated for presence of thrombus.

Peritoneal Fluid (Ascites)

Evaluation for ascites should include documentation of the extent and location of any fluid identified. Assessment for ascites should include limited images of the pelvis.

Longitudinal and transverse images should be obtained in the right upper quadrant looking for fluid around the periphery of the liver, in the subhepatic space, and in Morison's pouch. Because fluid will collect laterally, it will be better seen on transverse images. Longitudinal and transverse images should be obtained in the left upper quadrant through the area of the spleen, with attention to fluid collections peripheral to the spleen, best seen on transverse images, and between the spleen and left kidney. Longitudinal and transverse images should be obtained in the areas of the left and right paracolic gutters for evidence of free fluid and through the pelvic region. A longitudinal image at the midline of the pelvis should be obtained to evaluate the cul-de-sac.

Guidelines for Performance of the Scrotal Ultrasound Examination

These guidelines have been developed to provide assistance for sonographers performing ultrasound studies of the scrotum and testicles. Ultrasound has its limitations and cannot allow visualization of all pathologic areas. It is the hope that following guidelines found on the American Institute of Ultrasound in Medicine (AIUM) website will maximize the probability of finding pathologic conditions that occur in the scrotum.

Guidelines for Equipment and Documentation

A high-frequency linear array transducer of at least 7 to 10 MHz should be used for scrotal and testicular ultrasound examinations. If the scrotum is very enlarged—for example, from a large hydrocele—a lower-frequency curved linear transducer should be used, employing the highest frequency possible that will provide the needed penetration. Standoff pads can be used as needed to improve the imaging just below skin level.

Guidelines for a Scrotal Ultrasound Examination

The testicles should be evaluated in at least longitudinal and transverse planes, with other planes as needed to fully evaluate the scrotum, testicles, and any pathologic conditions. Transverse images should be obtained in the upper, mid, and lower portions of each testicle. Transverse and anteroposterior measurements should be taken at the widest mid-pole area. Longitudinal views should be obtained from midline, with a measurement of length and the medial and lateral aspect of each testicle. The head, body, and tail of the epididymis should be evaluated, with the head evaluated in both longitudinal and transverse planes. The size, echogenicity, and blood flow of each testicle should be compared with the contralateral side. This is best accomplished with a side-by-side transverse image at the mid-pole with and without color Doppler. Some departments may require a side-by-side image of the epididymal head with and without color Doppler. The scrotal wall should be evaluated and measured on each side. If one or both testicles cannot be found within the scrotum, the inguinal canal should be scanned to look for an undescended testicle.

If the indication is for a palpable lesion or area, that area should be directly imaged in at least two planes. When there is a suspicion for a varicocele, a Valsalva maneuver can be performed to look for retrograde flow in the pampiniform plexus. For patients with acute scrotal pain, color and/or power Doppler will be required to make the distinction between torsion and inflammation. At least one side-by-side image comparing both testicles using identical Doppler settings should be obtained to evaluate for symmetric flow. An absence of flow in one testicle is suggestive of testicular torsion, and the Doppler settings should be adjusted to try to elicit any flow. In patients who have solid testicular masses, the retroperitoneal lymph nodes should be evaluated for enlargement. Enlarged nodes from testicular cancer will be found around the aorta and inferior vena cava at the level of the renal veins.

Guidelines for Performance of the Female Pelvis Ultrasound Examination

The following is based on the proposed guidelines provided by the American College of Radiology, American College of Obstetricians and Gynecologists, American Institute of Ultrasound in Medicine, Society of Pediatric Radiologists, and Society of Radiologists in the Ultrasound Practice Parameter for the Performance of Ultrasound of the Female Pelvis. For the complete document, visit http://www.aium.org.

These guidelines have been developed to provide assistance to sonographers performing ultrasound studies of the female pelvis. Ultrasound has its limitations and cannot allow visualization of all pathologic conditions. In some cases, additional imaging examinations may be necessary, such as magnetic resonance imaging or sonohysterography. Although it is not possible to detect every abnormality with ultrasound, adherence to the following guidelines may maximize the probability of detecting most of the abnormalities that occur.

Equipment

Ultrasound examination of the female pelvis should be conducted using a curved linear array transducer between the frequencies of 3 and 5 MHz. A lower-frequency transducer, such as a 2–3-MHz sector/phased array, may be needed in larger patients or patients with a fibroid uterus. A transvaginal (TV) transducer with frequencies between 5 and 10 MHz is used to increase the resolution of the pelvic organs and structures. All TV transducers must be high-level disinfected (HLD) and covered with a protective sheath before insertion. After the examination, the sheath should be disposed of properly and the probe must be HLD according to the manufacturer's guidelines.

The following guidelines describe the examination to be performed for each organ and anatomic region in the female pelvis. All relevant structures should be identified by an abdominal or vaginal approach, although in most patients both approaches will be performed.

General Pelvic Preparation

For a transabdominal (TA) pelvic sonogram, the patient's urinary bladder should be full, although some departments will use how full the bladder is at the time of the examination. For a TA-only sonogram, the patient's urinary bladder should be full, with the tip of the bladder extending past the fundus of the uterus. If the patient has an overdistended bladder, it may make the examination difficult, and the patient should partially empty her bladder. For a vaginal sonogram, the urinary bladder should be empty.

The vaginal transducer may be introduced by the patient, the sonographer, or the sonologist. It is highly recommended and mandatory in some departments for a TV sonographic examination to be chaperoned, even when the sonographer is a woman. The chaperone can be of either sex and must be an employee of the hospital or office. Family members cannot be used as a chaperone. The main purpose of a chaperone is to protect the sonographer from a legal situation. Usually the name or the initials of the chaperone is documented in the appropriate place. It is important that the patient understands what will happen with a transvaginal examination and an interpreter provided if there is a communication problem to explain the procedure.

Uterus

In evaluating the uterus, the following should be evaluated and documented: the size, shape, and orientation of the uterus, the endometrium, the myometrium, and the cervix. The vagina should be imaged and can be used as a landmark for the cervix and lower uterine segment.

Uterine size can be determined using a TA or TV approach. The longest length of the uterus is evaluated in a long-axis view from the fundus to the cervix, or to the external os, if it can be identified. The anteroposterior (AP) dimension of the uterus is measured in the same long-axis view from its anterior to posterior walls, perpendicular to the length. The maximum width is measured in the transverse or coronal view. Abnormalities of the uterus should be documented in at least two planes.

The endometrium thickness should be measured and the presence of any fluid or pathologic area documented. The thickest part of the endometrium should be measured in the AP dimension from echogenic to echogenic border and is usually best measured by a TV approach. The thickness of the endometrium will vary depending on the phase of the menstrual cycle.

The myometrium and cervix should be evaluated for contour changes, echogenicity, and the presence of any masses.

Adnexa, Ovaries, and Fallopian Tubes

The ovaries are situated anterior to the internal iliac artery, also called the hypogastric artery, which can serve as a landmark for their identification. The size, shape, echogenicity, presence of follicular cysts, and their position relative to the uterus should be evaluated and documented. The ovarian size can be determined by measuring the length in long axis with the AP dimension measured perpendicular to the length. The ovarian width is measured in the transverse or coronal view. A volume can be calculated by the unit if required. In some patients one or both ovaries may not be identified, especially before puberty and after menopause.

The normal fallopian tubes are not commonly identified. This region should be surveyed for abnormalities, particularly dilated tubular structures.

If an adnexal mass is noted, its relationship to the ovaries and uterus should be documented. The size and sonographic characteristics should be documented.

Cul-de-sac

The cul-de-sac, also known as the rectouterine pouch or pouch of Douglas, is the extension of the peritoneal cavity between the rectum and the posterior wall of the uterus. It is the lowest point in the pelvis and a good place for fluid to accumulate. The cul-de-sac should be evaluated for the presence of free fluid or masses. If a mass is detected, its size, position, shape, sonographic characteristics, and relationship to the uterus and ovaries documented. Seeing peristalsis of an area will differentiate a mass from bowel.

Three-dimensional (3D) ultrasound can be used in certain situations, such as intrauterine device (IUD or IUCD) identification. 3D should be used as per the department's protocol.

Doppler may be used when it is important to evaluate blood flow. Some departments may routinely obtain an arterial and venous signal from each ovary. For the suspicion of ovarian torsion, color and spectral Doppler is mandatory to evaluate the presence or absence of flow. Color and spectral Doppler should be used as per the department's protocol.

Guidelines for Performance of the Antepartum Obstetric Ultrasound Examination

The following guidelines are based on the American College of Radiology, American College of Obstetricians and Gynecologists, American Institute of Ultrasound in Medicine, Society of Pediatric Radiologists, and Society of Radiologists Practice Parameter for the Performance of Standard Diagnostic Obstetric Ultrasound Examinations. For the complete document, visit http://www.aium.org.

These guidelines have been developed to provide assistance for sonographers performing obstetric ultrasound studies. Although it is not possible to detect all structural congenital anomalies with diagnostic ultrasound, it is the hope that following the guidelines found on the AIUM website will maximize the possibility of detecting many fetal abnormalities. In some patients, additional and/or specialized examinations, such as amniocentesis or magnetic resonance imaging, may be necessary to determine a diagnosis.

A limited examination may be performed in clinical emergencies or if used as a follow-up to complete an examination. In some cases, an additional and/or specialized examination may be necessary. Although it is not possible to detect all structural congenital anomalies with diagnostic ultrasound, adherence to the following guidelines will maximize the possibility of detecting many fetal abnormalities.

Equipment

Obstetric ultrasound studies should be performed using a curved linear array transducer with frequencies from 3.5 to 7 MHz. The transducer should be the highest frequency that allows proper penetration. A 5–9-MHz vaginal transducer can be used when better resolution is needed, especially in the first trimester. All transvaginal (TV) transducers must be high-level disinfected (HLD) and covered with a protective sheath before insertion. After the examination, the sheath should be disposed of properly and the probe must be HLD according to the manufacturer's guidelines. The sonographer should use the lowest possible acoustic output that allows good visualization of the fetus and uterus.

Guidelines for First-Trimester Sonography

Both transabdominal (TA) and TV scans are typically performed in the first trimester. A standard examination should include evaluation of the presence of a gestational sac and the location, size, and number of gestational sacs. A mean diameter of the gestational sacs can be used to document gestational age. The gestational sac is examined for the presence of an embryo and/or a yolk sac. A measurement should be taken when an embryo or fetus is found with cardiac activity noted and, if possible, measured. When the fetus is large enough, the crown-to-rump length (CRL) should be obtained and measured. Cardiac activity can be documented with M-mode or a video clip. Color or spectral Doppler should not be used because of the higher output power generated. The uterus, cervix, ovaries, adnexa, and cul-de-sac should be examined and any pathologic or abnormal findings documented.

When the fetus is of appropriate size, the fetal head, abdominal cord insertion, and presence of limbs should be demonstrated and documented. A nuchal translucency measurement should be performed when indicated.

Guidelines for Sonography in the Second and Third Trimester

A standard fetal examination would include documentation of the presence of cardiac activity and a measurement of the fetal heart rate. Again, the use of spectral or color Doppler is discouraged because of the increased acoustic output.

Fetal measurements should include biparietal diameter, head circumference, femur length, and abdominal circumference. The amniotic fluid volume should be documented either qualitatively or using a semiquantitative method. The placenta location, its appearance, and its relationship to the cervical os should be documented. The placental cord insertion should be documented when seen. The number of vessels in the umbilical cord should be documented. The uterus, cervix, ovaries, and adnexa should be evaluated for any abnormalities or pathologic condition.

The following structures should be documented as part of the fetal anatomic survey, understanding that fetal age, fetal position, and maternal abdominal wall thickness may make some structures difficult to completely evaluate. A more detailed fetal anatomy scan may be needed when indicated.

The structures from the head, face, and neck include the lateral cerebral ventricles, choroid plexus, midline falx, cavum septi pellucidi, cerebellum, cisterna magna, and upper lip. Some protocols may also require a fetal profile. A measurement of the nuchal fold as required per protocol.

The structures from the chest include fetal heart size and position, four-chamber view, left ventricle outflow track, and right ventricle outflow track. If the area can be visualized, a three-vessel view and three-vessel trachea view can be included.

The structures in the abdomen that should be evaluated include the stomach, including size and situs; kidneys; urinary bladder; fetal umbilical insertion; and umbilical cord vessel number.

The cervical, thoracic, lumbar, and sacral spine should be fully evaluated in both longitudinal and transverse planes.

The presence of arms and legs and hands and feet should be documented.

When indicated, the fetal external genitalia should be documented.

When multiple gestations are seen, it is important to document the chorionicity, amnionicity, comparison of fetal size, amniotic fluid volume in each sac, and fetal genitalia when seen.

When required, a detailed fetal anatomic examination would include the images in the following lists.

Fetal head and neck images would include the third ventricles, the fourth ventricle, the lateral ventricular wall integrity, contour and ependymal lining, cerebellar lobes, vermis, cisterna magna, the corpus callosum, integrity and shape of the cranial vault, brain parenchyma, neck, fetal profile, nasal bone at 15 to 22 weeks, and a coronal face image demonstrating the nose, lips, lens of the eyes, palate, maxilla, mandible, tongue, ear position, and size and the orbits.

The fetal chest would add images of the situs aortic arch, superior and inferior venae cavae, ductal arch, and interventricular septum; three-vessel view and three-vessel and tracheal view; and lungs, integrity of the diaphragm, and ribs.

Images of the fetal abdomen would add the small and large bowel, adrenal glands, gallbladder, liver, renal arteries, spleen, and integrity of abdominal wall.

Fetal spine images would include demonstrating the integrity of the spine and overlying soft tissue and the shape and curvature of the conus medullaris.

Images demonstrating the number, architecture, and position of the fetal extremities and the number and position of the digits of hands and feet would be added.

Additional images of the placenta would include documenting any masses, accessory/succenturiate lobe with location of connecting vascular supply to the primary placenta and internal cervical os, and the implantation site with evaluation for abnormal adherence.

The following additional fetal measurements that would be needed include the cerebellum; the inner and outer orbital diameters; nuchal fold thickness when the fetus is between 16 to 20 weeks; and the humerus, ulna and radius, and the tibia and fibula.

Guidelines for the Performance of Lower Extremity Venous Doppler Examinations

These guidelines have been developed to provide assistance for sonographers performing venous Doppler studies of the lower extremity to evaluate for deep vein thrombosis (DVT). Ultrasound has its limitations and cannot allow visualization of all pathologic conditions. It is the hope that following guidelines found on the American Institute of Ultrasound in Medicine (AIUM) website (http://www.aium.org) will maximize the probability of finding pathologic conditions in the lower extremity veins. Guidelines are also available from the Intersocietal Accreditation Commission - Vascular Testing at https://www.intersocietal.org/vascular/. As a reminder, the superficial femoral vein is now called the femoral vein, and the greater saphenous vein is now called the great saphenous vein.

A good article to read is "Ultrasound for Lower Extremity Deep Venous Thrombosis" by the Multidisciplinary Recommendations from the Society of Radiologists in Ultrasound Consensus Conference. It was published in volume 137, number 14 of *Circulation* in April 2018. The lead author is Larry Needleman, MD, and the article can be downloaded at no charge. This article covers a lot of clinical information pertinent to a venous duplex study for DVT.

Equipment

A linear array transducer of at least 5 MHz should be used for venous Doppler examinations. If the leg is swollen or large, a curved linear transducer should be used, using the highest frequency possible that will give the needed penetration. A curved linear array transducer may be needed to evaluate the external iliac veins when required and may make scanning the popliteal veins easier because the curve of the transducer will fit into the popliteal fossa. It may be necessary to switch between the two transducer types during the examination to provide a complete diagnostic examination. For example, a linear array transducer is used to evaluate the common and proximal femoral veins, but because of the size of the mid-thigh, a curved linear array transducer with a lower frequency is needed.

Because the vein will be going deeper as it courses to the popliteal fossa, the overall gain, image depth, focal zone placement, and other image settings will need to be optimized with respect to the depth of the vein.

Guidelines for a Lower Extremity Venous Doppler Examination

The scan is done with the patient in the supine position, with the knee bent and the leg rotated slightly outward to allow better access to the inner thigh and popliteal area. The head of the stretcher may be slightly elevated using a semi-Fowler position, to help distend the veins by pooling blood in the legs. A towel may be tucked under the edge of the patient's underwear to protect it from gel. If the underwear makes it difficult to evaluate the groin area or is constrictive, it should be removed and the patient appropriately covered.

Compression of the vein is the main diagnostic criterion to verify the absence or presence of a venous thrombosis. The goal of compression is to see that the vein walls touch or coapt. If the vein walls touch and the vein compresses, that implies that there is nothing in the vein. However, if the vein walls cannot touch or the vein cannot compress, this implies that there may be a thrombus in the vein. Therefore, the most important part of any venous duplex study is careful compressions of the vein from the common femoral vein, above the saphenofemoral junction to the popliteal vein or calf veins, depending on the protocol being followed. Venous compression is performed every 2 cm or less in the transverse plane with enough transducer pressure on the skin to completely obliterate the venous lumen. The vein is evaluated carefully so as not to miss any segment of the vein, because clots may be smaller than the width of the transducer and could potentially be "skipped" over. Compression can be documented using ciné clips recording the entire length of the vein, with or without documenting with still images, or with just still images. If documenting with still images, transverse gray-scale images with and without compression must be obtained from the following areas: common femoral vein, saphenofemoral junction, proximal deep femoral vein, proximal femoral vein, mid-femoral vein, distal femoral vein, and popliteal vein just proximal to the tibioperoneal trunk. If the calf veins are included, images of compression of the posterior tibial veins and peroneal veins are included. Only one image of each set of calf veins needs to be documented, and it is suggested that the image be near the tibioperoneal trunk. The compression view of the proximal deep femoral vein and the proximal femoral vein may be included in the same image. If the patient has a duplicated femoral vein, each vein must be evaluated. If compression is difficult, place one hand under the area to be compressed and press toward the transducer while simultaneously pressing the vein with the transducer. This can be an especially helpful technique when compressing the femoral vein in the adductor canal, which is also known as Hunter's canal.

Scanning of the popliteal fossa can be performed with the patient in the position as described previously, with the sonographer placing the transducer behind the knee, or by having the patient roll onto the side placing the "up" leg in front of the leg being scanned. This will have the patient in an anterior oblique position.

The calves can be scanned in the same position as the thigh. Another position is to have the patient bend the knees and put the feet on the stretcher because this allows blood to pool in the calves and fill the veins. Another method to scan the calf veins is to have the patient sit on the edge of the stretcher and dangle the legs over the edge. This position may present some ergonomic challenges. Only the posterior tibia and peroneal veins need to be evaluated, because there is no documented evidence of isolated anterior tibial vein thrombosis.

Color Doppler is used to demonstrate that the vein is widely patent, to demonstrate flow through a nonocclusive thrombus, or demonstrate flow that is reconstituting through a complete thrombus. The proximal deep femoral and proximal great saphenous veins should be examined using color and spectral Doppler. Some laboratories may also require a color and spectral Doppler image of the external iliac veins. A curved linear array transducer is typically used to evaluate the external iliac veins.

Spectral Doppler is used to evaluate for spontaneity and phasicity of flow. Spectral Doppler waveforms are obtained from the long axis of the vein and should include signals from the common femoral and popliteal veins. Augmentation is no longer required. In a unilateral study the contralateral femoral vein should be evaluated with spectral Doppler to compare the signal characteristics of both femoral veins looking for symmetry. If both femoral veins have lost phasicity, the inferior vena cava should be evaluated for a central obstruction. If one femoral vein has lost its phasicity, the ipsilateral external iliac vein should be evaluated for thrombus.

AIUM: American Institute of Ultrasound in Medicine

ALARA: As low as reasonably acceptable

ANT: Anterior

AO: Aorta

ART or A: Artery

AVF: Arteriovenous fistula

BIF: Bifurcation

BPD: Biparietal diameter

CBD: Common bile duct

CCA: Common carotid artery

CD: Common duct

CFA: Common femoral artery

CFV: Common femoral vein

cm: Centimeter

COR: Coronal

CRL: Crown rump length

C-SPINE: Cervical spine

DECUB: Decubitus

DPA: Dorsalis pedis artery

DST: Distal

ECA: External carotid artery

EPI: Epididymis

ER/TR: Endorectal/Transrectal

EV/TA: Endovaginal/Transvaginal

FV: Femoral vein

GB: Gallbladder

GS: Gestational sac

Hz: Hertz

IAC-VT: Intersocietal Accreditation Commission Vascular Testing

ICA: Internal carotid artery

INF: Inferior

IVC: Inferior vena cava

KID: Kidney

LAT: Lateral

LLD: Left lateral decubitus

LPO: Left posterior oblique

L-SPINE: Lumbar spine

LT: Left

LVOT: Left ventricular outflow tract

MHz: Megahertz

ML: Midline

mm: Millimeter

MSK: Musculoskeletal

OBL: Oblique

OV: Ovary

PANC: Pancreas

PFV: Profunda femoris vein

POP: Popliteal artery or vein

POST: Posterior

PROX: Proximal

PTA: Posterior tibial artery

PTV: Posterior tibial vein

RI: Resistive index

RLD: Right lateral decubitus

RPO: Right posterior oblique

RT: Right

SAG: Sagittal

SFA: Superficial femoral artery

SMA: Superior mesenteric artery

SUP: Supine

SUP: Superior

SV: Seminal vesicle

TRV: Transverse

T-SPINE: Thoracic spine

UT: Uterus

V: Vein

VAG: Vagina

Index

Page numbers followed by f indicate figures; t, tables; b, boxes.